The Book of Birth

—————— VOLUME I ——————

A Sevenfold Approach to Your Ideal,
Perfect Conception, Pregnancy, and Birth

by MariMikel Potter, CPM, LM, RN-BSN

DEDICATION

I dedicate this book to the incredible women, men, and families
that I have had the honor of serving over the course of my career.
Much of what I share with you in this book comes either from
them directly teaching me new ideas and concepts or from research
they inspired me to do so I could help them.

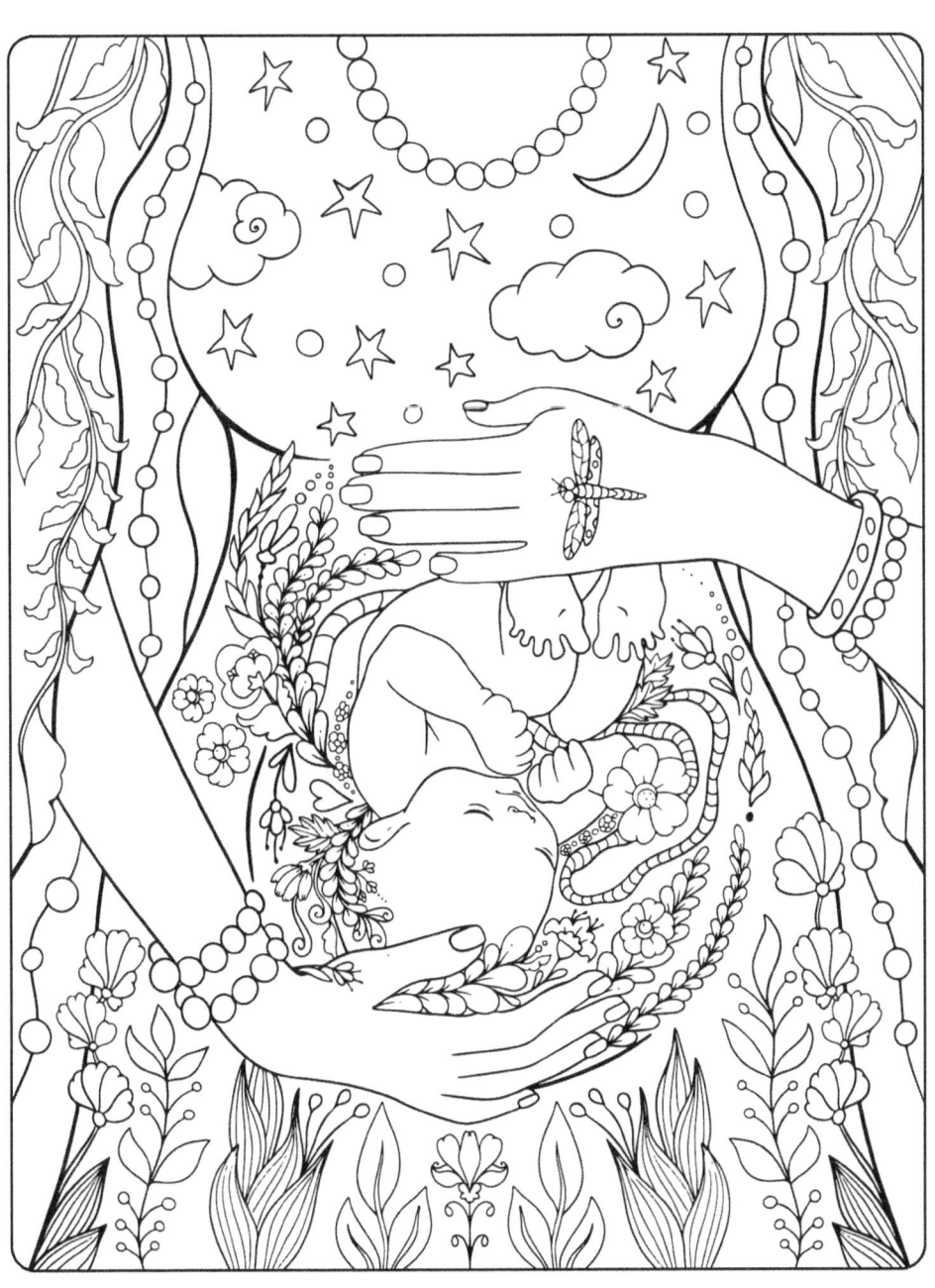

TABLE OF CONTENTS

INTRODUCTION 1

Why I Became a Midwife 4
   Hospitals, Birth Centers, and Home Births...........................8

Ideal and Perfect 10
   Ideal...10
   Perfect 11

A Sevenfold Approach 12
   1. Nourishment..12
   2. Hydration 12
   3. Movement 12
   4. Emotional/Spiritual..12
   5. Knowledge..13
   6. Rest...13
   7. Joy 14

How to Use This Book.. 15
   Where to Start...15
   When to Finish...15
   How to Find More Information 15
   Take What Works for You...15
   Birth Stories..15
   When and How to Prepare for Postpartum 16
   Midwives and OB/GYNs..16

CONSCIOUS CONCEPTION **17**

Introduction 18

Nourishment 22
   Be a Conscious Consumer 23
   Carbohydrates and Low Carb Diets..................................24
   Protein 25
      Seafood 25
      Poultry 27
      Beef & Pork...27

Gluten 28

Phytoestrogens 28

Processed Food Alternatives 29

Tools for Assessing Your Diet 30

    Protein Counter 30

    Glycemic Index 33

    Apps for Nutritional Information 34

Meal Planning 35

    Getting Started 35

    Meal Planning Tool 36

Supplements 39

Can't I Just Take a Prenatal Multivitamin? 40

Supplement Recommendations 40

    Morning 41

        400-Unit Mixed Tocopherol Vitamin E 41

        1,000 mg Ester-C 42

        Probiotics 43

    Lunch 43

        NaturesPlus Ultra-Mins 43

        B Complex 45

        Folic Acid/Methylfolate 46

    Dinner 47

        400-Units Mixed Tocopherol Vitamin E 47

        1000 mg Ester-C 47

        Beta Carotene 47

        Omega-3s 47

        Vitamin D 48

Supplement List 49

When Should I Stop? 49

Getting Your Partner on Board 49

Natural Medicine Chest 52

    Warning Labels 52

    What to Get 52

        Echinacea 53

        Oil of Oregano 53

        Astragalus 53

        Grapefruit Seed Extract (GSE) 53

        Oscillococcinum 53

Clay Powders 54

Cranberry Extract (pill form) & D-Mannose.......................... 54

Colloidal Silver 54

Tea Tree Oil 54

Castor Oil.. 54

Pepto-Bismol 54

Arnica (gel, cream, and pellets).. 54

Aloe Vera 54

Elderberry Syrup 55

Xylitol 55

Rescue Remedy 55

Tobacco Products 55

Alcohol 57

Cannabis...57

Drugs 58

Epigenetics 58

Hydration 60

Introduction...60

What You Need...60

Improve Your Tap Water 61

Electrolytes 61

Caffeine 62

Movement.. 64

Introduction..64

Walking...65

Swimming...66

Weight Work 67

Yoga 68

Your Weekly Routine..68

Partners Need to Get in Shape Too...68

Emotional/Spiritual 69

Introduction...69

Preparing for Baby...69

Birth History Questionnaire 70

Develop Your Intuition..71

Affirmations...72

Journaling...73

Knowledge **76**

Building New Habits 76

When to Start Your Family 77

Preparing for Changes at Work 78

Anatomy & Physiology of Conception....................................79

    Your Body's Reproductive System 79

    Your Cycle and Conception..80

    Spindle Mucus/EWCM..83

    Use an Ovulation Kit 84

    Chart Temperatures to Track Ovulation 84

    Conceiving with a Retroverted Uterus 84

Toxins to Avoid..86

    Mercury..86

    Glyphosate 86

    Bisphenol A 86

    Toxins in Beauty Products 87

    Pesticides 87

    Lead..87

    Pollution, Solvents, and Radiation 88

Mayan Abdominal Massage or Abdominal Massage Therapy......88

Timing Your Conception...89

    Flying in Early Pregnancy 89

    Solar Activity and Excess Gamma Radiation 89

    Aim for a Time of Low Stress 90

    Herpes 90

    COVID-19...91

    Get Off Anti-Depressants 91

    Getting Off Birth Control 92

Immunizations...93

Sperm Health...94

Influencing the Baby's Gender 94

Infertility and What to Do About It..95

Early Signs of Pregnancy..97

Initial Thoughts on Choosing a Care Provider 98

Rest **99**
    Remove Stressors 99
    Pay Attention to Sleep Hygiene 99
    Other Kinds of Rest 100

Joy **101**
    Stress Reduction 103
        The Stress Cycle 103
            Triggers 103
            Immediate Relief 103
            Handling Residual Stress 104
    How to Boost Your Joy 105
        Journal for Joy 106
        Be Kind to Yourself and Others 107
        Focus on What You Can Control 109
        Take Refuge in Nature 110
        Sing, Dance, Listen To, and/or Play Music 110
        Mindfulness, Meditation, Prayer, and Noticing & Gratitude 111

FIRST TRIMESTER **115**

Introduction 116

Nourishment 117
    Nourish Your Baby! 118
        Healthy Weight Gain 118
        Food Aversions 119
        Digestive Sensitivities 119
        Hormonal Imbalances 120
        Eating to Combat Morning Sickness 120
        Protein 122
        Be a Snacker 123
        Eat Your Veggies 123
        Healthy Fats 123
    Vitamins and Supplements 125
        Evening Primrose Oil 125
    Natural Medicine Chest 126

Hydration 127
   Overheating.. 127
   Pregnancy Tea.. 128

Movement.. 130
   Build Up Your Core 131
   Practice Getting Up Properly for Late Pregnancy 131
   Take Care 132

Emotional and Spiritual 133
   Your Partner's Role.. 135
   Strategies for Navigating Emotional Turmoil..................... 136
      Noticing 137
      Think Positively 137
      Breathe Deeply... 137
      Counseling.. 139
      Avoid Sources of Fear and Images of Violence.............. 139
      Access Your Intuition 140
      Affirmations... 141
   Timing Your Announcement... 141
   When Will My Baby Be Born? 142

Knowledge 144
   What's Going on in My Body?... 144
   Uterus Retroversion 146
   Implantation Bleeding.. 147
   When Can I Hear My Baby's Heartbeat? 147
   Flat or Inverted Nipples... 147
   Considerations for Choosing a Care Provider.................... 148
      Hospitals.. 148
      Freestanding Birth Center.. 154
      Home Birth with a Midwife 155
   Choosing a Care Provider 168
      It is Your Choice 168
      Questions to Ask a Potential Provider............................. 169
      How to Find a Midwife 171
      What Will it Cost? 172

Demystifying Pregnancy Dos and Don'ts 173
    Myth: You Can't Have Sushi 173
    Myth: You Can't Get in a Hot Tub 174
    Myth: You Can't Have Soft Cheeses & Lunch Meats 174
    Myth: Don't Drink Any Alcohol, Ever 174
    Myth: Sex Will Hurt the Baby 175
    Myth: You Can't Lie on Your Back 176
    Myth: Once a Cesarean, always a Cesarean 177
    Truth: You shouldn't Wear Thong Underwear 179
Handling the Common Discomforts of Pregnancy 179
    When to Call Your Midwife 179
    Morning Sickness 180
    Headaches 180
    Migraines 180
    Constipation 181
    Herpes 183
    Pregnancy Brain 183
    Uterine Cramping and Spotting 184
    Bleeding 184
    Leg Cramps 184
    Pain from Ligament Stretching 185
    Varicose Veins 185
    Acne 186
    Nosebleeds 186
    Bleeding Gums 186
    Dizziness 187
    Yeast or Bacterial Infections 187
Miscarriage 187
    When to Go to the Hospital 189
    Miscarriage at Home 189
    Emotional Aftermath 190
    When to Try Again 192
Natural Remedies for When You are Sick 192
    Preventative Measures 192
        Wash Your Hands 192
        Don't Sleep in a Bed with Sick People 192
        Additional Best Practices 193

Steps to Take When You Feel an Illness Coming On 193

    The Remedy Shot...194

    Fever/Pain...195

    Respiratory Infection 195

    Flu...196

    Stomach Viruses...196

    Bladder Infection 197

    Cough, Cold, or Sore Throat...197

    Allergies..198

    Ear Infection/Pain 198

    Asthma..198

What if It Doesn't Work? 199

10–12 Week Genetic Screening...199

Pets 201

Rest 202

Feeling Low Ebb is Common 202

Know Your Rights 202

Babymoon Vacation...203

Start Preparing for Your Maternity Leave 204

Joy 205

Creating a Positive Birth Experience 205

Be Kind to Yourself...206

Focus on What You Can Control.. 206

Connect With Nature 206

Spend Time with Your People 207

Pamper Yourself...210

Sing, Dance, and Listen to Music 210

Gratitude Practice..211

THE SECOND TRIMESTER.. 215

Introduction 216

Welcome to Your Halcyon Days! 216

Nourishment 217

Weight Gain Window 217

If You're Struggling to Gain 217

If You're Still Struggling with Nausea 218

Satisfying Your Sweet Tooth 218
Supplements 218
    Add an Ultra-Mins to Prevent Muscle Cramps 218

Hydration 219
Alternative Methods of Hydration 219

Movement...220
Considerations for Exercising While Pregnant 220
    Yoga 220
    Swimming 221
    Impact Exercise 221

Emotional/Spiritual 222
Bolster Your Body Image 222
Connect with Your Baby..223
Develop Your Intuition..224
Affirmations...225
    Sample Affirmations for Pregnancy 225
Noticing..225

Knowledge 226
What's Going on in My Body?..227
    Uterine Contractions 227
    Ligament Stretching 227
    Placental Growth...228
    Baby's Movements 229
    Pelvic Floor...229
Finding Out Your Baby's Gender..231
Cord Blood Banking..233
    Why do it?...233
    How Does it Work? 234
    How Much Does It Cost? 234
    Private versus Public Stem Cell Banks 235
Handling the Complications and Common Discomforts of Pregnancy........235
    Anemia 235
    Back Pain..237
    Congestion..238
    Cramping and Spotting 238
    Fatigue 238

Gestational Diabetes 239

Hemorrhoids 240

Herpes 241

Indigestion 241

Ligament Stretching Pain 242

Pregnancy Brain 243

Varicose or Spider Veins 243

Vaginal Infections 244

Other Helpful Practitioners 248

Acupuncturist 249

Chiropractic Care 249

Naturopath 251

Abdominal Massage Therapist 252

Counselor 252

Dentist 252

Doula 253

Homeopath 254

Massage Therapist 255

Repatterning Practitioner 255

Educate Yourself 255

Rest **257**

Joy **258**

Self-Care in the Second Trimester 258

Prenatal Massage 258

Manicure and Pedicure 258

Facial or Skincare Routine 258

Hydrotherapy 259

Stretch Your Pampering Dollars 259

Meditation and Mindfulness 260

Connect with Nature 260

Nature Hikes 260

Nature Photography 261

Nature Inspired Arts and Crafts 261

Camping or Glamping 261

Outdoor Sports and Water Activities 262

Nature-Inspired Journaling 262

Sunrise or Sunset Appreciation 262

Build Your Support Network 262
Birth Plan 262
    What to Put in Your Birth Plan 263
    Surrender 265
Build Up Your Emotional and Spiritual Health 265
    Avoid Negativity 266
Sun Your Belly 266
Babymoon Vacation 267
Take it All In 267

THIRD TRIMESTER 269

Introduction 270

Nourishment 271
Supplements 271
    Borage Oil, Evening Primrose Oil, or Black Currant Oil 272
    Herbal Blend for Birth Preparation 272
Preparation for Postpartum Nutrition 273

Hydration 275

Movement 276
Exercise 276
    Swimming 277
    Walking 278
    Squatting 278
    How to Squat 279
    Weight Work 279
    Continue Abs Work 280
    Prenatal Yoga 280
When to Stop 280
Rise Carefully 281
Breathing Techniques & Relaxation Exercises 281
    No Single Way 281
    How Often to Practice 282
    Partner's Role 282
    Breathing Exercises 283
        Deep Cleansing Breath to Kick Things Off and Wrap Things Up 283
        Focus 283

Deep Breathing 284

The Pant 284

The Pant-Blow 285

Practice Relaxation 285

Emotional/Spiritual 288

Fear and Spirituality 288

Components of a Holistically Safe Birth 289

Intuition 291

Affirmations and Visualizations 291

Combatting Fear 291

Noticing 293

Whom to Invite to the Birth 293

Energy in the Birthing Room 293

How Many People to Invite 294

Harmonious and Private 295

Inviting Your Mother 296

Watch Birth Videos 297

Sibling Preparation 297

Co-Sleeping and the Family Bed 299

Friend and Extended Family Preparation 299

An Advocate 300

Boundaries and Difficult Situations 300

Going Radio Silent 301

Continue to Avoid Negativity 302

Partners, Help Now 302

Knowledge 303

What's Going on in My Body? 303

Ripening and Softening 303

Preparing to Breastfeed 304

Your Baby is Growing 304

Why am I Peeing so Much? 305

Handling the Common Discomforts and Complications
of the Third Trimester 305

High Blood Pressure 305

Don't Cross Your Legs When Sitting 305

Swelling 305

Herpes 306

Glucose Screening..306
Pregnancy/Mommy Brain 307
Wanting Your Partner to Understand What You're Going Through 307
How Big Will My Baby Be?..........................308
28-32 Weeks...308
   Belly Support..308
   Childbirth Classes...................................309
   Babyproofing 312
      All Over the House!..............................312
      Baby's Nursery 313
      Test Small Objects...............................314
      Kitchen...314
      Bathroom...314
      Living Room...314
      Laundry Room 315
      Create a Safe Play Spot 315
   Eight to Twelve Weeks Before Your Due Date 315
Weeks 32 to 34 315
   Do What You Can and Rest 315
   Education and Reading List 315
   32-Week Exam 316
   Prepare for a Hospital Birth 317
   Prepare to Cease Working 317
   Keep Up with Childbirth Classes 317
   Belly Support System 318
   Kick Counts... 318
   Contractions..320
   Six Weeks Before Your Due Date 320
Weeks 35–36 320
   Vaginal Culture & Bacteria Screen 320
   Blood Draw...321
   Partners, Clean Your Environment 321
   Practice Your Breathing.......................... 323
   Purchase Your Nursing Bras................... 323
   Diapers..324
   Pack/Prepare Your Birth & Postpartum Supplies 326
      Supplies for All Births........................326
      Supplies for a Home Birth...................327

    Supplies for a Birth Center Birth..333

    Supplies for a Hospital Birth..333

    Mitigating the Cost of All This New Stuff..336

Perineal Massage 336

Castor Oil Packs 337

Air Filters..337

Pets...338

    Sleeping with Pets..338

    Dogs..338

    Cats...339

Choose a Pediatrician 339

Assessing the Baby's Position 340

    What to Do...342

    External Version..343

    Breech Birth..344

Four Weeks Before Your Due Date 345

Week 37 345

Preparation Postpartum Nourishment..345

Preparation for Postpartum: Room Setup 346

Preparation for Breastfeeding 346

Three Weeks Before Your Due Date 348

Week 38 349

Stop Working If at All Possible 349

Assessing Baby's Position...349

    Breech and Other Less-Than-Optimal Positions..349

Set Up Your Birth Pool (Optional)..349

    Select a Location for the Pool...349

    Inflating and Cleaning the Pool...349

    Filling the Pool...350

Two Weeks Before and Until You Go into Labor 350

Signs of Impending Labor..351

Hormonal Surge 351

Ripening 351

Increasing Contractions...352

Engagement...352

Cervical Effacement 353

Cervical Dilation..353

Change in Maternal Activity Levels 354
Change in Fetal Activity Levels 354
Vaginal Discharge 354
Meteoric Emotions 354
Cramping 355
Nausea 355
Diarrhea 355
Mucus Plug 355
Warm-up Labor 356

Rest **357**
The Four-Hour Rule 357
Rest and Decreasing Stress 357
    Alleviating Hip Pain so You Can Sleep 358
Stop Working by 36–38 Weeks 358
How to Sleep During Warm-Up Labor 361

Joy **364**
Boosting Joy in the 3rd Trimester 364
    Have Lots of Sex 365
    Spend Time with Your People 365
    Pamper Yourself 366
    Connect With Nature 368
Focus on What You Can Control 369
Baby Shower Ideas 370

THE BIRTH PROCESS **373**

Introduction 374

39–42 Weeks **376**
What to Do While You're Waiting for Labor to Begin 376
    Distract Yourself with Projects 376
    Have Patience 377
      A Message for Women Planning a Hospital Birth 378
    Shift Your Energy Toward Your Ideal, Perfect Birth .. 378
    Movement 380
    Sex 380
    Rest 380
    Engage Your Spirituality 381

Signs of Actual Labor 381

    Bloody Show 381

    Quality of Contractions 381

    Other Signs...383

When to Call the Midwife... 383

What Your Partner Should Do When Labor Starts 384

When Your Water Breaks..388

Sterile Technique..390

TO DO 391

Keep in Mind 392

Get the Support You Need 392

Take a Nap 393

Use the Trick..393

Mechanisms of Labor 394

Stages & Phases of the Birth Process 398

  Stage 1: Dilation 1–10 cm...398

  Stage 1 Pre-Labor 398

    Keyword: Discouragement..398

    What To Do When Pre-Labor Starts...399

    Stay Nourished 399

    Stay Hydrated.. 400

    Take a Shower 400

    Revisit Your Affirmations.. 400

    Rest...401

    What to do for Nausea/Vomiting 402

  Stage 1—Dilation Phase I: Early Labor 1 –4 cm................................402

    Keyword: Excitement 402

    Joy During Early Labor 403

    Rapid Birth 403

    Early Labor at the Hospital... 404

    Early Labor at a Freestanding Birth Center................................405

    Early Labor at Home—Midwife's Role 406

    Early Labor Anywhere 410

    Partner's Role.. 416

  Stage 1—Dilation Phase II: Active Labor 4–7 cm 416

    Keyword: Serious 416

    What to do to Support Yourself in Active Labor 418

Water in Birth...419

Partner's Role...420

Squatting...420

Aid in Relaxation...420

How to Help with Back Pain..421

Midwife's Role at a Home Birth..421

Hospital Birth..422

Birth Center Birth..423

Stage 1—Dilation Phase III: Transition 7–10 cm.............................423

Keyword: Psychedelic Discouragement 423

Partner's Role..427

Midwife/Home Birth Experience...428

How to Get in the Zone During Labor at the Hospital...........................428

Stage II: Pushing...429

Squatting..430

What to Do..431

Getting Back in Bed for Birth 432

The Umbilical Cord..434

The Moment Before Birth 435

Birth...435

The Ring of Fire...436

Baby Arrives and Goes Skin to Skin...436

Birth Stories..438

Hospital Birth: Sarah's Story...438

Hospital Birth: Penelope's Story... 441

Birth Center Birth: Juliana's Story...446

Birth Center Birth: Monica's Story—a Journey of Love and Empowerment.......451

Birth Center Birth: Justus's Story..453

Home Birth: Aleah's Story...454

Home Birth: Sheryl's Story 460

Home Birth: Andrea's Story..460

Newborn Pictures..464

42 Weeks 466

Ultrasound..466

Pumping and Herbs..466

Breaking Waters 467

Other Methods..467

Complications and Interventions 468
    Oxygen.. 468
    Sutures for Tearing or Lacerations 469
    Breaking the Waters.. 469
    Suctioning.. 470
    Stripping the Membranes 470
    Stimulating the Cervix/Cervical Massage......................... 470
    Administering Fluids Intravenously................................... 471
    Episiotomy 472
    Herpes in Labor and Delivery 473
    Hospital Transfer 473
        Reason for Hospital Transport: Non-Progression of Labor 474
        Reason for Hospital Transport: A Blood Pressure Problem 475
        Reason for Hospital Transport: Fetal Distress 475
        Reason for Hospital Transport: Bleeding.................................. 476
        Reason for Hospital Transport: Placental Problems 476
        Reason for Hospital Transport: Infection 476
        What to Expect at the Hospital.. 477
        Epidural 478
        Other Methods of Pain Management... 479
        Caesarean Section (C-Section).. 479
        When Are Interventions a Good Idea? 481
        The Mindset to Adopt if You Transport.................................... 481
        How Long You'll Be There 482

What to Do in the Case of Sudden Childbirth 483
    Important Steps for the Partner to Take............................. 484

Before I Leave You 488

Epilogue... 490

Acknowledgements... 492

APPENDICES.. i
    Appendix A: Product Recommendations & Vendors ii
    Appendix B: Recipes and Tips... v
    Appendix C: Medical Questionnaire...................................xlv
    Appendix D: Resources for Miscarriage and Grief li

Appendix E: Organizations lii
Appendix F: Book Recommendations...liii
Appendix G: Tracking Contractions...lvi

Glossary lvii

Credits.. lxxiv

Endnotes.. lxxxii

Index ci

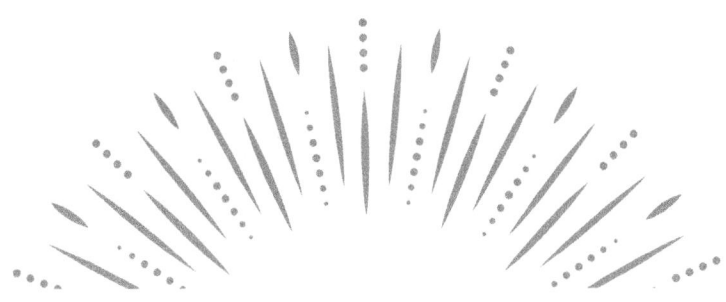

INTRODUCTION

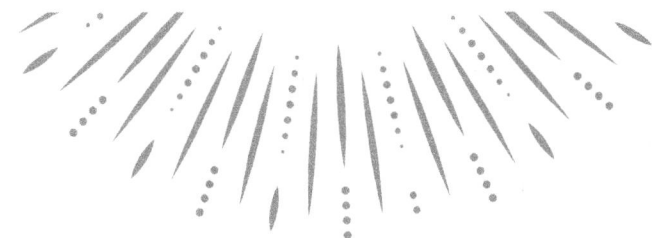

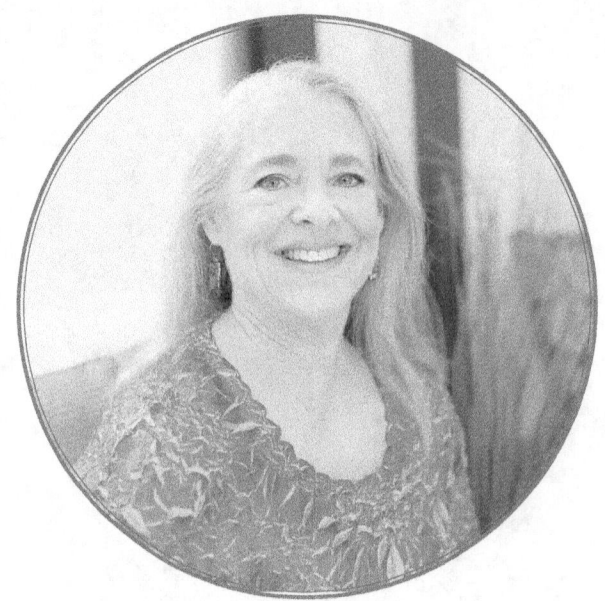

MariMikel

Hello my dear,

If you are reading this book, it is likely you are either wanting to or expecting to welcome a baby into your life. I hope that with this book I can be at your side, sharing my knowledge, wisdom, and experience as one of the guides on the path to your ideal, perfect birth.

Let me introduce myself. My first name sounds like Mary Michael, but it's all one word—M-A-R-I-M-I-K-E-L (Thanks, Mom and Dad!)—and Potter is my last name. I'm the owner and director of New Life Birth Services[1] in Austin, Texas. I have a Bachelor of Science in Nursing from The University of Texas at Austin, and I've never done anything but be a midwife.

I started attending births before I ever even got out of nursing school, and I've been a midwife here in Austin for nearly 50 years. I've attended well over 3,000 births and I have handled every situation in the birthing room you can possibly imagine and many I'm certain you can't.

I have great safety statistics, which I will speak about later in this book. I have a great rapport, relationship, and reputation with the medical community here in Austin, which means that I have wonderful medical support and backup from every kind of healthcare provider you can imagine.

I've had six children of my own. My oldest child is now 54 and my youngest is 36. I had my first three births in the hospital and the last three at home. Two of my hospital births were transports from planned home births. I have learned so much and seen so much in my practice over the years that I wish I could share with all pregnant woman everywhere, but I am just one person. This book gives me the opportunity to help so many people, and I hope you will be among them.

I have put absolutely everything I could into these pages. My deepest desire is that you will find this book to be a compassionate resource with which to supplement your provider's care. No matter your question, I want you to be able to find an answer in this book, and that is why I have written the most comprehensive guide I possibly could.

I want you to have your ideal, perfect conception, pregnancy, and birth. I want you to be empowered in your life—in all aspects of your life, but empowerment in pregnancy is imperative to the safe and joyous birth you want to achieve. I want you to fully understand your options and choices so you can make the very best decisions for you and your family.

In these pages you will find the framework of my Sevenfold Approach to Your Ideal, Perfect Conception, Pregnancy, and Birth, and at each phase of your pregnancy I will use this framework to help provide you with the information you need to make the choices that are best for you and your baby.

Blessings and light,

Marimikel Potter

Why I Became a Midwife

This story has a sad beginning, but a joyful ending. When I was in my second year of nursing school, I went through a period of great loss. My grandmother and father both died in a short span of time, and my second pregnancy ended in stillbirth. I was 20 years old, and I'd never really experienced loss before. I struggled with that pain for a very long time.

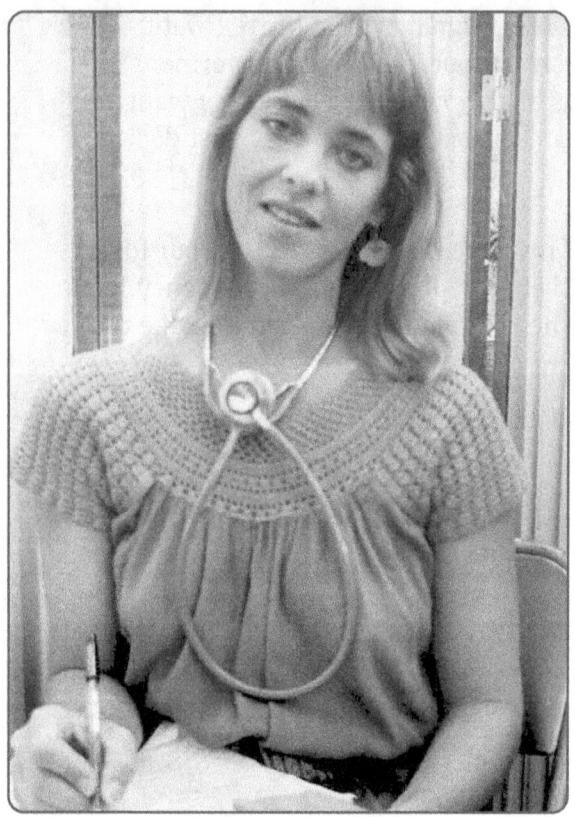

MariMikel in the early '80s

Some members of my family told me that my baby's death was a punishment from God because I was not married. I didn't really believe that, but it sure got into my heart in a hard way, and I went through a long questioning of the divine.

After much soul searching, I finally answered my own questions and realized that God does not do things to me. I am not a puppet. God has given us free will. We were created in the image of the divine as creators. We create our reality, and we are in charge. The divine is there to give us strength and guidance when life goes amok, but not to push buttons, make things happen for us, or punish us. I believe that even the most horrible things I experience are opportunities for me to learn from. It never feels like that at the time, though, and sometimes it takes me years to recognize what I gained from the trauma I went through.

When I returned to nursing school, I was by chance put on a labor and delivery rotation. My heart was so wrenched open and raw from my loss, and being present for these mothers and babies filled that hole. I had been studying to be a psych nurse, but my focus changed as I became more and more fascinated with mothers and birth. I felt like every birth was such a miracle and cried tears of joy at each one. The other nurses thought it was a little odd that I was so

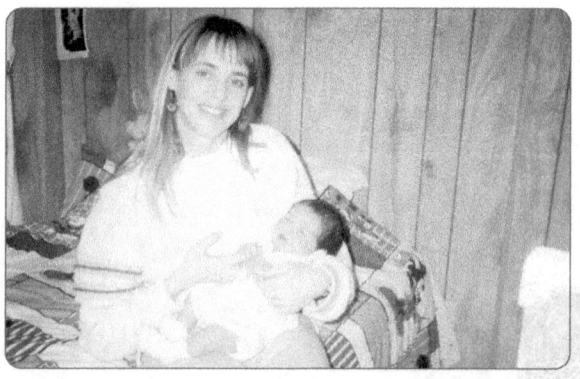

MariMikel with a Client's Baby in the '80s

affected. But I was. It was absolutely mind boggling to me how much participating in the birth process filled my heart with such joy.

One day, during one of my electives at the hospital, the nurses were talking with great shock. They were passing around an article in the *Austin American–Statesman* about people having their babies at home without a doctor present.

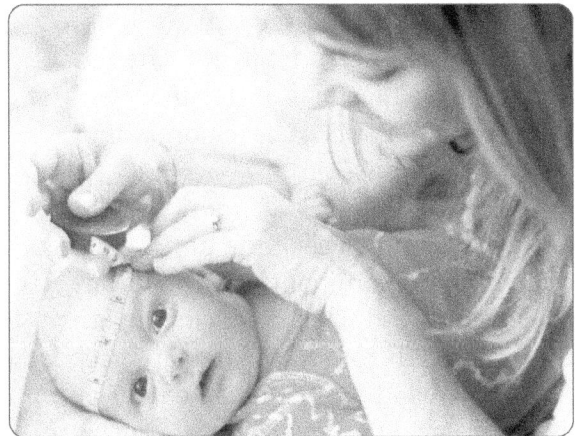

MariMikel Conducting a Newborn Checkup in the Late '80s

I said, "Oh, let me see that," and the article happened to have the contact information for a couple who were helping people to have home births. I reached out and had the absolute joy of meeting Niki and David Richardson. They were working with some incredible women, Jane Goehring and Allison Nash, and I came and sat in on their meetings. I had lots of medical information, but absolutely no knowledge of the spiritual side of birth. I told them that I was a nurse and they welcomed me into the fold.

I graduated from nursing school at a time when Scopolamine and Demerol were routinely administered to almost every

laboring mother, whether she wanted them or not. You may have heard of twilight sleep. Also, every baby was removed from the mother the moment after birth and kept from their mother for between four hours and sometimes as much as twelve hours, just for observation. The mothers were all medicated, and as a result not in any shape at all to take care of their newborn babe or do anything, really. It was a vicious circle, and I had pregnant friends who told me, "I'm not going to do that. I'll take my chances at home. But it would help if you were there with me, MariMikel. You could listen to the baby's heartbeat and take my blood pressure." I realized if I was there, it would be better than if I were not, so that's how I got started.

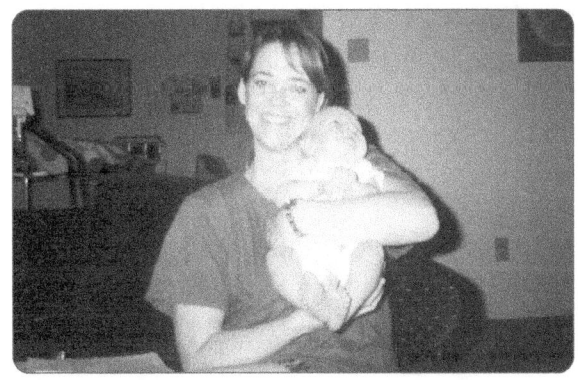

MariMikel in the Early '90s

By the time I graduated from nursing school, I had attended more than 100 births. In the hospital there was no room anywhere for or acknowledgement of the sacred and spiritual side of it. But these people I'd met who were helping families to have home births were very sacred in their approach to birth. It was an absolute eye-opener for me. We joined forces and started the Austin Lay Midwives Association (ALMA). We stayed together for many years, and I attended hundreds of births with them.

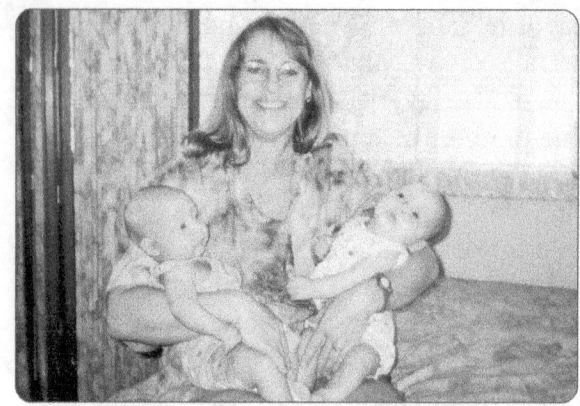

MariMikel in the Late '90s Reuniting with Twins She Caught

Ten years after she passed, I dreamed about my baby, the one I told you about at the beginning of this story. She appeared to me as a ten-year-old. We were in a big field, and I could see her, and I knew it was her. She ran to me, and I ran to her. I saw that she was perfect. She didn't have any of the birth defects her body had been born with, and she was so incredibly happy and filled with joy.

In the dream she told me there is no death and there are no dead. Death is an illusion we grapple with in this place. We are in a big learning ground to experience some massive spiritual lessons about the illusion of separation, of duality, right and wrong, good and bad, up and down, light and dark, etc. Each of these are constructs we have created to experience this reality, but she told me *she* was in the real world, and we were in a learning place. Everyone I'd ever loved and lost and everything I'd ever loved and thought I'd lost were there with her. She told me we will all be connected again because time is also an illusion.

When she was born, I'd been studying to become a psych nurse. Well, that wasn't the

path I was supposed to travel, obviously. In that dream, my daughter told me she'd volunteered to come in and head out in order to transform my path, and it had worked splendidly. I have to agree; her time here with me *did* open my heart and direct me on a new path.

When I began attending home births in the early '70s, the only certification available to midwives in the US was a certified nurse-midwife (CNMs) credentialling program. To become a CNM, you first earn a registered nurse license, then attend graduate school and receive a master's degree in Nurse Midwifery. In the US, the majority of CNMs work in hospitals.

Non-nurse midwives at the time I started midwifing predominantly learned from one another and from practicing together. I branched off from ALMA to start a school for midwives in 1980 and named my practice New Life Birth Services. This was the first out-of-hospital (freestanding) birth center licensed to a non-doctor in the state of Texas.

Throughout much of the '80s and '90s I worked with many other wonderful women to further midwives' professional standards. I served as a board member, represented my state or region, and participated as a member in several different professional midwifery associations like the Midwives Alliance of North America (MANA) and North American Registry of Midwives (NARM). I was a frequent speaker at conferences for midwives.

In the early '90s I served on the Board of Directors of MANA. At that time, MANA formed a separate body to research, write, and offer a national exam to test the empirical knowledge of midwives. That separate body became known as the North American Registry of Midwives (NARM). I participated in the process that established what is now known as NARM's Certified Professional Midwife (CPM) process.

MEAC is an organization that credentials midwifery training programs and schools. After midwives are trained through a MEAC-accredited school, they are then eligible to sit for the NARM examination to be credentialed as a CPM.

This process of education, clinical, and birth experience, followed by the NARM CPM exam is now widely used to certify a midwife's credentials and has been since the early '90s. I sat for and passed the exam in 1992.

I also later became a Licensed Midwife (LM) in the state of Texas through the Texas State Health Department when that was offered as a certification. The state of Texas utilizes the NARM CPM process as the requirement for midwives to be licensed. Certification standards vary by state.

I wanted to share these qualifications to show the rigorous standards midwives are held to and how we receive our certifications and licensing. CPMs and CNMs are trained, educated, and experienced professionals entirely focused on the pregnancy and birth experience.

I maintained my birth center for 35 years before deciding to let the center go. I just didn't want to work that hard anymore. I attended six to twelve births a month for a very long time. I now maintain my practice

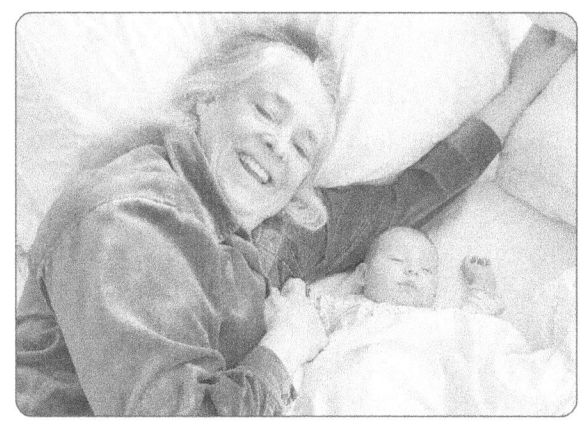

MariMikel with Her Granddaughter Téa

out of my home and attend two to three births a month, and I still have apprentices learning the craft at my side. If the idea of being a midwife appeals to you, I hope you will take steps to explore that path. I believe strongly that the world needs many more midwives and doulas.

I chose to move onto a new path that changed my life and a lot of other lives as well. I never did become a psych nurse, but I have had the pleasure and privilege of helping women and attending the births of thousands and thousands of babies. So, sometimes the very hard things we deal with in life can work for good if you trust, have faith, and allow time to reveal your true path.

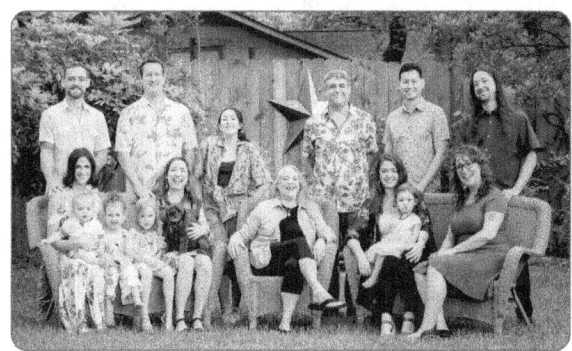

MariMikel with Her Children and Grandchildren

Hospitals, Birth Centers, and Home Births

The one thing uniting every single human on the planet is the primordial experience of birth. This foundational experience we all share is incredibly impactful and substantial in its lifelong effects. We can't afford to be thoughtless, mindless, or disinterested in our approach to birth. When there are people present who consciously welcome your new baby into the world with great love, I believe that compassionate giving, loving, joyful energy flows into the baby at the moment of birth and affects who they're going to be.

You have choices when it comes to where you give birth, and many women have access to at least a few different options. In major metropolitan areas it is very likely you will have multiple hospitals, freestanding birth centers, and midwives who can help you with a home birth. These are very different options, with obvious differences, myths, and misconceptions surrounding each of them. I'll share a lot about each option in detail in the First Trimester chapter, so you can make an informed choice about where you would like to give birth. No matter what you decide, implementing my Sevenfold Approach will help you achieve a better outcome in *your* conception, pregnancy, and birth.

Before you become pregnant is a great time to start exploring and familiarizing yourself with the different options available to you for your baby's birth. By far the most common choice is a hospital delivery (98 percent in the US). A much smaller percentage of women opt for a home birth (about 1.5 percent). An even smaller percentage of women opt for a birthing center (0.5 percent of all US births).[2] I would absolutely love to turn these numbers on their heads, and I want you to have a deep understanding of why I feel this way. Of course, I am biased, but I have absolutely the best reasons for this bias, and I will share them with you.

Now, I do not want in any way to denigrate hospitals. Two of my own births were planned home births that ended up having complications. So, those experiences really made me more appreciative of how great the hospital is when you *need* to be there. They serve a wonderful purpose and are absolutely lifesaving. But I'd like you to consider that perhaps they shouldn't be where you start out, only where you end up if you must (unless you are at high risk for certain complications).

I also want to say just a little here about the experience of giving birth. Birth is a deeply sexual experience—albeit a painful one. It is on the continuum of sexual experiences that you have in life. Because it is a deeply sexual experience, where you are comfortable having sex is where you're going to be comfortable giving birth.

Think about this scenario: "Feeling a little amorous tonight, dear? Let's go to the hospital. There'll be lots of strangers around with masks on, and real bright lights, and nobody we've ever seen before. There'll be a little tiny bed ..." This does not sound at all sexy, and that's a problem. Your body will likely feel stressed in that environment, not safe. Where you feel sensual is where that primal energy and hormonal rush floods you with support to help you give birth in a more natural, more organically human way. Stress can shut down the process of labor completely, just as it could a sexual moment.

You know, when sex is wonderful and orgasmic, it's transcendental. You are in a completely other space. You feel a sense of expansion and oneness with the universe. It's transformational. You go to a state beyond words and beyond everything— and that's the state you achieve with an unmedicated birth. I call it *the zone*. We have all had times when we were composing a grocery list during sex, but those are not our best moments. It's the same thing with birth. You don't want to be making a grocery list while it happens to you; you want to be in the zone. I'll talk a lot more about this later.

In a hospital, women in labor are slated into an assembly line process. It's almost like they're in line to have their oil changed. There's not a whit of sensuality or spirituality to the process. You may have heard the adage that to a person with a hammer, every problem looks like a nail? Well, similarly, to the majority of hospital practitioners, the pregnant woman looks like someone who must be managed and shuffled through their process. If her labor doesn't move along according to their schedule, they will manage it through medical intervention(s), so that it does. There are a few reasons for this, which I'll mention briefly here and we'll explore in more detail in The First Trimester chapter.

I know I can come across as anti-hospital. The truth is I am exceptionally pro-hospital. I am so grateful for our wonderful hospitals here in Austin. When a pregnant woman needs to be there because of

complications, they are there for her and her baby, and they save lives every single day.

Also, I don't want to sugar-coat it. I want you to know the environment you are likely facing if you choose a hospital delivery. Hospital maternity wards are absolutely deluged with patients. They must move laboring women through the labor and delivery process or they will be stretched too thin. For example, currently in Austin, Texas, every hospital is doing 200–800 births a month. It's hard on them. My heart goes out to them for how hard they work and how much they give. For what they capably handle, we should be bowing down in honor of them. But this overwhelm also means is that women must conform to their vision of the birthing process and enter the hospital assembly line, so they can handle so many babies and mommas every single month.

This does have an impact on the level of care they can provide. The hospital practitioners can't really get to know people individually when they're dealing with so many patients. An OB/GYN may only have ten minutes for you at your prenatal visit, because they have to see so many other women. There is no real connection when you, as a woman giving birth, are dealing with strangers.

I am here to promote a different way of giving birth.

What the world desperately needs is more midwives, doulas, and birth centers, and we'll talk more about that later as well. For now, I want you to know that you have options, and that we'll dive into them more deeply in the chapters to come.

Ideal and Perfect

Ideal

What I am presenting to you in the pages of this book is my Sevenfold Approach to an Ideal, Perfect Conception, Pregnancy, and Birth. I want to take a moment to talk about the words *Ideal* and *Perfect*.

The first thing I want to say is that there is no single ideal way to give birth. Every birth worker's core goal is for you to have a birth that results in a healthy baby and a healthy momma. My Sevenfold Approach describes optimal behaviors at every stage, what you can be doing to be your very healthiest, happiest self throughout your pregnancy and beyond.

Optimizing your mental, physical, and spiritual health puts you in a position to have the birth that you want to have, *your* ideal birth. It does not in any way guarantee that your ideal birth will manifest, but when you take strides to optimize your health, it certainly moves you more in that direction. After that, surrender is critical. Trust that things are unfolding the way they're supposed to.

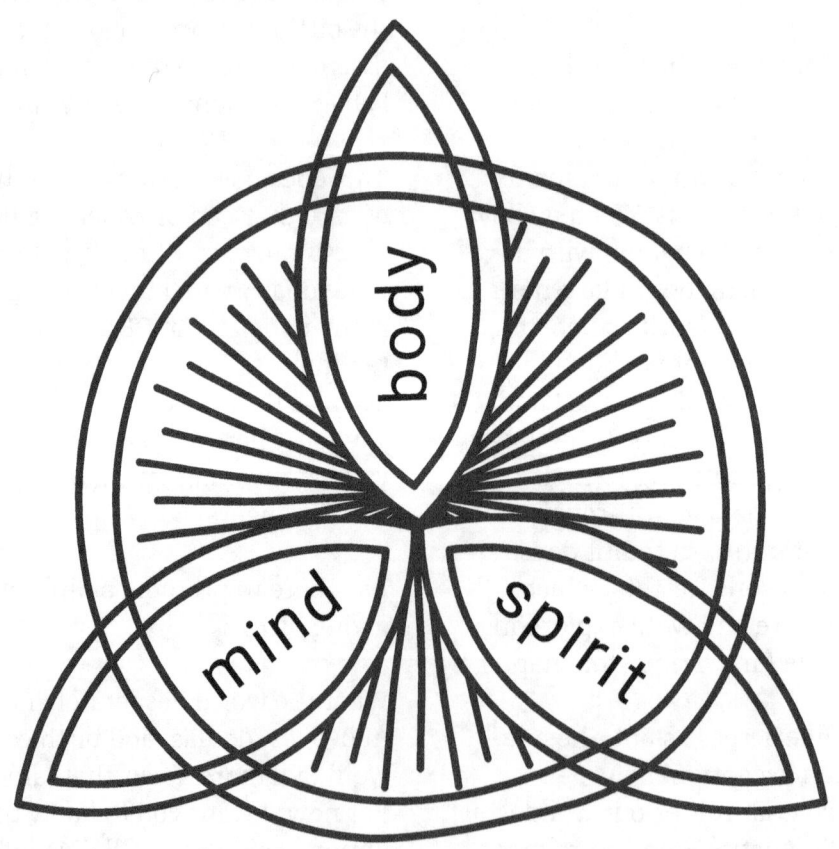

I want to also recognize that we are all human, and it's difficult to implement drastic lifestyle changes. Work toward the ideal and know that every step you take in pursuit of it will have a wonderful, positive impact on you and your baby.

Now, it is easy to talk about the ideal and perfect birth when you are in the dominant stratus of culture and society. I'm talking about middle- to upper-class white women in this country. White women have it easier than our Black, Brown, and Indigenous American sisters who are marginalized by our healthcare systems far too often[3]. And if you live in poverty or in a food desert, even talking about all the great ideas surrounding nutrition can possibly even be hurtful. If you do not have the financial wherewithal to get quality vitamins, and all the good things that we all know are helpful, this can feel hurtful too. Throughout this book I'll share any tips I have on how to make this journey less financially burdensome.

It is not my intention to denigrate in any way the people who experience pain and suffering caused by racism, discrimination, and the marginalization of People of Color in our society. We as a society have to figure out a way for there to be a better path for all women and families. The fact that the statistics are so abysmal for Women of Color in the US is beyond abhorrent and must be addressed by each and every responsible person out there. It has to be in our minds and in our hearts that we must help our Sisters of Color any way that we can to have the opportunities that upper- and middle-class white Americans have and take for granted. That would truly be ideal.

We must all band together as women, people, and communities to change this. The ability of every mother to access quality care is important to the health of each family and to the health of our nation. We must rise up and stand as one to help those in need, to find ways to give on every level, so we elevate our sisters, until they have at least the support that we may have. We can make a difference by starting food pantries for pregnant women in our community. We can create communities that reach out to those in need, and we can give philanthropically.

Perfect

Perfection is also not singular. There is no one perfect way to give birth. I read Voltaire's *Candide* when I was very young, and one of the key thoughts that stuck with me is that this existence, as it is unfolding, is absolutely perfect just as it is. It's perfection. Maybe it's not ideal. Maybe it's not even okay. We don't have to like it. We don't have to want it. We don't even have to agree to it; our reaction belongs to us. But what is unfolding is perfection. If you've got to go through difficult things in life, why not have a philosophy that says that's okay? For me, this helped a lot. I was able to find a way to be alright with the messiness of life with this approach.

I also need you to know that you can do absolutely everything perfectly and still have things turn out differently than you expected or wanted. Surrender is key in these moments, and I will talk a lot about that over the course of this book.

A Sevenfold Approach

My Sevenfold Approach is practical and spiritual; it is scientific and deeply personal. In this book I'll cover each step of this approach in each phase of your pregnancy, from conception through birth.

Number one—the most important thing— is **nourishment**. Two is **hydration**. Three is **movement**. Four is the **emotional and spiritual** component; it's profound and deep and sacred. Five is **knowledge**. Six is **rest**; we do not do enough of that, and last but not least is **joy**. When you wholeheartedly adopt my Sevenfold Approach, you will absolutely increase the probability of experiencing *your* ideal, perfect birth. Let's talk about each of these a little bit.

1. Nourishment

Food and minerals and vitamins are your first medicine. We'll discuss optimal diet choices, supplements, and everything you need to fully nourish yourself and your baby at each stage of your pregnancy. I'm going to spend a lot of time and energy talking about nutrition and vitamins, because I believe they are the first key to a healthy pregnancy, baby, birth, and life.

In a nutshell, we need to eat lots more vegetables, lots more good quality protein, fewer carbohydrates, and less sugar. Prenatal vitamins are dandy in the beginning of the pregnancy, but I just don't think there's enough in them, and I think you need a lot more than what is offered out of a prenatal vitamin alone. In these pages

you will find my recommendations for supplements and herbal remedies. I've been prescribing this regimen for 35 years, and I swear by it.

2. Hydration

All kinds of studies have shown that a huge percentage—75–85 percent—of all Americans are deeply, chronically dehydrated. Drinking enough water is one of the easiest things you can do to improve your health. In this book, you'll learn how much water you need to drink every day and why, because it's just so important.

3. Movement

Evolutionarily speaking, it is only very, very recently that we humans have shifted to a more and more sedentary lifestyle. Sedentary lifestyles are a leading cause of disease. They cause our bodies to hold onto detrimental stress chemicals and contribute to a less than optimal birthing experience. You'll learn how much and what kind of exercise you should be doing at every phase before and during your pregnancy.

4. Emotional/Spiritual

Often unacknowledged but absolutely vital to recognize are the emotional and spiritual components of your birthing experience. The birthing room is sacred space. At the moment of birth, you can feel the veil lifting in the room; you can feel the energy pulsing and coursing. The light is a different color. It's one of life's most profound experiences, and I believe it helps to acknowledge that this is a spiritual experience and treat it as such. I will help you to encourage and support the spiritual aspect of your birth experience.

I've worked with spiritually disparate people in my practice. I've helped fundamentalist Christians, Buddhists, Jews, Muslims, Hindus, Pagans, atheists, and every shade in between. A good midwife has to meet people where they are and find a way to support them spiritually because this is the most sacred space I have ever witnessed. Throughout this book I'll share ways that you can honor the sacred path you are on, whatever that path may be.

5. Knowledge

We are all so heavily bombarded with media and information technology data points. We are under a constant barrage of frightening and stressful information. Our minds are absolutely riding on high alert and that makes it difficult for us to get out of our heads.

Birth is an experience of the body and spirit. There's very little room for the mind in the birthing room, but in order for you to fully relax and allow your body and spirit to take over, your brain has to have enough information to understand what's going on. When the brain can calmly assess the situation and understand what is happening, it is able to let go and relax, so your heart, spirit, and body can take over. The body feels safe when it understands what is happening and what could happen.

If you're a first-time mother-to-be, there will be a lot of new and unfamiliar experiences that might freak you out a little and bring unnecessary stress into the process. When you've got enough information going into the birthing room, your mind will relax, and your body will follow its own mystical lead automatically.

In this book I will share what you need to know to quiet that monkey brain. There is a lot of information to absorb, and trying to learn it all at once will simply overwhelm you. We'll take it chunk by chunk, so you don't get overwhelmed.

6. Rest

We are so incredibly Type A obsessive compulsive and just driven in this culture to *do do do, go go go*. This is part of the Judeo-Christian work ethic, which says you are not valuable unless you are producing, it is more blessed to give than to receive, and you must keep doing more or you're not okay. I believe that babies are designed to not be so pushed, and I think when they are pushed in the womb, they become more anxious, more tense, more pushed people.

There is no such thing as one-sided generosity. Giving and receiving are necessary to one another.
—Toko-pa Turner

It's not valued in this culture for you to rest, say, "no," or do less, and I think this is a serious problem. It sure was for me, and I very slowly learned that it is as much a blessing to receive as it is to give. If there's nobody receiving, no one can give. I learned to slow down, to not be so type A and driven, and everything in my life changed. Rest is an important component of pregnancy and life. We'll explore different methods for you to increase the amount and quality of rest you're getting.

7. Joy

Joy is almost the inverse of stress. The more joyful times you have—the more fellowship, good friends, wonderful food, music, song, dance, and all of these things—the more you will build joy in your biochemistry, which is showered on your baby. I believe these biochemical states create joyful babies. We'll talk about different methods and ways you can bring more joy into your life.

Over the years I've come to believe that Joy deserves its own category, separate from Emotional/Spiritual. While joy is contained in emotions and often provoked by spiritual endeavors, the emotional/spiritual work that I explore in this book tends to be heavy at times. It is where you dive deep, whereas joy is always uplifting. As humans, we are hardwired to be on the lookout for danger and to pay attention to stressors. Our brains pay more attention to negative input than to compliments. We must strive especially to incorporate joy into our lives and to amplify the good vibrations.

My Sevenfold Approach does take dedication, discipline, effort, and attention. I'm not saying that this is easy, but neither is parenthood. If you wholeheartedly adopt this approach, you will find yourself living a healthier, happier life, and your pregnancy and birth experience will be the best it can possibly be.

How to Use This Book

Where to Start

You may already be pregnant and feel inclined to skip the Conscious Conception section of this book. That's completely fine. In subsequent sections, I'll let you know when you need to refer back to it. Dive in where you are in your pregnancy, and you can always refer to earlier sections when you need to.

When to Finish

I do suggest reading the whole book by Week 32 of your pregnancy, so you can prepare yourself, your family, and your environment for what's to come.

How to Find More Information

Throughout this book I touch on many subjects repeatedly, so I can provide you with information relevant to that stage of pregnancy. At any point you can refer back to the Table of Contents or Index to see where you can find more information on a subject that you're interested in. There are important topics, which I cover repeatedly and in great detail, and other topics that are interesting, and I want you to know about them, but I'm not going to dive deep. Please always feel free to supplement my information with your own research if something piques your interest.

Take What Works for You

I want to acknowledge that not everything I write about in here is right for everyone. Maybe most of it resonates, but a few things just don't jive with you. That's okay. Learn in life to take what works for you and let go of what doesn't. But don't miss out on the glimmers of knowledge and benefits you may receive from those things that do resonate. This is your journey.

Birth Stories

I'd also like to introduce you to Aleah, Robbie, Justus, Sheryl, Juliana, Monica, Sarah, and Penelope, who share stories about their pregnancies and births with you in these pages. Their stories run the gamut from hospital to freestanding birth center to home birth and include a variety of experiences. I like to say that birth is as unique as women are, and I hope these stories help to illustrate that. Aleah is my daughter, and I had the immense pleasure of serving as her midwife for her two

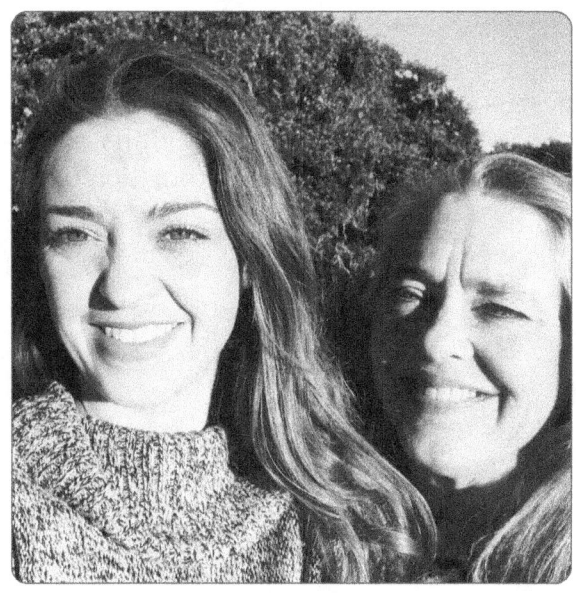

Aleah and MariMikel

beautiful daughters. I have been so honored and joyful to have been the midwife for all six of my grandchildren, five girls and one boy.

When and How to Prepare for Postpartum

I also strongly suggest that you read all of *The Book of Birth Volume II: Your Postpartum Journey through the Fourth Trimester* before you enter your third trimester. It will help you to prepare for the initial postpartum period and set you up for success with your new baby and with your own healing process. Our culture as a whole is far too dismissive of the postpartum period and the amazing development, healing, and bonding work that happens in those first months after birth. I've dedicated an entire book to it because it's just that important.

I had initially conceived this as a single volume that would cover everything from conception through postpartum and beyond, but when the book reached 650 pages and I hadn't yet finished telling you all I wanted to tell you, I realized you would be best served by having the information in two volumes. That way, you won't have to lug around the pregnancy information once

you no longer have need of it. Those first few months with your infant are so very important, for you and your baby. Please prepare yourself for them ahead of time.

Midwives and OB/GYNs

Throughout this book I often suggest that you contact your *midwife*. I understand that you may choose to work with an OB/GYN as your primary care provider. Know that when I use the word "midwife," if you aren't working with one, substitute "primary care provider" or "OB/GYN" in its place. I have always absolutely admired, respected, and appreciated doctors, and the role they play. That said, if a midwife isn't the first person you think of as a primary care provider for pregnancy and birth, I'd like to help to change that. A trained and educated midwife ably serves in that role, and many women would be benefitted from the level of care midwives provide.

Any time in your pregnancy is the right time to pick up this book, but if you aren't yet pregnant, that's absolutely the best time, because you can do so much to set the foundation for an excellent pregnancy in your pre-conception period. Turn the page to find out how.

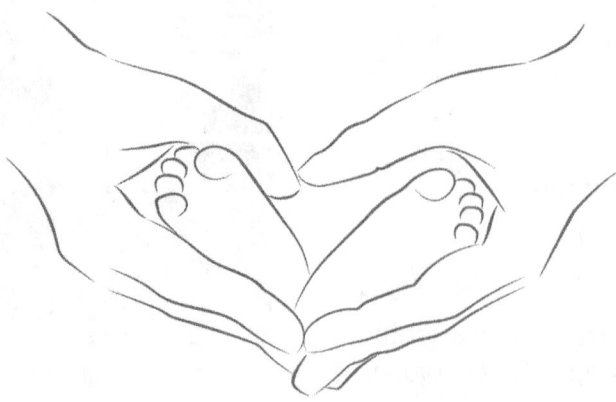

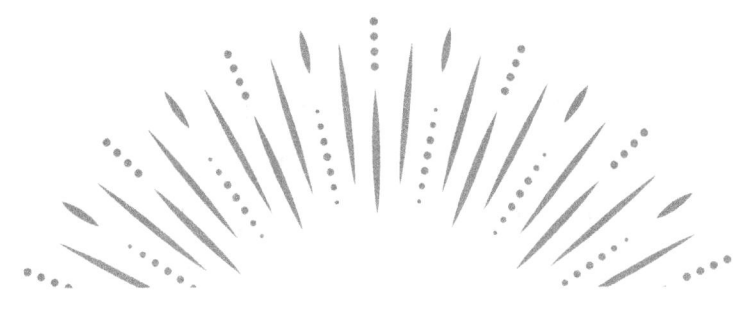

CONSCIOUS CONCEPTION

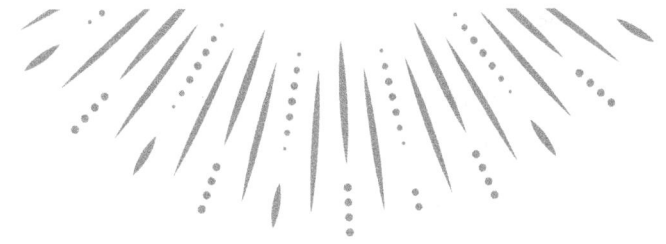

Introduction

Conscious Conception is much more than just getting pregnant. It is a conscious, mindful approach to every aspect of your mental, physical, and spiritual health in preparation for embarking on a new life path. When we take a conscious or mindful approach, we become more aware. We open our eyes to more of what is going on around us. We dig deeper into our psyches and become more willing to understand the psyches of others, their motivations, their needs, and their humanity. Consciousness and mindfulness go hand in hand, and anything that you can study about these tenets is going to help you to be a better person, partner, and parent.

We will take a holistic perspective, which recognizes the wonderful circle of mind, body, and spirit, and acknowledges that you cannot divorce any of these facets from the others and still have a healthy process. They are completely intertwined in an unbreakable way. When we shower attention on all three aspects—intellectual, physical, and spiritual—we find our best selves and our best journey through pregnancy. Your conscious approach to conception will provide the foundation for a healthy pregnancy, family, and life.

Deciding to have a baby should require a tremendous amount of thought, attention, and planning, as it is one of the most profound experiences in anyone's life. Most people do not realize how much you can affect the pregnancy, birth, and baby by what you do in the prenatal period and before. It is very possible to affect these outcomes in really positive ways, but doing so requires work on your part.

This Sevenfold Approach to Your Ideal, Perfect Conception, Pregnancy, and Birth might feel overwhelming. There's a lot to pay attention to. Don't worry. I'm here to help you implement each of these components step by step. They build on each other, and as you implement one in your lifestyle, the others become easier to incorporate. Just do the best you can.

Making the decision to have a child—it's momentous. It is to decide forever to have your heart go walking around outside your body.

—Elizabeth Stone

If it's too much in its entirety, take it one part at a time. Something is better than nothing.

 Let me tell you, people have never taken this optimal approach as a society. We are shooting for the moon with this approach to pregnancy. We can absolutely get there, but it's quite a journey. You are not alone, and it will help considerably if you can get the support of those around you, most importantly, your partner. Whatever you are able to implement will impact you and your family for the better. Throughout this book I'll highlight sections that are essential for your partner to read with the icon you see at the start of this paragraph. Also, while I recognize that not all partners are male gendered, I chose to use the pronoun "he" when referring to your partner as it is representative of the masculine role they play in the pregnancy and birth process.

This, of course, assumes that you have a partner, and not every woman does. I have attended many, many births for single moms and they have had wonderful, complete, and happy experiences. Most single-mommas-to-be do have some sadness at not having someone to share their journey with, but not having a significant other does not preclude you from a perfect, ideal experience. You just may have to work at it. I do suggest that you ask a family member or friend whom you trust and can count on to support you throughout the process, to be with you during the birth, and to stay with you for the first couple of weeks postpartum. We'll talk more about this later.

Pregnancy requires a tremendous expenditure of the body's energy and resources. If you're thinking about getting pregnant, you want to factor in how much it takes from your body. In our society, most people have no idea of how hard it is to be pregnant. Women make it look so easy, complain so little, and are acknowledged so rarely that the information is just not out there. The process can be quite difficult in the early part and at the end of pregnancy. Not every woman is affected to the same degree by pregnancy. There is a bell curve from not much different to absolutely altered and unable to function. You never know in advance which one you're going to be. Even if you've had a child before, this pregnancy may be very different from your previous experience. So, you at least should anticipate that it could be more difficult than you think.

There is tremendous external and internal pressure on people to procreate. I think that the first drive of humanity is survival—food and shelter—but boy, just after that is the drive to procreate. It is genetic and instinctual. When I say drive, I mean humans are *driven* by their need to procreate.

I believe there are a lot of things that can stand in the way of the process unfolding easily. One of the biggest obstacles is stress. When you are planning for a pregnancy do everything in your power to ease the path. Give yourself the expectation that it will take time for this process to unfold. Give yourself a year. A lot of people get pregnant on the very first try, but for many it takes a while. Too much pressure to conceive can be a barrier to conception. There are many anecdotal stories of women who struggled to conceive, were unsuccessful, adopted, and then got pregnant. I believe these women let go of their attachment to the outcome and let go of their stress relating to conceiving. Once they had a child, some deeper part of them let go so things could happen naturally.

On the flip side, I talked to someone not long ago who told me they were expecting to have fertility issues, so they started trying to conceive with the preconceived idea that they would struggle and would probably need to consult with fertility specialists. When they got pregnant almost immediately, they were unprepared for it because they had already decided that they weren't going to be successful. I suggest that you remove any preconceptions you have around how long it may take to conceive, be they long or short. Give yourself the grace of an expectation-free conception.

The more pressure you feel to conceive, the more barriers it installs; conversely, the more you can relax, the better it goes.

After the death of my baby, I wanted to get pregnant again immediately, but it took almost a year and a half to conceive. I believe this was because my deepest self knew that I was not ready. I needed to process my loss and grief. You cannot replace loss; you cannot replace the loss of a child or a pregnancy by having another one. You can add to your life, but you cannot take away loss. I was very young, and I did not understand this yet. I eventually got pregnant at the time that I was ready—or mostly ready.

I need you to really understand that if you are having a seriously hard time in your relationship, having a baby is not going to fix it. If your relationship is foundering, if you are struggling with your partner, having a baby is not going to bring you closer together. It sure can load additional stressors onto the situation, though. Wanting a child to fix your relationship is an exceptionally poor reason to have a child. Fix your relationship before you attempt to welcome a child into your family.

Another tremendous issue is how hard we all work now. Pretty much everyone I know works. Women are stretched very thin. Having a baby and parenting a child is a full-time job and trying to fit a pregnancy, baby, and child into a 40–50-hour work week is not a recipe for success. No one will get everything they need this way.

The idea of having a few weeks with your baby after the birth and then going back to work is so very sad to me. I don't ever see anyone thrilled with having to go back to work. A lot of times financially you're just not able to do anything else. I understand. I was a single mom with three kids, and I had to work. Luckily, I had a job where I could take my baby with me, but most do not have that luxury. Daycare is just that. They will *care* for your baby. The sign doesn't say Day *Love* it says Daycare. The studies about what babies require to be healthy individuals are absolute and unequivocal.[4]

Babies need love. If there's any way that you can take plenty of time off after the birth to bond and be with your baby, plan to do that. I fully believe that six months is a minimum. I know this goes against the grain; most women in the US only get 6–12 weeks.

If you don't already have kids, it's easy to think they're just going to kind of fit into your life and you're going to get up in the morning and hold the baby on one hip and check your phone and drink your coffee with your free hand. This is not reality for most people. Your lives are upended with a newborn. Eventually the baby requires less of you, and you have more and more time to get back to the routines that you love, but if you don't go into this with the idea that it will change your lives, you are

mistaken. I hope you will do the very best job you can with this to give it your all. Your baby deserves it, our society deserves it, and our world deserves it. We need to create healers and people who are going to bring peace to the planet, people who have been raised in ways that are spiritually, emotionally, intellectually, and physically empowering.

Suffice it to say, while motherhood has brought the greatest joys of my life, having a child is no small endeavor and it's not for everyone. Make sure it's right for you. If this is a life path you are 100 percent committed to, then wonderful! Let's begin.

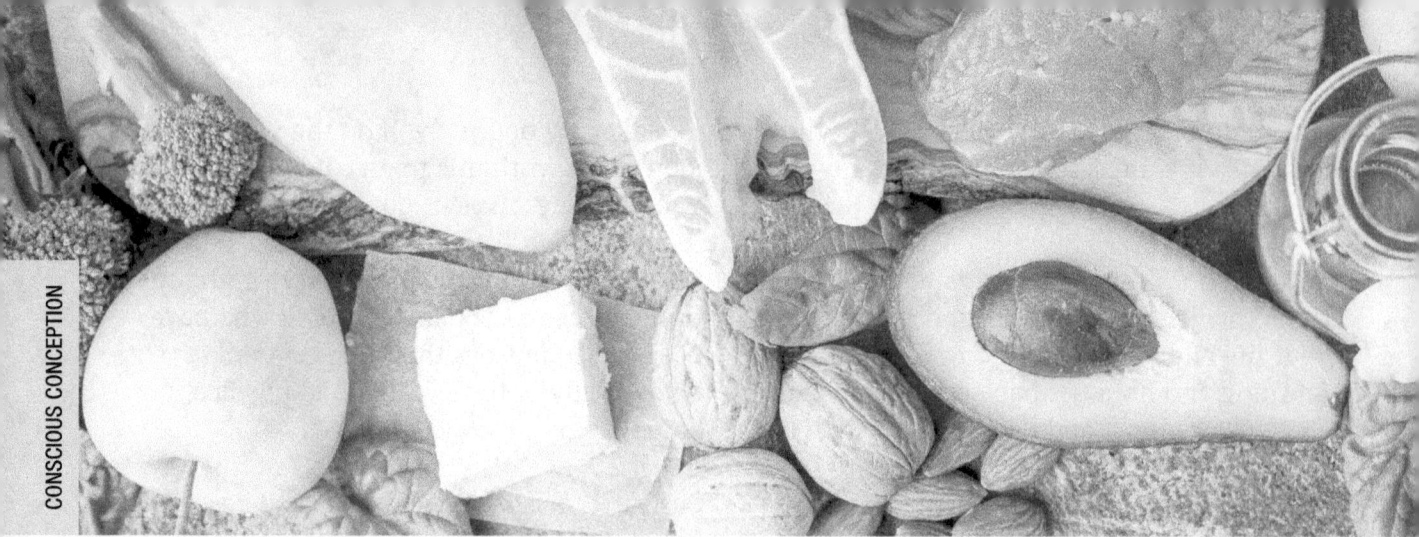

Nourishment

Let food be your first medicine. You want to eat lots and lots of vegetables. You want to eat as much organic or all natural, whole foods as possible. Do your best. While I provide you with lots of information and guidance in this section, my overarching guidance is this: Experiment until you find out what works for your body. Once you find that rhythm with food you can relax into it and not stress so much about watching every detail. For example, I try to eat organic produce as much as I can, but I do not eat 100 percent organic, and that's okay.

> Experiment until you find out what works for your body. Once you find that rhythm with food you can relax into it and not stress so much about watching every detail.

The standard American diet (SAD) is way too high in wheat, conventionally raised meat, conventionally raised dairy, funky fats, preservatives, chemical food additives, and it's super high in carbs/sugar. This is not a healthy way to eat. Your body isn't going to work optimally if you feed it poorly. There will be all kinds of problems as a result that you may think are due to something other than the fact that you are not eating well.

There are vegetables and fruits that you need to eat 100 percent organic or do your best to not eat them. They're known as the Dirty Dozen. The corresponding list is the Clean Fifteen; these are the fruits and vegetables that are less likely to cause harm if you select conventionally grown produce. Although potatoes don't currently appear on these lists, I recommend buying organic potatoes as much as possible. This list does change from time to time, but at the time of this writing, what's shown in the sidebar is accurate.

It is very important for most people to cut back on all conventionally grown wheat

DIRTY DOZEN

1. Strawberries
2. Spinach
3. Kale, Collards, and Mustard greens
4. Nectarines
5. Apples
6. Grapes
7. Bell and hot peppers
8. Cherries
9. Peaches
10. Pears
11. Celery
12. Tomatoes

CLEAN FIFTEEN

1. Avocados
2. Sweet corn
3. Pineapple
4. Onions
5. Papaya
6. Sweet peas (frozen)
7. Asparagus
8. Honeydew melon
9. Kiwi
10. Cabbage
11. Mushrooms
12. Cantaloupe
13. Mangoes
14. Watermelon
15. Sweet potatoes

What's an excellent breakfast? It is not a carton of yogurt. It's not an orange. It's definitely not a bagel and coffee. It is something more like two eggs and a few corn tortillas with some cooked, shredded chicken and spinach piled on top. You should be eating vegetables with every single meal.

Whenever you do eat something that's maybe not as ideal nutritionally as it could be, but it's going to taste so good—bless it. Visualize it being wonderful and empowering to you. It's okay to indulge once in a while. It's not okay to beat yourself up about it. Relax and enjoy the occasional treat.

> It's okay to indulge once in a while. It's not okay to beat yourself up about it. Relax and enjoy the occasional treat.

Be a Conscious Consumer

There are over 10,000 chemicals approved for use in the food and drink of the United States and the FDA has admitted that over 3,500 of them have not been tested.[5] Many studies have shown that the rampant use of preservatives, colorings, and food additives have harmed us on a lot of different levels, from learning disabilities to ADHD to reproductive problems and even questions about birth defects.[6] You have got to read labels and not buy things with chemical names in them. If it's got polysorbate 80 and sodium benzoate, don't buy it. You can find an alternative.

products, commercially processed meat, conventionally produced dairy, sugar, and salt. I'm not telling you to be a teetotaler when it comes to these foods. You can have all of them; you just need to be minimal to moderate with them. Do your best and don't stress the rest. I do my best: I eat perfectly twice a week. I eat exceptionally well two times a week. I eat okay two times a week, and once a week I may not eat as well.

It is also critical to look at the ingredients of all products that you purchase. All ingredients should be things you can pronounce and know what they are, if you can't pronounce it or it looks like the name of a chemical, it probably is, and I suggest you don't buy it. There are great substitutes these days for many of the products you may be eating that contain ingredients that can be harmful.

Seek out these more natural products, which are much better options for you because they do not contain the additives and chemicals. For example, you can substitute coconut aminos for soy sauce, which has less salt and no wheat in it, and provides that umami taste that we all love. There are a lot of good gluten-free cracker options these days like Nut-Thins, Mary's Gone Crackers, Simple Mills Almond flour crackers, or other rice or almond flour options. These can be better for you and have a higher quality food content than traditional crackers. No matter what you choose, make sure to look at the ingredients. Avoid eating crackers made with traditionally grown American wheat, which usually has glyphosate used on it. I'll tell you more about this in a bit.

It does take a little time to look over the ingredients list in items you buy, but I encourage you to be a conscious consumer and know what is in the food you ingest.

Carbohydrates and Low Carb Diets

You should limit and count carbs for a little while until you figure out what is an appropriate amount for you. You may have to experiment for a short while to find a really great diet that works for your body. You may have to learn how many grams of protein, carbs, and fat are in your food so you can create a diet that is balanced. An excellent way to eyeball it is to have half your plate filled with vegetables, a third of your plate with protein and the rest of your plate with carbs and fat.

A lot of Americans are also on some form of a low-carb or carb-free diet. There may be a place for a Keto diet or a carb-free diet, but it's not during pregnancy or preparation for pregnancy. The human body needs carbs. I think that our response to our inability to control ourselves and our rampant desire for carbs, from fruit to pasta to bread, potatoes, rice, etc., has gone too far the other way. That being said, I have to note that whenever somebody is gaining too much weight almost inevitably it's because they've chosen to eat a lot of carbs and fat. So, balance and information are imperative. Work to include healthier carbs in your diet, like vegetables.

Carbohydrates are important in pregnancy. The problem for most of us is that we're getting the wrong kind of carbs. Where

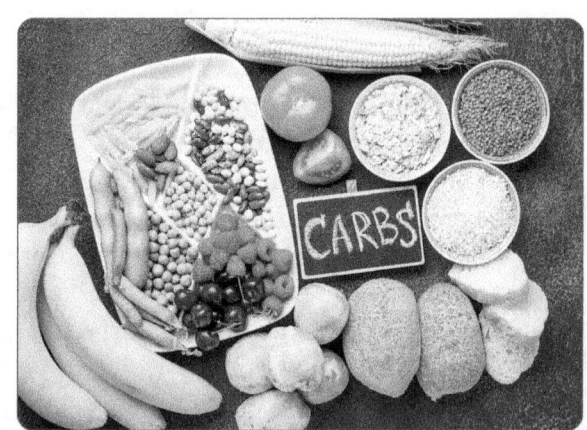

you can, switch out grains for nuts or vegetables. For example, use cucumber slices instead of crackers for dips. I love KIND Bars because they are usually lower in sugar, grain free, nut-based, and delicious. If you have a granola bar habit, try KIND Bars, Larabars or EPIC Bars instead. KIND Bars are nut-based instead of grain-based (look for the varieties with 5g of sugar or lower), Larabars are date-/nut-based, and EPIC makes delicious snacks primarily from grass-fed, pasture-ranged animals with other natural ingredients like fruits and nuts.

On that note, I'd like to say that one reason many Americans dislike vegetables (my favorite carbs—eat as many as you like!) is that they've been prepared poorly. Boiled to death. When preparing vegetables, raw, roasted, or steamed is best for flavor and nutrient preservation.

Protein

You want to eat good quality meats, poultry, and pasture-raised eggs. The Recommended Dietary Allowance for adults is 0.36 grams of protein per pound of body weight. This usually equates to 50–100 grams per day. (This goes up in pregnancy.) Look for farm-raised chickens, turkey, and other fowl. Seek out a relationship with a local rancher and it's likely you'll pay better-than-retail prices for excellent 100 percent grass-fed meat. If you are unable to find grass-fed meats locally, it is possible to find ranches that offer amazing meats, poultry, and fish, and ship across the contiguous US. Order in bulk for discounts and store in your freezer.. See Appendix B for a list of suppliers you might try.

Seafood

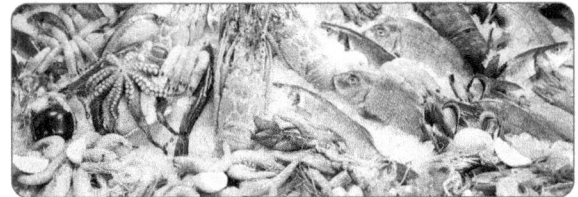

I encourage you to include lots of low-mercury seafood in your diet. There are plenty of fish that are healthy and provide important nutrients for your brain's health and for your baby's developing brain. Our ancestors evolved near sources of water—oceans, rivers, lakes, ponds, creeks, etc.—and they took advantage of the enormous amounts of fish that were in these waterways. I believe that we evolved with a great need for the omega-3 fatty acids found in seafood. This is a critical nutrient, and we now ingest a lot less fish in our American diet than our ancestors would have. I also have to make a plea at this point to not deplete the wild stocks of fish any more than we already have. There are sustainable sources of fish that we can be confident about eating without harming the environment. That being said, please eat more fish. It will help with the brain development of your baby and keep your brain healthier as you age.

We know that seafood can be very nutritious and are packed with great nutrients such as omega-3s, B vitamins, and lean protein. But unfortunately, fish can also have some unhealthy contaminants. Mercury is a contaminant found in fish that can affect brain development and the nervous system. The FDA has released guidelines for children, women who are pregnant, and women who are trying to become pregnant.

These guidelines state that no more than 12 ounces of "low" mercury fish should be consumed weekly. The "high" mercury fish should be kept to only three 6-ounce servings per month and the "highest" mercury fish should be avoided altogether.

What does this mean for women who are pregnant but also trying to get some of their much-needed nutrients from the critters of the sea? It is all about moderation. You want to eat lots of good quality protein, including fish, avoiding the fish that are high in mercury. Remember that a 4-ounce serving of meat is a healthy portion.

While I believe you should eat lots of fish in pregnancy, there are some you should avoid and some you should consume less of.[7] Use these lists as your guide.

Least Mercury

Enjoy these fish without worry.

- Anchovies
- Butterfish
- Catfish
- Clam
- Crab (Domestic)
- Crawfish/Crayfish
- Croaker (Atlantic)
- Flounder
- Haddock (Atlantic)
- Hake
- Herring
- Jacksmelt (Silverside)
- Mackerel (N. Atlantic, Chub)
- Mullet
- Oyster
- Plaice
- Pollock
- Salmon
- Sardine
- Scallop
- Shrimp
- Sole (Pacific)
- Squid (Calamari)
- Tilapia
- Trout (Freshwater)
- Whitefish
- Whiting

Moderate Mercury

Eat six servings or fewer per month of these fish.

- Bass (Saltwater, Striped, Black)
- Buffalo fish
- Carp
- Cod (Alaskan)
- Lobster
- Mahi-mahi
- Monkfish
- Perch (Freshwater)
- Sheepshead
- Skate
- Snapper
- Tilefish (Atlantic)
- Tuna (Canned chunk light, Skipjack)

High Mercury

Eat three servings or fewer per month of these fish.

- Croaker (White Pacific)
- Halibut (Atlantic, Pacific)
- Mackerel (Spanish, Gulf)

- Perch (Ocean)
- Sablefish
- Sea Bass (Chilean)
- Tuna (Albacore)

Highest Mercury

Avoid these fish altogether.

- Bluefish
- Grouper
- Mackerel (King)
- Marlin
- Orange roughy
- Shark
- Swordfish
- Tuna (Bigeye, Ahi/Yellowfin)

Poultry

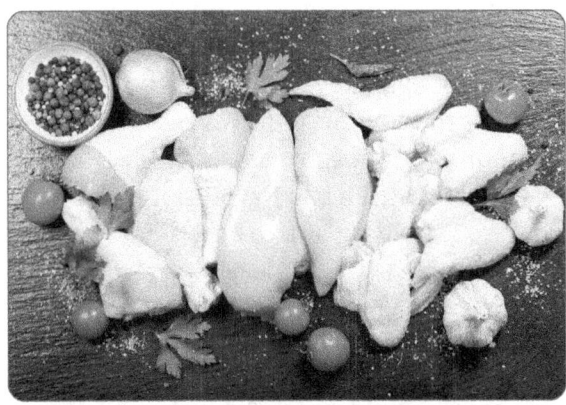

Poultry is another excellent protein to include in your diet. This includes things like chicken, turkey, etc. I do caution you to buy organic or pasture-raised organic if you can. There are health and environmental concerns relating to factory raised chicken, as there are for beef and pork. Pasture-raised chicken is higher in omega-3s than its factory raised counterparts.

Beef & Pork

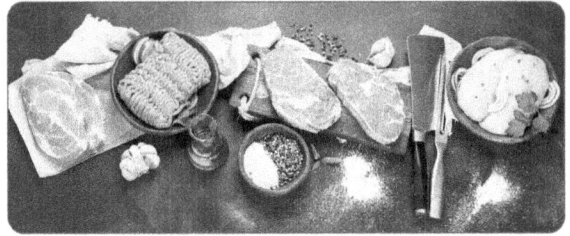

I personally do not digest beef and pork very well, so I keep those to a minimum in my diet. I also find that emotionally I am more okay with processing and eating poultry than I am cows and pigs, but that is a personal choice, and everyone should make their own personal choices. If you want a good beef or pork burger you should have that. I want to provide you with ways that you can eat less conventionally grown meat, but in no way am I telling you to eat none. Make the choices that are right for your body.

In my twenties I read a remarkable book called *Diet for a Small Planet* by Frances Moore Lappé. It was absolutely life changing for me. It described the impact of the factory farming of beef and pork in the United States. One of the facts that it made me aware of was that it takes 1,800 gallons of water and 2-½ pounds of grain to make 1 pound of beef.[8] This is not ecologically sound or sustainable. Also, the amount of methane that is produced by factory farming is unsustainable as well. We need to eat less commercially raised beef and pork. It doesn't have to be none, but my family ate far too much beef and pork as I was growing up, and it was not a healthy diet because of the large amount of cholesterol and saturated fats.

While I prefer to not consume red meat, I know there are women who thrive on it. If you like to eat red meat, seek out sustainable sources raised by small farmers who have their cattle on pasture, and choose to eat it less often. The composition of grass-fed meat is different from factory-raised meat, higher in omega-3s and lower in omega-6s (it's better for you).[9] I have some more tips for you in Appendix B.

Gluten

Many people are sensitive to gluten and don't know it, and many people are specifically sensitive to the gluten found in US-grown wheat. I suggest if you eat wheat, look for products like bread and crackers that use whole (not refined) grains and have product labels that say 100 percent whole grain. I also suggest that you only eat pastas produced in Italy or alternative pastas (grain or gluten-free pastas, spaghetti squash, etc.) and do your best to avoid anything made with conventionally grown wheat, which is grown in fields treated with the herbicide glyphosate, a product known to have carcinogenic or cancer-causing effects that is restricted in the EU, Canada, and Mexico.[10]

Phytoestrogens

I am often asked whether we should be limiting our intake of soy and other fruits and vegetables that contain phytoestrogens. Phytoestrogens are plant compounds that have a similar structure to estrogen, a sex hormone. There are two main types: isoflavones and lignans. Isoflavones are found in soy and other legumes, while lignans are found in flaxseed, whole grains, and fruits and vegetables.

Scientific studies on phytoestrogens have shown both benefits as well as drawbacks. Some of the potential benefits of consuming phytoestrogens include reducing the risk of heart disease, breast cancer, and osteoporosis, improving menopause symptoms, as well as protecting against Alzheimer's disease.[11] Some of the potential drawbacks of consuming phytoestrogens include interfering with a baby's development in utero, reducing sperm count in men,

Penelope: I had been struggling to lose the last of my baby weight and decided to try Keto, which required me to give up wheat. Over the next six months I steadily lost about three pounds a week and found that I felt great. I had more energy and was less bloated. I had battled depression throughout my life and when I gave up grains, I lost the depression too. There is some correlation between the inflammatory properties of gluten and depression, so learning this was a massive game-changer for me.

A few years later I heard people talk about how they didn't have the problems with gluten in European-grown wheat that they did in the US. I knew about the differences in our domestically grown wheat compared to theirs and decided to start ordering organic flour from Italy (on Amazon) to see if I could tolerate it. It turned out that I could. I don't eat bread every day, but I do enjoy it a few times a week now, and as long as the wheat wasn't grown with glyphosate, I do fine with it.

causing thyroid problems, and interacting with certain medications.

Obviously, one of the most important risks to consider during pregnancy is the impact it might have on your unborn baby.[12] One study, published in the journal Human Reproduction in 2010, found that women who consumed the highest levels of phytoestrogens during pregnancy were more likely to have daughters who had delayed puberty. Another study, published in the journal Environmental Health Perspectives in 2012, found that women who consumed the highest levels of phytoestrogens during pregnancy were more likely to have children with cognitive delays. It's important to note that these studies are observational, meaning that they cannot prove that phytoestrogens caused the health problems observed in the children. I believe that more research is needed before we can confidently determine whether phytoestrogens are truly harmful to pregnant women and their babies.

That said, I think it is prudent to be conscientious when consuming phytoestrogens in pregnancy and to limit your consumption of them. The American College of Obstetricians and Gynecologists (ACOG) similarly states that there is no need for pregnant women to avoid all phytoestrogens and recommends that pregnant women limit their intake of soy products that are high in phytoestrogens.

Processed Food Alternatives

I think what I'm trying to get at is that our bodies simply function so much better when we nourish them with whole, real foods.

These are the things you buy on the edges of the grocery store, typically the produce, meat, and dairy aisles. I would also include the oil and spice shelves in this category. It is so beneficial to buy *ingredients* and make your own meals.

One of the food items I suggest you limit tremendously is processed foods. This includes fast food restaurants, most packaged foods with ingredient labels containing multiple ingredients, frozen meals, frozen pizzas, canned foods, etc. All of these have a lot more preservatives, chemicals, sodium, sugars, and questionable fats than foods that you healthfully prepare for yourself do.

I'm going to especially call out diet soda drinks here as something to avoid. Researchers have just shown that the consumption of diet sodas and aspartame-sweetened drinks daily in pregnancy is linked to an increased incidence of autism in their male offspring.[13]

When you process and package foods, their vitality decreases. What you get out of a fresh apple that you chew up and swallow is completely different than when you eat applesauce, which has been killed and is in a jar. It still has nutritional value, but what we don't talk about enough is vitality or the energy of food, the *chi* of food, and how when these foods are processed the *chi* is diminished or destroyed.

When I started getting serious about my health, I was able to find an alternative to everything terrible for me that I loved. My favorite snack foods were a chemical nightmare, and now we have many all-natural, healthy, and even organic substitutes that are perfectly fabulous and tasty and will meet every need you have without the chemical pollutants.

There are so many chemicals used in our foods these days, especially in processed foods, fast food, and sugary drinks. Some of the most commonly used chemicals in food have been linked to health problems. I suggest you choose not to purchase food products with the following ingredients:

- Polysorbate 80
- Sodium benzoate
- Sodium nitrate
- Potassium nitrate
- Sulfur dioxide
- High fructose corn syrup
- Cellulose
- Artificial colors and artificial flavorings, including aspartame.

Always read food labels and stick to buying as many products as you can that use whole food ingredients.

Tools for Assessing Your Diet

It may seem overwhelming to be asked to assess your entire diet and experiment until you find what works for you, so let me give you some tools to help you. I'd like to suggest that you keep a food diary for a week. Write down absolutely everything you eat, and also track your mood and energy levels. Notice any symptoms you might display, like feeling bloated, passing gas, diarrhea, etc.

At the end of the week, review what you're consuming daily in terms of carbs, fats, proteins, and sugar. Here are some tools to help. In the next section, we'll talk about what to do from there.

Protein Counter

I don't want you to be put off by the idea of having to count everything you're eating in terms of grams of protein, sugar, fat, etc., but I do want you to have these tools so you can use them to help you understand what you're eating and then notice how those foods affect you. It helps to count until you get a good idea of the amounts you need to eat without counting. You only really need to count until you have a feel for it. The same thing goes for counting calories.

There is no one perfect diet for everyone, but there certainly are guidelines that can help channel us into a healthier diet. If you already have a sense of how much protein is in the food you eat, great! No need to start counting again. If you have no idea, this chart will help.

Protein Rich foods	Protein	Measure	Typical Serving
Almond butter	21 grams	100 grams	2 tablespoons = 7 grams protein
Almonds	21 grams	100 grams	1 ounce = 6 grams protein
Bacon (cooked)	37 grams	100 grams	1 slice–3 grams protein
Beans (cooked legumes)	8.7 grams	100 grams	1/2 cup = 7 grams protein
Beef, ground (95 percent lean)	27 grams	100 grams	3 ounces = 23 grams protein
Beef, steak (sirloin)	27 grams	100 grams	3 ounces = 23 grams protein
Cashew	18 grams	100 grams	1 ounce = 5 grams protein
Chia seeds	17 grams	100 grams	1 ounce = 4.7 grams protein
Chicken breasts	31 grams	100 grams	4 ounces = 36 grams protein
Chicken thighs	24 grams	100 grams	4 ounces = 28 grams protein
Cottage cheese (2 percent fat)	12 grams	100 grams	1/2 cup = 13 grams protein
Edamame (cooked)	11 grams	100 grams	1 cup = 17 grams protein
Egg whites	11 grams	100 grams	1 large = 3.6 grams protein
Eggs	13 grams	100 grams	1 large = 6 grams protein
Fish, Cod	18 grams	100 grams	3 ounce = 15 grams protein
Fish, halibut (cooked)	23 grams	100 grams	3 ounce = 19 grams protein
Fish, salmon (cooked)	24 grams	100 grams	3 ounce = 21 grams protein
Fish, Tilapia	26 grams	100 grams	3 ounce = 22 grams
Hemp seeds	30 grams	100 grams	3 tablespoons (30 g) = 9 grams protein

Protein Rich foods	Protein	Measure	Typical Serving
Peanut butter	22 grams	100 grams	2 tablespoons = 7 grams protein
Peanuts	25 grams	100 grams	1 ounce = 7 grams protein
Pine nuts	14 grams	100 grams	1 ounce = 4 grams protein
Pork chops (lean, cooked)	21 grams	100 grams	3 ounces = 18 grams protein
Pork, tenderloin	27 grams	100 grams	3 ounces = 22 grams protein
Protein powder (whey)	78 grams	100 grams	38 grams (1 scoop) = 30 grams protein
Pumpkin seeds	19 grams	100 grams	1 ounce = 5 grams protein
Refried beans	5 grams	100 grams	1/2 cup = 7 grams protein
Ricotta cheese (part skim)	11 grams	100 grams	1/2 cup = 14 grams protein
Shrimp (cooked)	24 grams	100 grams	3 ounces = 19 grams protein
Sunflower seeds	21 grams	100 grams	1/4 cup = 6 grams protein
Tempeh	19 grams	100 grams	1 cup = 31 grams protein
Tofu	8 grams	100 grams	1/2 cup = 10 grams protein
Tuna	28 grams	100 grams	3 ounces = 24 grams protein
Turkey breast	29 grams	100 grams	3 ounces = 26 grams protein
Turkey, deli meat	18 grams	100 grams	4 ounces = 20 grams protein
Turkey, ground (93 percent lean)	19.5 grams	100 grams	3 ounces = 16.5 grams protein
Yogurt (low-fat, plain)	6 grams	100 grams	1 cup = 11 grams

Glycemic Index

The glycemic index is a wonderful tool for you to use to understand how much sugar you're eating. Foods that have a very high glycemic index require more insulin for your body to metabolize, and if you tend to eat a lot of those foods it can put you at risk for Type II diabetes. I'm providing the following chart[14] to give you a broad sense of the food groups and where they fall; you might find some of the values surprising.

Note that meat tends to have a very low glycemic index. Please do dive deeper on your own and investigate the foods you consume regularly.

KEY:
Low = 55 or less
Medium = 56–69
High = 70 or more

Glycemic Index

Grains/Starches		Vegetables		Fruits		Dairy		Legumes	
Rice bran	27	Asparagus	15	Grapefruit	25	Low fat yogurt	14	Peanuts	21
Bran cereal	42	Broccoli	15	Apple	38	Plain yogurt	14	Beans, dried	40
Spaghetti	42	Celery	15	Peach	42	Whole milk	27	Lentils	41
Corn, sweet	54	Cucumber	15	Orange	44	Soy milk	30	Kidney beans	41
Wild rice	57	Lettuce	15	Grape	46	Fat-free milk	32	Split peas	45
Sweet potatoes	61	Peppers	15	Banana	54	Skim milk	32	Lima beans	46
White rice	64	Spinach	15	Mango	56	Chocolate milk	35	Pinto beans	55
Couscous	65	Tomatoes	15	Pineapple	66	Fruit yogurt	36	Black Eyed beans	59
Whole wheat bread	71	Cooked carrots	39	Watermelon	72	Ice cream	61		
Muesli	80								
Baked potatoes	85								
Oatmeal	87								
Taco shells	97								
White Bread	100								

Apps for Nutritional Information

There are several apps that can scan products to check their ingredients and safety. Some of the most popular apps include:

1. Chemical Cuisine is a free app developed by the Center for Science in the Public Interest (CSPI). It is a searchable database of over 130 food additives, including descriptions, safety ratings, and sources. The app also includes a barcode scanner that allows you to scan the ingredients of a product and get information about the additives it contains.

   The Chemical Cuisine app was created to help consumers make informed choices about the food they eat. It provides information about the safety of food additives, so you can decide whether you want to avoid them. The app also includes a list of "best avoided" additives, which are those that have been linked to health problems.

2. Yuka app for scanning products

   This app is available for both iOS and Android devices. It scans the barcode of a product and provides information on the ingredients, including their safety rating. Yuka also recommends similar products that are better for your health.

3. Think Dirty: This app is also available for iOS and Android devices. It scans the barcode of a product and provides information on the ingredients, including their safety rating and potential health risks. Think Dirty also recommends similar products that are cleaner and safer.

4. EWG's Healthy Living: This app is available for iOS and Android devices. It scans the barcode of a product and provides information on the ingredients, including their safety rating and potential health risks. EWG's Healthy Living also includes a database of over 100,000 products, so you can search for products by brand or by ingredient. www.ewg.org

It is important to note that these apps are not perfect. They may not have information on all products, and their safety ratings may not be accurate. It is always best to do your own research before buying a product.

Here are some other tips for using these apps:

- Scan the barcode of the product before you buy it. This will give you the most accurate information about the ingredients and safety.

- Read the ingredient list carefully. Even if the app gives the product a good safety rating, you may still want to avoid products with ingredients to which you are sensitive.

- Use the app as a tool, not as a replacement for your own judgment. The app can give you valuable information, but it is still up to you to decide whether a product is safe for you to use.

Meal Planning

Now that you have a clear picture of what I recommend and are keeping a diary of how you have been eating, it may be time to improve your nutritional game. If you are eating in alignment with these ideals already, that is so wonderful. You're winning the game. If not, this section includes a menu planning tool with several ideas for healthy options for breakfast, lunch, snacks, dinner, and dessert.

One of the best benefits of meal planning is that you will likely drastically cut back on the amount of food that goes to waste in your kitchen. Meal planning helps you decide exactly what you will need over the coming week, so you are less likely to overbuy and thus overspend on food. Also, when you cook at home you usually spend less per meal than if you were to get takeout or processed/frozen meals. Use these savings to buy better ingredients for your home-cooked meals.

Getting Started

Here's an approach I recommend:

1. Make a weekly plan for what you will eat. Make sure you cover a big, healthy breakfast, a morning, afternoon, and evening snack for each day, a big, healthy lunch, and a small, healthy dinner. Generate a grocery list that covers all these items.

2. Clean out your pantry. Get rid of absolutely everything that you shouldn't be eating. Seed oils. Trans fats. (See page 124 for more information on these two). Candy. Processed foods. Snacks high in refined grains. Make a lovely donation to your local food bank, then head to the grocery store with the list you generated in Step One. If you can, treat yourself to a healthy meal out as a reward for your hard work.

3. On the next day, prepare any foods that you can. For example, you might want to roast a chicken, prep salad toppings, and have lettuce ready to go for a large chicken salad at lunch for a few days. If there is other prep work you can do in advance to lighten the coming week's cooking load, do that too!

TIP: Get your partner to help. If you don't have a partner or if meal preparation feels very daunting to you, there are often companies that offer meal preparation kitchens in metropolitan areas that provide a fun group environment, as well as guidance from professionals to help you out on this journey. Look for one near you! Alternatively, you can try out some of the meal prep services that allow you to choose your meals and provide exactly the ingredients you need along with directions shipped to your door. There are nationwide chains, but many cities have local options that may be more appealing to you.

Your initial grocery trips may be more expensive as you stock your pantry with healthier foods and replenish less healthy staples, but over time you'll find that this investment in your health far outweighs the monetary costs, and that with time and a dedication to preparing your own healthy meals, you'll find that you can have a very manageable food budget. Keep up your meal planning and shopping, and this part of your life will fall into place. It helps so very much to have a set time each week where you plan what you will eat and make your grocery list, and then do the shopping that day or the next. Consistency really helps.

TIP: To avoid the temptations at the grocery store, take advantage of online shopping and curbside pickup if you can. At the very least, eat a good snack before shopping to cut down on less healthy impulse purchases.

Dedicate several hours during your free time to prepping meals for the week. Put it on your schedule and make it a regular part of your weekly routine. This might include chopping ingredients, preparing breakfast muffins or Mimi's Special Spinach, or even just planning and shopping for the week so you have what you need on hand to prepare healthy meals at home. When you are pregnant it can be difficult to get enough to eat. You are often tired and don't want to cook in the moment. Take advantage of a higher energy time to prep as much as you can for those low ebb spells.

If you are unsure of yourself in the kitchen and have any questions about what to do, YouTube is your friend. You can find a reference to just about anything there.

You don't have to stick to my suggestions. Feel free to personalize your diet. Add your own favorite, healthy recipes. If you don't like something, substitute something else. Add more fat (like grass-fed butter or cheese) if you're struggling to gain weight

or take some fat out if you're working to not gain as much.

Keep the season in mind when you are eating and take advantage of fresh, local produce from your local farmer's market. You may want to go a little lighter in the spring or summer and have heartier options in the fall or winter to follow your body's normal biological rhythms and wants/needs.

 I really hope that if you are not already comfortable in the kitchen, you will work to develop this skill. If you're used to microwaving a quick meal or grabbing takeout cooking from scratch may seem intimidating at first, but I think you'll find yourself having lots of, Oh, that's all I have to do? moments. Involve your partner. Build menus together, share the shopping load, and ensure that both of you have the opportunity to provide wonderful meals for your family.

Meal Planning Tool

The following two pages contain my meal-planning suggestions in a menu-like format.

When you are doing your meal planning, choose one from each main meal category for each day of the week and have several options available to snack on so you always have something healthy on hand. Reserve the dessert category for when you really need it, or maybe plan on having a weekly dessert. I've also included several of my own personal favorite recipes for you to explore in Appendix B! I've denoted these with an asterisk on the menu pages. (My grandchildren call me "Mimi," hence the inclusion of "Mimi's" in several recipe titles.)

BREAKFAST

MORNING SMOOTHIE*

Egg Dishes

CHICKEN OR TURKEY OMELET
WITH CHEESE & MUSHROOMS
OR VEGETABLES

MIMI'S SPECIAL SPINACH* AND
CHEESE OMELET

SCRAMBLED EGGS WITH
TURKEY, SPINACH, & ONIONS

SCRAMBLED EGGS WITH
CHEESE & TURKEY BACON

EGGS HOW YOU LIKE THEM
WITH AVOCADO AND CHEESE

BREAKFAST TACO*

EGG MUFFINS*

MIGAS* WITH REFRIED BEANS
& TORTILLA CHIPS

Open-Faced Sandwiches

EGGS ON TOAST W/HAM,
CHICKEN, OR TURKEY,
ARUGULA, & CHEESE

POACHED EGGS ON ENGLISH
MUFFIN W/ AVOCADO & TOMATO

FRIED EGG WITH MAYO OR
BUTTER & NUTRITIONAL YEAST

POACHED EGGS ON AVOCADO
TOAST

AVOCADO TOAST WITH
SMOKED/ROASTED TURKEY

Grain-Based Options

FLAX WAFFLES WITH:
- BUTTER & FRUIT
- NUT BUTTER & CHOPPED
  PECANS
- APPLE BUTTER & CHOPPED
  APPLES OR
- MAPLE SYRUP & BLUEBERRIES

CHIA SEED PUDDING W/ FRUIT,
WALNUTS, & MAPLE SYRUP

OATMEAL W/ WALNUTS & FRUIT
WITH PARMESAN TOAST

GRANOLA W/NUTS & SEASONAL
FRUIT AND/OR GREEK YOGURT

LUNCH

Sandwiches

TUNA SALAD* W/SIDE SALAD

MIMI'S NUT BUTTER* & JELLY

TURKEY WITH LETTUCE,
TOMATO, AND AVOCADO

TURKEY BACON, LETTUCE, AND
TOMATO WITH CHIPS & SALSA

Soup & Salad

ALEAH'S EVERY DAY SALAD*

SOUP OF YOUR CHOICE & SALAD

International Cuisine

TOSTADA OR CHALUPA W/BEANS,
CHEESE OR AVOCADO, LETTUCE, &
TOMATO OR TACO MEAT WITH SALSA
AND LETTUCE

CHICKEN WONTONS IN BROTH WITH
SCALLIONS

MIMI'S PASTA SALAD*

DINNER

SHEPHERD'S PIE* WITH
STEAMED BROCCOLI

BAKED SALMON WITH SALAD
AND MASHED POTATOES

BAKED OR GRILLED CHICKEN
W/LOADED BAKED POTATO &
SAUTEED VEGETABLES

CHICKEN, SHRIMP, OR TOFU
STIR FRY* WITH VEGETABLES
SERVED OVER BROWN RICE

PECAN CRUSTED FISH WITH
MASHED POTATOES AND
STEAMED BROCCOLI

CHICKEN-FRIED CUTLETS*
W/MASHED POTATOES &
SAUTEED SQUASH MEDLEY

ALEAH'S RAINBOW BOWL*

DINNER

BAKED OR GRILLED CHICKEN
SALAD WITH STRAWBERRIES,
FETA, AND WALNUTS

VENETIAN STUFFED CHICKEN*
W/BROCCOLI & RICE MEDLEY

BAKED FISH WITH WHITE WINE
SAUCE,* QUINOA, & STEAMED
CAULIFLOWER

CHICKEN TIKKA MASALA* WITH
SALAD AND RICE

CHICKEN, TURKEY, OR BEAN
TACOS W/ CHEESE, LETTUCE,
TOMATO, ONION, AVOCADO, &
SALSA

CHICKEN OR VEGGIE
ENCHILADAS WITH RICE,
BEANS, AND MIMI'S SALAD

TURKEY BURGERS* WITH
BAKED FRIES AND SALAD

SALMON BURGERS W/ HOME
FRIES & STEAMED VEG OR
SALAD

SAUTEED SHRIMP SERVED
OVER PASTA OR BROWN RICE
WITH VEGETABLES

MIMI'S SPAGHETTI* W/CRUSTY
GARLIC BREAD & SALAD

GARLIC LEMON CHICKEN WITH
ROASTED VEGETABLES*

COUNTRY CAPTAIN CHICKEN*

MIMI'S CHICKEN SOUP* WITH
MIMI'S SALAD*

CREAMY COCONUT CHICKEN
SOUP*

CHICKEN TORTILLA SOUP

KING RANCH CASSEROLE*

TOODLE OODLE CASSEROLE
(TUNA)*

MEXICAN CASSEROLE*

*Denotes recipe in Appendix.

DESSERTS

ANGEL FOOD CAKE WITH
STRAWBERRIES AND WHIPPED
CREAM

MIMI'S FRUIT SALAD*

KOZY SHACK RICE OR TAPIOCA
PUDDING WITH FRUIT

GREEK YOGURT WITH HONEY
OR MAPLE SYRUP AND FRUIT

A SMALL PIECE OF DARK
CHOCOLATE WITH NUTS,
COCONUT OR NUT BUTTER

DATES (HALVED & SEEDED)
STUFFED W/NUT BUTTER & SEA
SALT ON TOP ("DATE BOATS")

AVOCADO PUDDING*

CHIA SEED PUDDING*

FROZEN YOGURT

SNACKS

Spring

SLICED BANANA WITH NUT
BUTTER

APPLES WITH CHEDDAR OR
NUT BUTTER

CELERY AND CARROT STICKS
WITH HUMMUS

DRIED CHERRIES & ALMONDS

GRAPES & CASHEWS

HARD-BOILED EGG WITH SALT
& PEPPER

1/2-1 CUP YOGURT WITH
GRANOLA, FRUIT, & NUTS

ORGANIC STRING CHEESE

MORE SNACKS

Summer

GUACAMOLE WITH CORN CHIPS
AND SALSA

PIMENTO CHEESE SPREAD
WITH NUT-THINS

ORGANIC STRING CHEESE

PEACHES & 2/3-1 CUP COTTAGE
CHEESE

CUCUMBERS & SALT

1/2-1 CUP YOGURT WITH
GRANOLA FRUIT AND NUTS

HARD-BOILED EGG WITH SALT
& PEPPER

2/3-1 CUP COTTAGE CHEESE W/
AVOCADO, TOMATO. & CORN
CHIPS

Fall

UNSULPHURED DRIED FRUITS

2/3-1 CUP COTTAGE CHEESE W/
AVOCADO, TOMATO. & CORN
CHIPS

2/3-1 CUP COTTAGE CHEESE
WITH HOT SAUCE AND CORN
CHIPS

CELERY FILLED W/NUT BUTTER
& TOPPED W/DRIED RAISINS
OR CHERRIES-ANTS ON A LOG

DRIED APRICOTS WITH NUT-
THINS AND NUT BUTTER

DATES ROLLED IN SHREDDED
COCONUT

1/2 CUP OF GRAPES OR
BERRIES OR AN APPLE, PEACH,
PEAR, OR NECTARINE-FRUIT IS
ALWAYS AN EXCELLENT
SNACK!

HARD-BOILED EGG WITH SALT
& PEPPER

ORGANIC STRING CHEESE

MORE SNACKS

Winter

TURKEY LETTUCE WRAPS-
OVEN BAKED SLICED TURKEY
BREAST WRAPPED IN LETTUCE
LEAF WITH THINLY SLICED
AVOCADO AND TOMATO AND A
SMALL SPREAD OF MUSTARD

NATURAL JERKY

HARD-BOILED EGG WITH SALT
& PEPPER

ORGANIC STRING CHEESE

CASHEW CLUSTERS

TURKEY PEPPERONI AND
ALMONDS

Anytime

TRAIL MIX

MIXED NUTS

POTATO CHIP ALTERNATIVES:
PIRATE BOOTY
PEA CHIPS
VEGGIE STRAWS
FREEZE DRIED VEGGIE CHIPS
SWEET POTATO CHIPS

KIND BAR, RX BAR, LARABAR,
EPIC BAR

RAW CARROT SALAD*

HYDRATION

PREGNANCY TEA*

FILTERED WATER

COCONUT WATER

FRUIT-INFUSED WATER

RECHARGE DRINK

HERBAL TEA

*Denotes recipe in Appendix.

Supplements

I want you to remember that the human body is an ancient organism developed by environmental pressures over hundreds of thousands of years to function in a particular environment. Now, suddenly (evolutionarily speaking), over the span of a few hundred years we have created a radically different environment for ourselves through technological advancement. We have both won and lost things in this transformation.

Supplementation should never take the place of food, but the unfortunate truth is that many of the foods most of us have access to are simply not as nutritionally dense as they were in times past.[15] Modern agriculture favors yield and appearance over nutritional density. The soils our foods are grown in arc not as mineral rich as they used to be. Conventional agriculture loads our fields with more and more pesticides and fertilizers to compensate for this, and these chemicals can be poison to our bodies.[16] In the 1970s, 40 percent of homes had kitchen gardens where they'd grow fresh vegetables for their families. That number has declined significantly in recent decades.[17]

Ancient peoples ate a lot of insects as a great source of protein, fats, and Vitamin E. It must've been much easier to knock over a termite mound and harvest that quality protein with a lot of fat than to try to run down antelope on the savanna. I don't know about you, but I'd rather not eat a bunch of bugs, thank you very much. We still need these nutrients in our diet, though, and I believe you must supplement.

Your growing baby will need abundant and available nutrients, and supplementation with a reputable brand is a good way to achieve that. If you become pregnant with a little girl, she will be born with every egg she will ever ovulate in her lifetime in her tiny ovaries, and therefore you are creating not just your child but your grandchildren as well. The nutritional needs of a healthy pregnancy cannot be overemphasized.

You never know when you will become pregnant, and you often don't know that you're pregnant for a few weeks after fertilization occurs, so it's important to supplement before you know that you're pregnant, so your growing embryo has access to those important building blocks.

Now, it's important to note that supplement companies are not regulated, and it's been shown that not all supplements are created equal in terms of bioavailability and certainly in terms of quality.[18] This is one place where it is worth it to spend a little bit more money, to do your research, and to be a conscious consumer. If you can't find the brands I recommend in Appendix A, look for a company whose products are independently certified to contain what they say they do. Look for a similar composition of vitamins and minerals to what I am recommending.

🔅 **TIP:** If you struggle to implement a regular vitamin routine, one thing that really helps is a vitamin box. You can get one with multiple compartments for each day. Load it up once a week, keep it near where you eat, and it will make remembering to take your vitamins much less of a hassle. Having to open a bunch of bottles each time you eat may prevent you from doing it.

Can't I Just Take a Prenatal Multivitamin?

While I do think that my vitamin regime is a lovely idea for all women—pregnant or not—I recognize that not everybody is going to be willing to incorporate all of it before getting pregnant. If this whole regime is too much prior to conception, then take a prenatal vitamin instead. There are a few that I recommend (see Appendix A).

Many of my other recommendations are for more easily absorbable varieties and for larger quantities than are typically recommended. The thing about prenatal vitamins is that they are the minimum daily requirement. They provide the least amount—what it takes to not die of scurvy or any of the other diseases that occur due to lacking a particularly important vitamin. Most Americans' diets are typically so poor that a prenatal vitamin may be saving lives, but more is often better. Your body will excrete or metabolize anything it can't use. Do note, there are levels at which some of these supplements become toxic to your body. This is not a license to take unlimited supplements.

So many prenatal supplements are lacking in both quantity and quality of the supplements. For example, most prenatals have 60–120 milligrams of Vitamin C in the form of ascorbic acid, which is seriously acidic, hard to digest, hard on your system, and hard to absorb.[19] In contrast I recommend 2000 mg daily of Ester-C with bioflavonoids, rutin, and hesperidin, which is buffered, incredibly absorbable, and not acidic. So, yes, if all you can do is take a prenatal vitamin, then by all means do that. But if you have the means to upgrade to the supplement recommendations that I'm about to share with you, then please do.

Supplement Recommendations

Rather than taking a prenatal vitamin, I recommend you follow the supplemental routine I'm going to describe in this section. Many studies have shown that you need lots more supplementation than a prenatal vitamin provides for optimal prenatal health, and that is what we are going for.[20] I have 50 years of experience and research to back up my claims that this creates healthy pregnancies, healthy babies, happier people, and results in fewer complications, diseases, and anomalies. I strongly suggest you follow this regimen.

I'm going to take a few pages to explain why I'm making these recommendations. If you find the information in the following sections to be too complex or overwhelming, you can just skip ahead to pages 50 and 51, where I provide clear lists of what I recommend you take and when. This will help you to make your supplement shopping list.

TIP: I recommend that you take your supplements with food. Eat a quarter of your meal, then take your supplements, then finish your meal. This will help your body to better absorb them, and they will be far less likely to make you feel queasy, or to sweat or burp them out.

Morning

400-Unit Mixed Tocopherol Vitamin E

Natural Vitamin E mixed tocopherols provides a full-spectrum, fat-soluble form of Vitamin E. Mixed tocopherols (and tocotrienols) are organic compounds commonly found in nuts, seeds, grains, legumes, some oils, and leafy green vegetables. They have antioxidant properties that are especially useful when added to fats and oils—protecting against oxidation, preventing rancidity, extending shelf life, and preserving taste.

I suggest taking a supplement that has both mixed tocopherols and mixed tocotrienols. I recommend that you take a 400-unit mixed tocopherol Vitamin E in the morning and in the evening. The one that I'm currently recommending is made by Jarrow Formulas, called Famil-E. Most prenatal vitamins only contain 40–60 units of d-Alpha tocopherol, and I want you to take 400 units in the morning and 400 in the evening of mixed d-alpha, beta, gamma, and delta tocopherols (the full Vitamin E complex). I think it's imperative.

If you are unable to obtain the brand I recommend, look for a natural, non-synthetic mixed tocopherol Vitamin E with tocotrienols.

The reason I recommend this much Vitamin E in your daily diet is because our ancestors had more Vitamin E in their diet due to eating insects frequently as part of their foraging.[21] Insects are incredibly high sources of protein and good quality fats. The Vitamin E present in insects is a mixed tocopherol of D-alpha, gamma, beta, and delta tocopherols. Most of the time the Vitamin E contained in a prenatal is just the D-alpha tocopherol because the original researchers decided that was the only one that was functional.

There are four main forms of Vitamin E: alpha-tocopherol, beta-tocopherol, gamma-tocopherol, and delta-tocopherol. Alpha-tocopherol is the most active form of Vitamin E and is the form that is often in supplements. Gamma-tocopherol is the second most active form of Vitamin E and has been shown to have multiple health benefits including antioxidant protection, immune function support, eye health, skin health, reducing the risk of heart disease and cancer, and reducing inflammation. Research on beta-tocopherols suggests that they may help with the absorption of minerals, including iron and zinc, and protect against the absorption of heavy metals, such as lead and cadmium. Delta-tocopherol is also a form of Vitamin E that is less active than alpha-tocopherol, but it still has benefits. Although tocotrienols are structurally similar to tocopherols, each has slightly different health properties. Experts believe that tocotrienols have many health benefits, some that are more powerful than those found in more common tocopherols. These include increased brain health and functionality, anti-cancer activity, and cholesterol lowering properties.[22]

You can get Vitamin E from food sources including:

- Extra virgin olive oil
- Nuts and seeds: Almonds, hazelnuts, peanuts, and sunflower seeds
- Leafy green vegetables: Spinach, kale, and broccoli

Although you can get Vitamin E from food sources, I highly recommend supplementing with vitamins and minerals to ensure optimal amounts for your health.

1,000 mg Ester-C

Vitamin C is absolutely essential for our health. It's critical in your immune system function and in cellular function for the transport of nutrients, oxygen, and carbon dioxide. There used to be a lot more Vitamin C in the human diet because we had vegetables and fruits that were very high in Vitamin C. Modern agriculture produces fruits and vegetables that are very flavorful,

disease resistant, easy to harvest, large, pretty, and easy to pack and transport, but the nutritional value was lost in the translation.[23]

When you take enough ascorbic acid (the most common form of Vitamin C available in the market) to actually benefit your body, it harms you by acidifying it. Linus Pauling, one of the most influential researchers of Vitamin C, searched for decades for a better way and developed the Ester-C process, which creates a form of Vitamin C that is 400 times more absorbable, 40 times more retainable by your body's tissues, and is not acidifying.[24] You always want to take a Vitamin C that has bioflavonoids, including rutin, and hesperidin (the C-complex). These bioflavonoids work synergistically with Vitamin C to enhance its absorption and biological activity. For example, hesperidin and rutin can help to protect Vitamin C from oxidation and prolong its retention in the body.

It's important to remember that almost all vitamins and minerals come in complexes, and for the body to absorb them optimally the full complex needs to be present. I suggest that you get a reputable brand of Ester-C in 500 mg tablets; there are many available. Take two to make 1,000 milligrams in the morning and again in the evening. This will boost your immune system and your cellular energy and will create more energy for you. One of the reasons I recommend taking this in the morning is so you can get as much boost as possible and get your day going without caffeine. This is gentle on your stomach and will not acidify your body.

I've had people ask me why I don't just recommend the 1,000 mg pill. First of all, it's a very big pill, and literally difficult to swallow. Also, if you are fighting an illness, I want you to take 500 milligrams of Vitamin C every four hours, so it's best to have the correct dosage on hand. I will talk about this in greater detail later.

Probiotics

You want a *good probiotic* with several strains—not just Lactobacillus, which is the bacteria found in yogurt. Lactobacillus it is a major gut bacterium, but there are approximately 600 different bacteria in the human gut and many of them are absolutely critical for your health.[25] A good probiotic will aid your immune system to be stronger and healthier, will keep the good bacteria colonies high enough to keep bad bacteria at bay, and will aid in the processing of the chemical components that your gut makes.

When you take antibiotics, you significantly deplete and may even destroy the gut flora. Some people never quite recover from this and have digestive issues for the rest of their lives.

Prebiotics are also wonderful to aid your digestive health and are often found in foods that are high in fiber, such as fruits, vegetables, and legumes. Some examples of prebiotics include:

- Inulin: Inulin is a type of fiber that is found in many fruits and vegetables, including onions, garlic, and asparagus.
- Fructo-oligosaccharides (FOS): FOS is a type of fiber that is found in many fruits and vegetables, including bananas, honey, and wheat.

- Galacto-oligosaccharides (GOS): GOS is a type of fiber that is found in many fruits, vegetables, and dairy products like milk, yogurt, and cheese.

Taking or eating probiotics/prebiotics can help to improve the balance of bacteria in the gut, which can lead to of health benefits[26] such as reduced inflammation and improved digestion. Pro-/prebiotics may help to reduce the risk of chronic diseases, like heart disease, cancer, and obesity. They may help to improve immune and cognitive functions by supporting the growth of beneficial bacteria in the gut. In other words, they can help you feel better and more "with it."

It has been found that excellent probiotics can help to replace the gut flora that may have been destroyed by antibiotics.[27] Some of your gut flora creates enzymes necessary for the human body to function. This is important stuff, people! I am now recommending Garden of Life probiotics; they make a bunch of different varieties and I recommend that you buy one that has many strains of bacteria and a large bacteria count. The one I take has 33 strains at a 100 billion count. These are easy to take in the morning.

Lunch

NaturesPlus Ultra-Mins

At lunch take a few bites of food, then **take two Ultra-Mins**. This is a mineral supplement made by NaturesPlus that I heartily recommend. It includes calcium, iron, phosphorus, iodine, magnesium, zinc, selenium, manganese, chromium, and potassium.

Minerals are key players in the vitality and health of your body. In nature, plants have strategies for seed dispersal (birds, wind) because if its seeds were to always fall straight down where the mother plant is, the ground would quickly be devoid of the resources the plant needs for sustainable growth. Modern agriculture and its practice of mono-cropping has depleted the soils of the minerals that would normally find their way into the produce. This is the reason we must supplement now with minerals; so many of them are no longer present or drastically reduced in the foods we buy.[28]

Without adequate and even abundant healthy minerals like calcium, magnesium, iron, manganese, potassium, sodium, and zinc your body doesn't function properly. These are all critical components for your body's function and health. When you get an abundant amount of minerals during your pregnancy not only do your teeth, hair, and fingernails thrive, but your baby thrives! They will have strong bones that will be much less likely to break when they fall off the playset at the park. Build healthy bones by doing as much dietarily as you can, but I don't think you can get all that you need that way. Ultra-Mins provides what you need in an easily absorbable format.

Chelation is also important. Minerals are absorbed in your intestines, which means they must survive the harsh, acidic environment of your stomach and make it to the intestines intact. Chelation is the process that coats the minerals, so they aren't broken down until they reach your intestine. If you don't choose to use Ultra-Mins, do look for a product that contains chelated minerals.

Calcium, magnesium, and iron are the most important minerals,[29] and I will go into a bit more detail about why.

CALCIUM

Calcium is the most abundant mineral in the body, and it is essential for bone health, muscle contraction, and nerve signaling. Magnesium is also essential for many bodily functions, including energy production, protein synthesis, and blood pressure regulation. Calcium and magnesium work together to support a variety of bodily functions. For example, calcium helps to transport magnesium into cells, and magnesium helps to activate enzymes that are involved in calcium metabolism. Additionally, calcium and magnesium can compete for absorption in the gut, so it is important to get enough of both minerals for the maintenance of healthy levels of either.

Pregnancy demands a lot of calcium from your body. Most women are getting calcium pulled out of their jaws and their bones. You need a lot more calcium than you think, and the ossification (or hardening) of the baby's bones is absolutely critical. Additionally, you must adhere to a rigid dental hygiene routine. At a minimum, brush, floss, and use mouthwash daily.

The dairy industry has rigorously marketed the idea that dairy products are a good source of calcium. There may be calcium in dairy products, but it is not as absorbable as you may have been led to believe.

I recommend 1,500 mg of calcium daily during pregnancy, whereas prenatal supplements usually only deliver 150 mg. You will get this from the Ultra-Mins.

Ground sesame seeds are a very high, non-dairy source of calcium. One tablespoon of ground sesame seeds has 105 mg of calcium. You can buy a small plastic grinder and then toast and grind your own, or use Gomasio, which is ground sesame seeds mixed with herbs and sea salt for a great salt substitute. Tahini is a fantastic sesame seed butter that can be used just like peanut butter.

Other calcium-rich food sources include:

- Almonds
- Bok Choy
- Black beans
- Broccoli
- Collard greens
- Cottage cheese
- Kale
- Kombu
- Milk
- Mustard greens
- Parmesan cheese
- Salmon
- Sardines with bones
- Seaweed
- Soy milk
- Spinach
- Spirulina
- Tempeh
- Tahini
- Tofu
- Turnip greens
- Yogurt

IRON

Iron is an essential mineral that plays a vital role in many bodily functions, including blood circulation, energy production in your cells, production of white blood cells for your immune system, and brain development. Getting more than the bare minimum daily requirement is extremely important during pregnancy. Don't sell yourself or your baby-to-be short here.

Good sources of iron include:

- Meat: Pasture-raised red meat, poultry, and fish
- Beans: Beans, lentils, and peas
- Tofu
- Nuts, such as almonds and walnuts.
- Seeds, such as pumpkin seeds and chia seeds.

B Complex

At lunch take 50 mg of a B complex vitamin. If you look at a typical multivitamin, the Vitamin B supplements are dosed at the 5–10 mg level. There's plenty of information out there that says 50 milligrams daily is a great idea, especially with stress.[30] I don't know very many people who haven't been stressed out for a long time.

If you take B vitamins in the morning, they may make you nauseated because you haven't had enough food to withstand that 50 milligrams of diesel fuel, and if you take them at night they'll give you a burst of energy that can keep you up, so take them with lunch when you've got a large meal to help with digestion and they can help power you through the afternoon.

This vitamin gives you 50 mg of all the Bs—B1, B2, B4, B6, and B12. Because it is a water-soluble vitamin, you will excrete anything that you don't need, but often your body will use it all.

Folic Acid/Methylfolate

It is critically important to be taking folic acid supplements prior to getting pregnant. Folic acid is the synthetic form of folate, a B vitamin that is essential for pregnant women. Methylfolate is a more bioavailable form of folate, which means that it is easier for the body to absorb. If you have the MTHFR gene, your body can't make full use of what you're getting from your diet, or easily absorb the regular folic acid found in most vitamins. Most people will not know whether they have this gene mutation or not and that is why I suggest all women who are pregnant or planning to conceive choose methylfolate, which everyone can metabolize. In most prenatals and B vitamins you will only see folic acid listed.

A study published in the journal "The Lancet" in 2011 found that women who took methylfolate had a 72 percent lower risk of having a baby with a neural tube defect than women who took folic acid.[31] A study published in the journal "Obstetrics & Gynecology" in 2013 found that women who took methylfolate had a 32 percent lower risk of having a baby with a cleft lip or palate than women who took folic acid,[32] which is why I now recommend you take methylfolate instead of folic acid.

This makes supplementing with methylfolate a better choice for pregnant women who are at risk of neural tube defects (NTDs) or who have difficulty absorbing folic acid. During the first few weeks of pregnancy the baby's neural tube develops. This is the closure of the skull and the formation of the spine, and if those don't go together properly, birth defects such as spina bifida and anencephaly can occur. Taking folic acid or methylfolate is a critical preventative measure, and it's absolutely essential that you start taking it daily prior to getting pregnant.[33] Taking folic acid before and during pregnancy has also been shown to reduce the risk of cleft palate by up to 70 percent.

During pregnancy folate plays a special role in the mom's health as well as in the formation of the baby's chromosomes and nervous system. Getting adequate levels can improve your egg quality, and can sometimes prevent miscarriage, as well as other pregnancy complications including preeclampsia (high blood pressure) and placental abruption (when the placenta separates from the inner uterine wall).

Methylfolate may also protect or reduce the risk of autism[34] by improving the methylation of DNA. Methylation is a process that helps to regulate gene expression and is thought to play a role in the development of autism. **To get these benefits, it needs to be taken in the first 28 days of pregnancy, so I suggest you start taking this before you get pregnant!** Folic acid/methylfolate may also protect against prenatal and postpartum depression in moms.

Take 800 mcg of **methylfolate (or folic acid)** at lunch time. There will be folic acid in your B-vitamin. Most of the time it is 400 mcg, but I believe you should be taking at least 800 mcg. If you are taking a standard prenatal supplement and can only find an 800-mcg folic acid or methylfolate, you can add it to your prenatal supplement for a total of 1200mcg daily. This is not too much. It will boost your energy in tandem with the B vitamins.

Dinner

400-Units Mixed Tocopherol Vitamin E

1000 mg Ester-C

Beta Carotene

Beta carotene is a type of substance called a carotenoid. Carotenoids give plants, such as carrots, sweet potatoes, and apricots, their reddish-violet colors. Beta carotene is a provitamin. This means it's used by your body to make Vitamin A. Vitamin A is metabolized by the liver. You need lots of Vitamin A during pregnancy to promote the development and function of good vision and eye health, a strong immune system, and for the growth and development of babies' organs and tissues. During pregnancy, Vitamin A is especially important for the development of the baby's brain and nervous system. Studies have shown that babies born to mothers who are deficient in Vitamin A are at increased risk of birth defects, such as neural tube defects.[35]

A woman's liver is really challenged during pregnancy. It's working very hard to metabolize your increased waste and all the metabolic waste from the baby. Beta carotene is a water-soluble precursor to Vitamin A that doesn't rely on the liver for metabolization. Since beta carotene is water soluble, if you have gotten enough Vitamin A in your diet, you will easily excrete any excess without taxing your liver. Many prenatal vitamins have Vitamin A palmate in them, but this is fat soluble, not excretable by the body, and must be metabolized by your liver to be removed from the body. Researchers have suggested that taking beta carotene is a much better

plan.[36] A great way to do increase your beta carotene is by consuming a raw carrot salad daily. (You can find a recipe in Appendix B.) I am hoping that you will include lots of colorful fruits and vegetables in your diet as well as supplementing with beta carotene to aid in getting all the Vitamin A that you and your baby need.

Omega-3s

Omega-3 fatty acids are healthy fats that can support your heart health. One key benefit is that they help to lower your triglycerides. They are an integral part of cell membranes throughout the body and affect the function of the cell receptors in these membranes, helping to provide structure and supporting interactions between cells. They provide the starting point for making hormones that regulate blood clotting, contraction and relaxation of artery walls, and inflammation. While they're important to all your cells, omega-3s are concentrated in high levels in cells in your eyes and brain. In addition, omega-3s provide your body with energy (calories) and support the health of many body systems including your cardiovascular and endocrine systems. They may also help to lower your risk of developing some forms of cancer, including breast cancer, Alzheimer's disease, ALS, MS, Parkinson's disease, senility, dementia, and age-related macular degeneration (AMD).

Omega-3s can also play an essential role in conception, and in the formation and development of the oocyte and embryo. Higher intake is associated with better ovarian reserve and higher rates of conception.

DHA and EPA are two of the most important omega-3 fatty acids, and are important for heart, brain, and eye health.[37] Your intake of DHA prenatally is also critical for your baby's brain and neurological development, and may prevent preterm labor, regardless of other risk factors. Interestingly, there have also been a few studies that have shown that DHA can improve stress resilience, even to severe social stressors, while EPA can prevent prenatal and postpartum depression.

I recommend a combined DHA/EPA, either from fish oil or a vegan source. I am now suggesting algae oil as the best form of omega-3s as it is the only plant-based source of DHA and EPA. DHA and EPA are made by certain types of algae, and they are then consumed by fish and other marine animals. This is why fish are a good source of DHA and EPA for humans. By taking algae oil instead, you can get the omega-3s through a more sustainable and ethical source. This also lowers your risk that your fish oil has gone rancid (it's estimated that 40 percent of the fish oils on the market are rancid on the shelf, which is worse for you than not taking them at all[38]). Two brands that I think are well sourced are IWI and Nordic Naturals, but if you cannot get those or are using another brand of algae oil, as with all products make sure it is safely manufactured and independently verified.

The amount of DHA and EPA in algae oil varies depending on the product. However, most algae oil products contain at least 200 mg of DHA per serving. Some products also contain EPA, but the amount is typically lower than the amount of DHA. I recommend you follow the dosage recommendation shown on the label of the product you buy. I suggest taking at least 200–300 mg per day, but there is some research that says taking 1,000 mg per day can be helpful to prevent the early onset of labor.[39]

Vitamin D

Vitamin D is a fat-soluble vitamin that is essential for many bodily functions, including bone health, immune function, and muscle function. You may think you can get enough Vitamin D from the sun, but it is very difficult to do so.[40] The bad UV rays are so high at this point that it puts you at risk of developing skin cancer to be in the sun without sunscreen. When you use sunscreen, as you should, you will not get enough Vitamin D naturally. The point of all of this is to say that you need to take Vitamin D supplements.

Most people are deficient in Vitamin D. This is especially true for older people, people who live in northern latitudes, or those who do not spend a lot of time outdoors.

Penelope: My last OB/GYN (who recently retired) told me that she tested absolutely every woman in her practice to see where their vitamin levels were. She said she found that only two women, in more than a decade of testing, had enough Vitamin D in their systems. Those women were both soccer coaches who spent all day, every day outside in the Texas sun. She also recommended that everyone supplement with Vitamin D (and everything else that MariMikel recommends).

Vitamin D is imperative in your absorption of calcium and without it you can develop osteoporosis, muscle weakness, and rickets, which is where you don't absorb calcium and it deforms your bones. Rickets was a huge problem in America until they started supplementing all milk in the United States with Vitamin D, which helped tremendously. Here are some of the benefits of Vitamin D:

- Improves bone health.
- Immune function—helps fight infection.
- Reduces the risk of some chronic diseases, such as multiple sclerosis and rheumatoid arthritis.
- Helps the body maintain muscle mass and strength. Deficiency can lead to muscle weakness and fatigue.

Vitamin D may also have benefits for other health conditions, such as depression, heart disease, and breast and colon cancer. However, more research is needed to confirm these benefits. It's become a topic of conversation amongst cancer researchers that a deficiency of Vitamin D seems to be present in a remarkable percentage of people with cancer.[41] Although it has not been fully established that taking Vitamin D helps to prevent cancer, I encourage everyone to take it daily. Yes, cancer prevention is good, but keeping your bones and your baby's bones healthy is essential, and Vitamin D is critical for that.

I test my clients' Vitamin D levels with their initial lab work, which is hopefully at the beginning of the pregnancy. I find most of my clients are deficient or low in Vitamin D, and when that is the case, I recommend 5000 ICU a day. If they have higher levels, I suggest 2000 ICU a day.

Supplement List

I've included a summary of my supplement recommendations on the following page for ease of reference. There's both a list for you to help with your shopping and a summary of what to take when.

When Should I Stop?

Stick to this regimen for your whole life. Even now in my senior years I take these same vitamins (plus some). I recommend that absolutely everyone take this regimen. Get your partner started on it, too!

Getting Your Partner on Board

None of these things ... regularly eating healthily, taking your supplements, exercising regularly, etc. ... are easily achievable unless your partner is on board. He needs to be adopting these changes for his own health and wellness, and for that of your baby-to-be. This is best when it's a joint venture, because almost all these lifestyle approaches or changes require participation from everyone in your home. You can't eat well if your partner constantly brings home indulgent foods. He needs to understand that his nutrition, lifestyle, and health make a difference in his sperm, and that he needs to be putting out the healthiest sperm that he can. This is not just your job. Additionally, lowering his stress level is important so your environment overall will have a lower stress quotient.

Throughout this book I'll talk more about lowering stress and how to prepare your

SUPPLEMENTS FOR CONCEPTION

1. Jarrow Formulas' Famil-E (Vitamin E)

2. Ester-C

3. Probiotics

4. Nature'sPlus Ultra-Mins

5. B-Complex

6. Methylfolate (folic acid)

7. Beta Carotene

8. Algea Oil (Omega 3 fatty acids)

9. Vitamin D

ONCE PREGNANT, ADD

10. Evening Primrose Oil

MariMikel Potter, CPM, LM, RN–BSN
The Book of Birth
IG: @marimikelthemidwife

SCHEDULE

*When amounts aren't specified,
take as directed on the package

Breakfast
·Famil-E – 400 IU
·Ester-C - 1000 mg – (two 500mg capsules)
·Probiotics*

Lunch
·Ultra-Mins– 2 tablets
·B-50 – 1 tablet or capsule or as directed
Methylfolate–800 - 1200 mcg

Dinner
·Famil-E – 400 IU
·Ester C – 1000 mg
·Algae Oil for Omega-3 fatty acids*
· Beta Carotene*
·Vitamin D3 –2000 - 5000 IU
·Once pregnant, add evening
 primrose oil at dinner*

Bedtime
·At Week 16 of your pregnancy
add 1 Ultra-Mins tablet

MariMikel Potter, CPM, LM, RN-BSN
The Book of Birth
IG: @marimikelthemidwife

family, friends, and colleagues so this process runs more smoothly.

Natural Medicine Chest

As a graduate of the University of Texas nursing school, I had a solid foundation in Western medicine. In the '70s more important information came out about alternative health care. As I studied, I realized there was much that Western medicine offered, but it was missing any kind of focus on preventative health care. I personally had health issues from a Standard American Diet (SAD) and lifestyle. When I began to take advantage of preventative avenues, including acupuncture, chiropractic care, massage, and naturopathic and homeopathic medicine practices and practitioners, I found that these things made a difference.

Western medicine is remarkable in its ability to perform surgery, assess lab work, and create and prescribe medications for existing illnesses, but alternative medicine is where we must turn for preventative health care. I have been using these methods personally and encouraging all my clients, friends, and family to use them as well because they are amazingly effective. The remedies that I most often share now comprise my natural medicine chest.

Now, this may feel a little airy-fairy hippie dippy to you, and I get it. It used to feel that way to me. I saw others around me using natural medicines with good results, and so I tried them and found they worked. I thought, Alright, well this is weird. Maybe there are some things that we just can't know yet and this might be one of them. But

they do work, and they won't harm you or your baby.

Many of the products I suggest you put in your natural medicine chest are herbs. Herbs are plants that have been used for centuries to treat a variety of health conditions. They contain active ingredients that can have a variety of effects on the body. For example, some herbs can help to reduce inflammation, while others can boost the immune system.

Warning Labels

Almost every product I see in the healthcare market has a disclaimer on it that says, "Do not take during pregnancy" or "Speak with your doctor before taking." This is because there are so few studies conducted on pregnant women. These remedies have been used in some cases for thousands of years. The products I recommend are useful, beneficial, and safe for you to use.

What to Get

These are the natural medicines I suggest trying for many ailments before you go to the doctor. In the First Trimester section I'll talk about common complications or issues during pregnancy and how you can naturally mitigate them. For now, I'd like you to start building your natural medicine chest, so you have easy access to these medicines when you need them. Some are quite affordable, but they do add up, so start buying a few at a time if your budget is already stretched. While I don't have brand recommendations for all of these, the brands I do recommend are listed in Appendix A.

Advice

Maria Sabina

Heal yourself with the light of the sun and the rays of the moon. With the sound of the river and the waterfall. With the swaying of the sea and the fluttering of birds.

Heal yourself with mint, neem, and eucalyptus. Sweeten with lavender, rosemary, and chamomile. Hug yourself with the cocoa bean and a hint of cinnamon. Put love in tea instead of sugar and drink it looking at the stars.

Heal yourself with the kisses that the wind gives you and the hugs of the rain. Stand strong with your bare feet on the ground and with everything that comes from it.

Be smarter every day by listening to your intuition, looking at the world with your forehead. Jump, dance, sing, so that you live happier. Heal yourself, with beautiful love, and always remember ...

You are the medicine.

Once you have the herbal remedies on hand, they should be stored in a cool, dark place.

Be sure to get the purest possible products. As many of these remedies have gained popularity in the mainstream market, it is easy to accidentally purchase something of compromised quality.

Echinacea

A natural immune booster. Great to use at the onset of or to ward off an illness. I suggest you get a tincture of echinacea, as it is more potent than capsules.

Oil of Oregano

A powerful antibiotic and antifungal. However, Oregano has many other benefits, and can help with digestive problems, migraine headaches, athletes' foot, sore throat, breathing problems, dandruff (and other skin problems).

Astragalus

Astragalus is used in traditional Chinese medicine for night sweats, diarrhea and for energy tonics that are taken daily at certain times of the year. It may also have mild antiviral activity and help with the prevention of colds. It may have a diuretic effect, which would lower blood pressure and it may cause blood vessels to relax.

Grapefruit Seed Extract (GSE)

Also contains antibacterial, antiviral, and anti-fungal properties. It has been recommended by some nutritionists for the treatment of candidiasis (yeast infection), earache, throat infections, and diarrhea.

Oscillococcinum

Oscillococcinum is a homeopathic remedy used for temporary relief of symptoms of flu such as fever, chills, body aches and pains. The flu (influenza) is a highly infectious viral disease. Homoeopathic preparations, such as Oscillococcinum or similar products, are often prescribed by homoeopaths for the prevention and treatment of the flu. Oscillococcinum is used by millions of people and recommended by doctors around the world. It can be found in many grocery stores' natural sections or online.

Clay Powders

Use white and green clay powders to draw out topical skin infections. Mix a few teaspoons with a small amount of water to form a paste. Apply to the infected area, allow it to dry, leave it on for 30 minutes to two hours, and then wipe off gently with a cloth soaked in cool to mildly warm water.

Cranberry Extract (pill form) & D-Mannose

Aids in healthy urinary tract function. Helps fight urinary tract infection. Taken in pill form.

Colloidal Silver

Powerful natural antibiotic. Use carefully as directed. This is another product that has differing opinions on safety. I think it is safe in small amounts for fighting an infection.

Tea Tree Oil

Tea tree oil contains constituents called terpenoids, which have been found to have antiseptic and antifungal properties. It can be used alone or in mixtures for many things including oral hygiene, skin problems, sinus problems, and household cleaning.

Castor Oil

Castor oil is a seed oil extracted from castor bean plant seeds. It has been used medicinally for centuries and is still used today for a variety of health conditions, including as a laxative, anti-inflammatory, antimicrobial, immune system support, skin care, such as for treating dry skin, eczema, and psoriasis, hair care, and as a poultice for chest congestion, coughs, and colds. It can also be used on the head for sinus congestion or on the eye for styes.

Castor oil is highly effective as a poultice applied to the perineum in the last month of pregnancy to help soften the tissues and prevent tears during the birth. To use, put the warmed oil on a piece of cloth (not terry cloth) and apply it to the area with either a hot water bottle or heating pad on top of the cloth to keep it warmed during the treatment. Leave on for 15–30 minutes.

Warning. Do not ever take castor oil internally during pregnancy unless under the direct supervision of your care provider to help bring on labor when you are significantly past the due range. Remember that castor oil taken internally can work on the baby as well you. I have concerns that it gives the baby gut cramps and I have seen meconium (baby's first poop) staining in the amniotic fluid after castor oil labor inductions.

Pepto-Bismol

Used to treat upset stomach symptoms such as diarrhea, nausea, and heartburn. This isn't totally natural, but sometimes it's totally necessary.

Arnica (gel, cream, and pellets)

Arnica is a homeopathic product that aids in healing minor skin injuries such as bruising, muscle soreness, back pain, carpal tunnel, or joint pain. It is essential to help reduce swelling of tissues of the mother and baby after birth.

Aloe Vera

Aloe is a wonderful skin soother used for burns, scrapes, and irritation. It can be taken directly from the leaf of the aloe plant or bought in stores. Look for 100 percent aloe and not something cut with alcohol. Aloe vera can be taken internally for chronic indigestion, Irritable Bowel Syndrome (IBS), and Crohn's disease.[42]

Elderberry Syrup

Elderberry syrup has been used for thousands of years to help knock back respiratory viruses and other illnesses. Elderberry is now recognized as nature's richest source of anthocyanins, a class of flavonoids that are thought to help stimulate the body's immune response. It has been suggested that elderberry syrup may be similar to the prescription flu medication Relenza.[43]

Xylitol

Xylitol is a sweetener used in oral products like chewing gum, mouthwash, and toothpaste. It has a powerful antimicrobial effect on the mucus membranes of the respiratory passages, making them less permeable to bacteria and viruses. It is wonderful to add to any gargle or mixture for nasal lavage.

Rescue Remedy

Rescue Remedy is a popular natural remedy that is used to relieve stress and anxiety. It is a combination of five flower essences that were developed by Edward Bach, an English homeopath, in the 1930s. The five flower essences are:

- **Rock Rose**—to help relieve terror and panic.
- **Impatiens**—to help relieve irritability and impatience.
- **Clematis**—to help relieve shock and detachment.

- **Star of Bethlehem**—to help relieve shock and trauma.
- **Cherry Plum**—to help relieve irrational thoughts and fears.

Rescue Remedy is available in a variety of forms, including drops, spray, and lozenges. It is typically taken when someone is feeling stressed or anxious. You can also take it before or during a stressful event, such as a job interview or a public speaking engagement.

Tobacco Products

Nicotine is such a highly addictive substance. I really feel for you if you have come under its compulsive sway. It is so very terrible for you and your baby, though, that you must give it up. Smoking a cigarette restricts oxygen to your baby by constricting blood vessels in the placenta; it can decrease the oxygen flow to your baby by as much as 60 percent.[44] This can result in adverse outcomes, including preterm delivery, low birth weight, stillbirth, and sudden infant death syndrome (SIDS). This is very serious. Fewer studies are available on vaping, but I suggest you play it safe and presume it's just as bad for your baby as smoking cigarettes (or cigars!).

There are many resources out there that can help with smoking cessation, and I strongly suggest you seek them out. Enlist the support of your family and friends. Use some of your daily affirmations to remind yourself that you are breathing fresh, clean air for you and your baby, and that you have the strength to claim your healthiest and best self. I'll talk more about affirmations soon.

This is a battle for your overall health. Tobacco use is the leading cause of preventable death in the United States. It is responsible for more than 480,000 deaths per year, or about one in five deaths. Secondhand smoke exposure can also cause death. It is estimated that secondhand smoke exposure causes about 41,000 deaths per year in the United States.

That being said, I want to lighten up just a tiny bit and also say that having a baby is

Aleah: I took up the unfortunate habit of smoking cigarettes when I was very young. It was one of those things that was still pervasive when I was growing up in the 'eighties and early nineties. We were bombarded with cigarette commercials—they were all over TV, movies, magazines, everything like that. Lots of actors smoked on screen for their roles. I saw a lot of my older siblings and kids in the neighborhood and kids at school smoking. I genuinely thought it was a cool thing to do.

I did not want to have kids in my twenties. I wanted to finish college and be more settled and financially ready and in a really loving, committed relationship. When I wanted to get pregnant in my early thirties, I'd been a smoker at that point for about 20 years. I'd tried a lot of different things to stop smoking—hypnotherapy, the patch, cold turkey—and I had been in a constant battle with my now-husband during our entire relationship to stop smoking. He was not a smoker. He hated it. We'd been together for over a decade when we were married and he was just done with it, and I knew he was right. I started going to counseling about six months before I got pregnant because I just couldn't understand why I was having such a hard time stopping smoking.

I understood the health ramifications and what I was risking by continuing to smoke, but to be honest, I liked it. It is really difficult when you like something that much to stop. Plus, it's one of the most addictive things on the planet. I'd been working with my counselor for almost six months, and I finally came to this point where I said, "Look I don't think there's anything that's going to help me stop smoking except for getting pregnant."

I remember so clearly her looking at me and saying "Okay, what's the problem with that? Maybe that's when you stop. Maybe that's okay. Maybe what you need to really look at it in a different way is for it to not be for you, but for someone else. Who's to say that that's wrong?"

I remember just thinking, *Oh yeah, maybe she's right. Maybe if that's the way I stop, then okay.*

Not four weeks later I went back for another session and told her that shortly after our last session I found out I was pregnant and had immediately quit smoking. I found it relatively easy to do. I had a little ritual for myself to say goodbye to the version of myself who was a smoker and I never looked back. I have not smoked since. I've been a proud non-smoker and yes, I did it for my kids, but also, by proxy, I did it for myself.

It was by getting pregnant that I was able to kick that habit. You can do it. For sure it is a difficult habit to kick, but I really believe in what MariMikel talks about—that it's something you must do for the sake of the baby. Even if it's something that you couldn't do before for yourself, you have to do it when you're pregnant. It's not just about you anymore, it's about the life that's growing inside you.

Penelope: I started smoking in Europe in my early twenties and was a light smoker through most of my adult life prior to becoming pregnant. As someone who had been infertile for so long, I had tried at various times to give up the habit to increase my fertility and health, but always fell back to it. Depression was another demon I battled, and I did find it easier to stop when I was on Wellbutrin for depression, which is also marketed as Zyban for smoking cessation. But I always started again. When I found out I was pregnant I wasn't expecting it at all ... I'd been without protection in a stable relationship for eleven years and figured I was the problem. When I became pregnant, I found that cigarettes were suddenly distasteful. It wasn't easy to quit. I was still addicted. But because they tasted nasty it was easier than it had been in the past. Like Aleah, there was no question of keeping up the habit once I was pregnant.

going to challenge everything in you to think about someone else before yourself, to make sacrifices, to be strong, to go the extra mile, and giving up something as unhealthy for you and the baby as smoking is wonderful practice for how incredibly hard it's going to be to be a good parent. If you are a smoker or use nicotine products, talk with your midwife about techniques and help for quitting. You don't have to be alone in this.

Alcohol

There is a serious stigma against alcohol in pregnancy in the United States; every restroom in every bar and restaurant that serves alcohol has warning labels advising against drinking it while pregnant. I'll talk more about this later, because the US is pretty puritanical in comparison with other developed nations, and I find there are times and places for the medicinal use of alcohol in pregnancy. In general, though, the heavy consumption of alcohol doesn't help your body prepare for pregnancy, and it's best to limit yourself to minimal consumption (a serving a week or less) while you're trying to conceive.

Cannabis

While I feel quite vulnerable sharing my true thoughts with you, I think it is important to talk about an elephant in the room, cannabis.

To date there have been some scientific, peer-reviewed studies conducted on the effects of cannabis in pregnancy.[45] Their findings point to some instances of lower birth weight possibly associated with cannabis use. My issue with these studies is that I have no idea how healthy the women in their test group were. Were all factors accounted for?

What I can offer you is my anecdotal advice from nearly 50 years of serving as a midwife and talking with thousands of women. I can tell you that approximately one-third of my clients used cannabis minimally to moderately throughout their pregnancies to combat stress, nausea, or both, and I have never seen a detrimental effect. If you choose to use this herb, do it in minimal amounts and in moderation.

The real killer is stress. Time and time again I have seen stress as a factor in a couple's inability to conceive, to miscarriage, and to babies with less-than-optimal birth weights or health indicators. Women turn to cannabis and alcohol to help reduce or relieve themselves of stress. I think if this is done in true moderation, there is absolutely nothing wrong with it.

The human body has receptors for THC, the active chemical component of cannabis,[46] which indicates to me that as a species we have been using this plant for a very long time.

There should be more research here, and I believe we'll see more and more studies on the medicinal properties and benefits of cannabis as it reaches legal status in more and more of the US.

If cannabis isn't yet legal in your state, or if you prefer not to experience the other side effects of cannabis, you may find CBD products to be a viable alternative for stress relief. Look for organic products that are independently certified.

If you choose to use cannabis, strive to use it medicinally, to combat stress, and do so in minimal amounts, occasionally.

Drugs

I hope it goes without saying that most recreational drugs, things like meth, heroin, MDMA (molly, ecstasy), LSD, cocaine, etc., must be completely avoided. Abstinence is the only acceptable approach here, for your own health and that of your baby-to-be.

Epigenetics

I have recently been fascinated by a new area of study called epigenetics, which looks at gene expression.[47] Basically, our genes are considered to "express" themselves when their code is used to generate proteins. Genes that are actively generating these instructions are considered to be "turned on." Genes that are not actively generating these instructions are considered to be "turned off." What this implies is that not all of our DNA code is active all the time. Epigenetics looks at behavioral and environmental triggers and their impacts on our DNA's gene expression. Specifically, these triggers include diet, exercise, stress, and environmental toxins, and they can influence our gene expression—for better or worse!

What we do to support our health during our lifetime, and especially in pregnancy, has long lasting effects. Without altering our DNA, gene expression can affect so many things, like physical appearance, behavior, and susceptibility to disease. Research has also shown that epigenetic changes can be passed down from parents to children. This is known as transgenerational epigenetic inheritance. It's thought that stress can lead to changes in the sperm and eggs of the parents, and this is how the gene expression is passed on. Researchers found that children of Holocaust survivors were more likely to express genes associated with a stress response, and more likely to develop PTSD, than their peers who were not born to Holocaust survivors.[48] Transgenerational epigenetic inheritance is thought to play a role in several health problems, including obesity, diabetes, and mental health disorders like PTSD.

All the eggs a woman will ever carry form in her ovaries while she is a four-month-old fetus in the womb of her mother.

This means our cellular life as an egg begins in the womb of our grandmother.

Each of us spent five months in our grandmother's womb, and she in turn formed in the womb of her grandmother.

We vibrate to the rhythm of our mother's blood before she herself is born, and this pulse is the thread of blood that runs all the way back through the grandmothers to the first mother.

—Romana Yesmin Sharna

More research is needed to fully understand the role of transgenerational epigenetic inheritance in trauma. However, the existing research suggests that these experiences can have a lasting impact on the health of future generations. While this might sound a little depressing, I think it's wonderful news. What epigenetics shows us is that our bodies respond to our lifestyles at a deep level. For example, a diet that is rich in whole foods has been shown to reduce DNA methylation in genes that are associated with chronic diseases. That means the triggers for those chronic diseases are turned off.

Importantly for you and your partner, your diet, exercise, and stress levels prior to conceiving can affect the epigenetic programming of your children. Research has shown that exercise reduces the gene expression in genes associated with developing cancer, whereas stress can increase the gene expression in genes associated with things like obesity, diabetes, and mental health issues. Environmental toxins can increase the risk of your baby's genes expressing cancer, heart disease, and neurological disorders.

I can imagine some of you feeling a bit anxious about this information. I'd love for you to shift that anxiety to excitement instead. What epigenetics shows us is that we have so much in our control! Epigenetic changes are not permanent, and they can certainly be influenced by our good choices. You can so very positively affect absolutely everything in your life and your baby's life with the tools in this book.

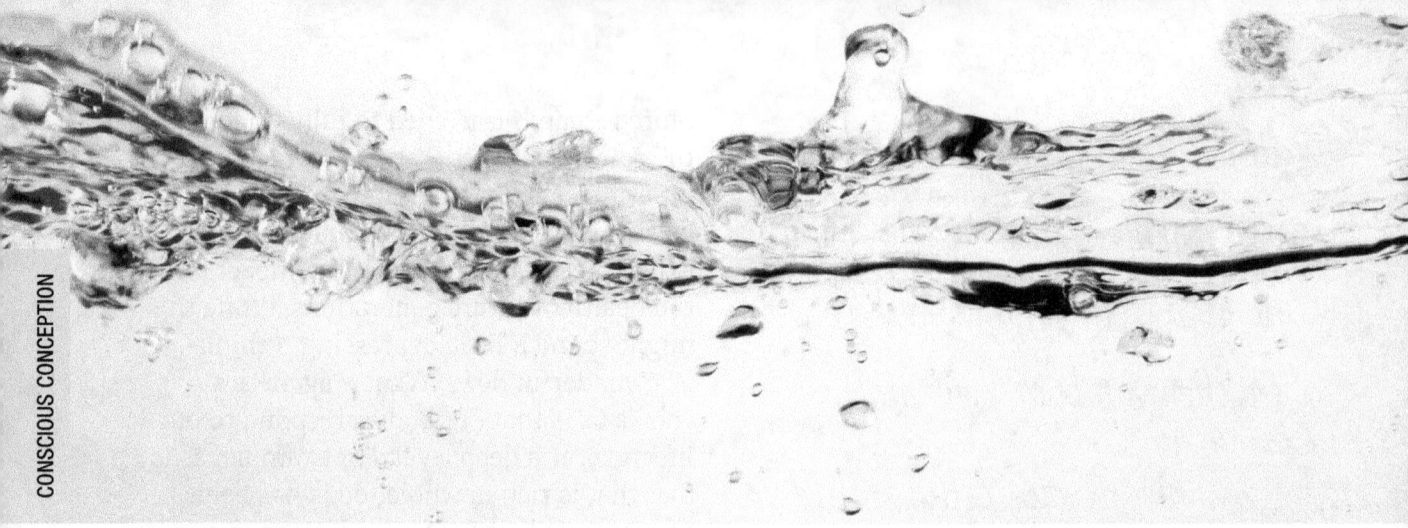

Hydration

Introduction

I was plagued in my youth with migraines, constipation, and bladder infections. I went to scores of doctors and not one of them ever asked me how much water I drank. When I finally went to a Doctor of Naturopathy, they asked how much water I drank. I said, "Lots!" and they asked how much "lots" was. For me at that time, it was two or three glasses a day. The doctor said, "I can't believe you're not dead! That is not okay." That conversation changed my life. It also changed my health. I am in my seventies now and I'm feeling pretty dang good for being really super old, and I contribute the vast majority of that to nourishment, hydration, movement, and emotional/spiritual work.

What You Need

Our bodies are composed of 60 percent water.[49] The vast majority of Americans are seriously dehydrated. You need to drink four quarts of water a day. Yes, that much. Yes, four quarts is a gallon. People go nuts when I tell them they need to drink a gallon of water a day. Think about this ... You're awake for 16 hours in the day; a gallon is 16 cups. That means you are drinking one tiny little eight-ounce measuring cup of water an hour. That one cup supports your bladder, your colon, your respiration, your kidneys, your liver, your circulatory system, your tears, your sweat, your saliva, your cerebral spinal fluid, your mucus—all of these are fluid-based systems and drinking one cup an hour while you're awake is not that much. You need it, and everybody needs it. Start right now.

Seriously. Right now. Go get yourself a nice big drink. I'll be here when you get back.

It may seem like such a little thing, but drastically improving your hydration can have an amazingly beneficial effect on your fertility and on your ability to conceive.

☼ **TIP:** You can set an alarm on your phone or smartwatch to remind you to get up and drink your eight ounces every hour (or sixteen ounces every two hours),

60 + THE BOOK OF BIRTH VOL. I: CONSCIOUS CONCEPTION

or you can use a gallon-size jug, fill it up in the morning, and drink from it all day. You could also use a half gallon and fill it twice a day, or a quart and fill it four times a day, but beyond that most people find they lose count. Try to drink half a gallon by 2 p.m.

Improve Your Tap Water

If your water is provided through a municipal water supply ("city water"), I highly recommend you get a water filtration system. If you don't know if you're on city water, you likely are. (You'll have a well or some other source of water if you aren't). City water is treated with chemicals like chlorine to ensure pathogens are killed.

I do not personally want to drink chlorinated water. I use a water filter to filter out the added chlorine in my city water. But I am thrilled that the water was chlorinated to begin with, and that I am filtering out the chlorine from pathogen-free water instead of having to deal with pathogens in my water.

I highly recommend the Frizzlife water filtration system. There are different models available online and at major retailers. It goes under the sink right next to the spigot and filters tap water. You do have to change the filters every few months, but this system is awesome, and I think the water it produces is delicious. It also puts minerals back into your water, whereas most filters remove everything. If you have a bottled water habit, this will be better for your bank account, better for the planet, and better for your health. If you don't have a bottled water habit, this will still be better for your health to remove chlorine and fluoride from your tap water.

I haven't always recommended a reverse osmosis (RO) system because many of them use two gallons of water (also called reject water) for every single gallon of water they produce. In this day and age, we simply cannot be that wasteful. However, there are some new RO filters on the market that use a variety of technologies to reduce the amount of water that is wasted, such as energy recovery devices and improved membrane materials. Look for these if you purchase a new RO system. If you already have or choose to get an RO system, make sure it includes an alkaline water filter. This will add a measured amount of minerals back into your water after treatment.

Electrolytes

Electrolytes are minerals that carry an electric charge. They aid the body to balance fluids, transmit nerve signals, contract muscles and regulate blood pressure. Active people with healthy diets often get enough electrolytes naturally, but during stressful times of your life (like pregnancy!), adding electrolytes to your water may help maintain optimal levels in your body. Several of my clients have reported that drinking electrolytes in their water helped them feel amazing. If you are drinking your daily gallon of water and still feel dehydrated, adding electrolytes is worth a try. I have found that I really enjoy the tiny change of flavor it gives to the water and crave it when I do not have it.

The most common way to boost your electrolytes and hydration is to add Celtic Sea salt, potassium citrate, and sodium bicarbonate to your drinking water.

Celtic Sea salt is mined from the Celtic Sea off the coast of France. Celtic Sea salt is a good source of sodium, chloride, magnesium, and potassium, all of which are important electrolytes. Celtic Sea salt also contains other minerals, such as calcium, iron, and zinc. It can be difficult to source, and if you can't find it, Himalayan salt is a good temporary alternative. Whichever you buy, make sure the package specifies the source of the salt and details the types and amounts of mineral content.

Potassium citrate is a form of potassium that is easily absorbed by the body and can help boost hydration.

Baking soda is a sodium bicarbonate that can be used to alkalinize the body and is sometimes used to treat or prevent dehydration, which can lead to electrolyte imbalances.

Directions

All you need to do is add a small pinch of each (Celtic Sea salt, potassium citrate, and baking soda) to a quart of water, then stir it or shake it in a closed container until it dissolves. Be careful not to add more than a tiny amount of salt as too much sodium can increase the risk of high blood pressure and other health problems.

Drink and enjoy your extra boost of hydration!

Caffeine

Most people throughout the history of the world ate a good breakfast right at dawn, ate the biggest meal of the day at midday, then napped during the hottest part of the day. Lots of people in Europe still sleep through the midafternoon. If you go to Spain or Portugal, you'll find there's not a lot going on between 1 and 3 p.m., and then they eat a very light supper around 9 p.m. I think that we've kind of lost our way and instead of taking our siestas, we're keeping ourselves going and messing ourselves up with caffeine.

I suggest that you do what you can to stay away from caffeine. It jolts the baby around in a really serious way. Your baby's liver is not as developed as yours, and consequently cannot process the caffeine as quickly. Caffeine stays in your system for about 10 hours, whereas the baby feels its effects for about 24 (depending on gestational age).[50] Consuming more than 200 mg of caffeine per day during pregnancy has been linked[51] to several adverse outcomes for the fetus, including:

- Low birth weight
- Premature birth
- Stillbirth
- Sudden infant death syndrome (SIDS)

Also, be aware of all the sources of caffeine. It's obviously in coffee and some teas, but also in chocolate, soda, energy drinks, and some medications and supplements.

Now, I am no saint. I had a caffeine addiction during my pregnancy that I believe I passed on to my baby. Caffeine doesn't transfer through breastmilk like it does to the baby through the placenta. So, I believe my poor baby came out and underwent caffeine withdrawals. She just cried and cried for the first few days of her life. She also had a rough time of it in labor,

I think, which may have contributed to her initial distress. As I like to remind you, every person is different. Your baby may not be affected like I believe mine was. At the very least, I suggest you strive to limit your consumption of caffeine to less than 200 mg per day.

How to Get Off Coffee

The best time to get off caffeinated coffee is before you get pregnant. The way to get off coffee (or a caffeinated tea habit) is to gently wean yourself from it.

Week Zero

Start by making sure that you eat something healthy before you down your first cup of caffeine. You need to teach your body that caffeine is not its first or most desired fuel to run on. This is really, really important.

Week One

If you're a coffee drinker, start by using 25 percent water-processed decaf to 75 percent caffeinated grounds when you make your coffee. If you have a single-cup coffee maker, you can brew a cup of decaf and use it over several cups of caffeinated coffee throughout the week.

Week Two

Switch to 50 percent caffeinated, 50 percent decaffeinated grounds.

Week Three

Switch to 75 percent decaf, 25 percent caffeinated.

Week Four

Switch to 100 percent decaf. If you don't care for decaf, if it's the zing of caffeine that's your sole reason for drinking coffee, start experimenting to find a morning or afternoon drink you do love. Maybe it's herbal tea or fruit-infused water.

If you cut back in this fashion, it will take a full month for the transition. You're not going to be in misery if you approach it this way. You'll avoid the withdrawal headaches as you gently exit the caffeine train. That's when you'll find your true energy levels.

It may be that you've been wired and running on adrenaline from the caffeine stimulus for so long that your body needs some time to learn how to optimally function again after you leave that addiction behind. Continue to give yourself true nourishment and give your body delicious, nutritious food and lots of water to support this new paradigm.

Take this same approach if you get your caffeine from soda. Slowly change out the soda you're drinking for drinks with a lower caffeine and sugar content.

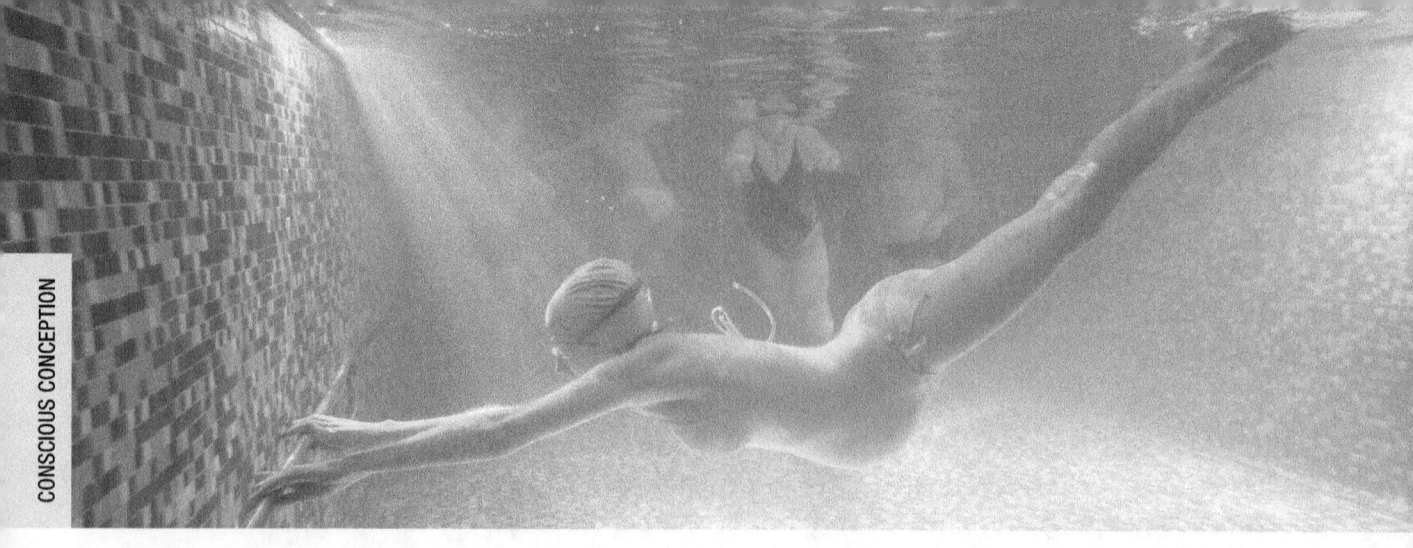

Movement

Introduction

Our ancestors were incredible athletes. They walked miles and miles every day, cut and carried all their firewood, carried all their water over distances, foraged for hours, spent many hours in the fields on their hands and knees picking bugs and pulling weeds, harvesting, and planting. They carried everything. Their lives were filled with aerobic exercise, and they were in different positions from dawn to dark every single day. And now with the wonderful labor-saving devices that we are all using, we are very sedentary in comparison. Birth for our ancestors was just another hard day's work, but now I believe that one of the reasons we have such difficulty with birth and such high c-section rates is that there are too many women who are simply unable to physically do the work of being in labor and pushing the baby out.

Everything that you can do to put yourself in a great position physically, emotionally, spiritually, medically, and intellectually is going to empower you to have a successful pregnancy. You want to get more sleep, you want to drink more fluids, you want to start taking vitamins before you get pregnant, and you want to be in the best shape you've ever been in before you get pregnant. If you're overweight, now is the time to lose that extra weight. Let me say this again. If you're planning a pregnancy and really thinking ahead, you want to be in the best shape of your life.

A woman who lives in a society where it's common to walk a lot doesn't have as many problems with muscle tone in her perineum as we do. We are generally so sedentary and so few people walk daily that, in general, our perineal and pelvic floors are simply not very strong. Pelvic floor exercises can help but the big factor is exercising regularly. All these things—walking, swimming, weight work, and yoga—help the perineal muscles to be strong.

Once you become pregnant, I advise you not to exercise in the first few months. I advise women to not push themselves. You're going to be exhausted. You're going to feel like all you want to do is sleep, and you should rest at that time because mystical, magical things are going on that sap your vital life force from your head to your toenails. But before that point, exercise is critical. You want to build your strength up with cross training now.

If you have a hard first trimester, that's a few months of inactivity. If you can go into that in good physical shape you can withstand it, but if you're not in great shape, that can really put you at a deficit when you enter your second trimester in terms of preparing for the birth. So, exercise beforehand to prepare yourself for the marathon of pregnancy. Work up to a balance of walking, swimming, weight work, and yoga.

Walking

If you are new to exercise, start with walking. I want you to walk at first light in the morning if at all possible. If you battle with depression or just generally find you have some blah moods, walking at first light has been shown to have beneficial effects, which I can attest to myself. When I was struggling with depression and didn't want to go on medication, a psychiatrist suggested I try walking in the morning. She told me it was based on the idea that every single human on the planet got up every morning of their lives and walked away from where they slept to go to the bathroom. They wouldn't have wanted to foul their nests.

Sleep studies have shown that the brain shrinks at night, opening a series of channels called the lymphatic system.

Scientists discovered that this was because the brain flushes out all of the waste from all of the enormous work the brain does during the day.[52] So, in the morning you are like a blank slate, chemically speaking, and when you get out and walk in the morning the particular angle of light and the movement of walking rocks the pituitary and jumpstarts the brain.[53] There is an amazing release of serotonin, endorphins, aldosterone, dopamine, and all of these happy chemicals that generally make our lives more wonderful. Best of all, if you take a walk in the morning, you'll feel the beneficial effects throughout the day.

I was not a morning person, but I committed to trying this approach. I'll tell you that after only two weeks, I was a different person. For one thing, I don't think I had been moving my body enough. I was overwhelmed and I wasn't giving myself enough care. I started getting up early enough to walk before the kids got up and everything got crazy, all of that. It made me feel so incredibly good, and gradually I was able to add other exercises to my routine.

If you don't walk, you may be a little bit limited in the brain chemistry department, so much so that depression and anxiety are often correlated with people not doing what their bodies were designed to do over millennia.[54] That is, moving. The simple act of walking every day can do incredible things to boost your mood.

Of course, if the morning is simply not an option for you, it's still going to be good for you to walk later in the day, but you're not going to get quite the same brain chemistry boost. If you are having any kind of emotional/mental difficulties, try walking in the morning and see what it does. It doesn't have to be a long walk. Even twenty minutes a day is enough.

Walk every morning. Walk at least five days a week. If you can build up to a couple of miles in 45 or 50 minutes, that would be really great. Remember to stay hydrated and avoid getting overheated.

Swimming

Swimming is wonderful for you. It is a true, full-body, cardio workout. It develops a full range of muscles and gives you so much stamina. It particularly helps with pectoral and front upper body muscles. If you're not already married to a particular stroke, do the breaststroke. I think it's easier to do and it uses a scissor kick or frog kick. It exercises muscles we don't often use— muscles that will come into play later in your pregnancy.

Many gyms and YMCAs have indoor swimming pools so that you can swim year-round. You might also have access to

a neighborhood pool or be lucky enough to have a pool in your backyard.

You'll want to wear a cap. A cap will protect your hair from the pool chemicals, and it will keep your head warm in the winter. It also will keep you from shedding into the pool, which is a courtesy you'll appreciate when other swimmers extend it to you. Put conditioner on your hair and then, if you have long hair, roll it up and put a cap on to protect it. You can't swim properly without putting your face down in the water, so I suggest you use goggles, too.

Swim Safely to Avoid Infection

Some people prefer to not swim in chlorinated water and don't like it on their skin because it is a chemical. But if you are going to swim regularly it behooves you to swim in a chlorinated pool to protect yourself. It is easy to get ear and sinus infections in unchlorinated water sources. Chlorine is a chemical element that is used to disinfect water and swimming pools. It is a powerful oxidizer that can kill bacteria, viruses, and other microorganisms that can cause various diseases. Chlorine is also used to remove algae and other organic matter from water. Algae can make water cloudy and unsightly, and it can also produce toxins that can be harmful to people and animals.

The use of chlorine in pools and water is generally considered to be safe. Some people may find that when chlorine is too concentrated, they may develop eye, skin, or respiratory irritations. Overall, the benefits of using chlorine in pools and water outweigh the risks. Chlorine is an effective way to prevent the spread of disease and to keep water clean and safe. I believe hundreds of thousands of lives have been saved by the careful use of chlorine to kill bacteria in water and to disinfect our homes and hospitals. The risks of chlorine exposure can be minimized by following these safety tips:

- Swim in pools that are properly chlorinated. The chlorine level in a pool should be between one and three parts per million (ppm).
- Avoid swimming in pools that are cloudy or have a strong chlorine odor.
- Rinse off with clean water after swimming to remove chlorine from your skin and hair.
- Avoid breathing in chlorine fumes. If you do breathe in chlorine fumes, move to fresh air, and get medical attention if you experience any symptoms.

TIP: It is a good idea to use SwimEar a few times a week. It's a product that is comprised of peroxide with a little bit of glycerin. Putting a few drops in each ear prevents ear infections by drying out the water, killing bacteria, viruses, and funguses, and it moisturizes the drying effects.

Develop Your Swimming Skills

If you're not a big swimmer and aren't all that good at it, use a mask and snorkel until you feel comfortable. If you don't know how to swim at all, take lessons! This is an important life skill as well as wonderful exercise.

If you need extra support as you build up your muscles, get a kickboard and swim a lap, then kick two laps with the kickboard so your upper body can recuperate. Then you can swim another lap and it won't be long before you'll be swimming two, kicking one, then swimming three, kicking one. Soon enough you'll be leaving that kickboard behind. You'll be able to slowly swim back and forth, and you will build upper body muscle, which you desperately need in labor and when you have a newborn.

Once you get your stroke down, then you want to take that snorkel off and add the proper breathing. Swimming is a lifesaving skill and one that's worth practicing. Plus, it is just fun. It is so awesome—it's so meditative and cooling. It's so weightless and can be so incredibly spiritual.

Work up to swimming two times per week for about 20 minutes per swim. You might only be able to do five minutes at first, and that's fine. But do start somewhere.

Weight Work

While swimming is amazing for upper body strength, stamina, and breath work, weight work is going to help you build muscle. Our ancestors carried everything, their firewood, water, and kids, everything they harvested, etc. They carried everything all day long and as a result had great upper body strength. You'll need that too once you start picking up your beautiful baby in their heavy car seat with a giant diaper bag laden with all your supplies. The demands of early motherhood will really knock your back and neck out seriously if you don't have some upper body strength.

Even doing something as simple as exercising with stretchy bands will help. But going to a gym and using the machines that are designed to help your body move correctly will be super effective. When you are exercising, you will not only increase your muscle mass, but because of the stress you put on your bones, you will build bone mass as well.

If you can't afford to join a gym, you can very inexpensively get hand weights, strength bands, and other such equipment. Try places like Craigslist, TJ Maxx, Marshalls, Ross, thrift stores, and yard sales. You can also find great free workout videos online or on YouTube to help guide you. Work up to doing weights twice a week for 20–30 minutes.

 TIP: Join a gym where you can work out on the machines and then swim.

Yoga

When you do weight work and then swim you will have a new body, one that is muscular and taut. Yoga is a critical component of a good exercise regime because it stretches out all the things that you're building and tightening, adding flexibility and resilience to your body. It can also stretch out muscles and ligaments in the pelvis to help you to push your baby out more easily when the time comes. I highly recommend this as the final component of your new workout routine. I suggest you do a 30–60-minute routine twice a week.

Your Weekly Routine

- I want you to walk five times a week for about 40 minutes each session.
- Twice a week I'd like you to swim for 10–20 minutes and do weights for 20–30 minutes.
- Twice a week I'd like you to be doing yoga for 30–60 minutes.

Partners Need to Get in Shape Too

 Partners, this advice goes for you too. If your woman has a natural birth, you are going to be by her side. It's very possible you will be helping her to stand and squat over and over again. Many women stand and squat for hours during their labors and births. You will be doing what is essentially repetitive lifting for a very long time, and you will need to be able to sustain the effort. You need serious stamina, and serious strength. This is no joke. Get training now if you aren't already!

I strongly encourage you to do everything you can to exercise together as a couple. This brings you closer together and fosters opportunities for you to talk on deeper levels, to connect on deeper levels, to feel each other's energy, and it positions you to be more supportive and loving of one another. So, exercising together is wonderful. Anything that you can do as a team, including exercise, is going to build your teamwork skills, which you're going to need in abundance for the amazingly wonderful yet arduous job of parenting together.

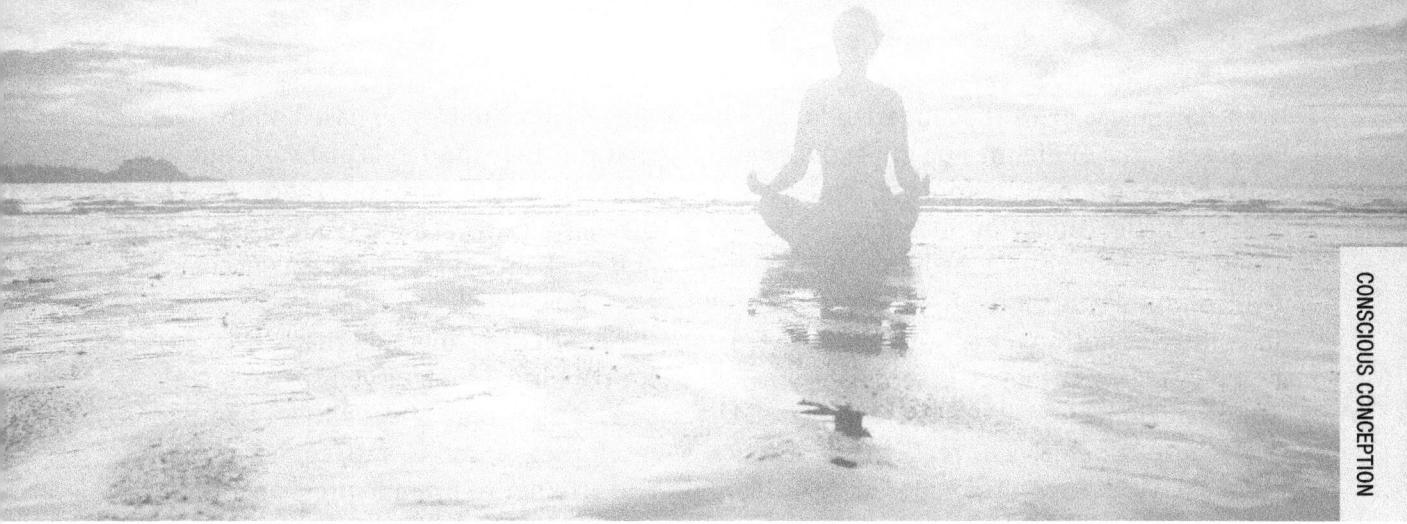

Emotional/Spiritual

Introduction

Taking time to care for your emotional health is such an important part of our self-care practices. You so often hear about taking care of your physical health—getting enough sleep, eating well, and being physically active—and more and more we're actively acknowledging that we need to improve and care for our mental health. But we don't seem to talk as much about the emotional component of our mental health, which is equally as important.

It can be so empowering to create space and focus time and energy on loving ourselves and building ourselves up with experiences that fill our emotional well. Pregnancy is a deeply emotional period in your life; work to prepare your emotional body as diligently as you do your physical body.

You can't take care of others unless you first care of yourself. Through acknowledging and expressing your feelings, practicing good emotional self-care, and connecting with yourself and others you'll be taking active steps to enhance and support your emotional self. The benefits can be palpable.

Preparing for Baby

New humans are very immature and require a tremendous amount of care and interaction to survive and thrive. I want to prepare you for this so you are aware and so you understand that this baby requires more from you than you might have thought, and you are going to have to find a way within yourself and your support network to give your baby what they need. Your life will not be the same. My children have taken more out of me than anything else in my life and have given me much more than they have ever taken.

 Because of this, you should be in the best emotional state with your partner before you get pregnant. Do not have a baby to fix or heal your relationship. Don't have a baby to get a partner to stay with you. That is a recipe for disaster. If you've got serious stuff going on with yourself, your family,

your partner, your work, your friends, or whatever area of life may be impacted, you must work on it now, before you conceive. A relationship counselor or couples therapist can serve as a mediator to help you communicate more effectively. Issues in your relationship are always exacerbated by pregnancy. Pregnancy is seriously emotional and puts all your emotional states into hyperdrive. It really helps if you can deal with your emotional issues through self-care, therapy, and other methods of well-being care before you get pregnant. You'll want to consider:

- Are we as a couple in a good place, a plateau, or a bad place? What do we need to do to get to a good place if we're not there now? Is it time for some quality couple time? Should we start couples therapy, so we have a space and place to talk about our future together and our future family?
- Is my partner supportive? Do they want a baby and all that goes along with that as much as I do?
- Am I ready for this massive life change? Do I really want a baby?
- How will another baby affect my older kids?
- Do I have a strong, local support network?
- Can I take time off? Will I be able to leave work two weeks before I'm due and stay home for several months after?
- Can our finances support this?

If you have had trauma in your life and been hurt a lot, you may have some PTSD and an inability to develop or a fear of developing a close relationship with your baby. There

may be a primal belief based on the fear that this new human is just someone else who is going to hurt you. There could be a barrier put up between the mother or father and the baby due to these unconscious anxieties, which would lead to a lack in the depth of connection that's necessary for bonding. If you or your partner feel these issues may affect either of you, this is another reason to seek counseling before you attempt to become pregnant.

Birth History Questionnaire

 I think it can be helpful and even important to gather information from you and your partner's parents about your own birth experiences. If your parents are unavailable, ask your aunts, uncles, grandparents, older siblings, or other family members who may have information on your birth. If you are orphaned, adopted, or don't have access to this information I don't want you to worry at all!

This information can be important and interesting because how you were born can affect how you view birth and how you give birth. Sometimes a perfectly fine birth can traumatize a person and sometimes a traumatic birth can leave them unfazed. If you start collecting this information and either you or your partner experience intense emotions, there may be something to look at and heal in your own birth story.

When a person is aware of issues in their mind, those can be healed and released, but being unaware leads to these issues affecting you on a day-by-day basis without understanding why you are mad,

> I'm sure you know that in forensics they often look at the teeth to assess how old a skeleton is. In some people, you can also see what is known as the *natal line*,[55] which is laid down in the teeth at birth. Birth is the most difficult thing that we ever go through, and that's why the natal line is so distinct. There's probably a reason we don't tend to remember the experience. Teeth continue to gain layers of what's known as *dentin* as children grow, and if the child experiences trauma or nutritional deficiencies, that trauma can also be indicated in the dentin.[56]

- Were forceps or vacuum extraction used on me?
- Was I born by cesarean?
- Was my mother drugged?
- Were there complications?
- Was there bonding after the birth?
- How old were my mother and father when I arrived?
- Were my parents getting along when I was born?
- Did I breastfeed soon after birth?
- If you weren't the firstborn child, what was your mother's first birthing experience like?
  - How long was she in labor?
  - If she had a vaginal birth, how long did she push?

sad, confused, irritated, etc. I believe it is always better to look at what is deep within us as opposed to being unconscious in life. Birth is one of the earliest and most intense experiences we go through, and it can affect your life profoundly. When you have gathered this information, sit with it, and look to see if it has any meaningful insights for you.

These are interesting and difficult questions to ask, and you may not have all the success you desire in getting answers to these questions. Don't stress out about it. Find out what you can and just let go of the rest. If difficult feelings come up for you, it is not because you asked these questions, but because these issues and feelings were already there. Here are some of the questions you might want to ask:

- Which baby was I?
- Was my mother early or late going into labor?
- How long was she in labor?
- How long did she push?
- Was my father involved and how?
- Was I a planned pregnancy?

Aside from emotional information, it's also important to gather your medical history at this time. There is a detailed medical questionnaire in Appendix C for you to use as a template to get the information that will be helpful to you and your midwife throughout your conception and pregnancy.

Develop Your Intuition

Intuition is a way of knowing. For thousands of years, it has been associated with a woman's way of knowing, and it is in alignment with prophecy and seeing into the future. I believe that intuition is a connection with your higher self, and that when you connect to your higher self you can get deeper messages from your body, your mind, your spirit, and the divine.

Intuition requires a certain amount of mindfulness. You have to think about what's going on and get deeper with your feelings to access the intuitive space within yourself. I believe that everyone has intuition, but some people feel more comfortable and connected to it. Others never speak of, acknowledge, or help it along and for them it is much harder to access.

I would like to help dispel the myth that you have to get all your information from Western medical healthcare providers. Most of the time these practitioners are too overwhelmed with the sheer number of patients they are seeing to give you the kind of information that you deserve. Not only do you need to investigate for yourself, but I hope you will also learn to feel what is going on in situations.

Learn to discern when something feels good and right and when it doesn't. Intuition can be developed and nurtured. First, trust that it's there, and second, create those quiet, still moments where you can hear your intuition coming through and then listen to it. I will be talking more about intuition in every chapter. I think it's so important that we're going to revisit it often.

Affirmations

Thoughts become things ... I believe we actively create our reality in any given moment, and we can do it consciously. If you want to create dynamic change in the actions you take or emotions you feel in your life, you can change your thoughts and accomplish that change! Affirmations are a brilliant way to consciously do this. An affirmation is a positive thought that you consciously choose to immerse yourself in, delivering a powerful message to your subconscious brain and rewiring your thought pathways to avoid fear and

negativity. Some of the issues people work on with affirmations include:

- Money mindset
- Prosperity and abundance
- Forgiveness
- Self-esteem
- Releasing fear
- Anticipating an ideal event, like a birth
- Safety and health

A technique that is sometimes used in therapeutic settings that has been shown to be effective and I believe is similar to the use of affirmations is Cognitive Behavioral Therapy (CBT). CBT focuses on the triangle of thoughts, actions, and emotions and is based on the idea that all three are interconnected. When we have negative thoughts, it can lead to negative emotions and behaviors and when we identify and challenge these negative thoughts and replace them with more realistic and helpful thoughts it can change our patterns of thinking and behavior. CBT tells us that when we dislike one aspect of ourselves on the triangle (e.g., the emotion of fear), we can change something else on the triangle (a thought or an action).

If you have social anxiety or a fear of being in social settings, a therapist might help the person to gradually expose themselves to social events and to develop coping skills to manage their anxiety while simultaneously encouraging them to increase their participation in activities that they enjoy and that are meaningful to them (Behavioral Activation). For example, you might have the thought, "Childbirth is going to be incredibly painful and I won't be able to handle it." You can actively challenge this thought by using the knowledge you are learning in this book to consider evidence for and against the thought and then develop more realistic and helpful thoughts about childbirth, such as, "Childbirth is a natural process and I am capable of handling it."

Remember that your thoughts are powerful, and you have a great deal of power within yourself to shape what you think, how you react to those thoughts, and subsequently how you feel.

I suggest you start with one or two affirmations. Select one that produces a kind of electric charge when you think about saying or believing it. That is, it might be a bit of a stretch for you to believe it. Think about what keeps you up at night, what your fears are, and dive in there. You might be afraid that you'll struggle to conceive, and so your affirmation might be, "My body readily and easily conceives. I am ready to be a vessel for new life."

You can say or write each affirmation 10–20 times. Writing is an extremely powerful technique for communicating with and rewiring your subconscious mind. You might also record them on your phone so you can listen to them with headphones when you are in a public place. Record each affirmation ten times, pausing between phrases, and talking slowly.

I'm going to revisit this topic in each trimester because it holds different weight throughout your pregnancy and may feel different while you are working toward conception versus in your first, second, or third trimester, and during the birth process itself.

Affirmations for Conception

Here are some affirmations you might try. You can always create one that delivers the message you need right now.

- My body works beautifully, and I conceive at the perfect time.

- I trust my body's ability to get pregnant.

- I am a spiritual being connected to health, love, and abundance.

Additional Tips

- Make a list of the affirmations that are most meaningful to you. Put specific names and situations into the affirmation.

- Say the affirmations to yourself in the first, second, and third person, as follows: I, MariMikel, am a spiritual being connected to health, love, and abundance. You, MariMikel, are a spiritual being connected to health, love, and abundance. MariMikel is a spiritual being connected to health, love, and abundance.

- Feel free to create new affirmations that are meaningful to you.

- It is useful to look into the mirror, say your affirmation aloud, and repeat it until you see yourself with a relaxed, happy expression.

Continue working with an affirmation until it no longer produces a charge for you. This usually means it has been integrated in your consciousness and you experience the intended results, such as no longer feeling anxious about getting pregnant. Then find a new affirmation to work with.

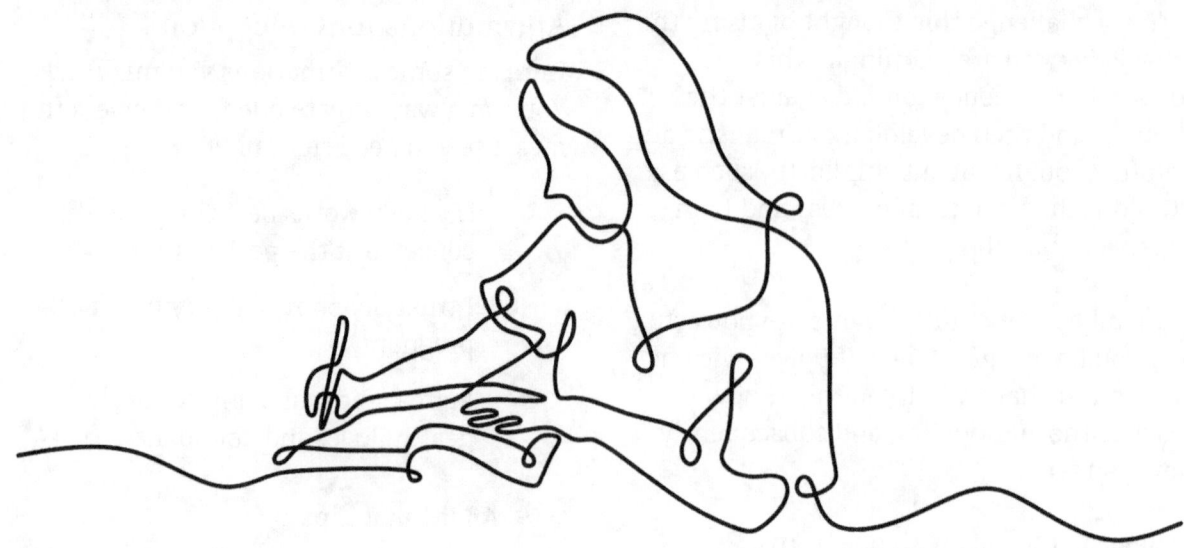

Journaling

Journaling can be a wonderful way to tap into your feelings. It helps to not ignore but acknowledge how you feel and to have an outlet to express and release your thoughts and feelings. It has also been scientifically proven to have direct benefits for our mental wellbeing.[57]

It is so normal to feel overwhelmed by the emotions and stress in our everyday lives. Journaling is one of the best ways to shed yourself of these lingering thoughts and feelings. Through the act of writing, we can put our thoughts and feelings onto paper, pour out our emotions, actively address our worries, and find a space to clear our minds. A self-care journal creates a safe space for us where we can unravel anything brewing inside of us without feeling judged or misunderstood.

Steps for Self-Care Journaling

Creating a regular habit of journaling can be a self-care routine that not only allows you to express your deepest thoughts and feelings but also can help to lend a sense of consistency and regularity to your life. Set aside a designated time for journaling, e.g., in the morning, before bed, or during your lunch break, to unwind and reflect. Commit to spending even just five minutes a day to reap the benefits. Maybe instead of crafting a social media post where you may be mindful of other people's approval, you spend a few uncensored minutes with yourself journaling instead.

Setting this time aside daily will really help; you'll come to relish it, too. You deserve this time for yourself. You have my permission to let go of doing a load of dishes or laundry to take care of yourself instead. Don't worry about "doing it wrong." That's impossible, as long as you're showing up to write and being honest with yourself when you do. You can write by hand, use full sentences or bullet points, type your entries on a computer, or use voice recordings to create an audio log. Don't worry about grammar or spelling. This is just for you.

Release Your Feelings

Sometimes, we just need a safe space to release our emotions, and journaling can be a fantastic way to do that. You can use your journal as a place to vent your feelings and frustrations without judgment or reprisal. This can be a cathartic way to work through any negative emotions and move forward with a healthier, more positive mindset.

Take Time to Process

Journaling can also be a way to slow down and process your thoughts, rather than rushing through life without reflection. It's a chance to let your thoughts settle, reflect on your experiences, and learn from them.

Try Guided Journaling

You might become stuck in a rut or feel bored with your current journaling practice. There are lots of ways to enhance your journaling practice, and guided journaling ideas or resources can help you explore different themes, prompts, and exercises. This can be especially helpful if you're struggling to find inspiration or direction in your journaling. You might try books with prompts for memoir writers to provoke an exploration of memory or guided self-care journals with writing prompts.

Be Grateful

Gratitude journaling can help you cultivate a more positive mindset, appreciate what's good in your life, and build resilience. I think it's such a good idea that we're going to dive deeply into this topic in the Joy section of this chapter.

Don't Edit

Lastly, when it comes to journaling, it's important not to censor or edit yourself. Your journal is meant to be a private, safe space free from judgment or fear of outside opinions. Allow yourself to write or speak freely and authentically, knowing that there's no right or wrong way to journal.

Taking time to care for your emotional health is such an important part of our self-care practices. It can be so empowering to create space and to focus time and energy on loving ourselves and building ourselves up with positive emotional experiences. I hope you will give yourself this gift.

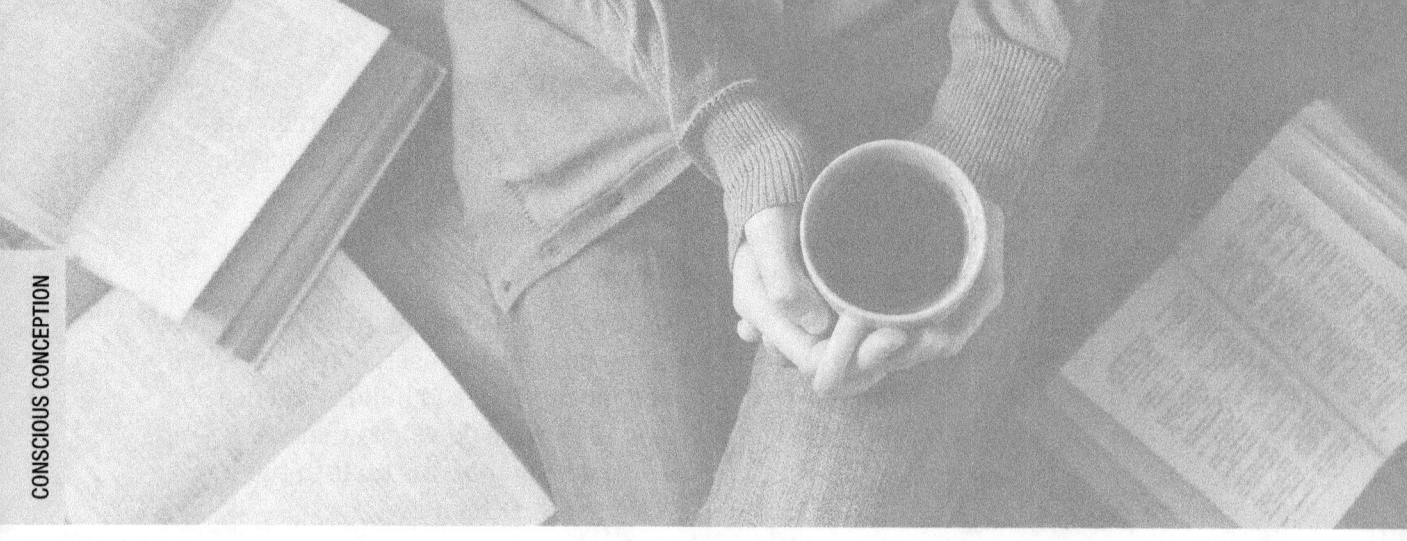

Knowledge

Building New Habits

I want to talk just a little bit about building new habits. Many of the behaviors I'm advocating in this book may be new to you, and I want you to have the tools on hand to implement them successfully. Building the good habits that support this new lifestyle is an excellent way to achieve what you want in your conception and pregnancy. Habit building is both an art and a science. You can use the science of habit building to engineer your life in a way that fosters and encourages success. I'll cover a few key ideas here, and if you'd like to learn more, I highly recommend James Clear's *Atomic Habits*.

At a basic level, we are hardwired to accumulate habits. They make our lives easier. We don't have to consider every single decision we make when we have a habit. For example, if we always hang our car keys on a hook when we get home, we'll always know where to find them when we're ready to go out again. Habits free up our mental load and give us the ability to be mindful of the moments that count.

There are three key concepts that I'd like to share with you that I think will help. The first is that *the habits we regularly engage with shape our identity.* If I want to be an artist, I need to be in the habit of creating art. If I want to be a healthy pregnant woman, I need to be in the habit of making the right choices for myself and my baby. Begin acting like a healthy pregnant woman before you are pregnant. Make the choices a healthy pregnant woman would make.

The second concept is that we are much more likely to implement a habit if we make a specific plan for *when* it will be executed, e.g., I will set an alarm on my phone to remind me to drink water *every hour.* I will go to the gym on *Tuesday, Friday, and Sunday afternoons after lunch.* Note that these examples are more specific than "on the weekend." They can be calendared. To make the new habit even stickier, you can link it with another behavior you already do on the regular. For example, *I will go for a 20-minute walk after I brush my teeth in the morning.*

The third concept is that we need to alter our environment, so our habits become easier to implement. If I am going to be a hydrated person who drinks a gallon of water every day, I need to have access to water all the time. I need to make sure that I always have water on hand. If I want to eat healthier, I need to remove the temptations from my pantry and work to make sure my meals are planned. If I want to exercise, I need to have the right clothing and equipment available.

Lastly, I encourage you to start with one or two habits at a time. These may be radical changes for you. Do them at a pace you can sustain.

When to Start Your Family

 For most of our existence, we human beings procreated starting at a very young age, as soon as we became sexually active, in our early- to mid-teenage years. In modern times, and with access to contraception, couples are more deliberately scheduling the growth of their families.

Nowadays, most women are delaying their childbearing years until they are more established in life. I see a lot of first-time moms in their mid- to late-thirties and even early forties. I think it can be a little bit of a struggle to suddenly push everything aside, all of your routines and practices, for the pregnancy and then for the new baby. But there are advantages. You are more patient, you are more mature, you are more educated and sometimes the older you are, the more disciplined you are, which really helps when making these changes. Often you are also more financially secure.

I've found that while your body gives birth and is pregnant more easily when you're young, you may not be the best parent in that phase of your life. Some mediation between the two is good. Typically, families that are older are a bit more patient and have a bit more equanimity about them, though I've also seen that some older families are more stable and established in their ways of doing things, and therefore more rigid as parents.

All this to say, there is no single, right answer, and also, don't wait too long. There is such a thing as too late. Maternal mortality rises after age 40.[58] Babies and children take a lot of time and energy. It helps to have the energy and vigor of your own youth on your side, balanced with the maturity of experience.

I want to take a moment to reinforce this idea: There is no mandate that says you must become a parent. Maybe it's just an idea you've had your entire life, a childhood dream. I want you to really examine that desire and be certain it is one you are willing to alter everything in your life for. Raising kids is no joke. This is hard work, people. This needs to be a "Hell, yes!" not just an "okay, I'll do it."

There is no mandate that says you must become a parent.

Most people are fairly shocked to find that a baby takes 16–20 hours of direct hands-on care every single day for the first four months. Then it is about 12–16 hours for the next four months, then 8–12 hours for the next four months. Childrearing is a very in-depth experience.

Most people are fairly shocked to find that a baby takes 16–20 hours of direct hands-on care every single day for the first four months.

As a midwife, I have seen thousands of women both before they have children, and in the days, weeks, and months after they give birth. I get lots of feedback about how hard it is to integrate this new person into their lives. This is something you should consider rather carefully.

Preparing for Changes at Work

Your pregnancy may also dramatically impact your work life. Hopefully your partner will be supportive in your personal life, and you will be further supported and encouraged by family and friends. But this still doesn't take into consideration your work responsibilities. When you're approaching conception consciously, consider what you can do to set your work up in such a way that you are supported through a potentially difficult first trimester. Once you are pregnant, you may not be able to go in as early as you could before. There's a possibility that you would have to leave early on a particularly bad day.

Sometimes I try to remember what I had thought being a mom would be like. And I think back to all the "just wait" comments I was getting while pregnant... yes, I sleep less. Much less. But they forgot to mention that the little person who keeps you up at night makes you feel the happiest you've ever been. That while you definitely have less time for yourself, you also realize how often you weren't fully present when you had all that time. Sometimes I catch myself watching him play with my hand for half an hour and it's probably as fascinating to me as it is to him. And yes, having a baby means a lot of sacrifice. It is a huge responsibility. It's work. It's challenging. It means sleepless nights. Being late. Chaos. It's stressful, scary, and sometimes really annoying.

But the love, oh the love will overflow. Your life suddenly has a new meaning. Priorities shift and you see the world in a different light. The joy you feel when you see your child smile or hear them giggle is on a level you didn't know was possible. And just wait, it only gets better.

It's hard to believe that he was once "my positive pregnancy test" and then the tiny dancer in my belly. With stepping into this role, I've definitely found a new sense of purpose and gratitude for life. Sure, the person I used to be maybe doesn't exist anymore. And yes, I miss her and those days sometimes. But as you might know I love to romanticize my life. And I choose to view this transition from old to new me as an upgrade. I'm evolving. We're evolving. And while it's not always easy, it is most definitely worth it.

—Jelena Weir

Prepare your workmates in advance and earn their support before you conceive (if possible—not all workplace environments are conducive to this.).

You and your partner will want to have discussions now about how your baby will be cared for. Will one of you stay at home? What is your philosophy about education? Do you have plans for childcare if you'll both resume your careers, and do you know what it will cost? These are fantastic things to discuss before you get pregnant.

Anatomy & Physiology of Conception

Your Body's Reproductive System

If you want to get pregnant, it helps to know about your body and its reproductive cycles. Let's start with your pelvic cavity. There's a lot going on in there.

The female reproductive system includes the vagina, uterus/cervix, ovaries, fallopian tubes, *perineum*, *introitus* (the opening of the vagina that leads to the cervical canal), clitoris, labia minora, labia majora, and rectum. At the opening of the small intestine and large intestine you have the appendix, the ileocecal valve (the valve in between the two intestines), and in women you have the fallopian tubes and ovaries. The entire reproductive system is located within the pelvic cavity. The uterus is below and behind your public bone in the pelvic cavity, where it is protected. The muscle of the uterus is called the myometrium. The cervix comprises a quarter of the uterus and is the opening to the uterus.

The actual opening of the cervix is called the *os*. There is an external os that leads into the vagina and an internal os that leads into the uterus. Between the two oses is the cervical canal. The top of the uterus is called the *fundus* and the bottom of the uterus is known as the *lower uterine segment*.

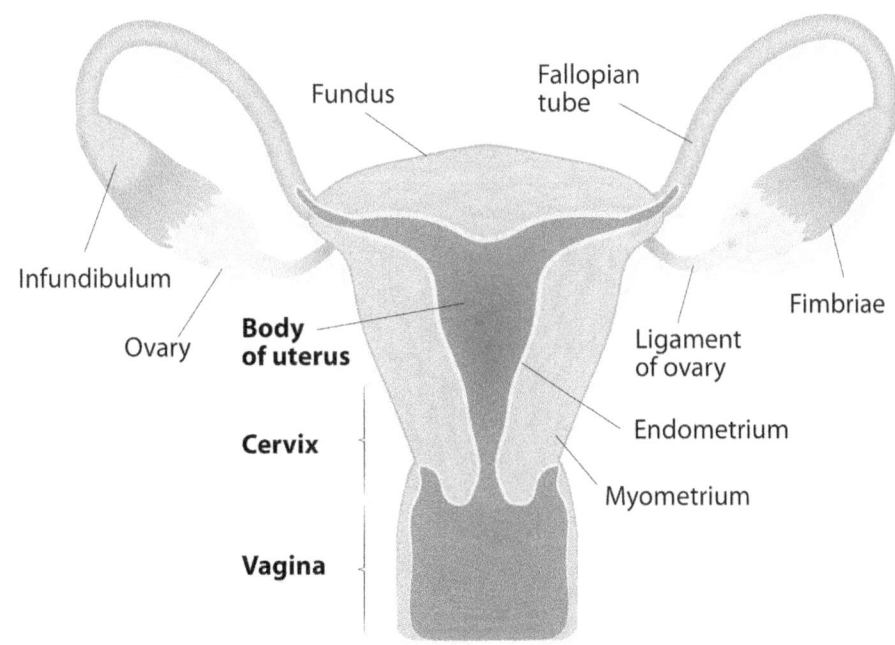

Female Reproductive System

The cervical canal does a lot of work. During pregnancy the cervical canal develops a mucus plug, which serves as its first line of defense against infection and anything foreign being introduced into the uterus and fetus. When you're not pregnant, the cervical canal produces a barrier of mucus that prevents the sperm from traveling up into the uterus easily when you are not fertile. But the body wants to conceive. It is a natural, primal drive.

The body wants to conceive. It is a natural, primal drive.

Your Cycle and Conception

The first day of a woman's period is considered Day One of her cycle. For most women, ovulation, where an egg is released into the fallopian tube, occurs about two weeks later, on Day 14. A blister forms on the ovary. That blister bursts and follicular fluid is released with an egg (or sometimes multiple eggs). That fluid irritates the end of the fallopian tube, which causes the tube to wiggle in response. The wiggling creates a kind of suction that draws the egg up into the fallopian tube. Small cilia also move to help the egg go into the fallopian tube, where, if sperm are present, fertilization can take place.

If sperm are waiting in the fallopian tube, conception occurs then or soon thereafter (when the sperm penetrates the egg). The egg only lives for 24 hours but sperm can live for four to seven days inside the woman's body. So, you can have sex before you are fertile, become fertile, and relatively quickly become pregnant. Sperm can also be introduced in that 24-hour period while the egg is alive. The sperm swim into the

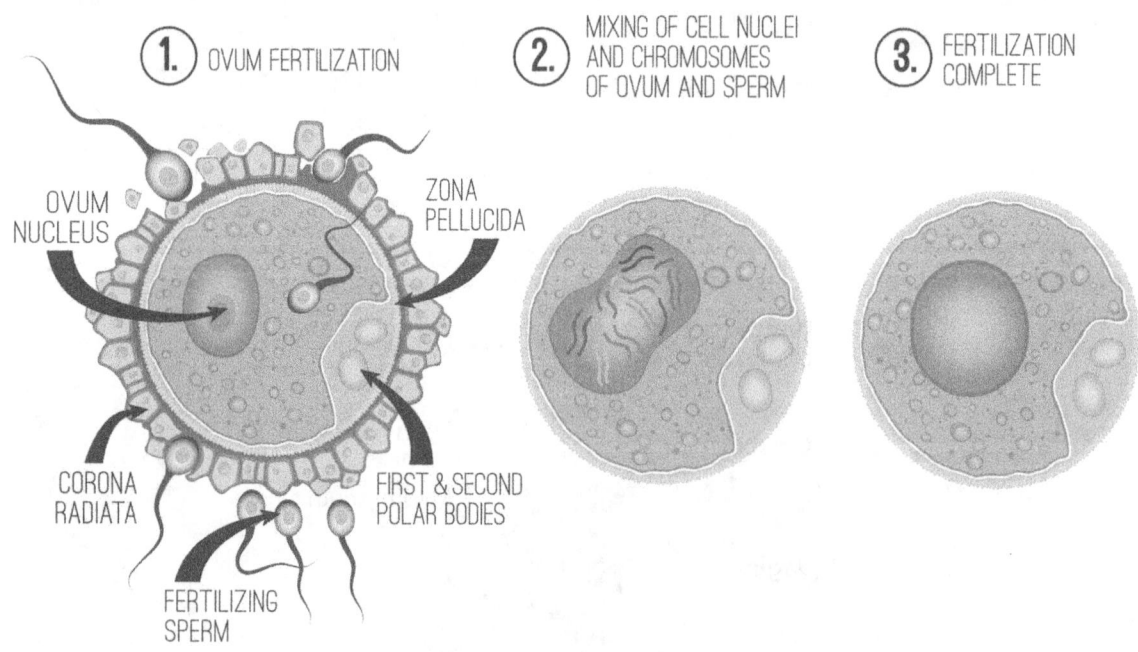

1. OVUM FERTILIZATION

2. MIXING OF CELL NUCLEI AND CHROMOSOMES OF OVUM AND SPERM

3. FERTILIZATION COMPLETE

OVUM NUCLEUS

ZONA PELLUCIDA

CORONA RADIATA

FIRST & SECOND POLAR BODIES

FERTILIZING SPERM

Fertilization

fallopian tubes where one lucky winner fertilizes the egg. Yet the egg has plenty of active agency in this fertilization process: it selects a particular sperm, draws it into its body, and then pierces its head, allowing the genetical materials in both egg and sperm to mix with each other, thereby creating a zygote that later becomes an embryo.[59]

If the sperm that was accepted was a female (X) sperm, the fetus will eventually become a girl. If the sperm that was accepted was a male (Y) sperm, the fetus will eventually become a boy. Science now recognizes

THE ZINC SPARK

When the egg cell is fertilized, it triggers a cascade of chemical reactions that ultimately creates a wholly new organism, your baby. One of these reactions releases zinc from the egg cell. When that happens, the zinc binds to small molecules called probes. In that moment of binding, they create a microscopic flash of light. It occurs within milliseconds of fertilization. This flash of light is known as a "zinc spark." This reminds me of The Big Bang. Isn't that fascinating?

You cannot observe this zinc spark with the naked eye, but it can be detected using special microscopes. Scientists have studied the zinc spark in a variety of animals, including mice, monkeys, and humans. They have found that the size of the zinc spark is a decent indicator of egg cell quality. They have found that eggs with larger zinc sparks are more likely to develop into healthy embryos.[61] This fascinating phenomenon is still not fully understood, but this flash of light plays an important role in conception.

many gender variations that are not accounted for in these two dominant gender manifestations.[60]

Once it is fertilized, the egg then takes four to eight days to slowly travel through the tube, dividing over and over. Implantation can occur six to twelve days after fertilization. This is when the embryo reaches the end of the tube, falls into the uterus, and attaches to a spot on the lining of the uterine wall, called the *endometrium*. The endometrium feeds the embryo (the collection of cells that will develop into your baby) until the placenta is in place. When the egg falls into the uterine cavity to implant, it has reached a mass of 288 cells, but only eight of those cells make up the embryo. The other 280 cells make up the support structures—the placenta, the amniotic sac, the yolk sack—all of which nourish the baby until the placenta is fully established.

Fraternal twins are conceived when the mother releases two individual eggs that are fertilized at the same time.

Identical twins are conceived when conception occurs and then a single egg divides into two genetically identical beings.

TIP: I find the Sprout Pregnancy app provides lovely, detailed information about the different stages of embryonic development.

The endoderm, ectoderm, and mesoderm are the three germ layers that form during the early stages of embryonic development.

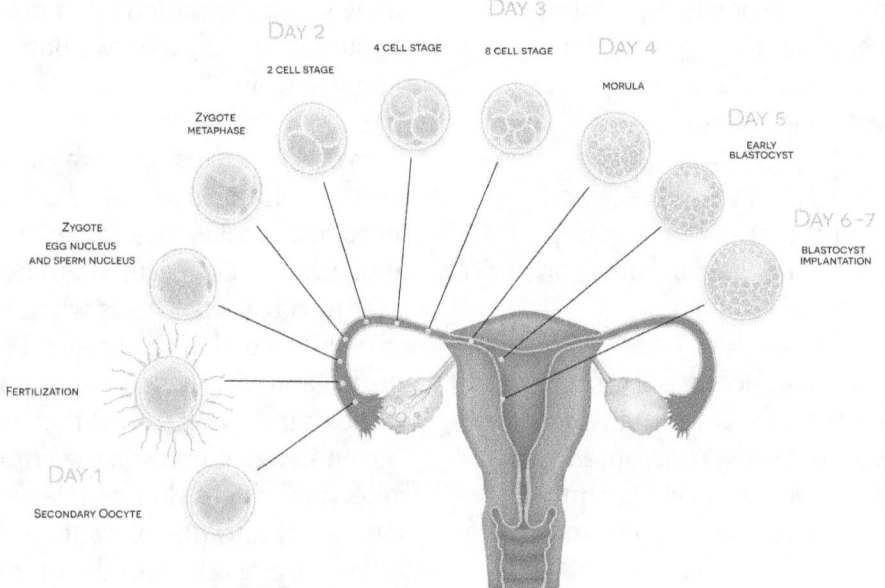

Human Development from Ovulation to Implantation

ONE LUCKY WINNER

In a recent fascinating study, researchers bred mice to try to trigger certain genetic traits so they could attempt to find treatments or prevention for disease.[62] In so doing, they were studying the fertilization of the egg. To date, the theory has been that the egg is fertilized when the first sperm breaches the *zona pellucida*, which then closes and prevents any other sperm from entering the nucleus of the egg.

Well, apparently this is not true, because the researchers found that the egg was *selective*. If the egg was a carrier for a disease, it would reject a sperm that was also carrier for the disease. So, the eggs were performing a sort of screening process for genetics that would result in an unviable pregnancy. The body is amazing, right? The egg actually chooses the sperm and will ward off the ones that are not ideal. Of course, it's not failsafe, but it is the first defense against an unviable pregnancy. These findings were in rat studies, but I believe they absolutely hold true for humans.

These germ layers give rise to all the tissues and organs in the body.

- The endoderm is the innermost germ layer. It gives rise to the lining of the digestive tract, respiratory tract, and other internal organs.
- The mesoderm is the middle germ layer. It gives rise to the muscles, bones, blood, and other tissues.
- The ectoderm is the outermost germ layer. It gives rise to the skin, nervous system, and other tissues.

The germ layers form during a process called gastrulation, which is a complex process that involves the folding and movement of cells. During gastrulation, the cells in the blastula, which is the early embryo, rearrange themselves to form the three germ layers.

The germ layers continue to differentiate and develop into specific tissues and organs

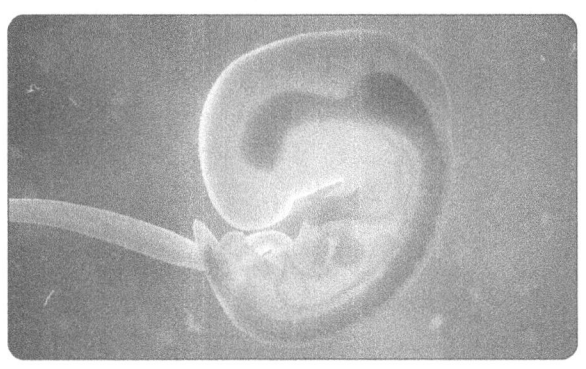
Embryo at Four Weeks

of form on opposite sides of the disc and then at this magical moment the disc folds like a taco onto itself putting everything where it's supposed to be on the fetal body. This is when neural tube defects and cleft lip and palate can happen, and one of the greatest preventions for those is taking methylfolate.

Spindle Mucus/EWCM

The vagina is very acidic and inhospitable so it can kill off the bacteria and viruses that might try to invade your body through the vagina, but it's also hard on sperm. A few days before you ovulate, your cervix changes the type of mucus it produces from barrier mucus—which keeps some sperm and bacteria from getting up into the cervix—to a type of mucus that aids the sperm to get to a more hospitable place.

throughout embryonic development. The endoderm, ectoderm, and mesoderm are essential for the development of a healthy embryo.

The three layers form what's called an embryonic disc. At a certain point in the pregnancy, the eyes, ears, arms, legs, and all the body parts that you have two

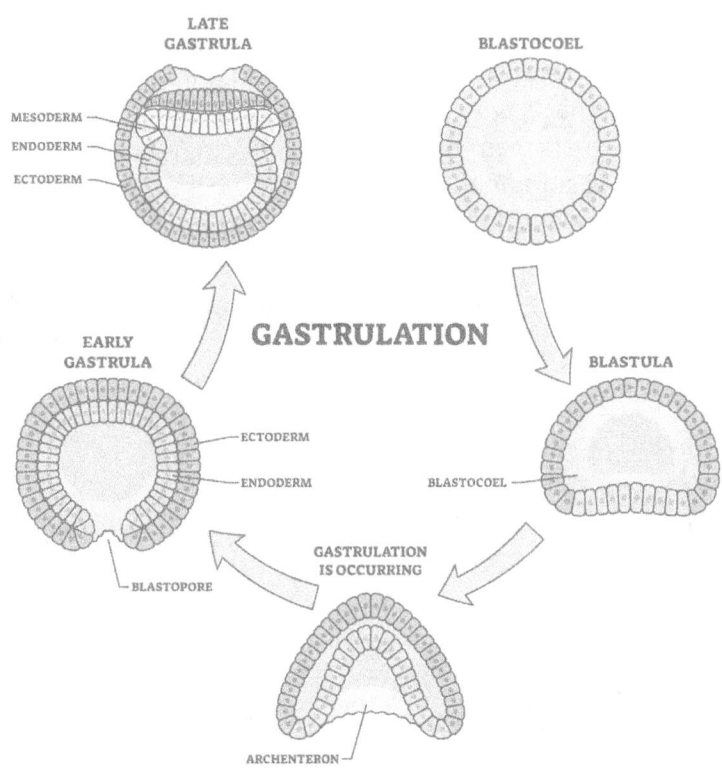

Embryonic Development of the Mesoderm, Endoderm, and Ectoderm

This is known as egg white cervical mucus (EWCM) or spindle mucus, because of its consistency and texture. Without the aid of this fertile mucus sperm tend to swim into the wall of the vagina and die.

During times of ovulation, the cervical canal produces a supportive mucus that instead aids sperm in their journey from the vagina to the cervix, uterus, and fallopian tubes so fertilization can take place.

Fertile mucus produces a thread that acts like a highway for sperm to more easily and with less energy swim up out of the vagina and into the more hospitable cervix and uterus. You can tell if you are getting close to ovulation and a fertile time of your cycle by putting your index finger all the way into the back of the vagina where the cervix is and collecting some mucus from your cervix. Pull your finger out and press your finger and thumb together, then pull them gently apart. If the mucus forms tacky little mountains on either side, that's barrier mucus. If it forms a stretchy thread that can span several inches, that is spindle mucus, which is fertile mucus, and your body is likely in a state of readiness for conception. If you are ready to welcome a baby into your life, go for it!

Fertile mucus produces a thread that acts like a highway for sperm to more easily and with less energy swim up out of the vagina and into the more hospitable cervix and uterus.

Use an Ovulation Kit

While for most women ovulation occurs on Day 14 of your cycle, it occasionally might begin as early as Day 10. However, if you're on a 32-day cycle, it may be as late as Day 18, 19, or 20. If you are having trouble getting pregnant, an ovulation kit can help pinpoint when you're ovulating, so you know when it will be most effective to have sex. That can be very helpful in terms of getting pregnant when you want to. These are widely available at grocery stores, pharmacies, or online.

Chart Temperatures to Track Ovulation

Charting your basal body temperature can help you to pinpoint ovulation and help to assure you that you are ovulating. Using a digital basal body thermometer, take your waking temperature before rising or doing anything at all. Chart your temperature. When you ovulate, you'll see a marked increase in your base temperature due to the increased flow of progesterone in your system. Your temperature will drop once your cycle begins. Doing this for a few months will help you to understand your own cycle better. Also, tracking your temperature and seeing that it remains high beyond when you would normally start your period can be an early sign of conception.

Conceiving with a Retroverted Uterus

Every picture you've ever seen of the uterus shows the uterus lying forward toward the pubic bone and over the bladder; it's called an anteverted uterus. But about 30–50 percent of women's uteruses do not lie

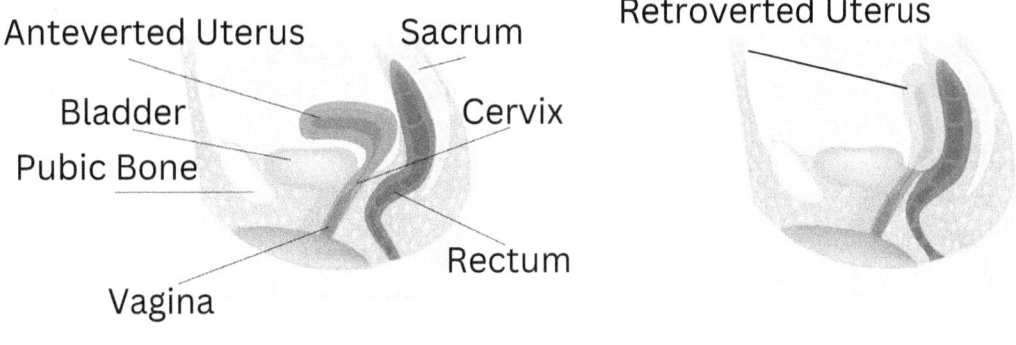

Anteverted Uterus   Sacrum   Retroverted Uterus

Bladder   Cervix

Pubic Bone

Rectum

Vagina

Uterine Positions

this way. They fall to the back toward your rectum in the sacral curve. These are called tipped, tilted, or retroverted uteruses.

Your midwife or OB/GYN can tell you which position your uterus is in.

If you have a retroverted uterus, you may have some difficulty getting pregnant. If your cervix is pointing up where the os is not in contact with the sperm, and you're always having sex on your back and staying that way afterward, it can be harder for the sperm to get into the cervix, and therefore more difficult for you to achieve conception. Try having sex from behind and then lying on your stomach for 15–20 minutes afterward to help the sperm to get into your cervix. This way, your partner will be more likely to ejaculate up against your cervix. If you lie in that position for a short while, rather than flipping over or running to the restroom right away, you'll increase your chances of fertilization.

Your Due Date

Most practitioners use a wheel to project a due date for your baby based on the first day of your last period. The idea

of a wheel being able to tell you a due date is misleading, given that there are so many variables as to when you could have conceived the baby. However, the common practice is to consider Day One of your last menstrual cycle before you conceived to be Day One of your pregnancy as well, regardless of how many days later conception actually happened, and for your due date to be exactly 40 weeks later. Once you have achieved conception, you are technically pregnant and in the first trimester. Congratulations!

Once you have achieved conception, you are technically pregnant and in the first trimester. Congratulations!

If fertilization does not take place and the egg passes through the fallopian tube unfertilized, the corpus luteum stops producing progesterone and you start your period on or about Day 28.

THE ORIGINS OF COUNTING

Anthropologists have discovered the earliest known counting sticks created by humans. One such marker is known as the Ishango bone. It was discovered in the Congo in 1950 and is thought to be 20,000 years old. Another is the Lebombo bone, which was discovered in Swaziland in 1973 and is thought to be around 35,000 years old. One bone had 28 notches and the other had 29. The researchers were puzzled at first ... until they realized the bones were likely created by women to track their menstrual cycles. Isn't that cool?

Toxins to Avoid

Many of my clients share concerns with me about exposure to everyday toxins, which are chemicals that we may encounter regularly at home and in the world at large. They want to know what they should really be looking out there and what's hype. While some toxins are relatively harmless to humans, others should be avoided because they can indeed be harmful to you and to your developing baby.

In addition to the toxins in food I mentioned earlier in the Nourishment section, the toxins I think you should work to avoid include mercury, glyphosate, Bisphenol A (BPA), chemicals in beauty products, pesticides, lead, air pollution, solvents, and radiation.

Mercury

Mercury is a heavy metal that can damage the nervous system. As we have mentioned previously, avoid exposure to mercury by being careful about the types of fish you eat (such as swordfish, shark, king mackerel, Bigeye tuna, and tilefish) and by avoiding dental amalgams, or silver-colored fillings, that are often used to fill cavities in teeth. A much better option is to use quartz composite fillings if you have a cavity.

Glyphosate

Glyphosate is the most commonly used broad-spectrum herbicide in the world and is regularly used to kill weeds on agricultural farms, and commonly used on American lawns by homeowners. Some studies have linked glyphosate exposure to cancer, birth defects, and other health problems. However, the World Health Organization (WHO) has classified glyphosate as "probably carcinogenic to humans," while the US Environmental Protection Agency (EPA) has concluded that glyphosate is safe when used as directed.

While more research is needed to determine the long-term health effects of glyphosate exposure, I believe fervently that you should choose to avoid eating foods that are likely to contain glyphosate residues. This includes but is not limited to foods such as US-grown wheat, soybeans, and corn. You can also choose to buy organic produce, which is grown without the use of synthetic herbicides. If you use herbicides on your lawn, have your partner check for glyphosate in the ingredient list and dispose of the herbicide responsibly if they find it.

Bisphenol A

BPA is found in many plastics and has been shown to disrupt hormone function, which can lead to health problems in both you as a pregnant woman as well as your developing baby. While the FDA has banned the use of BPA in baby bottles, sippy cups, and infant formula packaging, these were previously manufactured with BPA (don't buy plastic containers secondhand). Additionally, around 15 US states also have their own laws restricting the use of BPA, mainly in food contact materials intended for children.

You can avoid exposure to BPA by limiting your consumption of canned foods and avoiding plastic food containers and plastic water bottles. Look for containers that are BPA-free or, even better, switch to using containers that are made from durable materials like glass, stainless steel, or food-grade silicone.

Don't use containers that are made from thin or flimsy plastic or containers with a recycling number 7 on the bottom, which means that the container is made of polycarbonate, a type of plastic that contains BPA. Always wash your containers thoroughly before using them, and never microwave in plastic containers as a rule of thumb, even if it says it is microwave safe.

Toxins in Beauty Products

Phthalates, parabens, formaldehyde, fragrances, sodium lauryl sulfate (SLS), sodium laureth sulfate (SLES), and triclosan are some of the more commonly used chemicals I suggest you avoid in beauty products. They each have different effects, but have been linked to issues like reproductive problems, hormone disruption, cancer, allergies, as well as skin irritation and dryness.

As with anything you put in or on your body, always read labels carefully to avoid chemicals and choose products that are labeled "natural" or "organic." It is also a great idea to test new products on a small area of skin before using them all over your body. Stop using them immediately if you ever experience any skin irritation or other discomforts.

TIP: INCI Beauty is an iOS app that scans the barcode of a product and provides information on the ingredients, including their safety rating and potential side effects. INCI Beauty also allows you to search for products by ingredient or by brand. incibeauty.com

Pesticides

Pesticides are chemicals that are used to kill pests and can be found in food, water, and soil. The best way to avoid exposure to pesticides is by eating organic produce whenever possible and by washing fruits and vegetables thoroughly before eating them. If you are a gardener, choose organic methods of pest control. If you use a pest control service, select one that uses organic or nontoxic methods.

Lead

Lead is a heavy metal that can damage the nervous system. You can avoid exposure to lead by staying away from lead-based paint, lead-contaminated soil, and lead-contaminated drinking water. If you live in an old house, you may want to check to see if the paint has lead (or if there is any potential for asbestos exposure) in it and, if you find it, get it professionally removed. Most drinking water you do not have to worry about, but if you live in industrial areas, it may be worth checking, and you can often ask the health department in your area to test water for lead contamination.

Pollution, Solvents, and Radiation

I also suggest limiting your exposure to air pollution, solvents, and radiation. Air pollution contains a variety of harmful chemicals that can damage the lungs and other organs. If you have the option, stay indoors on days when air quality is poor, and avoid taking busy roads if possible.

Solvents are chemicals that are used to dissolve other substances. They can be found in a variety of household products, such as paints, thinners, and cleaning products. You should avoid exposure to solvents by wearing gloves and a mask when using these products and only use them in well-ventilated areas. Radiation from X-rays, CT scans, and other medical procedures should also be avoided when pregnant unless absolutely necessary, as radiation can be harmful to developing babies.

I know this is a lot to think about but remember that the knowledge I share with you in this book is here so you can make informed decisions in your life. If you don't know something is bad for you, you probably won't work to avoid it. That said, toxins are literally everywhere. It is impossible to completely avoid all exposure to chemicals and toxins during pregnancy, so it's best to not let it scare you but rather empower you. Do what you can to avoid these toxins when possible and then surrender, knowing you are doing your level best. Every single improvement you choose to make to live a healthier life positively impacts you, your ability to conceive, your growing baby, and your family as a whole.

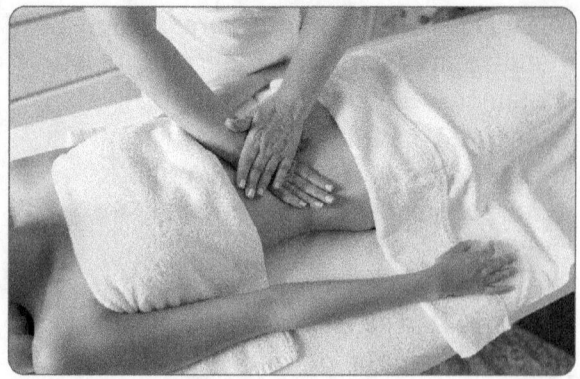

Mayan Abdominal Massage or Abdominal Massage Therapy

Abdominal massage is a marvelous practice that I think can be of great benefit to women and especially helpful to begin prior to conceiving. Mayan abdominal massage or abdominal massage therapy is a gentle, non-invasive massage technique that focuses on the abdomen and pelvic organs. It is based on the traditional Mayan practice of *sobada de matriz*, which means "massage of the womb."

Abdominal therapists may use a variety of techniques, massage, energy healing, and herbal formulas to support the body to release physical and emotional congestion, to bring about better circulation of arterial blood, venous blood, nerve supply, lymph, and energy, which the Maya call *Chu'lel*.

The massage is done using a combination of long, sweeping strokes and deep, circular movements. The therapist applies pressure to specific points on the abdomen, using their fingers or thumbs. The goal of the massage is to help the organs return to their proper alignment and function more effectively.

Mayan abdominal massage is thought to be beneficial for a variety of conditions, including:

- Infertility
- Menstrual problems such as menstrual cramps, pain, and other symptoms of PMS
- Digestive problems
- Pelvic pain, including pain caused by endometriosis, fibroids, and other conditions
- Stress and anxiety

If you are interested in finding a practitioner in your area, check out the Abdominal Therapy Collective's directory. www.abdominaltherapycollective.com.

Timing Your Conception

 I recommend that you establish this new Sevenfold lifestyle as a couple for two to three months prior to attempting conception. Give your body a strong foundation for conception and pregnancy. When you're ready, consider some of the following factors when timing your conception.

Flying in Early Pregnancy

There are higher than normal rates of radiation on airplane flights. There's nothing to do about it—the planes are not shielded; you'd have to skin them in iron, and so we don't really talk about it a whole lot. However, I have had a number of clients who worked as flight attendants who have had miscarriages, and I believe it was because they were flying frequently in the developmental part of the process, in the very beginnings of embryonic development.

Before I formed you in the womb, I knew you; before you were born, I sanctified you.
—Jeremiah 1:5

I can't know this for certain, but I think that it can occasionally be a problem, so you don't want to willingly fly when you are in your early pregnancy (the first 10 weeks) if you can avoid it. If you must, you must. I mean, if somebody dies or something happens and you need to be there, then go. This is not a guarantee of miscarriage, but rather an increase in risk.[63]

This is something to keep in mind, as you may not want to conceive, especially if you fly frequently.

Solar Activity and Excess Gamma Radiation

I do think that one of the causes of miscarriage is gamma radiation, and the highest levels of gamma radiation occur in solar flares, which produce intense solar activity. There is not very much literature around the human experience, though a few studies do support this idea.[64] And yet I see it absolutely correlates. When one of my clients has a miscarriage, I look back and see if there was solar flare activity and so often there was. Then I look to see if there are other women who became pregnant around that time and wait for the other shoe to drop, because it's more typical another of my clients miscarries than not. I want to say it here now, and I will revisit this topic in the First Trimester because it's so important to understand this. Miscarriage is an incredibly common, incredibly normal (although often sad) experience.

As I mentioned before, when the egg falls into the uterine cavity to implant, it's comprised of 288 cells, but only eight of those cells make up the embryo. All the rest of the cells make up the support structures—the placenta, the amniotic sac, the yolk sac—all of which nourish the baby until the placenta is fully established. These support structures are obviously super important. But this means there are only eight cells that make up the embryo when it begins to implant, and so if a gamma ray hits one of those eight cells, it's over. It's done right then. When this happens, it's called a blighted ovum. In my own miscarriages I never saw an embryo; I never saw a little pink thing; it was always a blighted ovum, and the embryo had been zapped at some point by something.

Again, this is a risk factor multiplier, not a guarantee of miscarriage. If you can manage your conception timeline so it doesn't coincide with heavy solar activity, I recommend it. Solar activity is predictable, and you can find forecasts for it. The Space Weather Live app is free if you'd like to track this on your phone.

Aim for a Time of Low Stress

If you can pick the timing of conception and birth, you don't want to be doing it when you are moving to a new place or remodeling your house. You don't want to be doing it when you or your partner's job is in jeopardy. You don't want to be dealing with a newborn when your two-year-old is getting their molars. If you can pick, pick wisely. Remember to consider how much flying you'll be doing and check solar flare forecasts. At the same time, if you wait for everything to be perfect you will never have any children at all, so don't wait for that dream raise, don't wait for all the stars to be in alignment. This is all just information to consider when timing your conception. You do your best to take in the information and then choose wisely, controlling what you can, and letting go of the rest.

Herpes

Herpes simplex virus type 1 is a virus that affects many, many people. It is also known as fever blisters or cold sores, and these typically break out on the face. Herpes simplex virus type 2 is genital and affects the labia, perineum, rectum, or vagina of the woman who has genital herpes—except when it doesn't. The blisters can migrate. You can have type 1 blisters on your genitals and type 2 on the mouth. I'll leave it up to your imagination as to how that might happen. You are very contagious when the blisters break. The fluid they release contains the virus. After they erupt, the blisters scab up and heal. If you have herpes blisters, you will need to have the blister fluid tested to know which type you have.

Type 2 is transmitted primarily by sexual contact. It is very contagious and if you have an outbreak, you must absolutely abstain from sex. You can give it to your partner, sometimes even while using a condom, so be very careful.

Herpes outbreaks are very typically brought on by illness, heat, stress, friction, and certain foods. One of the reasons it's known as fever blisters is because running a fever often results in an outbreak. Most people have what are known as prodromal symptoms before the outbreak occurs. These can include buzzing, tingling, and an uncomfortable feeling in the area where you have had an outbreak before. If you can learn to recognize those prodromal symptoms, you can take steps that will often minimize it or stop the outbreak altogether.

The first thing you do is avoid getting hot. Don't take a hot shower, don't take a hot bath, don't get in a hot tub or sauna, don't exercise, don't work in the yard, etc. Friction creates heat, so you want to avoid tight pants, tight underwear, etc. Sex is obviously going to create a lot of friction, so definitely avoid sex when you have an outbreak or feel those prodromal symptoms. You must understand that you can give herpes to your partner, and if ever decide to roll the dice and have sex around the time that you think you could be getting an outbreak or obviously have one, you need to use condoms.

It is far better to not have sex when you're having an outbreak. You do not want to pass it on to your partner.

After friction and heat, the next helpful thing to avoid is arginine, an amino acid found in meat (beef, pork, turkey, chicken), fish, nuts and seeds, legumes, whole grains, watermelon, eggs, chocolate, spirulina, and dairy products. Avoid consuming these foods when you feel the prodromal symptoms coming on.

Lysine is an amino acid that some studies have shown to mitigate or prevent an outbreak. You can buy lysine in supplement form. Because they are both amino acids, many of the foods that contain lysine also contain arginine, so if you try this, I suggest the supplement. Take 1,000–3,000 mg a day. Talk with your midwife before starting this supplement to make sure it's right for you.

In general, lower your stress and work to tune into those prodromal symptoms so your incidence of outbreaks can be greatly lessened.

COVID-19

A recent study[65] found that semen quality in unvaccinated men who contracted COVID-19 remained poor three months after the illness abated. They observed declines in sperm count, concentration, motility, and seminal volume, among other things. It may take six months or more for sperm quality to return to normal. Knowing this, you may want to delay attempting conception if your partner has recently had COVID.

Get Off Anti-Depressants

In my practice I have had many women who came to me taking one form or another of antidepressants. I have heard that these medications have been found in the bloodstreams of babies. I feel that as the baby's emotional spiritual and intellectual self is being developed, antidepressants may not be good for them.

I have asked every single one of my clients to stop taking antidepressants for the duration of their pregnancies and none of them have had problems. One of the things that's been pointed out to me is that these women have me consciously stewarding them through their transitions. I care for and love them. I am always available to them by phone. I interact with them about their emotional, spiritual, and intellectual lives every time they come to my office. I give advice. I help them, and I am very supportive. If you do not have that kind of support, it may be difficult to make this work for you. It doesn't have to be a midwife who helps you. It could be a partner, therapist, or doctor.

If you are on anti-depressants, this is important for you to think about. There are no real studies yet on pregnant women and antidepressants and the long-term effects on the baby, so if you can make it work without them, I suggest that you do. If you need to get back on them as soon as the baby's out, that is absolutely fine, but do consider this seriously.

If you choose to go this route, make sure that you have a strong partner or friend who will check in with you daily, especially in those first several weeks to months, and who will be able to help you suss out any red flags. If it doesn't work out, you can start back on the anti-depressants.

Getting Off Birth Control

All methods of preventing conception are birth control, but it's easier to remove some barriers than others. For example, if you use condoms and spermicide, when you are ready to try to conceive, just stop using them! Other methods take some consideration.

I generally do not suggest hormonal birth control ("the pill") because of the potential detrimental side effects. I am especially unhappy with hormonal implants, as I think they are much harder on your

---

Penelope: My OB/GYN advised me to get off the Wellbutrin I was taking for depression when I became pregnant. I was a single mother-to-be and I had only recently moved to the city, so I didn't have a strong, local support network. I did it anyway, and it was rough.

What I know now that I wish I'd known then is that had I also cut out conventionally grown grains, I could have kicked both the depression and the meds at the same time. Taking gluten out of my diet really worked for me. I have now gone more than a decade without experiencing a major depressive episode, and I am certain it is due to this dietary change. If you struggle with depression, I suggest you try it. Maybe it will work for you, too, and bring the relief that it did for me. The dietary transition can be eased by drinking a cup of hot bone or chicken broth (like tea) if you experience flu-like withdrawal symptoms.

If I relapse or am "gluten bombed" unknowingly with US-grown wheat, the symptoms are noticeable. At the risk of sharing too much information, I'm talking bloating, diarrhea, wicked mood swings, and minor depressive episodes that show up within 24 hours of that first bite, even if I only take one bite. I've made the choice to consciously indulge often enough that I know this is guaranteed to be the price I pay for eating that birthday cake, and so I do it less and less often.

system and have been shown to have more significantly negative side effects than other birth control methods.[66] I do believe the pill is an excellent form of birth control for young women who are sexually active, but as soon as a woman is in a stable relationship, I believe it's best to switch to a barrier method of birth control (e.g., condoms, diaphragm, cervical cap, vaginal contraceptive film). These aren't as detrimental to her hormonal system.

For a huge percentage of women, getting off the pill seriously jars their hormonal systems. They often experience depression, headaches or migraines, skin eruptions, and hormonal vagaries that are very unpleasant. It's important to get off the pill for at least a few months (but ideally six to twelve months) prior to attempting conception, so your body can find its natural hormonal balance and homeostasis again. Once you stop taking it, you will need to use another method of birth control until you are ready to conceive. The pill convinces your body that you are pregnant. It mimics pregnancy with surging progesterone levels, and when you come off of it, your body needs time to heal and to find its normal hormonal cycle again.

If you have an IUD in place as your form of contraception it is imperative to take it out and allow the lining of your uterus to heal before you start trying to conceive. You need to go to a care provider capable of pulling your IUD out. It is a relatively easy process as there is a string that comes out of the uterus so it can be identified as being in the right place. Your provider will pull this string slowly and gently with forceps until the IUD comes out. Again, I highly recommend that a healthcare professional do this for you.

Immunizations

In my practice, after seeing several babies die of diseases they could have been immunized for, I am a believer in the benefit of immunizations. It needs to be understood that immunizations do not prevent you from getting the disease, being very, very sick with the disease, or even dying from the disease. What they do is dramatically increase your chances of not getting the disease, not getting terribly sick, and not dying of the disease. Immunizations give your body a blueprint of the disease so they can learn how to fight it, were you ever to contract it.

Immunizations have been instrumental in handling some of the world's most difficult diseases. Smallpox is estimated to have killed 300–500 million people in the 20th century alone. In 1970 over 700,000 children a year died of measles worldwide; by 2010 it was closer to 200,000. Immunizations have made all the difference around the world in reducing the incidence of measles, German measles, polio, pertussis (whooping cough), tetanus, and many more. Because we have collectively been immunized for so long, some people have come to believe the need for immunizations is nonsense and even that immunizations are dangerous.

The truth is that billions of people have been immunized and immunizations have saved hundreds of millions of lives. The WHO estimates that immunization currently prevents 4–5 million deaths every year and an additional 1.5 million deaths could be avoided each year if global vaccination coverage improves.[67] There are so many more people damaged and dying from diseases than are damaged or dying from immunizations—the number is minuscule in comparison. In *The Book of Birth Volume II: Your Postpartum Journey through the Fourth Trimester* I will share what I believe a good immunization schedule is for your baby.

Before pregnancy, it is important for the mother and father to be immunized against tetanus, diphtheria, and pertussis (with a single DTaP vaccine), and to get the most current flu and COVID vaccines. I have had clients who had bad cases of flu during their pregnancies, and it damaged the baby in some instances. In 2022 I had a *horrible* year. There were several women in my practice who contracted COVID-19, and I believe it damaged their placentas, resulting in placental insufficiencies, and impacted the babies in serious ways. I had the highest hospital transport rate ever in my career, and I believe nearly all that increase was COVID-related.

I understand that this is a thorny issue for some people, and, again, you have the right to make your own decisions about your body and your life. But you have turned to me for guidance, and in this book, I'm doing the very best I can to give you the best information I can. I want you to take charge of your bodies and your processes. Information is power. This is how you can make good, informed choices. The scientific data makes it clear that it is important for both you and your partner to be immunized and being immunized prior to conception is ideal.

Lastly, I do not recommend getting multiple immunizations at once. The DTaP forces you to have three at once; that's the only

way you can get it, but space the others out by two to three weeks. I don't think the human body mounts as strong of an immunologic response when you do multiple vaccines at once.

Sperm Health

Your partner has just as many reasons to adhere to this Sevenfold Approach as you do. He needs to be well fed and to take his vitamins. He needs to be working out and getting stronger, too. His role requires him to be as dynamically healthy as possible, and when he is, it changes the energy around conception. Energy is real. Even though it can't be measured we can all feel it, and when he is healthy, that energy is going to be better, and conception is more likely to happen easily and at the right time.

It is important to note that excessive use of cannabis can lower sperm motility and sperm count, as can the excessive use of alcohol. I advise minimal usage to abstinence here for both partners while you attempt conception.

Influencing the Baby's Gender

While there is no 100 percent, works all the time method of influencing your baby's gender, there are some things to consider.

Manage Your Stress

One recent finding is that elevated levels of cortisol in the mother—women who conceive with higher amounts of stress hormones—are more than twice as likely to have a girl. If you are trying for a boy, you may want to first look to making sure you're reducing your stress.[68]

Timing

Some studies show male (Y) sperm move ever so slightly faster and are a teensy bit larger than female (X) sperm.[69] Other researchers who studied this found no difference. More research needs to be done, but if you want to skew your chances of one gender or another, you can consider timing sex based on these factors. Sperm can live three to seven days! (Remember this when trying to prevent pregnancy.)

Here's the thought process: when you have sex a few days before ovulation, Y sperm are going to arrive first but die off, while the X sperm will still be alive to penetrate the egg when it arrives, increasing your chances of having a girl. If you want to have a boy, wait to have sex until you think you're ovulating, and then it's likely the Y sperm will arrive at the egg first, increasing your chances of having a boy.

Diet

A recent study conducted on mice showed that people—especially fathers—who consumed a diet high in iron and zinc prior to conceiving were more likely to have a boy, whereas diets higher in saturated fats more often produced a girl.[70]

Infertility and What to Do About It

Infertility is defined as the inability to conceive despite frequent and unprotected intercourse for at least a year.[71]

There are many causes of infertility, including mechanical problems such as blocked fallopian tubes from infection, pH abnormalities between the mother and father, and non-ovulation due to hormonal irregularities or stress. Another issue that can affect fertility is unresolved emotional trauma in your own life or in your relationship. There was a time in my life after I'd lost my baby where all I wanted to do was to conceive again. I was trying to push through, ignoring my emotional wounds. I tried and tried and couldn't conceive. I eventually turned my lens inward and worked on my own healing. Once I had done the work, I easily conceived a baby. You may think that's correlation, not causation, but I am certain it helped tremendously.

Being overweight can also make it difficult to conceive. One of the things that researchers have found is that excess fat on the body acts as another endocrine system.[72] Hormones that are supposed to attach to other sites sometimes attached to fat cells instead, so being markedly overweight can decrease the hormonal equilibrium necessary for pregnancy to occur. I am not saying this to shame anyone. It can be a factor, though.

Conversely, I have also seen lots of underweight women who have had difficulty getting pregnant. I think that this is a biological safety mechanism from our ancient past. If there's not enough food, your body stops ovulating or does not prepare hormonally for the process to unfold. If you're not getting enough food, it's hard for the embryo to develop properly and it's hard for the fetus to be nourished.

Penelope: My husband and I didn't use birth control, ever. I figured I would conceive in a year and when I didn't, I started reading books about conception and women's hormones and educated myself to the best of my ability. Still, no conception. I was pretty sure I was ovulating, so we just kept on trying. Finally, after years, we saw a specialist who ran a battery of tests and said nothing was wrong, maybe the sperm count was slightly low, but everything looked good. They suggested we try artificial insemination. We tried a few times to no avail, and it was just too expensive to keep trying. Years passed and that marriage fell apart.

In retrospect, I think being underweight is what kept me from conceiving all those years. I lived on coffee in the morning, maybe ate lunch (maybe), grabbed a handful of nuts and more coffee to get through the afternoons, and ate a substantial dinner. My body was in a constant state of starvation. When I did conceive, it was after living with a roommate who ate three squares on the regular and often included me in her meals. I had put on close to 20 pounds and was much more fully nourished at the time.

The body is so brilliant. If it perceives any threat to the mother, it doesn't support procreation.

The very first instinct of the human body is for survival and fortunately the body is not about to have a baby if it perceives there's not enough food to sustain the mother. Being underweight may send alarm bells throughout your body that this is not the time for pregnancy because there's just not enough food.

There is no one-size-fits-all answer to the question of what the right weight is or how much is the right amount to gain in pregnancy. This is such a thorny issue to discuss in our culture. I have many challenges with my clients in discussing weight gain. I have had many clients who really struggled to not gain too much weight or to gain enough weight. Not everybody is supposed to weigh the same and your BMI (body mass index) can be misleading. If you have more muscle and bone than other body types, it can seem like you are overweight when you're not. The same goes for being underweight. If you have a very slight build sometimes it can seem like you are underweight when really, you're just fine.

We all have to struggle against the cultural pressures of looking a certain way. We all do not need to look the same, but I do see more complications in women who are significantly overweight or significantly underweight. It benefits you to figure out what's right for you.

If you're experiencing infertility, it always makes sense to start by ruling out mechanical trauma like blocked fallopian tubes, low sperm counts or motility, and endometriosis. If you have been adhering to the recommendations in this book and after twelve months have not yet conceived, it is time to see a specialist who can help you to figure out what's going on.

Early Signs of Pregnancy

Some of the longest weeks of a woman's life when she wants to be pregnant are the two weeks while she's waiting for the result of pregnancy test to be accurate. (Testing too early can produce false negatives, meaning the test can say you are not pregnant when you really are!)

The most predominant sign of early pregnancy is missing your period, but you can miss your period because of stress, illness, travel—all kinds of things.

In the sacred journey of pregnancy, a woman becomes a conduit for the divine forces of life and creation.

—Osho

The next most common sign is breast tenderness, although this is also a symptom of an impending period.

The next most commonly occurring symptom is fatigue. Many women start experiencing fatigue at about four or five weeks of pregnancy. Remember that since the first day of your last period is considered the beginning of the 40-week pregnancy process, but conception doesn't usually take place until the end of Week 2 typically, so when we say that somebody's a month pregnant, the truth is they conceived only two weeks earlier. Breast tenderness usually starts occurring around the time that the period would have been missed, and the fatigue starts about a week later. You just start feeling really tired all the time, compelled to nap.

You could have what's called implantation bleeding. This usually occurs about three weeks into your pregnancy. It's usually just a very small amount of spotting from when the embryo burrows into the lining of the uterus.

Then at around Weeks 6 and 7 a lot of women experience nausea. I believe that it's because you must eat more frequently, very small amounts, even during the night. I'll describe this more thoroughly in the First Trimester chapter. It can also be caused by a reaction to the hormonal changes in your body.

There are some interesting/odd ways of experiencing pregnancy. One is an increased gag reflex. Another is a salivating reflex.

A lot of women develop food aversions. There are some visceral, primal revulsions to food and to some smells, especially tobacco, coffee, dogs, and cooking meat.

Mood swings are extremely common. Many women start developing some hypersensitivity where they easily swing from anger, to joy, to irritation, to laughter, to tears for any number of reasons. Everything is just meteoric and that's completely normal. If you have serious mood swings with your periods, I think you are more prone to having mood swings in pregnancy.

Penelope: I had been wanting to be pregnant for so long that every month was a scientific investigation. *Were those period cramps or pregnancy cramps? Were my breasts extra tender? Was this it?*

When I did finally conceive the change in my body was undeniable. For me the two major signs were hunger and fatigue. I, someone who was never hungry, was suddenly ravenous. I could not eat enough. It was very unlike me. I was also exceptionally tired and took naps for the first time in my adult life.

Many women experience cramping in the first month to two months of pregnancy. The uterus starts out the size of a plum and immediately starts to grow and enlarge. By the end of your pregnancy, it will be closer to the size of a cantaloupe. It's an amazingly mobile organ. It wiggles around and does all kinds of interesting things. When it orgasms, it actually pulses, and of course there's labor, where it contracts and pulls the cervix open. The enlarging of the uterus in the first few weeks of pregnancy can be a crampy bit of business.

If you suspect you may be pregnant you can always check with a store-bought pregnancy test kit. Remember that they are not as accurate in the immediate aftermath of conception; it can take a few weeks for your body to generate pregnancy hormones at the levels the kit is able to detect.

Initial Thoughts on Choosing a Care Provider

Now that you are attempting to get pregnant, it is a great time to familiarize yourself with the options available to you for pregnancy care and to begin to think about what kind of support you would like when you conceive. I encourage you to do some research and find out what's available in your immediate area. Depending on where you live, you may have access to a hospital, midwife, freestanding birth center, or all three. I often travel an hour or more to my clients' homes to attend their births, so if you wish to work with a midwife and the closest one you can find is a little out of range, contact her and see if you're in her delivery area. You will want to consider that you'll likely be travelling to her for prenatal appointments.

I don't want to pay too much attention to this topic just yet. You have enough to think about. Rest assured; I'll cover this topic in great detail in the First Trimester chapter.

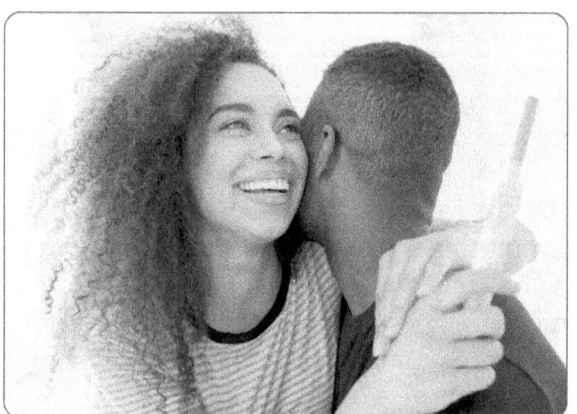

Getting Some Good News from a Storebought Pregnancy Test

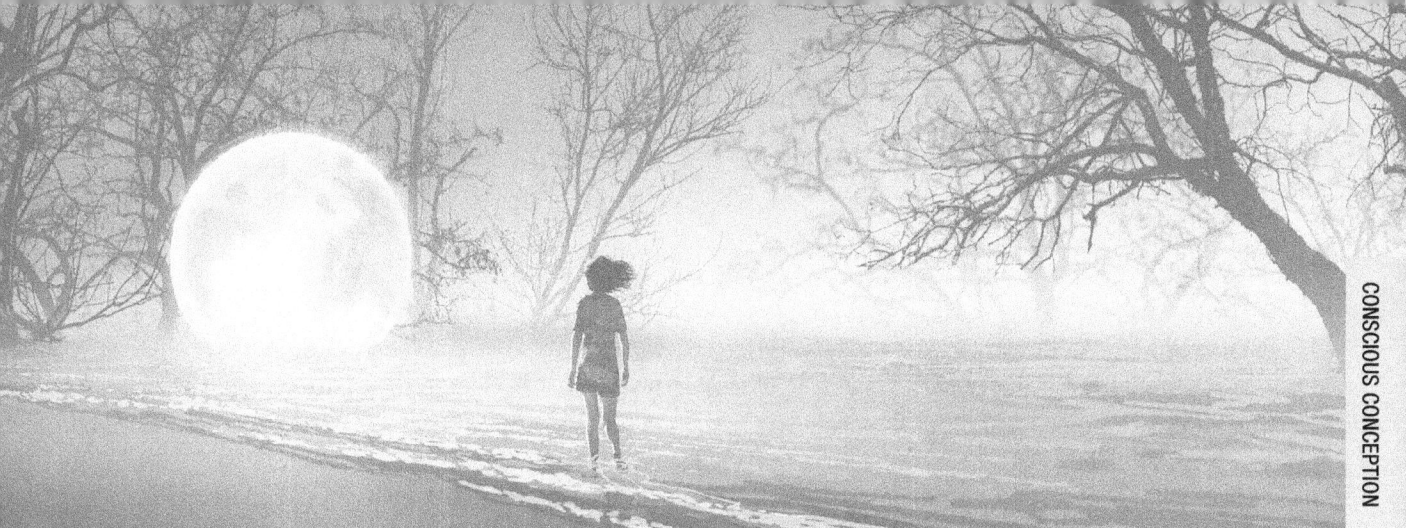

Rest

Remove Stressors

Preparation is everything. You never know if you're going to get pregnant at the time that you choose; it could take you six months to a year or even longer to get pregnant and that is all still normal. Often when you're not conceiving, it's because there are factors that you don't understand but that are seriously important and still at play.

So, if you're in a difficult job with a lot of stress, if you have older kids who create a lot of stress, if you've got school, financial, work, or marital problems—these are issues that are going to elicit biochemical responses in your body that could affect your body's willingness to get pregnant.

Deal with these issues now and lower the stress you experience in your life. Find an easier, more forgiving work environment if you need to. Get help with your other children if you have them. Ease the burden of your daily situation so you will have the space to welcome new life. Take the time needed for the work it takes to create a healthy pregnancy, birth, baby, and

postpartum experience. I'll talk more about this in the Joy section of this chapter.

Pay Attention to Sleep Hygiene

When you are well rested, you are going to have an easier time getting pregnant, being pregnant, going through labor and birth, breastfeeding, and caring for a newborn. When you are well rested everything goes better, and you'll find that you can handle just about anything for short periods of time. In contrast, when you are sapped, you may find you can't do much of anything anymore; even fun things are no longer fun when you're exhausted. Make it a habit in your life to get adequate sleep and relaxation. It's so important to rest to enhance mindfulness, gentleness, kindness, gratitude, and forgiveness; these gifts come to us from restful states, not from agitated, intense, and stressful states.

- Pay attention to your sleep hygiene.
- Do not watch TV or look at your phone in bed.

- Avoid blue light (from a TV, phone, or computer screen) for half an hour before bedtime.
- Choose a regular bedtime and implement a regular bedtime routine.
- Use blackout curtains if necessary to block ambient light.
- White noise helps many to fall and stay asleep.
- Earplugs or an eye mask may be helpful for you.

There are a ton of free sleep apps that can be an aid to your rest protocol. You may find earplugs or an eye mask helpful. Earplugs may take some initial adjustment as you acclimate to them, but after a short while you'll likely find them indispensable. Establish a healthy routine now and it will carry you through your pregnancy.

Don't stay up too late! You need to actually go to bed. Your body has a unique circadian rhythm, and you can reinforce it or fight against it. If you are in bed on time to fall asleep in concert with this rhythm, you are more likely to get a good night's sleep. While this is not the same for everyone, for many women this time falls between ten and eleven o'clock. When you learn to listen to your body, you will feel a natural pull to sleep at a regular time. If you fight to stay awake past that time, your body will release stress hormones like cortisol and adrenaline to help you stay awake.[73]

It will then become difficult for you to fall asleep until those hormones have abated, usually a few hours later.

Other Kinds of Rest

Sometimes people get enough sleep, but still don't feel rested. If this is you, pay attention to whether you are getting emotional, spiritual, and intellectual rest as well. Listen to your intuition and see what it feels like you need a break from right now.

- When you rest **emotionally**, you disengage from people and situations that provoke drama, tension, or stress.

- When you rest **spiritually**, you meditate, pray, and practice mindfulness and breathing techniques.

- When you rest **intellectually**, you take things off your mental decision-making list, you read less, you consume less content and less media.

Sometimes the body is not the only part of ourselves in need of rest. Pay attention to the whole and see if there are parts that need extra attention. These are all things you can be working on during your preparation for pregnancy, so these practices, techniques, theories, and paradigms will already be in place when you need them.

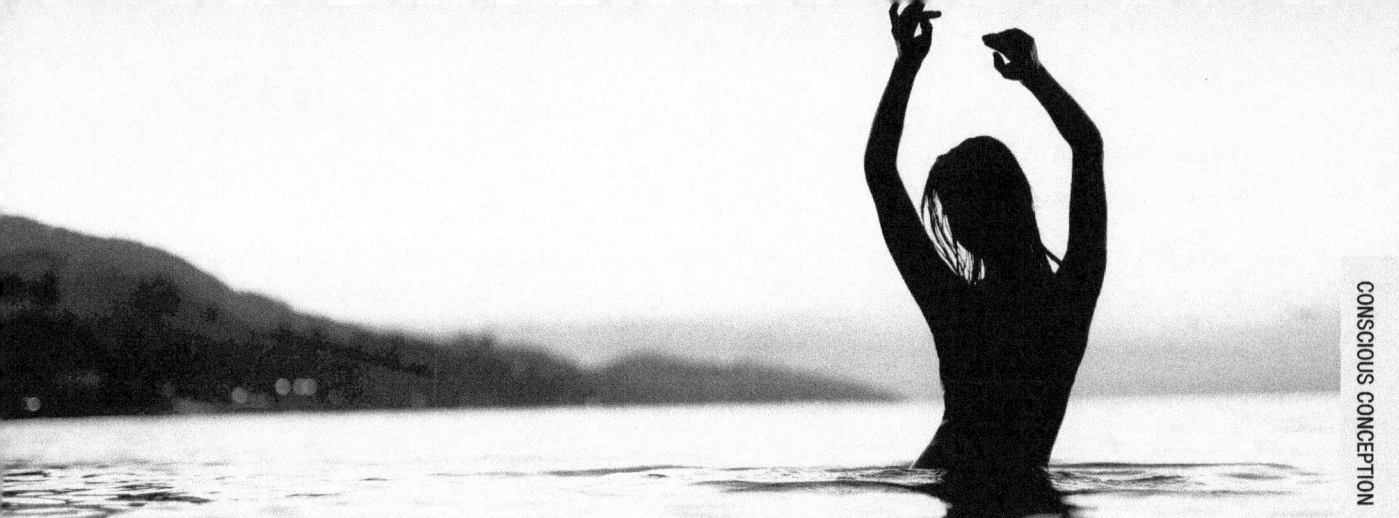

Joy

The more you seek out and create situations where joy can flow, the more expansive and open and joyful your life will be. I truly believe the cultivation of joy in your life can have a profound effect on your ability to conceive a baby. The use of mindfulness, affirmations, visualizations, positive thinking, and your relationship with the divine are all worthy of spending as much energy on as you do hydration, nourishment, movement, emotional work, building your knowledge base, and resting.

I want to take a moment here and address what kinds of activities and things actually bring joy. Trust me, it's not a big expenditure like a brand-new car—those big things bring their share of headaches (though you may feel joyful at first). Joy comes in the little moments, in the attitude shift, in the reframe. It comes in the tiny choices we make about how to think about things. Do you have to make dinner, or do you get to prepare a wonderful meal for you and your partner? The choices we make about how we approach life make all the difference in our day-to-day outlook.

We must find joy in the little things, in our day-to-day lives, because most of us don't have the budget to continually splurge for those big things.

Studies have shown that positive emotions can have positive effects on physical health.[74] Joyful experiences and positive emotions are associated with better immune function, reduced inflammation, improved cardiovascular health, and overall well-being.

Joy works to create positive change in your life, and it is particularly important during conception and pregnancy for so many reasons. We humans are engineered to be on the lookout for danger. We're very receptive to stress. We need to actively work to incorporate moments of joy in our lives because our primal drive will have us in a constant mode of stress in our modern environment if we don't actively work to counter it. When you experience joy, you are more likely to have a positive outlook on life, cope better with challenges, and maintain healthy mental and emotional states.

ON EXPERIENCING JOY

Watch the ducks. Feel the cool breeze. Listen to the grass swish.

That's what I just did, ... But as I was standing on my deck, watching the ducks swim, and feeling the breeze on my face, I realized I was feeling "joy," but I wasn't "happy" per se.

Because the feeling of joy isn't the same as the feeling of happy.

Joy, for me, is connection. Deeply belonging. Love. Peace.

I worry that when we talk so much about joy, people who aren't naturally happy by nature will feel like I'm engaging in toxic positivity. ("Pretend nothing is wrong because we aren't allowed to feel hard things.") And not everyone should be happy as a default setting. No.

But in the middle of body pain and stress and transition, I had a moment of standing on the deck and feeling like I was deeply connected and at peace for just a moment. That joy made all the other feelings go away, just for a second. I wasn't happy, though. I've been doing emotional work for 20+ years and I have a very fine-tuned sense of what happiness feels like.

This moment of joy was just a deep and abiding sense that everything was going to be okay. And even though I was also feeling stress and pressure and disconnection and fear the moment before that, that tiny "glimmer" as some would call it ... of the world being as it should be... it just set things back to the reminder that everything was going to be okay.

It's not happiness. It's just peace.

And every single person experiences joy in a different way. For some of us, joy is the release of stress, and for some of us, joy is happiness, and for some of us, joy is gratitude, or it's quiet, and for some of us, joy is loud and boisterous and celebratory. (And probably, at different times, it's different things for each of us.)

But this was on my mind today as I was thinking about joy. Joy is just the absence of fear. That's all it is. And most of us, when we're feeling fear, we don't know it, because we're so hard-wired to feel it all the time. (And that's our biology. It helps us survive. It doesn't do a great job of helping us thrive, though ... to thrive, we need to let go of the fear.)

So, ... I'm taking a moment to intentionally feel the moments of joy that are already present. The ducks are already swimming outside. The breeze is already blowing. I just had to step out of my stressed-out brain and connect with that tranquility, and then I could go on about my day ... and be good.

What moment of peace/content/joy/happiness/comfort have you had today? What one moment can you make for yourself right now?

—Becca Syme

Joy helps you to cultivate a positive mindset and builds your resilience, which are important qualities during pregnancy. Positive thinking and resilience enable you to adapt to changes, cope with challenges, and maintain a hopeful and optimistic outlook. Frankly, you just feel better when you are fully nourished, fully hydrated, and full of joy. When you face the world with this positive mindset you'll make better decisions, be more open to seeking support when you need it, and the transformative journey of pregnancy will be easier to navigate.

I'm going to talk about the different ways that joy is critical for you, your conception, and your baby, but don't worry. After that I'll provide you with lots of ideas for how you can incorporate more joy into your day-to-day life.

Stress Reduction

Joy has a powerful effect on reducing stress and promoting relaxation. As I've mentioned before, joy is nearly the inverse of stress, and many of the activities you can do to bring more joy into your life have the added benefit of reducing your residual biochemical stress. That's pretty fantastic! Dropping or lowering stress in your life is absolutely one of the best ways to help your body move into a way of being in which it can more easily conceive and carry a baby to full term.

The Stress Cycle

There are two components to stress—the external trigger and the internal lingering biochemical results in our bodies. The trigger is anything stressful: thoughts of an upcoming exam, the evening news, narrowly avoiding a collision on the road, crunch time at work, negative interactions with other people online or in person ... Any stress-inducing event triggers the release of stress hormones in the body, especially adrenaline, cortisol, and epinephrine.

Triggers

Let's deal with triggers first. I want you to work to minimize these triggers in your life. What stresses you out and can you mitigate it? Is traffic obnoxious for you? Can you carpool or take public transit or a different route? Are you working too hard? Can you find a way to excuse yourself from especially stressful work projects? Is drama that belongs to other people filling your life with unnecessary negativity? Can you work to set boundaries so toxic relationship drama is no longer welcome in your life? Is it all just too much? Can you get help with the tasks that are overwhelming you?

Immediate Relief

That's proactively handling stressors. But what about when you get stressed out? What do you do in the moment? When you've had a stressful encounter, there are a few practices you can employ to help the adrenaline stop flowing so freely through your body.

Grounding

Take your shoes off and go barefoot in the grass or dirt. When you do this, your vibrational self connects to the vibrations of the earth and the higher powers. It is very powerful, very healing, very cleansing of the spirit, and very supportive of your nervous system. It doesn't take long; if you've only got five minutes, that's fine. If you've got fifteen, even better, but take time to take your shoes and socks off and get some primal nurturing from Mother Earth, the mother of us all.

Breathing

Take a few deep, cleansing breaths. Make sure that the exhale is longer than the inhale, if possible. This serves as a signal to your nervous system that the danger has passed, and you can relax now. (That's why singing can be a stress relieving activity!)

Handling Residual Stress

Our ancestors became stressed when their lives were in danger. They'd see a large predator, be flooded with adrenaline, and have the extra boost they needed to run away quickly and for longer than normal. This movement, the running, helped the body to quickly shed the extra stress chemicals in their bloodstream. Exercise is a fantastic way to shed your residual stress.

In our modern world, most of us no longer have a physical release after a stressful event. Many of us are carrying layers and layers of stress in our bodies that have never been properly shed. This is another reason that regular exercise is so healthy and good for you. It is a massive stress chemical shedding mechanism. But there are other ways to relieve stress when you don't have time for a workout (or when you conceive, and I advise that you take two or three months off from your exercise routine).

Shaking

If you've ever seen a deer startled in the woods and stayed to watch them recover, you'll see them recover from their freeze position, and then they start to shake all over. After this, they get up and move around normally, calmly. The danger has passed, and the shaking got rid of their stress.

You can mimic this for a similar effect. Lie down on your back on your bed and start by shaking each foot as fast as you can, then move to each leg, each hand, each arm. Stand up and shake your torso and head. Finish off with a full body shake. This takes no more than 30 seconds and afterwards you will feel calm and gentle. Almost all mammals shake or shudder after birth as the experience of birth is so intensely stressful.

(Once you are pregnant, do not do this if you have cramping or bleeding. Instead, call your midwife.)

Laughter

Deep belly laughter provokes a stress release response as well. Get together with friends who never fail to make you laugh. Watch your favorite funny movie or a stand-up special by a comedian you love. Try some Try Not to Laugh challenges on social media. Try laughter yoga. Laughter is a primal signal to your body that you are safe, and the physical component of a deep belly laugh helps the body to shed those stress chemicals.

Crying

Like laughter, crying can provoke a cathartic, stress-relieving response in our bodies. The stress in your life may give you obvious reasons to cry, and you can draw on those emotions to provoke this response. You may or may not be a crier. It may or may not feel good and natural to you. If you're not a crier, if you're someone who maybe likes to schedule your cries so as not to disturb your life too much, know that there is no shame in this cathartic release, and there is no demand for you to have this experience publicly. The shower is a great place for a nice, extended, ugly cry. You may find it easier to cry once you are pregnant, as pregnancy does have a way of tearing down our emotional barriers.

Many women really struggle to let themselves cry. It can be so hard to cry, even if you need to. When you feel yourself on the verge of tears, you can encourage the tears to come by thinking of sad things from your past, like lost loved ones or pets so you can cry yourself out thoroughly. I always feel deeply cleansed and calmer after a good crying session. It is okay to cry. Let yourself have this cathartic release when you need it.

> **THE COMPONENTS OF TEARS**
>
> Researchers have studied the components of tears. They stimulated some people to create tears by using onions or other eye irritants, and they compared those tears with tears stimulated by people who were sad, upset, or frustrated. They found different chemicals in the tears depending on what the stimulus had been.[75] They found lots of interesting chemicals in tears, especially tears of sadness. The theory is that your tear ducts work to filter out the chemicals that build up in your system when you're upset, and the reason that you feel better after crying is because the act of crying has actually filtered out chemicals that cause you emotional pain. So don't hold back on crying. Crying is a very healthy release and possibly an amazing filter.

Dancing

Dancing makes us feel good. Find some music that you can't help moving your body to and let yourself go, even for just a few minutes. Once you are pregnant, I don't want you to overdo this, but if you're feeling it, go for it. This acts much like shaking to release the stress in your body.

Stress is a barrier to conception, so if you are struggling to conceive, amp up your joy! Once you've done your best work to reduce the major stressors in your life, you can work to incorporate even more joy in your life.

How to Boost Your Joy

Building joy into your life is more than just stress relief. It can be so empowering to create space and focus time and energy on loving ourselves and building ourselves up with experiences that fill our emotional well. It can make such a difference and it costs us nothing but a bit of time.

The following are some ideas for activities that can help you to focus on your emotional health and enhance your joy quotient. I'll talk more about most of these in a moment and save a few for you to explore in the chapters to follow. I encourage you to read this whole section, but it may feel overwhelming to try to incorporate all these ideas into your already busy life. This is meant as inspiration, not as a giant to-do list. Pick one and add it to your schedule for this week. See how it feels. Did you love it? If you did, do more. If you didn't, switch it up the following week and try something else.

- Journal for joy.
- Be kind and gentle to yourself and others.

- Focus on what you can control and release what you can't.
- Pamper yourself.
- Connect with nature.
- Spend time with beloved family and friends.
- Sing, dance, and listen to music.
- Use mindfulness, meditation, noticing, prayer, and gratitude to keep you grounded.
- Build community.

You can't take care of others unless you first care for yourself. By acknowledging and expressing our feelings, practicing good emotional self-care, and connecting with ourselves and others, we build up our joy quotient, and the benefits can be palpable.

You can't take care of others unless you first care for yourself.

Journal for Joy

Journaling can be a powerful tool for self-awareness and shedding negative emotions, but it can also be a tool for creating an awareness of joy. Here are a few ways you might structure a journaling session to increase your awareness of the moments of joy already in your life.

Joyful Moments Journaling

Record moments of joy and happiness that you experience throughout the day. Write about the activities, interactions, or experiences that bring you joy. By capturing and revisiting these moments, you can cultivate a greater sense of appreciation and

happiness as well as having a better idea of what works to bring you joy.

Future Dreams and Goals Journaling

Write about your dreams, aspirations, and goals. Visualize and describe in detail what brings you joy and fulfillment. Use your journal as a space to explore possibilities and create a vision for the joyful future family you want to create. This can be especially helpful when visualizing and affirming conception, your pregnancy growth and development, as well as your ideal labor, birth, and postpartum experiences.

Reflection and Growth Journaling

Reflect on past experiences, lessons learned, and personal growth. Write about moments of resilience, strength, or positive changes in your life. Celebrate your growth journey and acknowledge the joy that comes from personal development.

Inspirational Quotes Journaling

Collect inspiring quotes that resonate with you and write about how they make you feel or how they relate to your life. Reflect on their meaning and explore ways to integrate their wisdom into your daily life.

Mindfulness and Present Moment Journaling

Use journaling as a tool to deepen your mindfulness practices. Write about your observations and experiences in the present moment, paying attention to the details and sensations around you. This practice can help you cultivate joy by fostering a greater sense of presence and appreciation for the here and now.

Remember, there are no rules or restrictions when it comes to journaling. Feel free to adapt these ideas to suit your personal style and needs. The goal is to create a safe and nurturing space for self-reflection, emotional expression, and the cultivation of joy in your life.

Be Kind to Yourself and Others

This is an essential aspect of self-care and can greatly contribute to your overall well-being, increase your happiness, and foster joy in your life. It is so important to treat yourself with kindness, compassion, understanding, and give yourself the same support you would give to others you love and care for. It is often easier for us to support others but more difficult to do it for ourselves. Acknowledge your struggles and setbacks without judgment or self-criticism. If this is something you struggle with, that's all the more reason to set an intention to actively participate in this type of work as part of your self-care regimen.

Set Healthy Boundaries

Learn to say no to things that drain your energy or overwhelm you. Respect your limits and make time for yourself without feeling guilty. Prioritizing your own needs is a necessary act of kindness for you and everyone in your life because when you have your needs met, you are more able to be your best self. Limit or eliminate the interactions with people who suck joy out of the situation. You don't have to set these boundaries immediately, all at once, but a little at a time, set and strengthen boundaries that protect you. This might look like saying, "no" to that volunteer opportunity, reining in the number of overtime hours you work, quitting

something you've been doing for a while but no longer really enjoy, not watching shows or movies that are disturbing or make you feel scared or threatened, etc. Listen to your intuition for guidance here.

Practice Positive Self-Talk

Replace self-critical thoughts with positive and affirming statements. Treat yourself with kindness in your internal dialogue and focus on your strengths and achievements.

For example, if your automatic thought is something like, *Why would you do that, MariMikel? You're so stupid,* remind yourself that you would NEVER talk to a friend that way. You need to love yourself enough to not talk to yourself that way either. When you catch yourself with these ugly thoughts, choose to replace them with kindness. Talk to yourself the way you'd talk to your best friend in the same situation. *It's okay, MariMikel. People make mistakes and this is not the end of the world. You can fix this.*

Forgive Yourself

Let go of past mistakes or regrets and forgive yourself. Understand that everyone makes mistakes, and these experiences are opportunities for growth and learning. You are human, and no human, not one of us, is perfect.

My wonderful minister of over 40 years, Dr. Landon Shultz said once that the word "sin" comes from a Greek word relating to archery that means "to miss the mark." Most of what we do wrong is not a heinous act to be shamed, but rather we have just missed the mark. Every day is a new day, and we can wake up and make different choices. Every day you can try again. Forgiveness is the first step. If you can't forgive yourself, you can't let go and move forward into better action. Be gentle and understanding with yourself. Whatever transgression you committed is in the past. Make whatever reparations you feel you need to, treat yourself with grace, and move on.

Take Care of Your Physical Health

Ensure you're getting enough sleep, eating nutritious food, and engaging in regular exercise. Nourishing your body is an act of self-kindness and promotes overall well-being. Remember, we are holistic beings of mind, body, and spirit. All three must flourish for our whole being to thrive.

Celebrate Your Accomplishments

Acknowledge and celebrate both big and small achievements. Recognize your progress and give yourself credit for your efforts and successes. *I swam for five whole minutes my first time out! I did great!!* or *I've only been doing yoga for two weeks and already I'm so much more flexible, wow! My body really responds to this stuff.*

TRY THIS

Next time you feel agitated or anxious, notice your breathing. Is it deep or shallow? Try to keep breathing that way consciously for one minute before changing the rhythm of your breath. How did that feel, and what changed when you breathed faster or slower?

Acceptance

Accept yourself as you are, embracing your strengths, weaknesses, and unique qualities. You are human. You are a gift from the divine. You are beautiful. Treat yourself with love, respect, and acceptance, fostering a positive relationship with yourself. Actively acknowledge your strengths and the gifts you bring to the world.

Look for Tiny Moments of Joy

Spreading acts of unexpected kindness reaps exponential rewards, in my opinion. I get such a boost from these tiny moments of joy, and I bet you do, too. Try to incorporate one extra kindness for others

Penelope: I was walking down the bread aisle at the grocery store when I noticed a loaf had fallen on the floor. I saw an elder gentleman a few steps ahead of me had also noticed it, because he was quite literally quaking with rage as he stooped to pick it up and put it back on the shelf. As I walked past him, I said, "You just passed the good person test." I took a few more steps, turned back, and said, "A plus!"

In that mere moment, all of his rage had evaporated. The expression on his face was naked and vulnerable and so grateful. "So did you," he said quietly.

I put my hand on my heart and said, "Thank you." We both had tears welling in our eyes. I felt like such a force for good in the world. In that tiny moment, I had moved mountains of emotions with just a few kind words. I think I probably got a lot more out of that experience than the gentleman did, because it's been more than a year ago now and I still get a happiness charge when I think of it, which is just about every time that I'm in the bread aisle, at a minimum.

in your day and you'll be astounded at how much of a joyous rush you get from it. Here are some things I love to do: leave a big tip, give and receive hugs, smile at a fellow gasser-upper, let someone in traffic into my lane, compliment a stranger, ask how the checker at the check-out counter is doing, and be kind to customer service reps and telemarketers.

Remember that being kind to yourself is an ongoing practice. It requires patience, consistency, and a genuine commitment to nurturing yourself. By putting your well-being first and treating yourself with kindness, you can cultivate a greater sense of self-love and fulfillment in your life. You are beautiful and you deserve this.

Focus on What You Can Control

Focusing on things you can control and consciously releasing feelings around things you do not have control over is a valuable self-care practice that can help reduce stress, enhance your overall well-being, and foster joy. Let's explore a few ways you can cultivate this mindset.

Identify

Begin by recognizing the aspects of your life that you can influence or change. These could include your thoughts, behaviors, reactions, choices, and the way you allocate your time and energy.

Accept

Understand that there are just some circumstances, events, and actions that are beyond your control. Acknowledge that you cannot change these things and that it is okay to let go of trying. This can be particularly useful during your conscious conception journey. Releasing expectations that revolve around getting pregnant and giving up control can have a significant positive impact on the process simply by taking off the pressure to conceive.

If you are actively trying to get pregnant, you do the work you need to do (hint: it's my Sevenfold Method) and then let nature take her course.

This is even more important when you are using techniques like in-vitro fertilization (IVF) or intrauterine insemination (IUI) to help with conception. The pressure is even more present if you have not been able to conceive without technological assistance, so taking conscious steps to release expectations can really help your body and mind to destress and instead focus on the things you can control (nourishment, hydration, emotional health, etc.).

Relax

Be kind and gentle with yourself when facing situations that are outside your control. Remind yourself that it is natural to feel frustrated, disappointed, or anxious, but also remember that you are doing the best you can. Allow yourself to feel your feelings, then try to release them and offer yourself words of encouragement to accept where you are in the here and now. Okay, this is happening. It's okay. I can deal with this as it is. I can meet this moment with grace.

Remember, letting go of what you can't control and focusing on what you can is a continuous practice. It takes time and patience to shift your mindset and release attachment to outcomes. By consciously redirecting your energy toward the things within your control, you can cultivate a sense of empowerment, peace, and resilience.

Take Refuge in Nature

Find your happy places and your happy people. Take refuge in nature's beautiful waters and springs. If you're near the ocean, get yourself to the beach. Spend time in forests soaking up the smells, sights, and sounds. Being in nature is really soothing and builds all these biochemical states that help you and your baby both. If the season allows, get in clean, natural water as often as possible. Take off your shoes and plant your feet in the dirt. Run your hands along the trunks of trees or crush leafy herbs in your palm and inhale deeply. Spend an hour in a hammock and let the breezes wash over you. Physically engage with the beauty of nature. It is so rejuvenating.

Sing, Dance, Listen To, and/or Play Music

Music can help you evoke and express a wide range of emotions and creativity. Singing, dancing, playing, or simply listening to music can provide healthy outlets for emotional expression. They allow you to connect with and process your feelings, whether these emotions are joyful, sad, excited, calm, or something else altogether. Through music, you can also explore your creativity and connect with your inner self.

Music can also help reduce stress and promote relaxation. It has the power to alter your mood, activate the relaxation response, and lower cortisol levels. It can serve as a form of therapy, helping you release tension and unwind after a long day.

Music has a direct impact on your mood. Upbeat, lively music can boost your energy and uplift your spirits, while soft, soothing melodies can calm and soothe your mind. By choosing music that resonates with you, you can intentionally enhance your mood and cultivate a positive state of mind.

Engaging with music requires that you be present and in the moment. When you sing, dance, or deeply listen to music, you enter a state of mindfulness, where your focus is solely on the rhythm, melody, and lyrics. This mindful engagement can help calm your mind, improve concentration, and promote a sense of inner peace.

Singing and dancing are physical activities that can contribute to your physical well-being. Singing exercises your lungs and diaphragm, improving breath control and lung capacity. Dancing is a form of exercise that promotes cardiovascular health, flexibility, and coordination.

Music is a powerful force for human connection. Singing or dancing with others can foster a sense of community and social interaction. Joining a choir, participating in dance classes, or attending music events can provide opportunities for social engagement, teamwork, and a sense of belonging. See what kind of musical activities or events are available in your area and try something new!

Music can transport you to different worlds and evoke a sense of escapism. It can provide a break from daily stressors and offer an enjoyable, immersive experience. Whether you're belting out your favorite song in the car, grooving to a beat, or getting lost in the melodies, music can bring joy, fun, and a sense of freedom.

Incorporating singing, dancing, or listening to music into your self-care routine doesn't require any special equipment or training. It can be as simple as playing your favorite tunes, having a dance party in your living room, singing along to songs in the shower, or creating personalized playlists that resonate with your emotions and uplift your spirit. For some people, incorporating music into their lives comes as easily as breathing. Others need to remind themselves to include it. If you're in that latter category, set reminders for yourself to play music while you're eating or to take a music break, so you build up this habit.

Mindfulness, Meditation, Prayer, and Noticing & Gratitude

Mindfulness, meditation, prayer, and noticing & gratitude are all practices that can be used to enhance joy in life by cultivating a sense of inner peace, presence, and a positive mindset. While they may have distinct origins and approaches, they are similar in that they ask you to focus your awareness and emphasize the importance of being fully present in the current moment. These practices concentrate on affirming and manifesting positive events, experiences, or emotions, and fostering a deeper spiritual connection.

As you try out these practices, I encourage you to observe your thoughts, feelings, and sensations without judgment or attachment. By practicing awareness and being present, you can cultivate a deeper appreciation for the joys and beauty in your life.

Mindfulness

Mindfulness asks that we become more conscious in our lives, our actions, our unconscious and subconscious drives, and conscious of others. This is critical to the furthering of humanity and our individual selves. When you are engaging in an activity or conversation, you want to bring your attention fully to the present moment. Everything you think, every interaction that you have with others … the more aware and conscious you are, the better all of this is going to go.

Put your phone down during meals. Better yet, leave it in another room. When you are talking with someone, don't also be conducting a conversation in your DMs.

Mindfulness is the practice of paying attention and being fully present in any given or chosen moment. The goal is to pay attention to what is going on both inside and outside of yourself (where you are and what you are doing), while calmly acknowledging and accepting your thoughts, feelings, and bodily sensations without judgement. I know it's hard, but strive to accept whatever happens, whether it's positive or negative, with an attitude of curiosity and non-attachment.

Start With Your Breath

Breath is a fundamental anchor for mindfulness practices. Get in a comfortable position, sitting or lying down, then close your eyes or gently focus on a spot at eye level. Take a few moments to focus on your breath, observing its natural rhythm. Notice the sensation of the breath entering and leaving your body as you breath in and out. Whenever your mind wanders, gently bring your attention back to the breath, using it as an anchor to be present in the moment. Always breathe in and out through your nose.

Engage Your Senses

Mindfulness involves fully engaging your senses in the present experience. Take moments throughout your day to notice the details of your surroundings. What does the world around you smell like, feel like, sound like, and what colors do you see? Engaging your senses helps ground you in the present moment.

Practice Body Scans

Set aside dedicated time for a body scan. Start from the top of your head and slowly move your attention down through each part of your body, noticing any sensations or areas of tension. Paying attention to your body in a non-judgmental way promotes self-awareness and relaxation.

Engage In Mindful Activities

You can inject moments of mindfulness throughout your day. Whether you're eating, walking, or doing chores, bring your full attention to the present moment. Notice the sensations, tastes, smells, and movements associated with each activity.

Use Guided Mindfulness Resources

If you're struggling to get started, try guided mindfulness/meditation apps, online videos, or audio recordings (you can search your favorite streaming service). These resources can provide structure and guidance for your mindfulness practice, especially if you're just starting out or prefer a more structured approach.

Put your hands on your heart and feel it beating for one to two minutes. You can make anything mindful by paying attention to it. Attention equals energy. When you pay attention to something, you are filling it with your energy.

Robbie: When my son Jason was around 2 years old, he would cling to my skirt and whine a lot while I was trying to cook dinner. I learned that if I stopped, got down on my knees, and gave him my full attention for just a few moments, he would get filled up with the loving energy that I was pouring into him and start happily playing with the pots and pans, leaving me free to finish cooking our family dinner.

Remember, mindfulness is a skill that develops over time with consistent practice. Be patient and gentle with yourself as you incorporate mindfulness into your self-care routine. I encourage you to keep it up. It will aid you to develop a deeper connection with yourself and those around you, reduce stress, and enhance your overall well-being and sense of joy.

Meditation

Meditation is the practice of sitting with yourself, paying attention to your breath and the present moment, and dismissing intrusive thoughts as they come up. It helps you to focus your attention on the present, allowing you to let go of regrets about the past or worries about the future, and to more fully embrace and appreciate the joys and beauty that exist in each moment.

Regular meditation practice can help you manage stress and negative emotions more effectively. By developing a state of mindfulness and non-reactivity through meditation, you can learn to observe negative thoughts and emotions without getting caught up in them. This allows you to experience more positive emotions and cultivate a greater sense of joy and well-being.

Meditation can also lend itself to the development of self-compassion, which I believe is an essential component during conception, pregnancy, birth, and postpartum. This self-care practice creates a nurturing environment within yourself, allowing joy to flourish. Meditation is a relaxing, tranquil activity. When the mind is calm, it becomes more receptive to experiencing joy. As you let go of distractions and mental traffic during meditation, you create space for joy to arise naturally.

To experience the benefits of meditation for enhancing joy, it's important to establish a regular practice. Start with short meditation sessions and gradually increase the duration over time. There are various meditation techniques to explore, including mindfulness meditation, loving-kindness meditation, and gratitude meditation. Explore meditation classes in your area, find an online group or guided practice, use an app, or read a book on meditation to explore different techniques. Find one that resonates with you and commit to incorporating meditation into your self-care routine.

Prayer

Many people find immense solace in prayer and communion with the higher powers they believe in. I am one of them. I find prayer to be a lovely way to connect with spirit, and it brings me joy. If this is you as well, I want to simply remind you of this practice and encourage you to find ways to incorporate more of it in your life. For example, I love to pray when I'm swimming. I find that environment to be so conducive for this communion.

Prayer and meditation are so similar. They are both ways of focusing our attention, energy, and encouraging deeper connection to the divine spirit. Feel free to call it whatever you want. You don't have to use the word "prayer" if that makes you feel uncomfortable. It's all about deepening and directing your spiritual energy.

Noticing & Gratitude

I encourage you to become more aware in every area of your life. I have spent decades trying to be more conscious, more aware, more connected, and to pay closer attention to what's going on with myself and with others in the present moment. This has led to more compassion for others and for myself, and more conscious actions on my part as opposed to reactive behaviors and acting out. It has also enabled me to better stand up for myself when I need to.

I'll talk about ways to increase your awareness through noticing what's going on in every chapter of this book.

Cultivating a daily gratitude practice is a great way to incorporate positivity into your everyday life. This is especially important during pregnancy as there are so many changes happening to you physically, intellectually, and emotionally/spiritually. For now, I'd like you to choose a daily time when you will commit to noticing five things that fill your cup and five things for which you are grateful. You might incorporate cues for additional practice, like thinking of three things you are grateful for when you make your morning tea, after you brush your teeth at night, when you sit down for lunch, when you hear an alarm go off, or when you are commuting.

Acknowledge and savor the positive experiences of your day, things that made you feel good, or people that lifted you up. These can be simple small things or larger things, it doesn't matter what you choose to focus on, just that it feels good to you.

You can visualize or list things in your head, write them in a journal, or make a video journal on your phone, whatever feels right to you. There isn't a right or wrong way to do this.

You might start a journal to keep these positive thoughts in. Don't let this become a burden or a heavy to-do; keep it light and fast. Some days I am grateful for my car, the hot water heater, the internet, the refrigerator, the sewage system, and my dishwasher. I'm not asking you to dredge the depths of your soul, simply start noticing the things that make your life better. As you move through your days, take time to pause and listen to yourself and your environment.

- *I am grateful for my bed, for running water, and my home that shelters us.*
- *I am grateful for my partner.*
- *I am grateful for my health.*
- *I am grateful for my family and friends.*
- *I am grateful for my job that helps to support my family.*

- *I am grateful for my body and all that it does for me and the baby I am inviting into my life.*
- *I am grateful for the food that nourishes me at each meal.*
- *I am grateful to the stranger who smiled at me today.*

Also taking the time to notice what filled your cup on the previous day can help you to really identify what impacts your mood and emotional vibration for the better. Did someone say something kind that made you glow? Did you stay hydrated and nourished and feel less jangly than normal? Did you make a positive connection with a friend or loved one? Tune in to your intuition when it is calling out to you. Listen to it. Notice. And take deep breaths!

If you're having a particularly difficult day, amplify your gratitude practice. Include one thing you're grateful about for each year that you've been alive. They don't have to correspond, but if you're 24, find 24 things you're grateful for. It can help if you include why you're grateful for each thing. Soak in the goodness.

A focus on gratitude and abundance opens you up to be more and more receptive to the simple and ubiquitous joys in life. It can rewire your mind for the better.

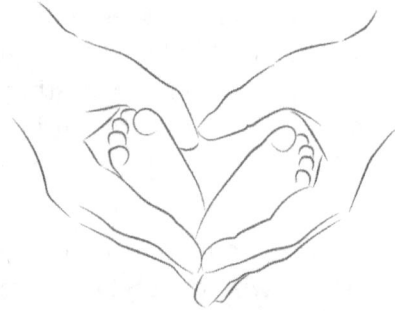

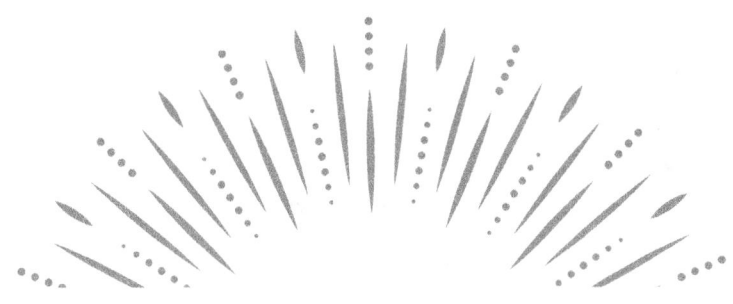

FIRST TRIMESTER

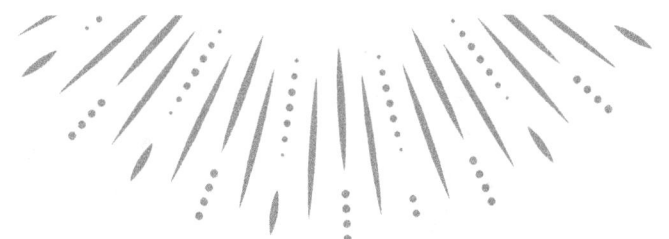

Introduction

Congratulations! You are now pregnant, and so you have embarked on what will perhaps be the most momentous journey of your life. You must be overjoyed! And terrified! And excited! And scared! And so, so happy! (Except, if occasionally, you are not!)

It is completely normal for these first few months of pregnancy to be an emotionally volatile time. In US society, we really don't give the difficulties of early pregnancy enough credence or support. Of course it's difficult and strange and puts you off kilter.

Your hormones are surging, your body is changing, and there's a small being inside of you demanding every last ounce of your energy. Of course you feel low ebb. But also, you're excited and scared and nervous and happy and just feeling all the emotions you can possibly feel.

Implementing my Sevenfold Approach to your first trimester will help you to better withstand any of the unpleasantness you might encounter in early pregnancy and help you continue to fully support and nourish yourself and your baby.

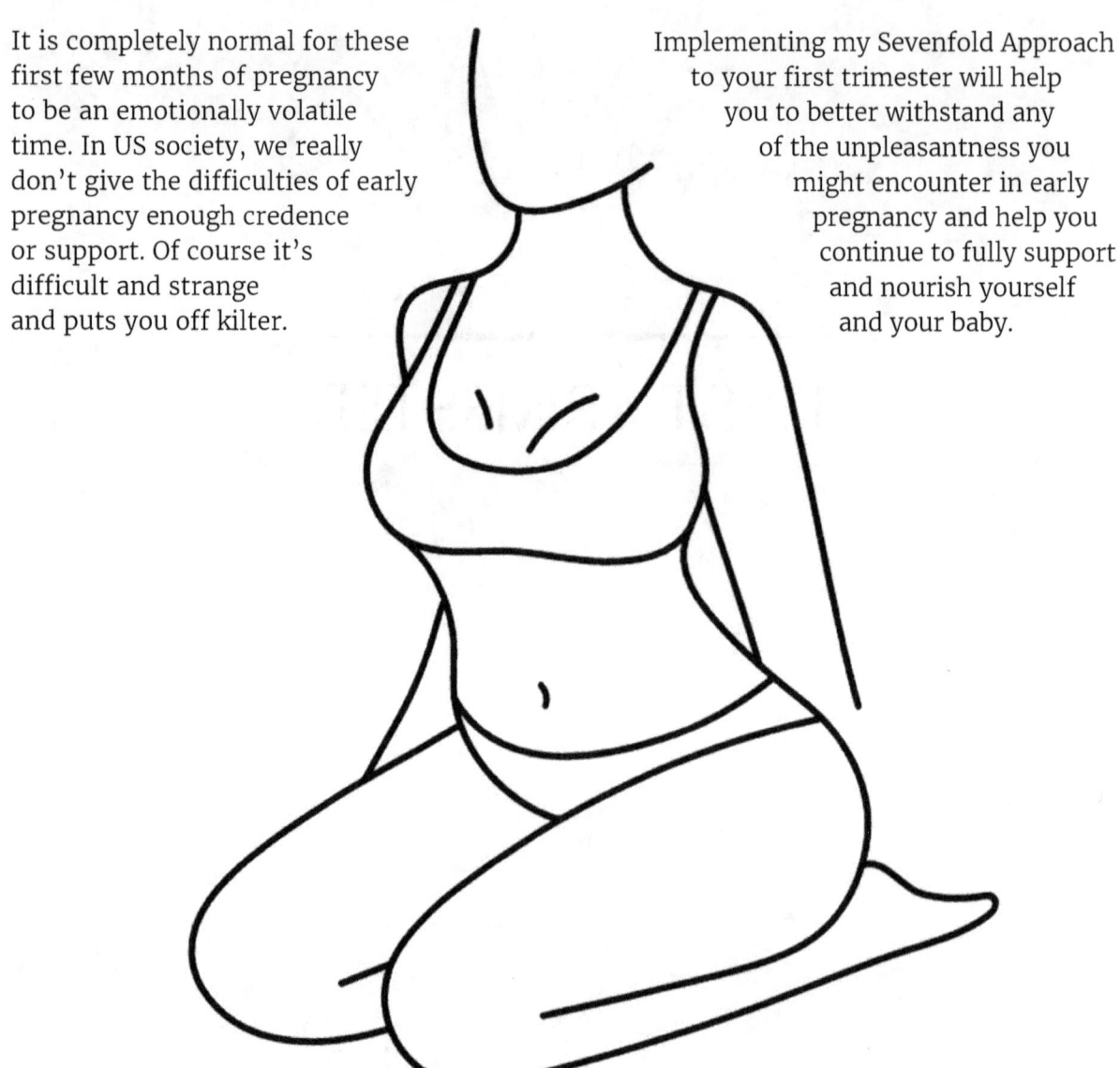

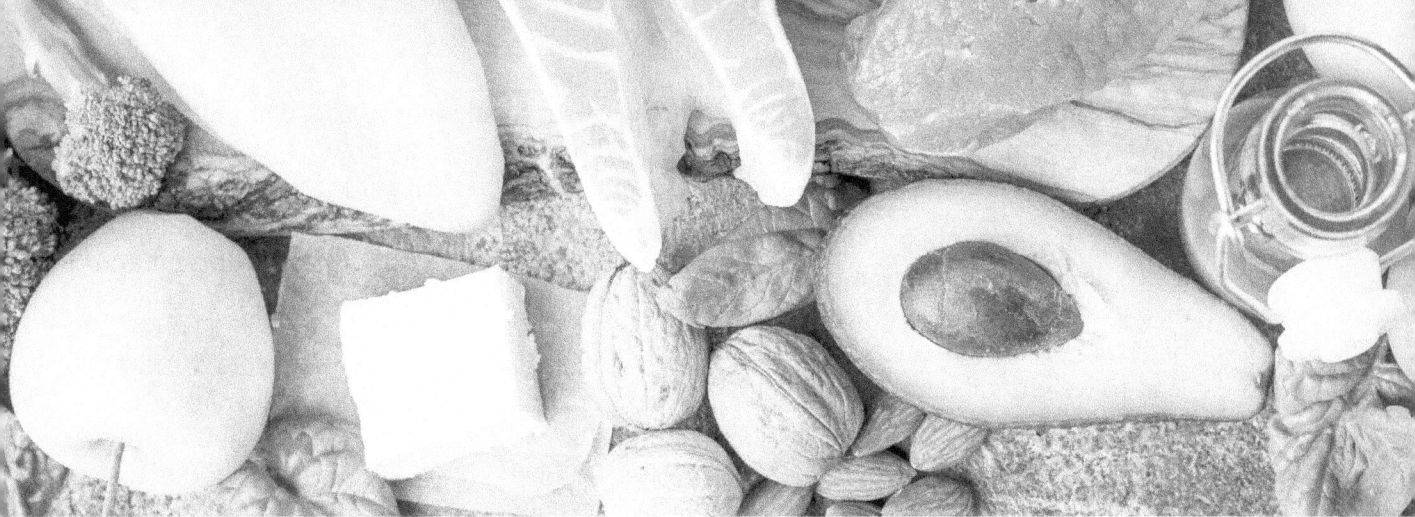

Nourishment

First of all, if you skipped right to this section because you're already pregnant and didn't think you needed to read about how to get pregnant, I'd like you to go back to the Nourishment chapter of the Conscious Conception section (see page 22), because you should implement all of those recommendations for dietary changes and supplements *immediately*. Start there, then come back here.

If you've already been following my Sevenfold Approach, I want you to continue to eat fantastically! Your diet should include lots of fresh fruits and vegetables—organic when possible. Continue to limit or eliminate processed foods. Here are a few things to continue to keep in mind as you prepare your frequent, healthy meals.

- Go to your local farmer's market regularly and include local, in-season produce in your diet.

- Eat lots of high-quality protein (less conventionally grown meat); try to buy non-contaminated, free range/ pasture-raised/grass-fed, or organic meats and poultry.[76]

- Eat lots of fish (pay attention to the mercury).

- Red meat is a good source of absorbable iron and protein, but it can also be high in saturated fat. Grass-fed and finished meat will have a better omega-3 count and lower omega-6 count than its conventionally grown counterpart.

- Gluten or conventionally grown wheat (that uses chemicals like glyphosate) can trigger an immune response in many people.[77] Buy Italian-grown, organic pasta or use pasta substitutes like spaghetti squash. If you continue to eat conventionally grown wheat products, choose bread, crackers, or other foods that contain 100 percent whole grains. Consider switching to gluten-free products.

- Dairy is a good source of calcium, but it can also be high in saturated fat and cholesterol. Limit your dairy intake and buy organic, pasture-raised, grass-fed dairy as much as possible.

- Limit your sugar intake. Sugar is a simple carbohydrate that can be easily digested and absorbed by the body. However, too much sugar can lead to weight gain and other health problems. Your body does need sugar, just not very much of it.

- Lightly steam veggies so you do not overcook them.

- Eat lots of seeds, nuts, and sprouts.

- Experiment with different types of seaweed, which are extremely high in calcium and other minerals.

- Take your vitamins and supplements faithfully.

Nourish Your Baby!

In the early days of your pregnancy, you may find yourself to be ravenous. Your appetite increases in pregnancy for a reason. You and your growing baby need those nutrients and calories! There is just so much going on in your body. Keep up that healthy eating you started during your conscious conception; it's more important now than ever before.

There is also a chance that you might not want to eat at all; if so, you will have to fight that tendency because you need food. We'll talk more about this later.

Healthy Weight Gain

When women ask me how much weight to gain, I generally tell them that I think around 30 pounds over the course of their pregnancy is ideal. If you're underweight, you might need to gain 40 pounds; if you're

over your ideal body weight you might only need to gain 20 or 25 pounds, but only you can decide what's right for you (with the guidance of your midwife) and you should gain that weight without shame or guilt and do your best to ignore cultural pressure.

It's also true that if you gain a lot of weight, especially at the end of your pregnancy, you increase your chances of having a really big baby. Nine-and-a-half or ten-pound babies are hard on your body and labor is hard on those babies. Gaining a lot of weight also increases your chances of blood pressure problems.

Conversely, the women in my practice who have had tremendous difficulty gaining an adequate amount of weight in their pregnancies have had a higher percentage of babies that were born early and were smaller than ideal. Rarely I have also seen miscarriages and stillbirths occur with significantly underweight clients and think this could be a factor at play. The fetus needs nutrition to be hearty and strong enough to withstand the rigors of labor and birth. All of this is exceedingly difficult to talk about and difficult to think about without triggering emotional distress for some women. What we really need here is body positivity and sensitivity and to know that we are all not supposed to look the same.

If weight gain stresses you out, know that a healthy approach to pregnancy and postpartum will lead to a quick and healthy weight loss on the other side. A woman will typically lose 10–15 and occasionally 20 pounds with the birth right off the bat. That weight loss initially comes from birthing the placenta and amniotic fluid, and of course, the baby. Then, when you breastfeed, your fat is all turned into the fat of the baby's milk. Your uterus shrinks back to its original size over the course of several weeks to a few months. The weight you've stored is melted off you and put into the milk you make for your baby. Your baby gets chubbier and chubbier while you get more and more slender. It's magic.

Keep all of this in mind and *nourish yourself* as much as you can. I've got some tips for you later in this section to help with that.

Food Aversions

Some women in early pregnancy find that they really can't eat a lot. You may have serious food aversions. This is an ancient biological safety mechanism to keep you from wandering out and trying a new mushroom or berry you've come across and finding out the hard way that it wasn't a good choice. These food aversions in pregnancy seem to almost always be related to vegetables, fruits, and proteins. It's okay if you don't eat perfectly. It's not okay to not eat. In these early days, find what you can eat and eat that. I know with some of my pregnancies there were only four things I could keep down early on, and they were all white: yogurt, mashed potatoes, rice, and pasta. Eat what you can for now, and once you can tolerate them, get back to eating lots of fresh, natural fruits and vegetables.

At this point in your pregnancy, whatever you can get in and keep down is fantastic.

Digestive Sensitivities

Anthropologists have shown us that we evolved as hunters and gatherers who grazed. They would find one thing and eat that, and then move on to the next thing and eat that, and then move on to the next

thing … usually consuming very small amounts of food very frequently.[78]

I believe that in pregnancy we revert to a very ancient way of being, biologically speaking, and that suddenly we cannot do three square meals a day as most of the world does. We have to eat very frequently, in very small amounts, like our ancestors did.

When I wasn't pregnant, I found I could eat those three squares, but when I was pregnant I could not combine all foods all the time. The big no-nos for me were starches and proteins, which just goes against everything in the American way. We love our meat and potatoes, but they were not good in combination for me. I could combine meat and vegetables, but I had to eat a baked potato while the chicken and squash and salad were being made. I could eat starches if I ate them 30 to 40 minutes before other foods. Not everyone is bothered by this, but some people don't realize it's a reason that they've had a lifetime of indigestion. If you find your meals make you uncomfortable, try separating your food groups and see if that helps.

- Start slowly with foods you know you do well with and gradually introduce new foods into your diet.

- Listen to your body and pay attention to how you feel after eating different combinations of foods.

- If you experience any negative side effects like bloating or indigestion, talk to a healthcare professional.

- Make sure you are getting enough fluids and fiber.

- You may want to talk with a registered dietitian or other qualified healthcare professional to make sure your diet is right for you.

Additionally, know that the benefits of food combining are likely to vary from person to person depending on your specific digestive patterns and nutritional needs. Ultimately, it is best to eat a varied diet rich in whole, organic foods and to listen to your body's signals of hunger and fullness to guide your dietary choices.

Hormonal Imbalances

You may really struggle with shifting hormones, and the two things you can do to support yourself through this turmoil are to eat and drink enough. You might choose to make three square meals a day, but if you do that, then take your time with each meal and eat each one over the course of several hours. Maybe have a third of each meal every 40 minutes. Frequency is as important as amount. You want to be digesting small amounts of food all day long. I know I'm starting to sound like a broken record, but it really is that critical. Nourishing food is the first foundation of a healthy pregnancy and a healthy life.

If you eat more frequently, you won't be as hungry when you get to the big meal, and that's a good thing. Do not let yourself get to the point of being ravenous. If you haven't eaten since noon and dinner's at 7:00, that is more than six hours to go without any food. You're going to be *so* hungry, and as a result your body is going to react hormonally in ways that make you feel off. It will be in a state of alarm and when you finally eat, it rushes to deliver the nutrients it's waited so long for to the places they're needed. You'll

likely feel faint or a bit jangly if you go that long without eating. Waiting too long to eat also leads to overeating because you waited too long and got too hungry.

Eating to Combat Morning Sickness

If you find that you experience nausea in the morning, it may be because your metabolism is surging, and your body is demanding calories during the night that simply aren't there. To combat this, prepare three tiny meals laden with complex proteins and healthy fats before you go to bed. It's important that these tiny meals are not just sugar-laden quick fixes. You should not just set aside three granola bars.

Consider making an extra portion of your dinner meal and portioning that into thirds. Eat one of the tiny meals just before bed, then set two alarms in the night. If you go to bed at 9:30, set your alarm for 1:30 a.m. and 5 a.m. Eat one of your prepared tiny meals at each of these times, so you are continually fueling your body with nourishing food. Most of my clients have found that this practice dramatically reduced or eliminated their morning sickness.

It's hard to wake up during the night. Most pregnant women are sleepy, they just don't want to get up. But I promise you, you are going to feel incredibly better if you make yourself do this. It is the key to not waking up feeling horrible in the morning.

This horrible morning sickness only lasts for about two months. Usually by the beginning of the second trimester you are over it and you can go back to your normal diet and your usual way of eating, and you

Aleah: I have had the great pleasure of having MariMikel, or "Mom" as I like to call her, as both my mother and midwife. She has also been one of the greatest teachers of my life and I have learned so much from her. I never thought I would follow in her footsteps but found myself drawn to work with her in my twenties. After a year of being her office manager, I realized I was missing all the most important, amazing, and interesting things that came with working for a midwife, so I started training as an apprentice midwife.

After an incredible five years, I chose to move in a different direction professionally and left my mom's practice to pursue a graduate degree in social work. I still work predominantly with women, children, and families. I always knew when the time came for me to have babies, it would be at home. My whole life I've been surrounded by information about pregnancy, labor, and birth. So, when I first got pregnant, I really thought that I would do so well. With my first baby I really didn't have any morning sickness. I was very lucky. It was an easy pregnancy, and honestly, enjoyable.

But when I got pregnant with my second it was super tough physically very early on for me. I had lost my social work job five days before I found out I was pregnant, which ended up being a gift from God, because within a week I was incredibly sick from the pregnancy to the point where I would not have been able to work for at least a month. I didn't necessarily throw up every day, but I felt so weak that I could barely move. It was incredibly challenging, especially with a two-and-a-half-year-old toddler at home. It was a physically and emotionally challenging time for me.

Of course, I knew what MariMikel would say about my morning sickness. I could hear her voice in my head every day. *You have to get up during the night and eat.* I understood her reasoning, but it sounded crazy to me. I already wasn't sleeping enough because I felt so bad, and she wanted me to set my alarm to go off two or three times a night, wake up when I felt terrible, and eat?! It sounded like torture. I dug my heels in the first few weeks, and I didn't do it. She'd check in on me and ask me if I was eating my tiny meals at night and I'd tell her "Yes, yes, yes, I'll do it I'll do it." But I didn't.

It got so bad that I finally said to myself, *Okay, nothing can be worse than this. I need to give mom's method a try.*

It pains the rebel in me to say it, but God she was so right. I remember starting to feel better within 24 hours. I would go downstairs, get the food, eat with my eyes half shut, and then within 5–10 minutes I was back upstairs in bed. I fell asleep again almost immediately. I have battled with insomnia for 20+ years, and I had worried that returning to sleep would be a struggle for me, but it wasn't. In the morning, like magic, I did not wake up feeling absolutely wretched. Other friends of mine and clients of hers have reported equally successful results with this method. I want to say that it's miraculous, but it's not. It makes sense. Twelve hours (from dinner to breakfast) is too long for a pregnant body to go without food. Those high hormones can really make you feel nauseated, especially if you're sensitive to them. It makes sense that you need to nourish yourself more often in the early months of pregnancy.

If you're feeling bad, it may feel a bit torturous to set your alarm clock and wake up in the middle of the night but take this advice and it will very likely help you too feel better too.

won't have to get up in the night, but right now, if you want to be okay, *you have got to get up in the night and eat.* If you eat at 7:00 p.m. and then you don't eat again until 7:00 a.m., that's twelve hours without any food. When you wake up in the morning and feel nauseated it's called morning sickness, but it's really hypoglycemia of pregnancy. The baby is taking so much out of you that your body can't keep up without frequent, small amounts of food. So many women wake up in the night and they think that because they can pee that they woke up because they needed to pee. The truth is that it's not about your bladder. It's about your baby being hungry and your body needing more nutrients to handle the needs of the baby, so let's make it easy.

I know it's hard to make yourself do this—no one wants to interrupt perfectly good sleep—but if you do, it will make an enormous difference in your morning sickness and your energy levels. Here are some tips for increasing your success in this endeavor. Have the food ready before you go to bed.

- You can have leftovers like I mentioned before.

- You could have brown rice or mashed potatoes cooked and left portioned out in containers in the refrigerator for you to quickly reheat. You can add cheddar and butter to the potatoes or butter and parmesan and tamari to the rice. This way your tiny meal will have the protein, fats, and complex carbs that you need to keep your blood sugar from dropping to the point where you feel nauseated.

- You could also have a sandwich prepared to eat a half or a quarter

of when you wake, but I don't recommend peanut butter, as it requires that you brush your teeth after eating it.

Brushing your teeth is a signal to your brain to wake up, so you don't want to brush your teeth during the night. I suggest you eat, swish your mouth with water, swallow it, and go back to bed. Try to keep the lights down low, don't turn on any music, and keep everything incredibly quiet. Do not look at blue light (i.e., cell phone, TV, computer screen). Eat quickly and return to bed.

This is the absolute trick to preventing morning sickness and it is imperative that you do it exactly this way. Again, it doesn't take very long before you're going to be past feeling like this and you won't have to do it at all, but right now eating to combat your symptoms is the key. You will sleep better. This method really works, but you have to make yourself do it. All right, good luck with this. You can do it!

Protein

You should be getting 75–100 grams of protein daily throughout your pregnancy. It helps to prevent blood pressure problems and is critical to the baby's muscle, organ, and brain development. Good sources of protein are grass-fed or pasture-raised meats, poultry, eggs, and dairy; low-mercury fish; nut butters; tofu and tempeh; and beans and rice in combination. I'm all for vegan, vegetarian, or macrobiotic diets, but it is more difficult to get enough protein to sustain your pregnancy on them. You do need to be very mindful.

One of the easiest ways to up your protein dramatically is to drink a protein shake every day. I suggest you start your day off with this special smoothie every morning.

I recommend NaturesPlus SPIRU-TEIN Protein Powder added to the smoothie (the vanilla flavor mixes well with berries, chocolate, and/or nut butters). All these ingredients are vital to your body, especially during pregnancy. They are also things that our diets are lacking even if you faithfully take vitamins every day and have the best possible diet. This smoothie gives you between 25–28 grams of protein and gets you off to a good start. Some of my clients love this as an afternoon snack, and that's perfectly fine as well.

Coconut oil contains medium chain fatty acids (as opposed to short or long chain fatty acids), which aid in digestion and are considered to be beneficial fats that enter your cells and are used immediately for energy as opposed to being stored as fat.[79] Buy cold processed, unfiltered, organic coconut oil. Costco is also a great place to find this.

Be a Snacker

I have a great idea to help you be a snacker. I want you to get up in the morning and put together a large smorgasbord of snacks to carry with you throughout your day. You never know what you're going to want. You can think *Oh, this will be great!* and then when it's time for a snack you can feel like *Oh my, I'll throw up if I even look at that,* so you want a smorgasbord of things so you can choose what's appealing to you in the moment.

Keep eating. Every 30 minutes to an hour put a few bites of something in your body. Not very much, just a few bites. You absolutely have to drag your smorgasbord of goodies around with you and eat something each and every hour. Again, it doesn't have to be much. Notice that it's important to combine your macros (if that works for you). Aim to have protein, carbs, and healthy fats in every snack. Check out the snack ideas in the Menu Planning Tool on page 38.

Eat Your Veggies

You want to get to a place by the end of your first trimester where a third of every meal you eat is made up of vegetables, including breakfast. There are lots of ways you can make this easier on yourself through advance preparation. Plan your meals and eat to your plan. For example, you can make my special spinach and store it in the fridge to add to a morning omelet or breakfast taco.

Healthy Fats

Fats are critical for you and your baby. Your brain is made of fat, every bit of it, and every nerve in your body is sheathed with a fatty coating called the *myelin sheath*, and so it is absolutely essential that you have good quality fats in your diet. What you want to avoid are trans fats and low-density fats. You also want to avoid vegetable oils, because they tend to oxidize at low temperatures, and oxidization is a factor in developing free-radical production in cells that can lead to cancer.

Sources of Good Fats
- Avocado oil
- Coconut milk
- Coconut oil
- Extra virgin, organic olive oil

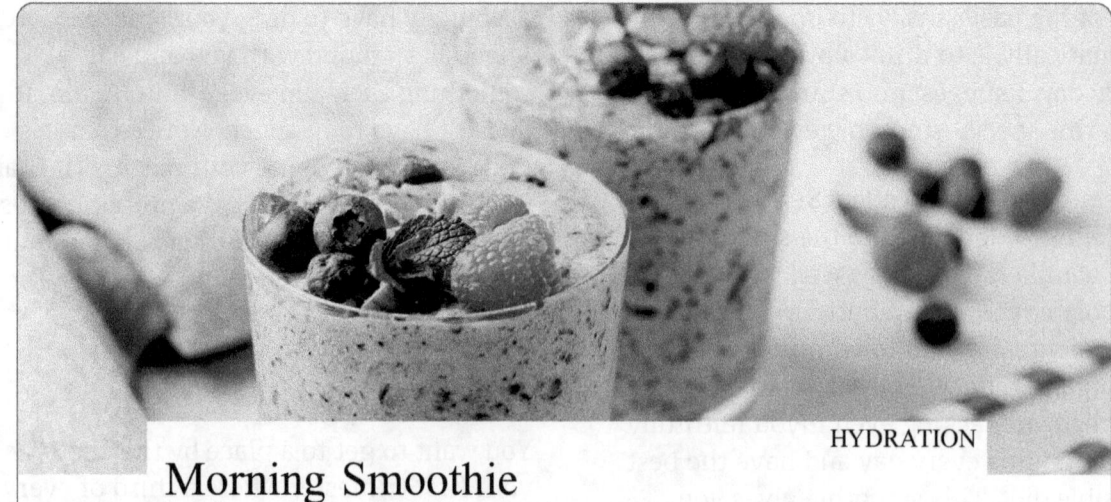

HYDRATION

Morning Smoothie

Once you are pregnant, I would love for you to start your day with this delicious smoothie.

INGREDIENTS

Organic milk/milk substitute or coconut water

1 ½ cups ice and 1 ½ cups fresh fruit
OR
3 cups frozen fruit

1 banana

1 Tbsp melted coconut oil
1 scoop protein powder (I use SPIRU-TEIN vanilla flavored protein powder)

For an added nutritional boost, add a scoop of Green Vibrance. It's so good for you and delicious, too!
Include your flax or chia seeds if you like as well.

DIRECTIONS

1. Mix all your liquid ingredients with ice and/or frozen fruit in the blender first, then, after they are fully combined, add your powders and the oil while the blender is still running. It is best to melt the oil before adding it to the smoothie so that it doesn't clump. Drink and enjoy!

Fruit can get expensive if you buy it fresh. Costco has an inexpensive brand of organic frozen fruit with blueberries, raspberries, and blackberries. It's difficult to wash pesticides off of berries, so make sure to buy organic whether fresh or frozen. Other fruits like bananas and oranges that you peel are usually okay to buy non-organic. Check the dirty dozen list before buying conventional fruits.

Sources of Fats to Use Moderately

These saturated fats used to be vilified, but science has not actually demonstrated a link between them and heart disease.[80] However, it is easier to put on excess weight by consuming too much of this kind of fat. All animal-based fats should be sourced from grass-fed, pasture-raised animals whenever possible. You can find resources for this in Appendix B.

- Grass-fed dairy
- Grass-fed butter
- Ghee
- Grass-fed lard
- Grass-fed tallow

Fats to Avoid

In general, you want to avoid trans fats and oils derived from vegetables and seeds with a few exceptions (see good fats, above). Trans fats are unsaturated fats that can raise your bad (LDL) cholesterol and lower your good (HDL) cholesterol.[81] An unfavorable cholesterol composition can lead to an increased risk of heart disease, stroke, and other health problems.

Seed and vegetable oils are often higher in omega-6 fatty acids, which can be harmful in excess, leading to inflammation.[82] That might sound tolerable, but inflammation is linked to a number of health issues like heart disease, cancer, depression, and autoimmune diseases. Seed and vegetable oils also are usually highly processed, meaning that they've been subjected to immense heat, pressure, and/or chemicals, which may damage the fatty acids and create harmful compounds.[83] These oils are also often made from genetically modified crops, and there is some concern that genetically modified foods may be harmful to human health.[84]

- Canola oil
- Corn oil
- Cottonseed oil
- Grapeseed oil
- Margarine
- Peanut oil
- Rapeseed oil
- Safflower oil
- Soybean oil
- Sunflower oil
- Animal fats from factory farmed animals (lard, ghee, tallow, butter, etc.)

Note that factory farmed animal fats will also have a higher omega-6 ratio than their grass-fed counterparts, which is why animal fats appear on two lists.

Vitamins and Supplements

I want you to keep doing exactly what you started in your conscious conception, plus one supplement, evening primrose oil. If you picked up this book after you became pregnant and you started with this chapter, read the Supplements section (starting on page 39), and immediately implement those recommendations.

Evening Primrose Oil

I started using evening primrose oil in my practice many decades ago when other, experienced midwives told me that it helps with labors that are seriously long due to the cervix not being fully ripe. If the cervix is not ripe/soft, it can make labor take days as opposed to hours. These midwives taught me that you can put evening primrose oil on the cervix to soften it. I began using it on my clients, and my gosh, it really worked!

Then I heard that evening primrose oil orally could help to soften a cesarean (or c-section) scar for a woman who was going to have a vaginal birth after cesarean (VBAC), and that it would help to prevent the very, very small risk of a uterine rupture during the VBAC, because the cesarean scar would have more give and stretchability.

I also heard that evening primrose oil orally would help to prevent the cramping of early pregnancy and most helpfully the cramping caused by the stretching of the round ligaments, which don't really do much in pregnancy besides stretch and cause discomfort for lots of women. And so, I started to have my clients who were experiencing ligament pain take it.

I then found that these women who took evening primrose oil in early pregnancy were more ready for labor, and had shorter and easier births, so now I recommend that all women take it throughout their pregnancies.

Unless you have bad hemorrhoids or serious varicosities, I'd like you to also start taking evening primrose oil now, at the beginning of your pregnancy. You can take it in capsule form as directed on the bottle. You'll likely start experiencing some cramping as your uterus grows and stretches in the early part of pregnancy. Evening primrose oil contains gamma-linolenic acid (GLA), an omega-6 fatty acid that softens those ligaments and the uterine muscle itself so there is less cramping

as you grow. It makes it so much more comfortable for you as it stretches. There is limited scientific investigation into evening primrose oil in pregnancy, but I have seen it help many hundreds of women personally with no adverse effects.

In addition to this early easing, the evening primrose oil will continue to help soften your vagina toward the end of the pregnancy, so you aren't as likely to tear, and the baby comes out more easily. It helps to keep the suture lines and fontanelle in the baby's head soft, so the head molds more easily to the shape of the pelvis and vagina, and it comes through without as much trauma to the baby.

If you have bad hemorrhoids or serious varicose veins, don't take the evening primrose oil until the end of your pregnancy. Consult your midwife or doctor. It may be that your cervix and vagina are soft already and you don't need assistance.

Natural Medicine Chest

During the early weeks of your pregnancy, I'd like you to work on completing your natural medicine chest so you have all the natural remedies on hand that can offer you relief during your pregnancy. Refer to the Natural Medicine Chest section on page 52 to see what's missing from your personal collection. You want to have these items on hand in case you experience the very common ailments and discomforts of pregnancy. It's no fun to be tracking down remedies when you're in pain or suffering through the worst of an illness. We'll talk about how to use the items you've been stockpiling in the Knowledge section of this and subsequent chapters.

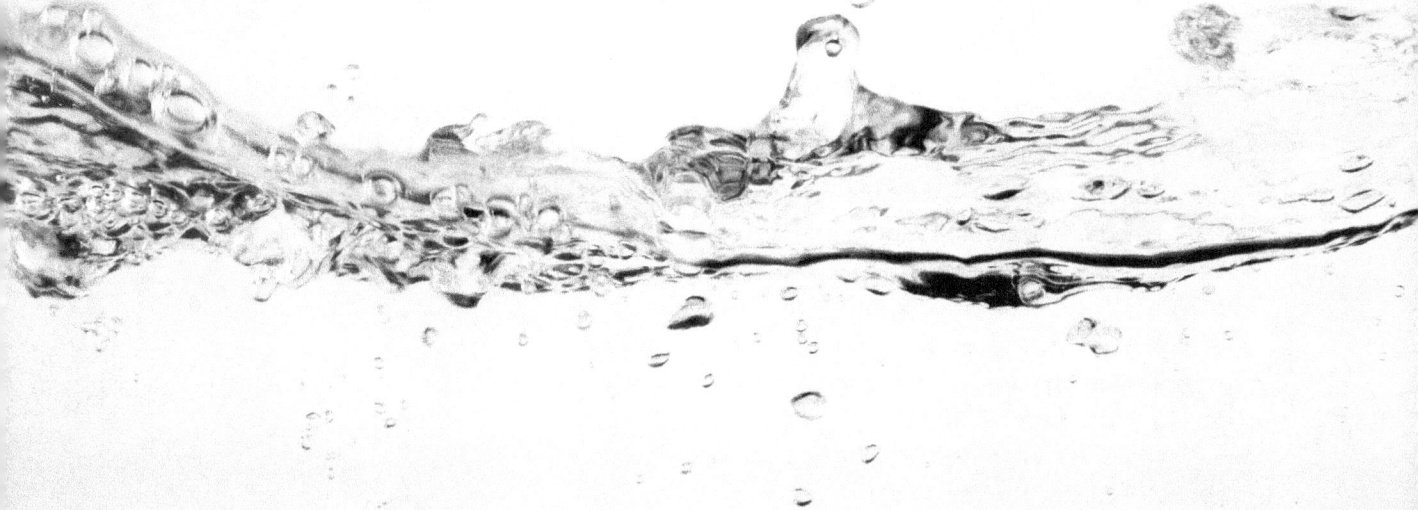

Hydration

 My recommendation for hydration remains constant. You absolutely need to be drinking four quarts of water every single day. Your baby needs it, too. So does your partner. Again, if you're picking up this book after you've conceived and you're starting here, go back to the Hydration section of the Conscious Conception chapter of this book to find my reasoning for this recommendation.

If you're struggling to implement this practice, set an alarm on your phone to go off every hour. Set sticky notes in places you visit often, like the bathroom mirror, your nightstand, on the refrigerator, at your desk, etc. Make sure you have something hydrating to drink close at hand at all hours of the day. It's easy to ignore the impulse to hydrate if you have to get up and go fill a glass in another room. Give yourself the right environment so that you are set up for success here.

Get your partner on board; they should be drinking as much as you are. Help each other. Remind each other. Encourage each other.

Overheating

You can easily get overheated by taking a shower or bath that's too hot, getting and/or staying in a hot tub that is too hot, going to a music or sporting event in the summer outside without enough hydration, working in the yard in the heat, or exercising in the heat. When you are pregnant you must not get overheated. You can damage the umbilical cord by getting overheated. Avoid situations where you might become trapped in a place that's too hot without respite.

When you are pregnant you must not get overheated.

Whenever you are in a hot situation, drink more fluids! Use a hat and umbrella for shade. Use sunscreen, too (that has less to do with overheating; it's just a good idea to help reduce your chances of skin cancer).

Penelope: I attended the Austin City Limits Music Festival when I was seven months pregnant with my first baby. I remember becoming separated from my friends and suddenly feeling overwhelmed by the crowd and the noise, and incredibly worried for my baby. I was worried about his poor little ears. I wrapped my arms around my belly and must have had an expression of panic on my face, because a darling woman tapped me on my arm and said, "Are you okay? I'm a nurse. I can help." I told her I was worried about my baby's hearing, and she told me confidently I didn't have to worry about that. She did say, "But you must stay hydrated and don't allow yourself to get overheated." Then she handed me a bottle of cold water.

There are definitely angels among us.

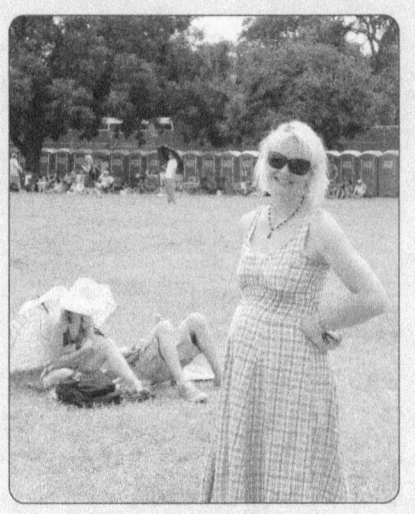

Penelope at ACL Fest

Pregnancy Tea

I'm including a recipe for Pregnancy Tea here that I encourage you to consume iced or hot as often as you like throughout your pregnancy. It is a uterine tonic that aids in building receptor sites for oxytocin in your uterus, so you can have an easier labor and birth.[85] Nothing in it will harm you or your baby when you consume it in greater quantities. It is mostly composed of red raspberry leaf and other natural herbs. Drinking a few cups a day will contribute to your gestational health and help lessen your pain and bleeding during birth. Keep some on hand in the fridge and drink it often throughout your pregnancy!

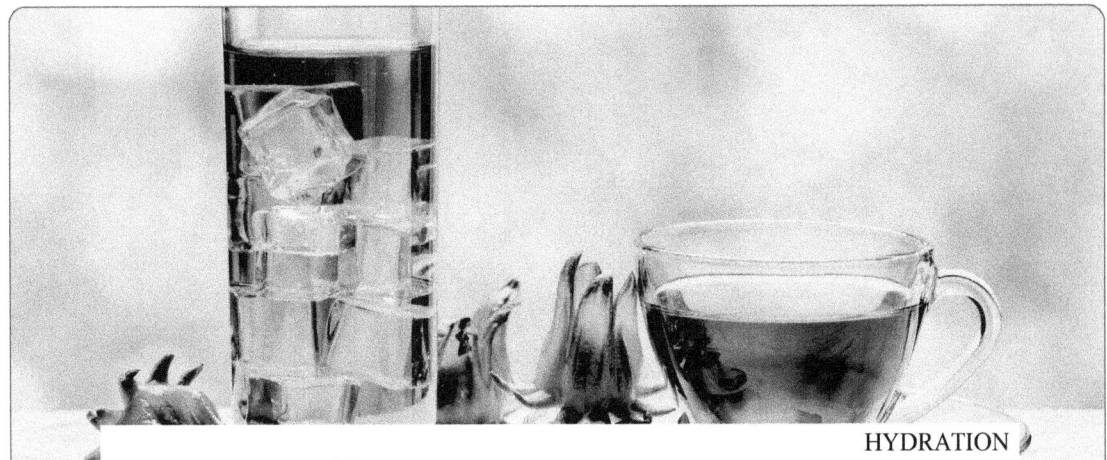

Pregnancy Tea

I have included a recipe below for Pregnancy Tea that you can consume iced or hot 2-3 times per day throughout your pregnancy. Red Raspberry leaf and pregnancy teas both tone the uterus and nothing here will harm you or your baby. Drinking a few cups a day will contribute to your gestational health and help lessen your pain and bleeding during birth. Keep some on hand in the fridge and drink it often throughout your pregnancy as well as postpartum to help build a healthy supply of milk!

INGREDIENTS

Red Raspberry Leaf
Contains vitamins A, B, and E, as well as calcium, phosphorous, iron, and is an acid neutralizer.

Stinging Nettles
Stinging nettles is a blood cleansing and blood building herb with high iron content. It is very nourishing to the kidneys and liver and will help relieve (or prevent altogether) vascular problems common during pregnancy. It also helps build a good milk supply.

DIRECTIONS

1. Combine one-part red raspberry leaf to one part stinging nettles.
2. Add some or all the optional herbs if desired.
3. A general rule of thumb is 1 tablespoon of herb to 1 cup water.
4. Place herbs in a non-metal container, preferably a half gallon mason jar, and cover the herbs with almost boiling water then cap tightly.
5. Let this steep for 4 to 6 hours. Pour mixture through a strainer and discard the herbs.

The tea will keep for up to 4 days if refrigerated. A small amount of fruit juice (grape, apple, raspberry) can be added as a sweetener if you like. There is no right or wrong way to make the tea. Experiment and find a mixture that works for you!

Add any of the following for variety:
Alfalfa: Contains vitamins A, B12, D, and E, as well as calcium and phosphorous. Great for the milk supply.
Rose Hip: Contains the entire vitamin C complex. Good for vascular problems (hemorrhoids and varicose veins) and to boost the immune system. Recommended for Rh negative women for fighting off infections.
Spearmint: Soothing to the stomach, helps digestion and lends a pleasant taste to the mixture. A little goes a long way. If you are taking homeopathic remedies, you should leave the spearmint out while the remedies are still active as spearmint can antidote some homeopathic remedies.
Red Clover: This blood purifying herb can be added from time to time. It is especially good during acute illness and for high blood pressure.

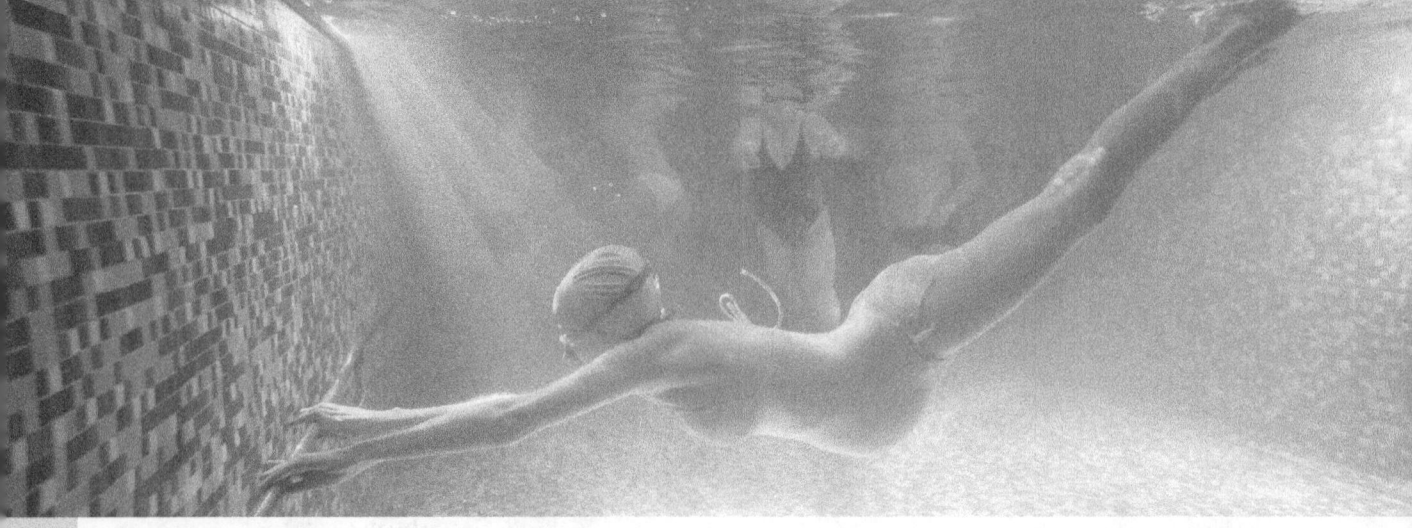

Movement

I advise that you **don't** exercise in early pregnancy. Yes, even if you are someone who absolutely loves to work out. I know that exercise is a fantastic and vital part of many women's lives, and an important part of a healthy self-care routine. If you are one of these women, I promise you we'll get back to it soon.

Most women experience some fatigue in early pregnancy, though, and they're what I often refer to as *low ebb*. Their energy is on the wane for now, and it's not going to get better for a short while. This common low-ebb state, I believe, is an ancient biological safety mechanism to prevent you from overdoing it and miscarrying. If you are too tired to get up off the floor of your hut to carry many pounds of water up the hill, you're less likely to strain yourself and lose your baby.

To compensate, the tribe stepped up to help their pregnant members. They helped during early pregnancy and took over some of the load, and then helped the woman at the end of the pregnancy and after she gave birth so she could rest and stay down while she healed and bonded with her newborn.

Now we don't even acknowledge that women *should* stay down after birth. I'm acknowledging it here and now. I'm introducing this to you early on because I want you to rest and stay down in your bed for two weeks after you give birth. It's helpful for you to know that now so you can begin to plan for it. You'll need physical support, meals on hand, and more. I cover this in depth in *The Book of Birth, Volume II*. For now, know that it is absolutely best that you stay down in your bed for at least two weeks after you give birth.

To sum up: do not exercise early on, in the first ten to twelve weeks. There is a very dynamic, mystical, magical creation going on in your body and it is taking a lot out of you. Rest and give over to it.

Breathe.

> To sum up: do not exercise early on, in the first ten to twelve weeks. There is a very dynamic, mystical, magical creation going on in your body and it is taking a lot out of you. Rest and give over to it.

Build Up Your Core

I do want you to build up your core so you can more effectively push your baby out and so you don't split your stomach muscles too far apart during the pregnancy. In the early days this won't seem to make a difference, but when you get really pregnant the stomach muscles may split some; you can mitigate this with preparation.

I'm asking for 30 seconds twice a day, morning, and evening. What you do is lie on your back, bring your knees up slightly pointed toward the ceiling with your feet flat on the floor, then rock your pubic bone up and tilt the bottom of your pelvis up to flatten your back against the floor as much as you can. Put each hand on the opposite side of your abs, pull them slightly to your center, and hold these muscles together.

It is important to keep your head and spine in alignment while you do these abdominal crunches. Do not try to jerk yourself up with your head. That would be a neck crunch, not an abdominal crunch. Your eyes should be looking up at the ceiling and should stay locked on a single point. This ensures that you are using your abs.

Once your hands are in place, use your stomach muscles to lift your breastbone, bringing your ribs toward your hip bones. You're just bringing your shoulder blades up off the ground and crunching your abdominal muscles. You do not have to rise up more than a few inches off the floor. Bring your clavicles (shoulder blades) off the floor. Then relax.

You can do 25 of these abdominal crunches pretty quickly. If you do 25 in the morning and 25 in the evening, that's 50 abdominal crunches a day. Girlfriend, do this every day and you are going to have abs of steel by the time you have your baby, and you are going to bounce back from the pregnancy quickly. The hard part is remembering to do it. I recommend putting a sticky note on your bedside lamp with "ABS" written on it to remind you or set a reminder on your phone to go off twice daily.

For those of you who might be a little bit addicted to exercise and are perhaps dismayed at my advice to stop for a few months, you might be excited to go above and beyond with this abs exercise and do more than 25 at a time. Do not do this. Respect that your baby needs that energy. Limit yourself to 25 in the morning and 25 in the evening.

Practice Getting Up Properly for Late Pregnancy

I want you to start getting up and down out of bed correctly now so by the time you are carrying serious weight, and your abs are beginning to separate, this practice will be natural to you.

When getting into bed, roll on your side using your arms to lower yourself down to your bed and then roll to your back.

When you rise, push off with your arms and use your arms to lift your body—not your stomach muscles. This motion is inconsequential at 9 weeks but by 20 weeks it's going to be really important for you to get up and down correctly, and if you begin to practice this movement now, it will be second nature when you need it.

Take Care

Avoid anything that causes an impact like jumping on a trampoline, jumping rope, snow skiing, snowboarding, waterskiing, jet skiing, horseback riding, jogging, running, rock climbing, and bicycling because of risk of injury due to a fall or collision.

Impact can dislodge the placenta and cause bleeding or even cause the loss of the baby. Avoid scuba diving due to the increased pressure experienced at depth.

Hopefully, you're seeing the pattern of no jumping. It can dislodge the baby and increases the risk of miscarriage. This doesn't mean a fall will automatically result in a miscarriage. I've known women to fall out of trees or ladders and then lost their babies, and I've known others who took similar horrible tumbles, and they and their babies were just fine. I've known women who've gone scuba diving before they knew they were pregnant, and their babies were just fine. You never know, so you want to be conscientious. Choose caution.

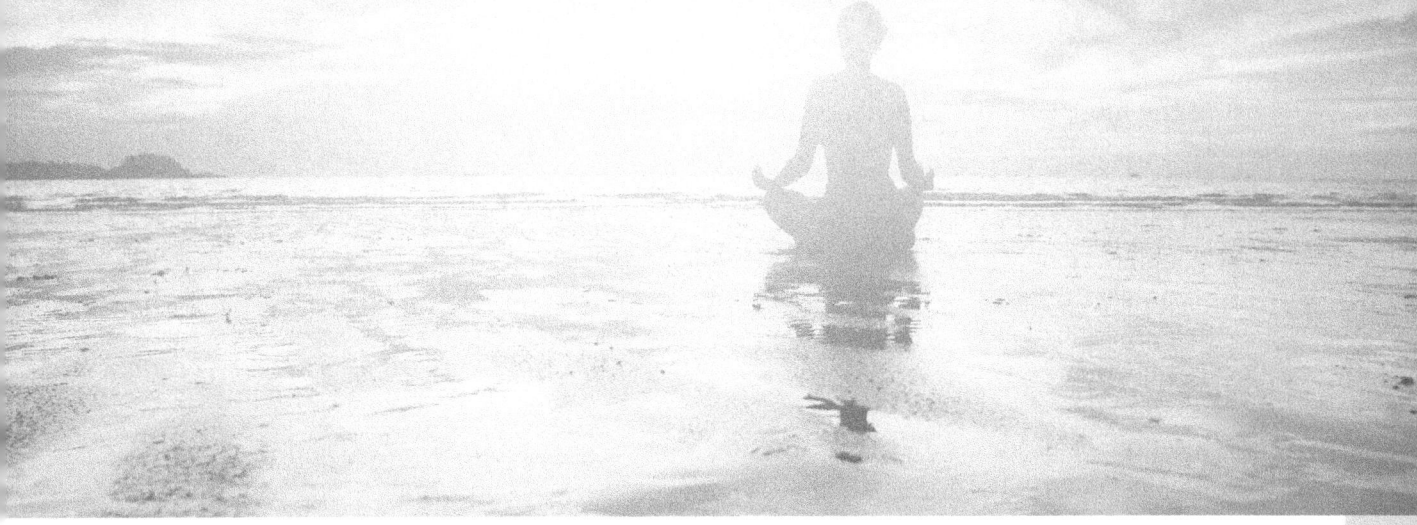

Emotional/Spiritual

In early pregnancy, your psyche pulls down all your defenses and suddenly you are very, very emotional, and very vulnerable, and very easily happy, irritated, scared, and on and on. I have seen it over and over again. Know that this is normal. Partners also especially need to come to understand this, because our society in general does not talk about early pregnancy (or women's issues) and what you may be going through. We need to do a better job of recognizing there's a reason for this storm of sensitivity.

The truth is that it is so hard to be pregnant. All your vitality goes to the growing baby and the body changes you're experiencing are enormous. This is a really big deal. Partners, give your woman a break! And women, do not use this condition as an opportunity to beat up your partner; it is not his fault. You want to build bridges, because you will be working together on all of this—during the pregnancy, during the birth, and very much while you raise

your child. Learning skills to navigate emotionally fraught times together will serve you well.

Once you are pregnant, you may burst into tears at the slightest provocation. This is so normal. It is a function of your body rebalancing itself. Many people think we cry only when we're sad, and of course this can be a reason for crying, but our tears are connected to our nervous system. They are a part of our body's natural ability to regulate itself. Researchers have found oxytocin and endorphins in tears.[86] Crying is a parasympathetic approach to leaving fight or flight and returning your body to a state of homeostasis. When your hormones are surging, crying is a natural response. It's almost like you're subconsciously seeking that release.

Pregnancy and birth can bring up deeper levels of your psyche for you to work on. We have powerful defense mechanisms that we unconsciously use to deal with trauma and confusion in our lives. Here's a list of the more common mechanisms we employ.

- Transference
- Sublimation
- Denial
- Repression
- Projection
- Regression
- Rationalization
- Reaction formation
- Compartmentalization
- Intellectualization

Your defense mechanisms create a sense of safety for you, but it's often a mask. With pregnancy's stripping of your emotional layers, you can go deep enough that you no longer have to hide from these issues or be tormented by them. This presents an amazing opportunity for healing.

This emotional turbulence seems to be a little bit more profound in the early part of pregnancy. Some of that is that you may be recognizing that your life is irrevocably changed, and you are going to be somebody's mommy. Everything will be different, and there's really no going back now. You know, that's wonderful and slightly terrifying at the same time.

It's natural for your mental monkey voices to freak out a little during this time. If you are a first-time mom, this is all brand new. Your body is doing things it's never done before, and on a subconscious level you may be crying out, *What is happening?* In these instances, talk to your nervous system as though it were a young child. "Thanks for letting me know how scared you are. I know everything's a little strange right now, but it's all going to be okay. Women have been

The universe conspires to create life through you, a vessel of divine expression, bringing forth the next chapter of existence.

—Deepak Chopra

doing this for millennia and this is my birthright. These strange feelings won't last forever. I can do this."

Remind yourself what the truth is, and how incredibly miraculous and wonderful it is that you're growing this baby. Know that you are doing an excellent job taking care of yourself and the baby. *Yes, it's new and different. Yes, it's all going to be okay.* This is a profoundly emotional experience, and you are riding its waves.

Accepting that this is a normal part of pregnancy is the first step. Keep strong with your supplement regimen. The B vitamins especially will help you to navigate the stress of these choppy waters.

Other natural aids include chamomile tea, passionflower tincture taken occasionally, and minimal amounts of lobelia and valerian are acceptable in pregnancy— moderate amounts occasionally. Each of these promotes restfulness. Consult your midwife or naturopath before using these.

If you struggle under the weight of these emotions and thoughts, seek help from a therapist, counselor, or repatterning practitioner. Pregnancy is a great time for healing, forgiving, and letting go.

Your Partner's Role

First, I want to acknowledge that it is not required that your supportive, wonderful partner in the birth process be your life partner, husband, or wife. You may have a partner who does not want to participate, is not available for whatever reason, or you may not have a partner at all. It's perfectly fine to have somebody else serve in this support role. This person could be a dear friend or family member who loves you and wants to be there for you through the pregnancy, birth, and early part of your postpartum period. It could be a team of a few of your closest friends.

All that matters is the person you choose is committed to helping you with this process, and that you feel safe, loved, and supported by them. The person you choose will need to be available to help you with childbirth classes, preparation for the birth, and be available to be at the birth whenever it happens! You also need support after the birth for a few days to a few weeks.

I also want to recognize that not all partners are male gendered. Because of this I have deliberately chosen to refer to your primary support person as "your partner" rather than as "the dad." We have chosen the pronoun "he/him" because of the masculine role this person plays, regardless of their gender. No matter what your gender may be, if your partner is pregnant and you are taking on the role as her main support person through the pregnancy, labor, and birth, and postpartum period these things apply to you as well. All families are beautiful, and I respect and support all choices when it comes to love. If you are both happy and healthy together, that is genuinely all I care about.

Throughout history, men have been sidelined (sometimes by choice) when it comes to pregnancy and parenting. In recent years we have been forging a new way for men, and all partners, to be a more integral and integrated part of the process. They are vital and important in the family. Partners are able to take on tasks and accomplish things within the family unit that might be more difficult (or even physically impossible) for a woman to do during pregnancy. We should respect each other, we should acknowledge each other,

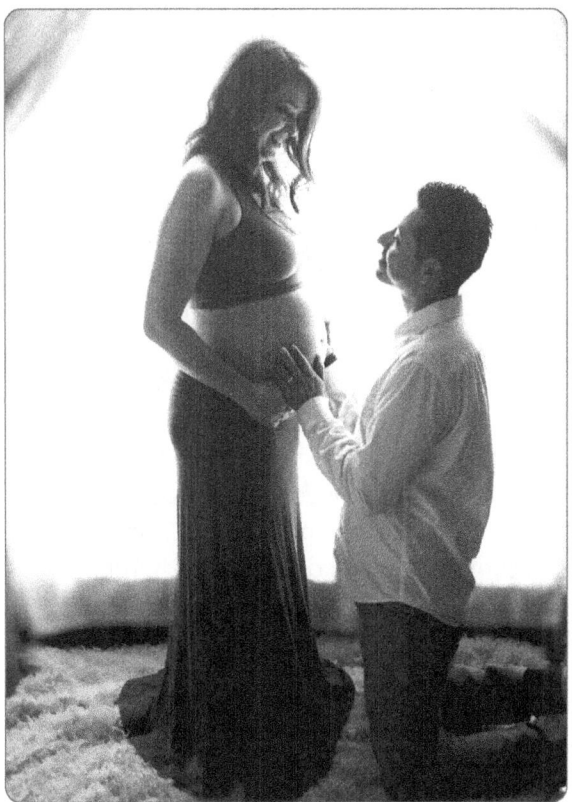

A Partner's Support Is Invaluable

we must hold each other in esteem and support one another. In this new, more egalitarian world, men (and all partners regardless of gender) deserve a role in the pregnancy and birth process. Lean on them; allow them to help you.

Partners, the caveat is that you have got to show up. You've got to be present and engaged in this process. Being pregnant is a two-person job. Whenever possible, I encourage you to attend prenatal visits together. Understand what she's going through. Read the books she's recommending. Ask her how she's doing and ask her what she's struggling to implement. Ask if you can help. Help her through it. Keep her nourished and hydrated. For now, find your better self, bite your tongue when you are frustrated, and be as supportive as humanly possible.

One of the reasons I ask that you both attend prenatal visits is that there is often an incredible amount of new information delivered during these visits, and it is a lot for one person to digest. Between the two of you, you'll retain more. Partners, it's important that you learn the information too. There's no way your pregnant woman is ever going to be able to convey everything that's going on at her appointments, and she needs your support. To properly support her, you need to be informed. Plus, there's something about an authority figure telling you what to do. Your midwife may be repeating exactly what your pregnant partner has been saying, but now you're somehow better able to hear the importance of it.

There is a lot to remember, and when you function as a team, you can make all these lifestyle changes happen, or at least a lot of them.

Remember, the more connected you are to one another, the better the birth will go. You must step into your role as her major support system and as a real partner in this process. It's especially important for you to work on your connection during the pregnancy, and I will give you tips for how to do that throughout this book. For now, work to attend prenatal visits with her. Read what she's recommending. Listen to her. Relieve her anxieties, her fears, her worries, and help with her pain. You are her rock.

Strategies for Navigating Emotional Turmoil

I want you to continue to combat the stress triggers in your life and engage in activities that shed your residual stress. Every emotional and physical state that we have has hormonal components to it, and these hormonal biochemical components imprint on your baby. Your body does not know the difference between bad traffic, demanding work projects, worldwide trauma, and the Mongol hordes marching up the valley to disembowel your tribe. To the body, stress is stress. You want to have less of it. It's super important.

During the COVID-19 pandemic, I had a 25 percent home-to-hospital transport rate, which was extremely high for me, the highest in fact it has ever been. I think that everyone was so collectively stressed out from what was going on in the world that their bodies generally had a harder time. There were more complications. It's so incredibly important to recognize and manage stress throughout your pregnancy.

Noticing

This is when you can start to pay more attention to what you are feeling in your body. Most women don't feel a thing until suddenly at Week 6 they are laid low. Pay attention to your body. Listen to when it's telling you that it's hungry or thirsty. Listen to when it's telling you that you need to rest, lie down, or sleep. Listen to when it's telling you it needs to stop whatever you're doing and do nothing or do something else.

Think Positively

It is important to expect the best. Some of the techniques you can use to change negative thoughts to positive thoughts are affirmations, visualizations, prayer, meditation, mindfulness, and conversations with family, friends, spiritual leaders, and caregivers. If you started with this chapter because you were already pregnant, you can revisit these sections in the Conscious Conception chapter of this book for a full explanation of any concept you're not familiar with.

Breathe Deeply

If we can control our breath, we can control our mind, and if we can control our mind, we can control our body. When we choose to consciously breathe slowly and in a controlled manner in through the nose, with full awareness of our lungs and body, we can then breathe out slowly through the mouth into relaxation and elevate our parasympathetic state. Each controlled breath that we take in through the nose and out through the mouth can reset some of the alarms in our nervous system. It can give us a sense of control and calm, as well as proper balancing of our oxygenating

Partners,

Your woman needs tenderness right now. Shower her with gentleness and love. Nurture her. Nourish her body, heart, and spirit. Understand that she is the vessel for a miracle, and miracles take energy.

I remember once, when my children were little and I was pregnant again, my husband turned to me and said, "You know what? You are just so mean. You're mean as a snake. I don't know what to do with you."

I took a moment to breathe and then replied, "I just want to point out that your body is not being occupied by an alien. You don't have to get stretch marks from your nose to your knees. You don't have to be completely crazy with hormones that you can't do anything about, and you don't have to have a cantaloupe come out of a hole that's normally the size of a penny. All you have to do is endure me and my mood swings. I'm doing all of this for us, and for all my sacrifices, you get progeny."

He looked at me and he said, "You know, babe, I had not thought about it like that."

So, no, your woman cannot do anything about the crazy. No, she doesn't like it. She would love to not be crazy, but for now, it is what it is. It will get better.

system. This control can take us out of the anxiety of living in a fight or flight state and give us the calm and comfort of living in a healthier balance with our state of rest and rejuvenation.

A nice, easy place to start is a slow breath in through the nose for four seconds with a slight pause at the top of the inhale, followed by a four second exhale with a slight pause at the bottom. Modify and repeat as necessary.

Practice deep breathing at least a few times a day. Use an app like Calm to guide you through a two-minute session in the morning and evening. As with all new routines, set a reminder on your phone or calendar to help you cement the practice in place.

I'm going to teach you a more in-depth breathing practice to help deepen your breath and let go of stress in your body. Find a comfortable, quiet place and start by taking a deep breath in through the nose and out through the mouth. Completely fill your lungs and connect the inhale to the exhale. Equalize the inhale and the exhale. Try to fully breathe into your diaphragm (below your chest/lungs and above your abdominal organs) and fully exhale each time. As you breathe in, your stomach should rise and your chest should stay still.

Once you have your breath down, envision a circle of white light coming in with every inhale and darkness, fear, tension, and pain leaving you with every exhale. Now we're going to work through your body and bathe you in this healing light. It can be helpful to introduce tension by clenching the body part on the inhale and then really let go and relax that part of the body on the exhale.

Start with your toes. Wiggle your toes. As you breathe in visualize white light coming in and bathing the tissues of your toes, the balls of your feet, and the soles of your feet, then your heels, the top of your feet, and your ankles.

Move on into your legs. Continue breathing in a deep, slow rhythm.

Relax your shins, relax your calves, relax the backs of your knees. Relax your kneecaps, your thighs, and the backs of your thighs.

Relax your buttocks, your vagina, your rectum.

Relax your intestines and the organs in your abdomen. Relax your stomach muscles and the intercostal muscles between your ribs.

Relax your fingers, the palms of your hands, the backs of your hands. Relax your wrists, arms, and elbows.

Relax your shoulders. Move your attention to your neck and move your head and shoulders until you can feel the muscles there. Let each of them go in turn.

Relax your chin, your jaw, your lips, your mouth.

Relax your cheeks. Relax your eyebrows, your forehead, your ears, your scalp.

When you get to the top of your head, envision the white light shooting out of it and your entire body bathing in the white light of divine love, peace, and goodness. Enjoy it. This is a lovely meditation. I have done it often enough now that even if I only have a very short time, I can ripple through this relaxation exercise. You will find that once you build this relaxation muscle memory, your results will also come in a shorter period.

i have been a thousand different women

Emory Hall

make peace
with all the women
you once were.

lay flowers
at their feet.

offer them incense
and honey
and forgiveness.

honor them
and give them
your silence.

listen.

bless them
and let them be.

for they are the bones
of the temple
you sit in now.

for they are
the rivers
of wisdom
leading you toward
the sea.

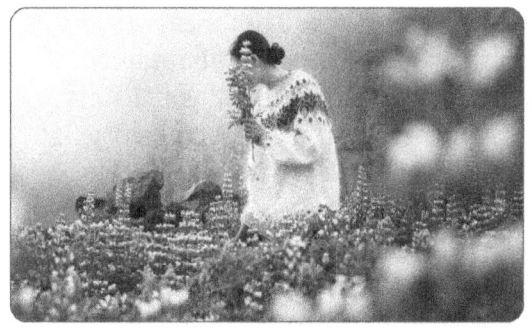

I Have Been a Thousand Different Women

Counseling

If you have any emotional or spiritual issues in your life or relationship, get counseling. Pregnancy is an amazing time for healing. It is easier to get to issues, forgive, forget, and resolve. These things can affect your pregnancy, birth, and postpartum experiences, and your relationship with the baby. If you are having difficulties in your relationship with your partner, that can be a big problem. Use this time to heal and move forward.

Avoid Sources of Fear and Images of Violence

Don't watch horror films or movies filled with violence and despair, and don't read scary books. I truly believe anything deeply upsetting can affect the baby, even if you think it's all in good fun. There is an energy to it that is not healthy for the developing baby. Many pregnant women find themselves more sensitive to violent content on TV, in movies, and on the news. Cut these out of your life for now. If you are a news junkie, ask someone you trust to tell you if something important happens, but otherwise tune it all out for a few months.

This goes for negative input from people, too. Every pregnant woman runs into friends, family, or acquaintances who want to tell them a terrible story about birth. When someone begins to tell you a story, stop them and ask if it's a happy story. If it's not, politely ask them to stop. Their story has *nothing* to do with your birth, and there's no reason to listen to it.

You are vulnerable in pregnancy, and you have to stop people from undermining your sense of confidence and peace in this process. The terrible things that happened to them may have happened because they didn't have enough information to make wonderful, informed choices and to implement practices in their pregnancy that might have ensured a different outcome. You are not them. Hold this boundary. Be firm!

People often tell you their stories about birth because they want validation. They want people to make the same choices they made so they can also feel good about what might not have turned out to be the best experience. They want reassurance that there couldn't have been another outcome. But their story is not your story. This is a boundary you need to set and hold, for you and your baby's sake.

Access Your Intuition

Merriam-Webster defines intuition as

1a: the power or faculty of attaining to direct knowledge or cognition without evident rational thought and inference

b: immediate apprehension or cognition

c: knowledge or conviction gained by intuition

2: quick and ready insight.

While I believe there is no single definition of intuition that is universally accepted, there are a few common elements that are often associated with intuition including non-conscious processing, rapidity, and accuracy. Intuition occurs without our conscious awareness. This is why we often say we have a "gut feeling" or a "hunch," as if the information is coming from a part of our mind that we are not consciously aware of. Intuition can also often lead to quick and decisive action. This is because we do not have to spend time consciously reasoning through the information. Instead, we can simply trust our gut and act on our intuition. Intuition can be surprisingly accurate as well, sometimes more accurate than conscious reasoning. It is important to use our intuition in conjunction with other sources of information to make the best possible decisions.

There is a growing body of research on intuition. Scientists are trying to understand how intuition works and how it can be used to make better decisions. Some researchers believe that intuition is based on pattern recognition. Our brains are constantly collecting and analyzing information, even when we are not consciously aware of it. This information is stored in our subconscious mind, and it can be used to make quick and accurate decisions. Other researchers believe that intuition is based on emotions. Our emotions can provide us with valuable information about the world around us. For example, if we feel a sense of danger, it may be because our intuition is telling us that something is wrong.

Whatever the mechanism behind intuition, it is a powerful tool that can be used to make better decisions. As you embark

Penelope: Intuition leads to flash insights that many would just call a gut feeling or hunch. The best description of this I've ever seen came from a fellow homesteader. She was walking in the fields one morning after a rainstorm and saw a cow's hoofprint. A chain of events flashed through her mind. The storm had knocked out the power. The electric fence went down. The cow got out. They needed to find her. All these insights hit her in a rush the moment she saw the hoofprint. She found the cow in a neighbor's field an hour later. Learn to listen to these insights.

on this spiritual journey to motherhood, engage your intuition. Listen to your inner voice. When you are making a decision, ask yourself, "What is my gut telling me?"

Affirmations

You can see my advice for implementing affirmations in your life in the previous chapter on page 72. Revisit your affirmations now that you are pregnant. Consider changing them to affirmations that will serve you now. Remember to choose something that you might not yet quite believe, something that is a bit of a stretch for you.

Sample Affirmations for Pregnancy

- Pregnancy is natural, normal, healthy, vibrant, and safe for me and my baby.

- My body is part of me and does everything in its power to support and protect me, therefore, my body is a safe place and a pleasurable place for my baby.

- I can communicate with the spirit that wants to come through me during my pregnancy.

- The universe loves me and supports me and my baby.

- Pregnancy is my birthright as a woman, and I fully nourish and support my body so my baby will be healthy and happy.

Timing Your Announcement

It can bring great joy to share the news of your coming newborn with your loved ones, but I encourage you to think a bit about when you will tell everyone that you're pregnant. With one of my babies, I had told everyone I was pregnant when I was six weeks along, and then when I miscarried it felt like the whole world knew I had been pregnant. Everywhere I went people would ask how my pregnancy was going, and it was a constant, painful reminder. I don't recommend that. I suggest you wait until you are at least 8–12 weeks along or you have heard the heartbeat—or when you feel ready—to announce to the world at large, social media, etc.

There may be a few key people you'll want to tell earlier, especially if early pregnancy is rough for you—like your boss and your other closest support people. Your boss will likely be more understanding of late mornings and earlier departure times from the office if they know you are pregnant. Your support people can and will up their game and help you out if you ask them to. Many women find it best to only share with family they are close with and their best friends at first. If they do miscarry, this circle of loving people can bring invaluable support.

When Will My Baby Be Born?

Birth Date and Due Range

Seventy percent of my clients give birth between Week 41 and 42, and some studies have shown that normal gestation can be as long as 42–44 weeks.[87]

The current insistence on a 40-week gestational period is another reason for our high levels of intervention in this country. You aren't "late" if Week 41 rolls around. You're very normal, and I want you to know that in your bones, so no one else's fear or ideas of "normal" can fill your mind at the end of your pregnancy.

In our society where nutrition is not supported, taught, and capitalism often drives down the quality of available food, the placenta may not be healthy enough to maintain the baby safely for 41 or 42 weeks. There is a small, increased incidence of stillbirth after 42 weeks, but you must take into consideration the mother's health and nutritional status. I trust that you are taking extremely good care of yourself, so your baby and your placenta are and will continue to be beautifully healthy.

The first day of your period is known as Day One of your cycle. Every doctor and app and pregnancy wheel in the world says that your

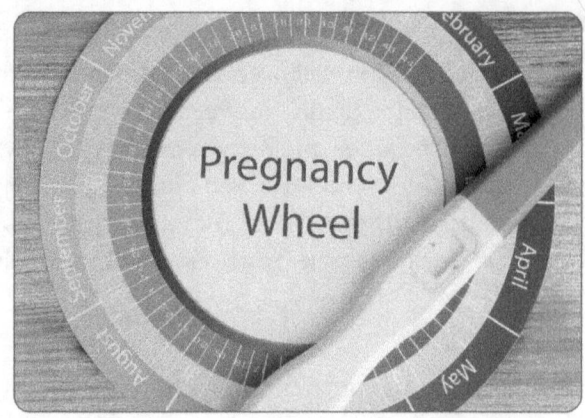

Due Date Calculator

due date is based on the misguided idea that every single woman on the planet will ovulate exactly 14 days after the first day of her period. Well, we know not all women's bodies ovulate this way. There are too many other factors involved: emotional, spiritual, intellectual, physical, and hormonal. So, assuming that the due date is correct just because the wheel or app says so is a big problem. It leads to an enormous amount of difficulty around the birth because of people not being willing to trust that the body knows what it's doing. Most healthy bodies know when to give birth.

When you do share your happy news, I highly encourage you to tell your friends and family that you are having the baby somewhere over a three-week period, from one week before the due date to up to two weeks after. It is a *due range*. Babies come on their birthday not their due date.

Babies come on their birthday not their due date.

Scientific research has finally shown what midwives have been saying for decades: when your baby is ready to be born, its body will send a hormonal signal to your body that will initiate your labor.[88] Not all babies gestate at the same rate. I have seen women who consistently gave birth at 38 weeks and their babies looked 41 weeks old. I have also seen babies who were born after Week 42 and looked to be about 38 or 39 weeks old. I like to tell these women that their oven is on a different temperature, and not every little muffin bakes at the same rate. The baby, the mother's body, and her psyche work together to pick the perfect moment for the baby to appear and it's not supposed to be scheduled—except when truly necessary.

When your baby is ready to be born, its body will send a hormonal signal to your body that will initiate your labor.

When armed with only a due date, people may begin to harass you if you have not produced the heir at the appointed moment and will call you incessantly, most of them very well meaning, asking you, "Haven't you had that baby yet? Is something wrong? Why hasn't the baby come yet? What are they going to do about it?"

It is already so hard to wait for your sweet baby, and it can be so much more challenging to hear things that make you feel like you are not performing to someone's expectations. If you do enough groundwork, you won't have this problem. Don't give in and provide people with a firm date. So, again, I urge you to tell people it is a due range, from one week before to up to two weeks after your due date, but (since you are taking such excellent care of yourself and your baby) much more likely in the two weeks after. At the perfect time.

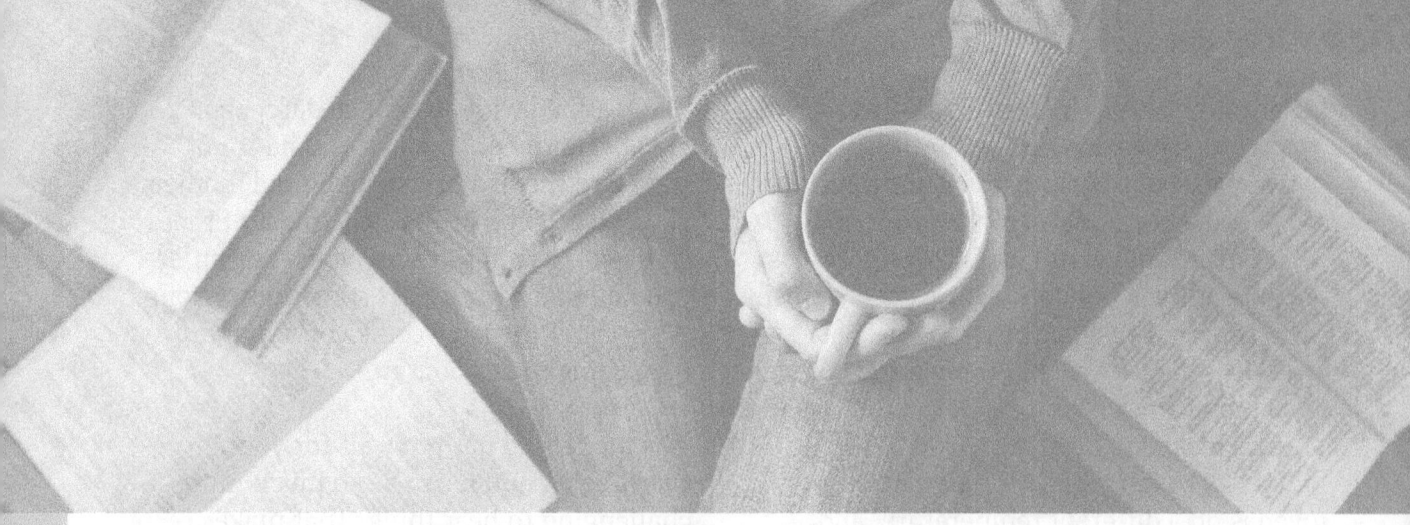

Knowledge

On the intellectual level, information that you gather ahead of time puts your mind at ease, so you can let go of your head and move into your heart and body, which is where labor and birth really happen. Knowledge helps to banish fear. Most people have so little information about what goes on in pregnancy and they are ignorant of how incredibly hard it is, especially in the beginning, at the end, and right after the

baby comes, so let's talk about what's going on in your body and how to mitigate the difficulties and discomforts of these early months.

What's Going on in My Body?

You begin having contractions from the moment of implantation and continue to

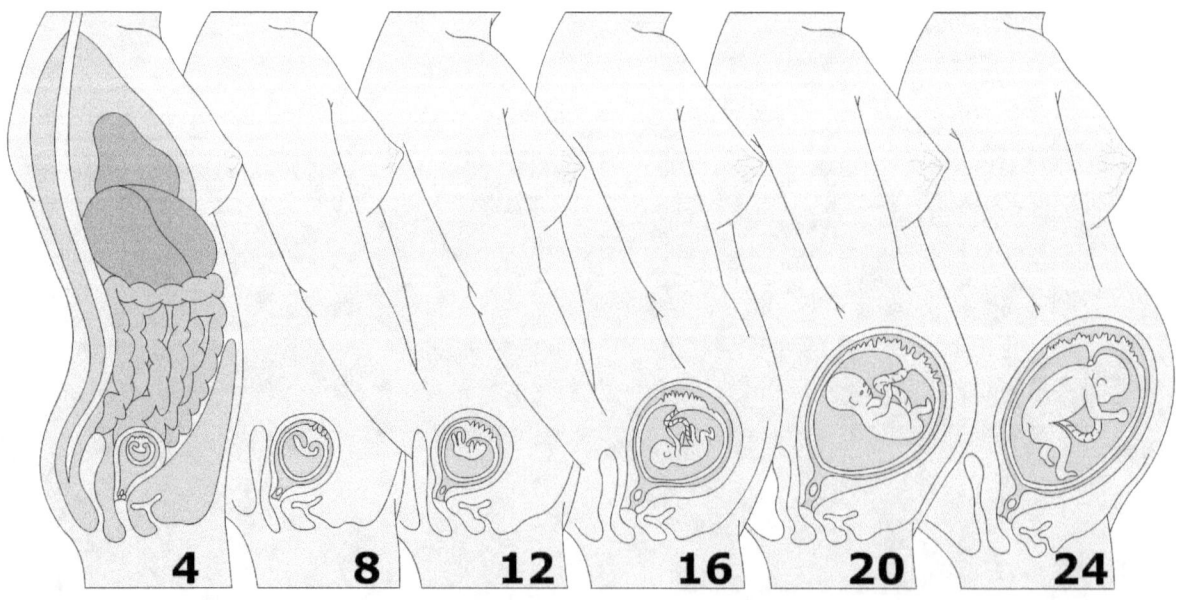

do so every five to ten minutes throughout your entire pregnancy. In the early days, your uterus tightens up, but there are no sensations from the contractions. It's usually not until later that you can really recognize contractions. If you have been pregnant before you may notice contractions as early as 12 weeks. With a first baby it may not be until 30 weeks that you notice them.

There's no pain with these early contractions, but they serve to prepare your body for birth. Over the course of your pregnancy, your uterus goes from being a six-ounce organ the size of a plum to four-and-a-half pounds (the size of a cantaloupe). These isometric exercises build the muscle mass of your uterus, so it can pull the cervix open and then push the baby through the pelvis and vagina.

In addition to preparing the uterine muscle, these contractions also prepare your baby

for the stress of labor. The baby needs to be gently and increasingly stressed through the whole pregnancy or labor would kill them. There is extreme force exerted on the baby during labor as your uterus contracts around the baby. It's tremendous pressure, and these practice contractions prepare your baby for that, too.

Very rarely, there can be problems with the fold during gastrulation, and cleft palate, cleft lip, and facial deformities can occur. This fold happens when you are four to five weeks pregnant—very early on considering that conception typically takes place at two weeks. As discussed in Conscious Conception, methylfolate supplements are your best defense against these deformities. Continue to take it throughout your pregnancy. Also, avoid the use of chemical agents or radiation, photography darkroom work laboratory work, x-ray work, and the like, especially in these early weeks.

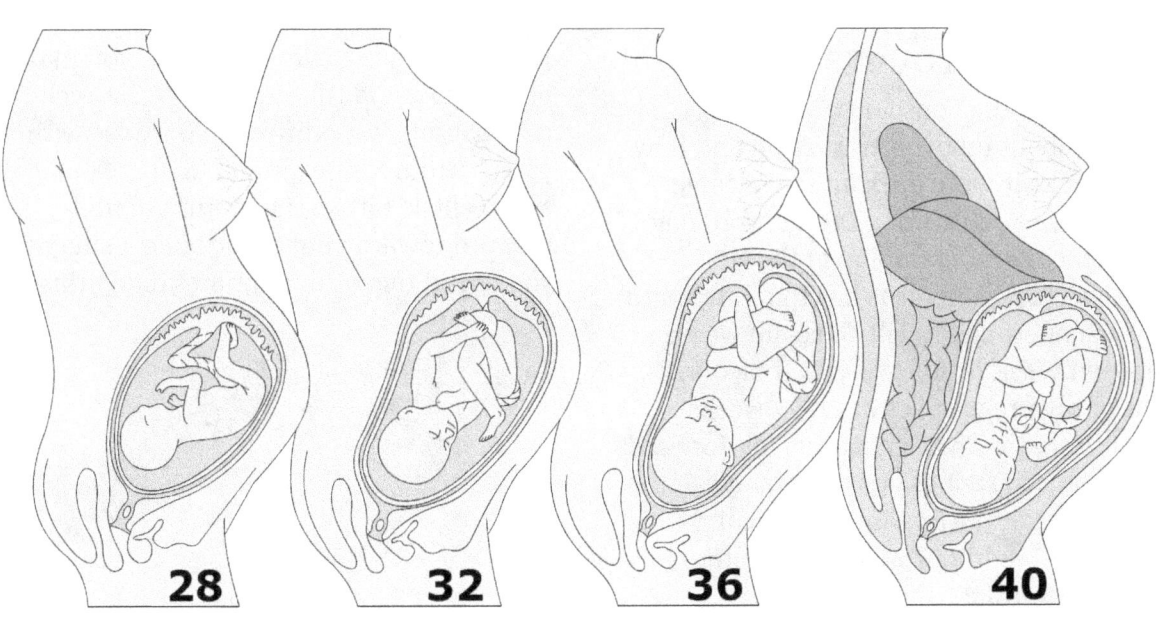

28   32   36   40

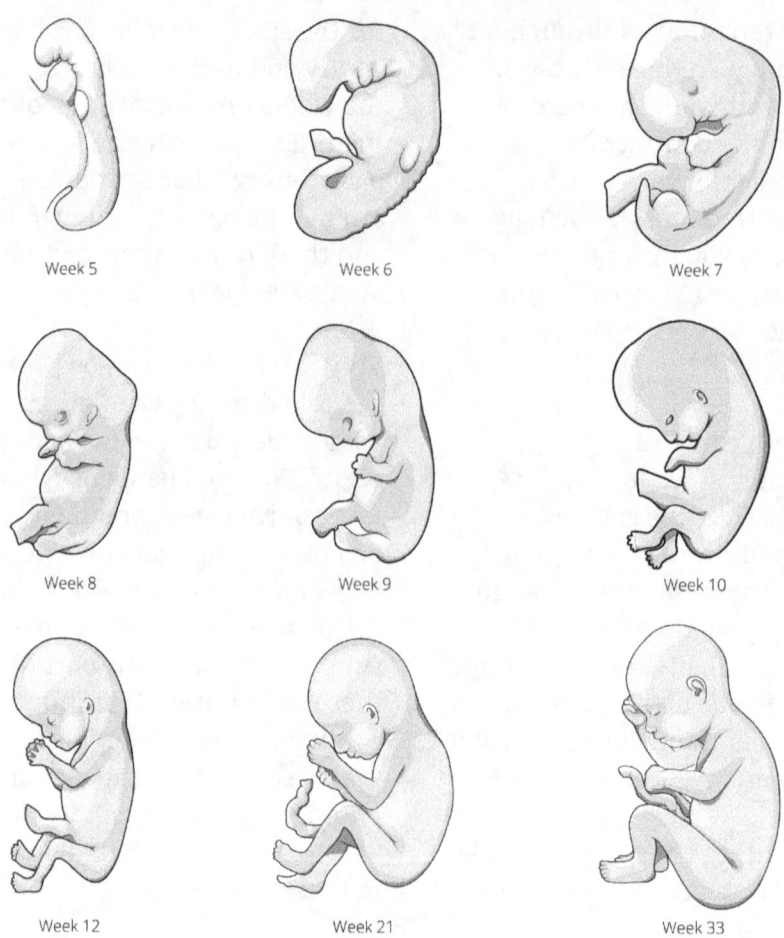

Fetal Development in the First 10 Weeks

Week 5 | Week 6 | Week 7
Week 8 | Week 9 | Week 10
Week 12 | Week 21 | Week 33

Uterus Retroversion

We talked in the Conscious Conception chapter about uterus retroversion and how it can make it more difficult to conceive. If you have a retroverted uterus, you may experience some cramping in the first 8–14 weeks. Your uterus has to fall forward in pregnancy, and it will do so anywhere between Week 10 and Week 14. I bled in four of my pregnancies at 12–13 weeks because that's when my uterus fell forward. I experienced serious cramping and each time I thought I was going to miscarry again. But I didn't. It was just my uterus falling forward.

If you have a retroverted uterus, you may be able to avoid this cramping. The trick is to get into a modified child's pose with your bottom in the air and then rock or sway a little bit, so the uterus will fall forward toward your pubic bone. I suggest you spend five or ten minutes doing this in

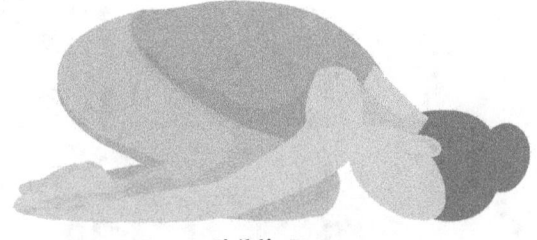

Child's Pose

the morning and in the evening, starting as soon as you know you're pregnant. Couple this with your ab work.

Implantation Bleeding

Implantation bleeding in pregnancy can occur when the egg burrows into the endometrium of the uterine lining. Occasionally this can cause a little bit of blood to pass. This usually occurs when you're 7–14 days pregnant. Occasionally you will think that your period is going to start, but then you only experience a single day of spotting and then it's gone. This is quite typical for implantation bleeding. Not everybody has this, of course, but if you do, take note. It can help your care provider to understand how far along you are in your pregnancy gestationally.

When Can I Hear My Baby's Heartbeat?

It is rarely but sometimes possible to hear your baby's heartbeat at eight weeks. By 10 weeks, 70 percent of babies' heartbeats can be heard, and by 12 weeks, 95 percent of babies' heartbeats can be heard.

Some of this depends on where the placenta attaches to the uterine wall. If the placenta is on the front (anterior) of the inside of the uterus, it can be much harder to hear the fetal heart tones. and can also delay when you can feel the baby moving. It can also be hard to hear the baby if your uterus is retroverted. Once it falls forward it's easier to hear the heartbeat.

Flat or Inverted Nipples

A percentage of women will anatomically have flat, very slightly protruding, or even inverted nipples. You can tell whether you have inverted nipples by pinching the areola with your thumb and index finger. If the nipple pulls in instead of pushes out, you've got them. In this society we start wearing bras at an early age, and I believe this practice presses the nipples down against the underlying breast tissue. Having these types of nipples can make it difficult for the baby to attach or latch to the breast and nurse effectively. The baby's mouth and sucking will eventually pull the nipple out, but this can take a while, and can be painful.

If your nipples are not prominent you can help this throughout your pregnancy by using several techniques. First, whenever you take a shower and have warmed your skin a bit, gently pull the nipples out. In pregnancy you are so soft that you can change your nipples by frequently pulling on them. Do not do this to the point of pain, but it should probably be slightly uncomfortable.

Second, you can use a breast pump on the gentlest setting for one minute a few times a week.

Lastly, there is a product called a breast shell, which is made up of two silicone or plastic parts worn inside the bra to help correct flat or inverted nipples either in preparation for or during breastfeeding. The inner section is disc-shaped, with a hole in the middle that encircles the areola, allowing the nipple to protrude through the hole. The outer piece protects the nipple from rubbing up against your bra. You wear it under your bra and eventually your nipple will protrude more. Breast shells are also used to protect sore nipples after birth, and they can be used to capture leaking colostrum or breastmilk.

Considerations for Choosing a Care Provider

Most women in the US automatically decide to work with an OB/GYN. Maybe most of them don't know there are other options available to them. I hope you will take the time to fully explore the options available to you.

Let's first talk about the options available to you broadly. In the US, depending on where you live, you have access to a hospital birth, a freestanding birth center birth, and a home birth with a midwife.

Hospitals

A hospital is a large organization full of modern medical equipment. Doctors work on a rotation, and the OB/GYN you select as your provider will be affiliated with a particular hospital and a particular group of on-call doctors, typically five or six others. So, any of those doctors could be on call when you go into labor, and you may or may not be attended by the OB/GYN you've been seeing throughout your pregnancy.

Birth Factory

Because hospital practitioners are overwhelmed, they're motivated to quickly move you through the birthing process, and if your labor is not conforming to their timeline they'll likely pressure you to succumb to intervention after intervention, each designed to accelerate the process.

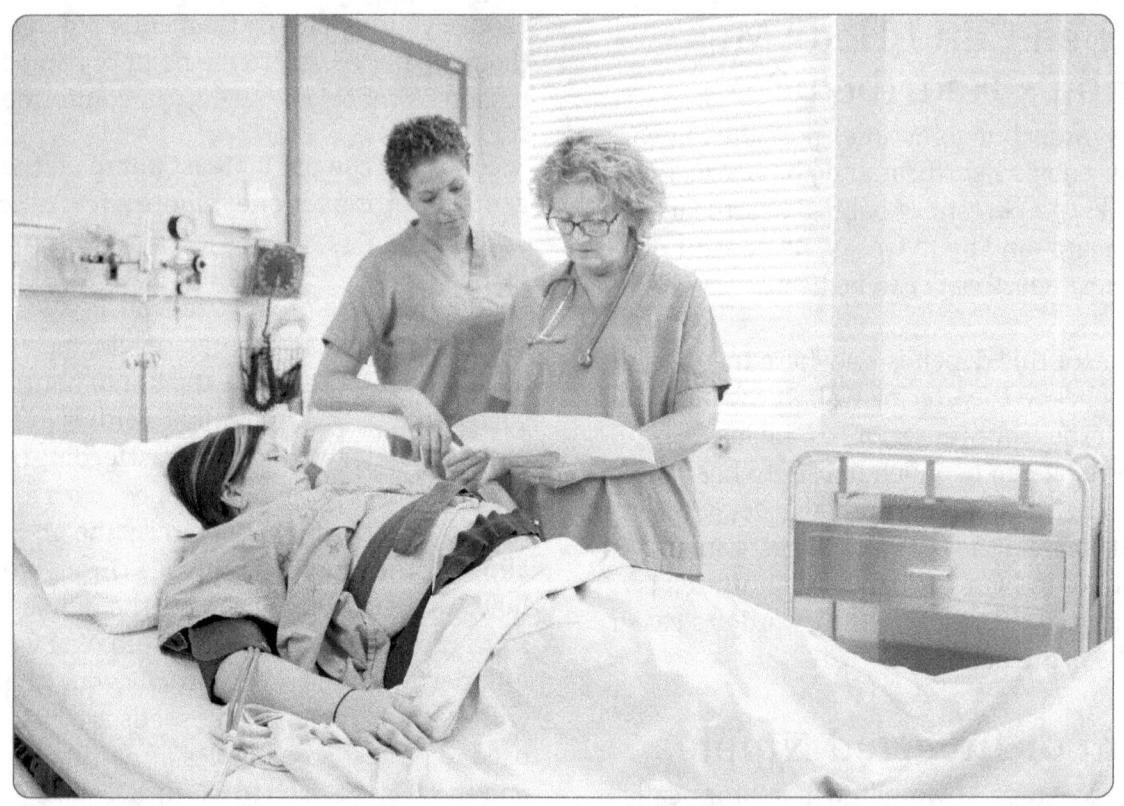

Hospital Environment

This all starts with the assertion that full-term gestation occurs at 40 weeks. This is simply not true. Most of my clients deliver between 41–42 weeks with no issues whatsoever. But if the medical industry can convince you that you are late if you hit 40 weeks and one day, then they can convince you to succumb to costly interventions that slate you into their assembly line.

Convincing women that they are late if they cross the 40-week threshold is one of the drivers behind the massive labor induction rates in the US. In Austin, Texas, where I live and work, OB/GYNs induce 50–60 percent of all labors. If they convince people that 40 weeks is when the baby should be out, they can get that many more women to agree to being induced, at a set day and time of the doctor's choosing, generally Monday through Friday from 8:00 a.m. to 5 p.m.

According to a 2018 study published in *Pediatrics*, approximately 17 percent of c-sections in the US are performed between 4 pm and 7 pm. The study also found that the percentage of c-sections performed between 4 pm and 7 pm has been increasing in recent years.[89]

Now, these drivers have produced induction and augmentation rates in hospital deliveries that simply would not be this high if more women had more agency in their birth experience. Early contractions can be misinterpreted as labor when they are still just warm-up labor. Doctors often act to speed up this warm-up labor instead of letting it progress naturally, and we call this augmentation. Here are 2022 statistics for augmentation and induction in the US, according to the Centers for Disease Control and Prevention (CDC).

- 60 percent of women in labor were augmented to speed their labor up with drugs like Pitocin.

- 25.4 percent of women in the United States had their labors induced. This means that their labors were started artificially, usually with medication (Pitocin).

- 81.5 percent of women in the United States had their labor monitored electronically. This means that their baby's heart rate and contractions were monitored with a device strapped to their abdomen. The data is transmitted to monitors in the room and at the nurses' station.

- 60.9 percent of women in the United States received epidural or spinal anesthesia during labor. This means that they received medication through a needle in their spine or back to numb or block the sensations of labor.

- 11.7 percent of women in the United States had an episiotomy during childbirth. This means that their doctor made a cut in their perineum (the area between the vagina and anus) to help the baby's head deliver.

- 2.8 percent of women in the United States had their babies delivered with forceps or vacuum extraction. This means that their doctor used a tool to help the baby's head deliver.

- 31.8 percent of women in the United States had a cesarean section (c-section). This means that their babies were delivered through surgical incisions in their abdomen and uterus.[90]

According to the World Bank, the United States ranked 36th out of 195 countries in infant mortality in 2022, and this is a marked improvement over prior years.[91] Even so, the infant mortality rate in the United States was 5.4 deaths per 1,000 live births in 2022, which is significantly higher than the average of 3.9 deaths per 1,000 live births for high-income countries. France, Sweden, Norway, Finland, and the Netherlands, where the vast majority of births are attended by professional midwives have cesarean rates around 19 percent. Even Bulgaria has better statistics than the US. I believe that induction and all the interventions that hospital practitioners rely on in this country also affect these statistics. So many babies come before they're ready, and that impairs early bonding and breastfeeding, which also impacts infant mortality.

The fetal mortality rate is the number of deaths of fetuses of 28 or more weeks gestation. The neonatal mortality rate is the number of deaths of liveborn infants within the first 28 days of life. The perinatal mortality rate is the sum of these two rates. The US ranks 35th out of 38 developed nations for perinatal mortality. Only Mexico, Chile, and Turkey rank worse.[92]

Modern doctors are incredibly overworked and underpaid for what they do. They're shouldering a monstrous load of debt when they leave med school, typically several hundred thousand dollars,[93] and they need to hit the ground running and start a practice quickly to make enough money to satisfy their debt and the monstrous insurance fees they have to pay. The debt pressure our doctors face is enormous, and so from the get-go they have to be focused on generating revenue through their practices. Birth has turned into a billion-dollar industry and somewhere along the way we have lost our connection to the sacredness of the experience. I believe that higher education and medical schools should be free of charge in the United States.

It is also important to know that it's the doctor who is in the delivery room when the baby is born who gets paid for birthing services, regardless of how many prenatal visits you had with your preferred OB/GYN. You can see why a doctor might be motivated to schedule your induction or c-section for the beginning of their hospital shift, so they can reap the reward of having worked with you over the course of your pregnancy.

Let me reiterate that. There is no incentive whatsoever for a doctor to encourage your baby to come on its own timetable. From the doctor's perspective, the baby needs to arrive while the doctor is there so they will get paid, and so they do everything in their power to have the baby arrive while they are still on the clock. If you are in labor and they are nearing the end of the shift, then all of a sudden, you're too big or the baby's too big or you're too small or the baby's too small or there's too much amniotic fluid or not enough … and it's time for a c-section. I have heard about this happening far more often than I would like to recount.

Induction forces the body into labor before it's ready. We are messing with an incredibly complex dynamic of layers and layers of physical, spiritual, emotional, and hormonal components, and it's all unfolding in a process that we don't fully understand intellectually yet.

Common Interventions

Frequent Ultrasounds

An ultrasound, also known as a sonogram, is a medical imaging technique that uses sound waves to create pictures of structures inside the body.

If a hospital experience is your choice, I want you to know that frequent ultrasounds are another way doctors make money. They over-recommend ultrasounds in the pregnancy and charge around $300 to your insurance for each of them. Multiply that by the six that they're typically recommending and there's an additional $1,800 in birthing revenue for them. The real villain here is the insurance industry, which often dictates prices for procedures and on the whole doesn't allocate enough money for the doctors, so doctors have to keep encouraging billable procedures in order to make enough money to keep their practice alive. I think that this is inappropriate, and mothers and babies are paying the price for it.

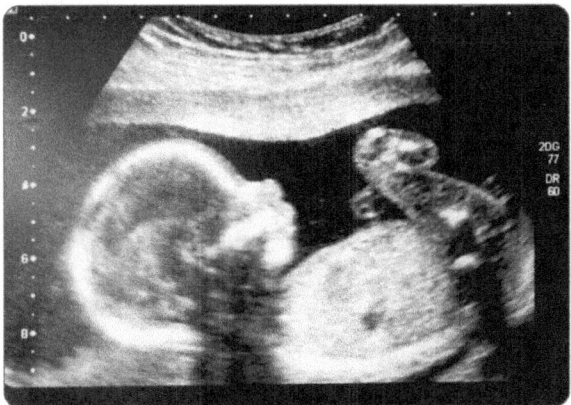

Ultrasound Image

There's a whole private industry promoting 3D ultrasounds, making it seem like it's baby's first portrait. These have nothing to do with prenatal care at all. I've seen women become very attached to these visual representations of their baby, so every time they go to the doctor, they want to see the baby. Nobody has told them that maybe that's not a great idea. I don't think it's going to cause miscarriage, but I don't think it helps the baby one little bit. I also think it sets you up for you for not listening to your intuition, for not nurturing that unseen connection. You don't need a picture to connect you to your baby. You connect to your baby through your heart, your spirit, and your emotional self.

Induction of Contractions with Pitocin

Pitocin is often used in hospitals to induce contractions. It's a drug that is biochemically similar to the natural hormone produced by the pituitary, oxytocin. It will induce labor. It will make your uterus contract.

Pitocin is a wonderful thing when you need it, so I don't want to throw the baby out with the bathwater; it's just overused. Pitocin is fantastic for women whose labor stalls out and they need some assistance. They've been laboring hard for a long time, and we go to the hospital and get that help. It is also a wonderful anti-hemorrhage medication to help your uterus to stop bleeding and to make it contract really hard after birth.

The contractions you feel on Pitocin are quite intense and they do not let up. It is a very different experience from natural labor with oxytocin; it is a relentless march up a very steep slope. It is brutal and painful, which is why many women opt for the next most common intervention, an epidural.

Epidural

Epidurals are a spinal pain blocker that effectively shuts out all feeling in the lower part of your body. In the US in 2022, epidural or spinal anesthesia was used in 68.5 percent of vaginal births and 86.7 percent of c-sections.[94]

Episiotomy

An episiotomy is a cut in your vagina to widen the vaginal opening and allow the baby to exit the vagina faster. Episiotomies were done on almost every laboring woman in the '60s, '70s, and even the '80s, but have fallen out of favor and fewer and fewer are done now. Episiotomies are absolutely lifesaving if the baby is in distress and the perineum is not stretching fast enough to get the baby out quickly. Helping that along can save the baby from oxygen deprivation.

Another situation where an episiotomy may be warranted is if your OB/GYN thinks that you are going to seriously tear. It is far better to make a small episiotomy off to the side than to let a big tear extend through the rectum.

Cesarean Section (C-Section)

A cesarean section, also known as a cesarean or c-section is a major abdominal surgery to remove the baby from your uterine cavity. My God, what wonderful things c-sections are when they're necessary. They can be absolutely lifesaving, but they are also overdone. Some women elect to have c-sections instead of attempting a vaginal birth. Maybe they haven't been told how much harder it is to recover from a c-section than from a healthy vaginal birth.

Now, all of these interventions have their places—induction or augmentation of labor with Pitocin is at times necessary and useful and good. Epidurals can help women to avoid traumatic pain. Episiotomies can help prevent massive tearing—but I have seen over and over again that early intervention in the birthing room leads to more and more intervention in the birthing room. The US has a 31.7 percent c-section rate[95] and there are places that have 50 percent c-section rates. Brazil has a 90 percent c-section rate in some parts of the country and an overall c-section rate of 56 percent.[96] In that country, the doctor is present for an hour from start to finish, and when it's all done, they make twice as much money and they have less liability, because everybody is ignorant of how much damage is done by the willy-nilly performance of c-sections. It's the wrong approach.

A c-section is not a great idea unless you really, really need it. I've heard women who are choosing to have a c-section say, "I don't want my vagina to change." I want you to know that your vagina does not have to become damaged as a result of a vaginal birth. You do have to do things to restore those muscles, but it's not a foregone conclusion that giving birth vaginally will irreparably alter your vagina. That is no reason to have major abdominal surgery.

Some people are also afraid of the experience of labor, and because of all the fear factor around it, they elect to have a c-section instead. I'm here to tell you, the pain of a c-section can be way worse than labor—*way worse*—I mean, it is a really big deal, and they don't tell you enough about it. "Oh, you'll be just fine," they'll say, but it's not just fine; recovery from major abdominal surgery while you have a newborn baby to care for is beyond difficult.

If you're approaching your due date, the doctor may employ my favorite manipulation tactic, "I may not be there if you don't select the day that you're going to have the baby. If you'll just sign up for Tuesday, then I'll be the one by your side when your baby arrives. You don't want to be pregnant anymore, do you? You're miserable, aren't you? Tuesday it is, then."

It doesn't take much to coerce uniformed women at Week 39, because by that point they are often so uncomfortable they'd almost let you take their leg if they thought it would bring an end to the pregnancy. All of this is compounded by the natural fears felt by a pregnant woman who is about to give birth and the myth that natural birth is dangerous and too painful.

The Patient Landscape

Now, doctors in this country are also dealing with a widespread health epidemic in that most of our population does not eat well or exercise at all. So many pregnant women do not eat properly to support their growing baby. Combine these factors, which can create poor placental health and promote stress in the baby, with a litigious society and it's no wonder that doctors work to exercise as much control over the process as they can.

A lot of the people who really struggle in pregnancy and birth are marginalized. They are not given enough information or enough opportunity to have healthy lives, and it is so much more difficult to have a healthy pregnancy, birth, and baby without having a healthy life. If you are desperately poor—no matter how good your intentions are—it is going to be really hard to eat well enough, to take the vitamins and supplements you need, and to get the care that you deserve. If you are a Woman of Color, you can sometimes find that you are offered only the dregs of care in institutionalized medicine.[97]

But I know that you are not going to be the typical, uninformed woman. I know that you, by the very fact that you are reading this book, are taking the steps you need to take to have a healthy pregnancy, and to do it in a better way.

Let me sum this up: A hospital is an excellent place to go when you have pregnancy or birth *complications* (My personal overall complication rate is 10 percent.). Hospital practitioners are well-versed in lifesaving techniques that can help you and your baby if they are necessary. The systemic issues of overworked and overloaded doctors, an on-call system, and saddling our new doctors with massive amounts of medical debt is a perfect storm that creates an intervention-prone environment, because medications and procedures are billable and create revenue. It's a birth factory, not a birth experience.

THE CASCADE OF INTERVENTIONS

You schedule your labor and are induced, which leads to great pain, so you get an epidural, but then there are signs of fetal distress, and all of a sudden you need an "emergency" c-section.

This is the cascade of interventions. It starts with something small, something you're told is completely safe and harmless. It will help because you have one of any number of concerns ... your baby is measuring big, your amniotic sac is looking depleted, your doctor is going out of town soon and they want to be around for the birth. "Aren't you ready to meet your baby?" They'll ask. You are! Of course you are.

Or maybe you go to the hospital thinking you're in active labor, but then it stalls or slows and the doctor suggests augmentation. You get the augmentation—an IV with Pitocin—and the pain is incredible. There's no break. The contractions are wicked and mean and they're right on top of each other.

"If you get an epidural, you can rest," they say. "It will take the pain away, and if you rest maybe you won't have to have a c-section." That sounds nice. You

need a break. You definitely don't want a c-section if you can avoid it.

And you get the epidural and you do get some rest, but then they tell you your baby is under extreme stress and the baby's heart tones are dropping. "We think we should get them out," they tell you. They mean surgery. You don't want anything to happen to your sweet baby. You trust the doctor to save your baby. You agree to the surgery.

Your family will be so grateful that you were in the hospital. "The doctors saved your lives! Thank God," they'll say.

Maybe the doctors did save these women. But if their labors had been allowed to progress naturally, would there have been anything to save them from? I hear this story all the time, and I want you to know this does not have to be your story. Some women recognize what was done to them, others don't. Either way, I have seen that this kind of birth is more likely to result in the women having to deal with depression, anxiety, and trauma from their birth experience.

While it's obvious that I feel strongly about natural birth, I want you to deeply trust your own self. If you choose differently, that does not make your choice bad or wrong. In fact, there are times I advise women to choose a hospital birth because I believe it will be the best choice for her situation. High risk births (e.g., breech, multiples) are often best attempted in a hospital environment. You are working toward *your* perfect, ideal birth. I only ask that you decide what your ideal, perfect birth looks like after you have complete information. Maybe you've known for years that you were going to go the hospital/induction/

epidural route. Allow yourself to revisit that choice as you continue to read.

Freestanding Birth Center

I am a firm believer in home birth, but there are plenty of people who are not yet comfortable with the idea. They feel they must be in a health care facility to be safe or feel secure. They are not yet ready to make the dive into what a home birth entails. A wonderful alternative to the hospital is a freestanding birth center, which is a birth facility that is not attached to a hospital.

A birth center is a facility that only deals with pregnant women. They typically have several birth rooms that are both spacious and intimate, designed to replicate a cozy home environment, and often with a bed and a very large birthing tub in the same room. The centers are often run by certified nurse midwives (CNMs) or certified professional midwives (CPMs), and it is very possible that you will see several care providers throughout your pregnancy, so you become familiar with everyone who might be in attendance when you give birth.

These centers offer you the ability to have a more natural experience, These practitioners will encourage and support you and they will allow your labor to progress naturally without unnecessary intervention. They will be there to help make you comfortable and to provide guidance when things get intense.

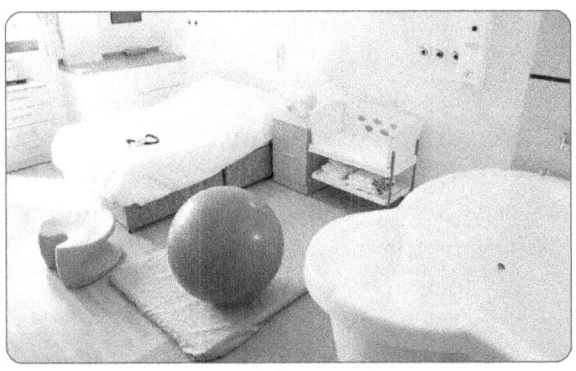

Typical Freestanding Birth Center Room

They will work with you to adhere to your birth plan and provide you an excellent experience. They are often situated near hospitals should the need for transport arise.

Birth centers are a fantastic option if there are no midwives available to you for a home birth, if your insurance will cover a birth center birth but not a home birth, or if you are simply not comfortable with the idea of a home birth. The only downsides I see to this choice for women are that their care providers are usually obligated by law to refuse to care for you if your pregnancy lasts beyond their 42-week deadline, there are times when transporting mammals in labor (and we are mammals) brings labor to a standstill, and it is harder to have to move back to your home after the birth than to already just be there. Regarding that second reason, on a primal level the body thinks something must be drastically wrong if you're moving during labor, and this can bring some women's labor to a dead stop. However, if you have familiarized yourself with the safe and comforting atmosphere of the birthing center, your body will recognize this and usually resume labor once you arrive.

Home Birth with a Midwife

The Experience of Laboring at Home

Let's get real about the pain of natural childbirth. It's true. It can hurt a lot! And for some lucky women it doesn't hurt much at all. There is a bell curve of experiences because some women are more innervated (have more nerve endings) in their cervix than others, so some women feel more, and some women feel less.

My mother told me that she was told that the pain of birth was a woman's punishment for Eve's original sin, and because women were so wicked, they were told they were going to have a hard time with birth forever and ever, which is just *absolute* hogwash. But this message is pervasive in our culture: *the pain of childbirth is a punishment.* We see it in movies and on TV. Because we perceive

MariMikel: Ages ago I showed up for a birth, and when I arrived the woman in labor came out to greet me. She was doing a little breathing, like a contraction was distracting her. I said, "What are you doing? Get back inside! Oh, my gosh!"

She said, "I'm fine. I'm fine," in a slow, sing-song-y voice.

Her husband and I got all my equipment unloaded and situated. This woman did not even seem like she was in labor. She seemed like she was just having a lovely day. I said, "Well, let's do an exam to see where you are in labor."

When I examined her, I said, "Oh my gosh! You're at nine centimeters! You are just about to have the baby!"

In her dreamy voice she said, "Oh my goodness. Nine centimeters …" She turned to her husband. "Isn't that amazing, honey? Nine centimeters." She had the baby about 20 minutes later.

While it can happen, I don't see a painless birth like that very often.

---

it as an unfair punishment, we may see no issue with using medication to assist with pain. But most women are going into the hospital and getting an epidural at four centimeters, and they do not feel anything at all. What they don't tell you—and may not even know—is that the sensations of birth are astonishingly transformative and can provoke a spiritual, life-altering state. They are worth experiencing.

> What they don't tell you is that the sensations of birth are astonishingly transformative and can provoke a spiritual, life-altering state. They are worth experiencing.

The pain of labor creates this crescendo, an *aha!* moment of glory when you realize it's over. When your baby comes into your arms, the experience you have both just gone through together facilitates a bonding moment that is much more difficult to achieve when you do not feel the sensations of labor.

I want you to know it is a pain you can handle, and it is a transformative experience you will miss out on if you're unable to feel because you've had an epidural and are passing the time watching the TV while Pitocin forces your cervix open. Your reproductive system is set up to *work*. Birth is an evolutionary process that was millions of years in the making. It wasn't designed incorrectly, and if you weren't supposed to feel anything, you wouldn't.

You want to feel it; it is worth it. Yes, it hurts, but it is a pain that is valuable. You grow out of that pain and your ability to handle the pain of birth makes you more likely to be able to handle other tough things in life. You have felt the power of being an Amazon woman. You won't just walk away from your relationships when things get tough. You won't just give up on your children because things are so hard. There are lots of benefits in your ability to go through this process and what you get out of it is spectacular and beyond my ability to communicate to you in words. The mysteries that unfold in your heart and life as a result of this process are incomparable.

There is what I like to call a zone in birth, like in sex. When sex is really wonderful, it is transcendental. You lose track of who you are and where you are, and you're no longer two, you are one. You inhabit a sacred, spiritual space and you're in an altered state. That same state is where you give birth easily, but you can't get to the zone if there's too much intervention.

As you experience natural labor your body will be flooded with oxytocin, which is an amazing hormone. It is often referred to as the *touch* or *love* hormone because it is released in any kind of physical interaction between people. When you touch someone's hand, you get a little tiny dose of oxytocin. You hug, you get more. You kiss, you get more. You have sex, you get *lots* more. Oxytocin is what makes people orgasm. Oxytocin is also the hormone that makes the mother's milk let down, and what makes women have their periods, so it is deeply intwined with all this sexual and reproductive activity. And, importantly for natural labor, oxytocin is the hormone that brings on uterine contractions. I think Pitocin (used in hospitals to stimulate contractions) blocks receptor sites in the brain that would otherwise be filled with oxytocin. When you have this big rush of

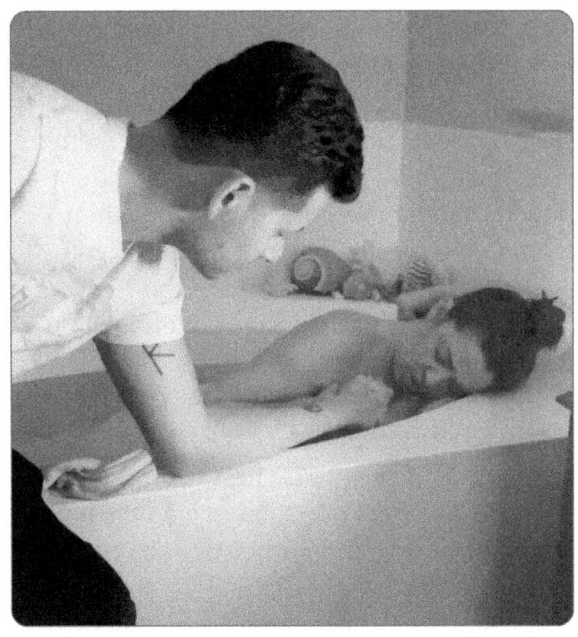

Aleah Laboring at Home

oxytocin flood your body at birth it is very orgasmic stuff. Meanwhile, nobody ever had an orgasm with Pitocin.

It is not the same experience at all as a woman laboring on Pitocin. Labor with oxytocin ebbs and flows. It'll take you up to the precipice, where you're struggling to breathe, saying, "Oh dear, oh dear," (or possibly something much saltier) and then it will level off and let you get used to the idea of that sensation before it escalates again. A lot of natural labor is spent resting in between contractions. Oxytocin-fueled contractions ebb and flow in this wonderful way like ocean waves, and you *can* handle it. *It is your birthright.*

If you are trepidatious about experiencing the sensations of labor and birth, know that you can always have an epidural. Even if you're at home to begin with. You can always go to the hospital and have an epidural. I've had it happen a few handfuls of times when a woman in labor told me she was done and didn't want to try anything else, she was ready to go, and so we went. No judgment, no delay. That has happened rarely, actually, because I teach my clients how to handle the sensations, and when women are educated about the positive impacts of natural birth, they *want* to experience it. In these pages I will teach you how to handle those sensations.

There are different levels of activity at the time of birth. The first is on the physiological level. If you were an ancient woman hunting and gathering, you had to do that every day or you did not eat. So, if you started having some pain you knew to go back to your nest and to prepare, because that's where you were going to be the safest. Your body recognizes when you are in a safe physical space and labor will progress more easily when you are.

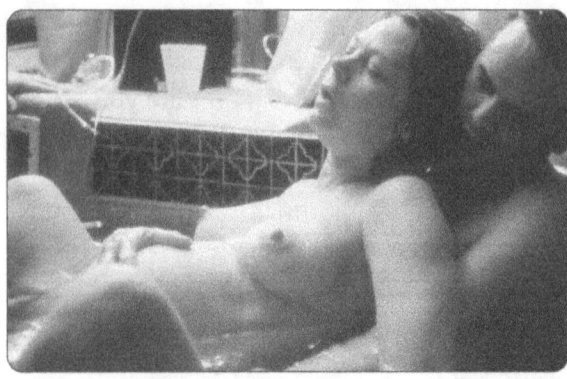

Robbie Laboring in Water

I have seen this happen with women who arrive at the hospital and are faced with strangers on call, and a new, loud, bright, and invasive environment. Their labor shuts down in the face of the hospital-induced environmental stress.[98] As mentioned earlier, studies have shown that moving mammals in labor can bring that labor to a

halt.[99] That, of course, makes it easier for the doctors to call for intervention with Pitocin to stimulate contractions and then they're off to the races. A safe space is conducive to a safe labor.

The second area of activity is on the emotional level. The process of giving birth is designed to open you emotionally so you bond deeply with your baby. No one gives birth with their mind. It is a body-spirit-heart-emotion experience and when you have an epidural, you are cut off from experiencing the sensations of birth. You're so disengaged you have to scroll through social media on your phone to have something to do while you're in labor. I'll just say that I never see the moment of birth in a medicated birth look the same as it does when the mother is unmedicated.

This is not an indictment in any way of those who have gotten an epidural. I just don't think a birth without the sensations leads to the same degree of bonding and heart opening that happens when the sensations are there. It doesn't mean everybody who's ever had an epidural didn't

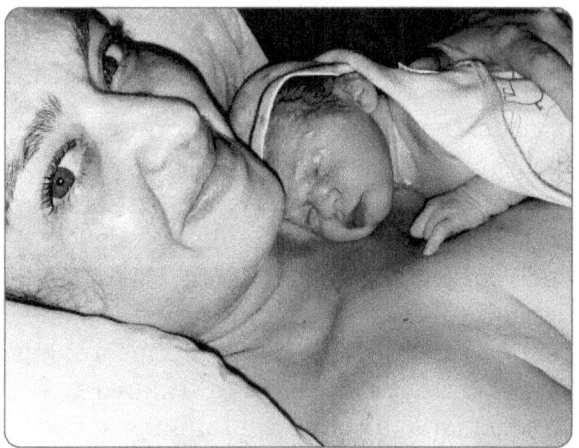

Aleah's Indomitable Spirit Shines after a Medication-Free Birth

bond with their baby. That's not it at all, but it's different in the immediate moment of birth. When I see a woman giving birth who is feeling the sensations she'll cry out, "Oh my God, oh my God. Oh my God! Oh my GOD! OH MY GOD!" and then as the baby emerges, she'll cry out, "My baby!" She's just in another world, and it's because of the rush of natural hormones.

Additionally, with a home birth you're in your favorite space, a private place of intimacy that you know well, surrounded by the people you chose to have with you, whom you know and trust and who love you, and in that space your body can relax and go to *the zone*.

One of my clients told me about how shocked she was when, during the birth of her first child in the hospital, a nurse came to her when her husband was out of the room and asked her if she was safe, and if she was making her own decisions or only being coerced by her husband. She was in a healthy, happy relationship, and her husband had been acting on her behalf. It rubbed her wrong for him to be treated with such suspicion, which is part of what prompted her to seek my care for the birth of her second child.

But as I've mentioned, the nurses at the hospital don't know you like a midwife and her staff would. They had to ask her if she was safe, because you would be shocked to know how many people *are* in a harmful position, and how many people nurses help when they ask discreetly. They ask that of every single woman when the husband is out of the room and 5 percent of the time the woman says, "I am not safe." This is a real thing.

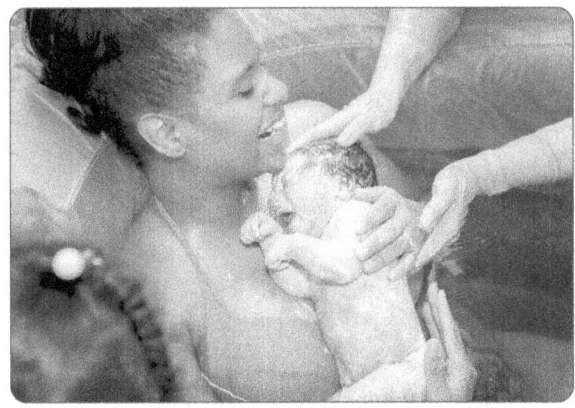

The Power and Joy of a Natural Birth

Nurses have to ask because they don't know their patients. To the nurse, the person acting as an advocate looks like they're calling the shots. Before you know it, the situation is adversarial, and the energy is all wrong for a birthing room.

Like all homebirth midwives, I know my clients; I would never have to ask. Over the course of a pregnancy, midwives build a relationship with every client through lengthy consultations. We want to get to know you well enough that we can help you have your ideal, perfect birth. We want to grow a bond of trust with our clients so when the time comes for you to

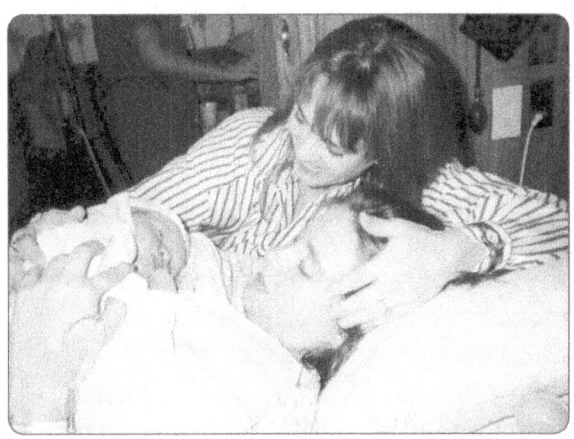

MariMikel with a Client and Newborn

experience birth, you can relax and sink into *the zone* because your midwife is no longer a stranger and hasn't been for quite some time if you've been seeing them for the duration of your pregnancy. This is the midwife's way.

> *The midwife considers the miracle of childbirth as normal, and leaves it alone unless there's trouble. The obstetrician normally sees childbirth as trouble; if he leaves it alone, it's a miracle.*
>
> —Sheila Stubbs

Is it Safe?

There is a pervasive myth in our culture that a home birth is unsafe, while a hospital birth is undeniably safe. This is simply not true. Your home can absolutely be a safe place to have your baby. Let's take a look at why. Statistically speaking, you are going to have fewer complications than you will in the hospitals. As I mentioned, the US is now 35th out of 38 developed nations in perinatal mortality.[100] We're in trouble in the United States with maternal and infant mortality rates, and, as I've mentioned, these are far worse for Women of Color than white women in the US. We've got to do something about it. All women deserve a better way, a better approach.

MIDWIVES MODEL OF CARE

The Midwives Alliance of North America's (MANA) Midwives Model of Care is a client-centered approach to pregnancy, childbirth, and postpartum care. It is based on the philosophy that pregnancy and birth are normal life events, and that women and birthing people are capable of giving birth naturally and safely. Midwives across the country adhere to these ideals.

Midwives are healthcare professionals who specialize in pregnancy, childbirth, and postpartum care. They are trained to provide comprehensive care, including:

- **Prenatal care:** monitoring the physical, psychological, and social well-being of the mother/birthing parent throughout the childbearing cycle.
- **Education and counseling:** providing individualized information and support to help women and birthing people make informed decisions about their care.
- **Labor and delivery:** providing continuous hands-on assistance during labor and birth.
- **Postpartum care:** providing support and care to the mother/birthing parent and newborn after birth.

The Midwives Model of Care emphasizes the importance of informed consent and shared decision-making. Midwives believe that women and birthing people should be active participants in their own care, and that they should have the right to make choices about their own bodies and their babies.

The Midwives Model of Care has been shown to have a number of benefits, including:

- Lower rates of c-section and other interventions.
- Better birth outcomes for mothers and babies.
- Higher satisfaction with care among women and birthing people.

The Midwives Model of Care is available in a variety of settings, including some hospitals, birth centers, and homes.

The Netherlands has one of the best maternal and infant mortality morbidity rates in the world.[101] The difference between the Netherlands and the US lies in the care. In the Netherlands, they have a 70 percent midwife-attended birth rate[102] and a 12.4 percent home birth rate. Dutch hospital intervention rates are also minimal. The results are far superior because of the type of care that midwives give and that OB/GYNs and nurses simply cannot afford to give in the US.

Many large-scale studies done in multiple high-resource countries have clearly demonstrated the safety of planned, midwife-attended home births.[103] All of these studies have shown that planned, midwife-attended home births entail very few interventions, result in healthier mothers and babies, have higher rates of breastfeeding, and carry the exact same risk of perinatal mortality for babies as low-risk hospital births: two baby deaths per 1,000 births. And in all these large-scale studies, the transfer rate from home to hospital ranged between 10–20 percent. These hospital transfers were mostly preventive—only around 5 percent of home-to-hospital transfers took place in emergency situations.

Over the many years that I have been in practice I've averaged about a 10 percent overall complication rate, about an 8 percent transport to hospital rate, and a 6–7 percent c-section rate for my clients. My episiotomy rate is 2 percent, and I've only done one episiotomy on anyone who's had a baby before. Most of the episiotomies I do are in order to relieve fetal distress or when severe tearing is imminent. I have an 80+ percent success rate with VBACs, which

is a vaginal birth after a cesarean. There are years where my complication rate has been much higher and years where it has been lower. In 2022 I had my worst year ever, statistically speaking, and I believe it was due to a lot of my clients having had COVID and the problems that can arise from the cardiovascular damage done by COVID. That being said, most of the time my complication rate has been low.

Compare the national averages between home births with midwives and hospital births so you can be armed with data when people come at you with the myth that a home birth is less safe than a hospital birth.

Many people are led to believe that it will be safer to have their baby in the hospital rather than at home because it will be cleaner. The truth is there are so many people going through hospitals, especially in labor and delivery units, and this high turnover rate of patients increases the number of germs and potential for infection to all patients entering the hospital.

A nosocomial infection, also known as a hospital-acquired infection (HAI) or healthcare-associated infection (HCAI), is an infection that is acquired while receiving medical care. Nosocomial infections are contracted after a patient has been admitted to a hospital or other healthcare facility. They can develop during hospitalization, during a healthcare procedure, or after discharge from the hospital.

According to the CDC, the overall rate of nosocomial infections in the US is about 3.2 percent of all hospitalized patients. This means that about 1 in 33 hospitalized patients will develop a nosocomial infection.

While hospitals do their absolute best and have significant systems to clean and sterilize, I believe if you follow my recommendations for preparation for birth you will be far better off in your own home. While there are germs present everywhere you go, those in your home you are already exposed to and very likely have already developed antibodies to them in your immune system.

Isn't it Messy?

I used to swim at the YMCA three times a week and one day an employee flagged me down as I came to the end of a lap and said, "There's a lady on the phone that really wants you."

I got out of the pool and took the call. She was one of my very pregnant clients and as I spoke with her, I realized, *Oh! It is on!* I hung up the phone, ran and grabbed my stuff, ran to my car, drove to my house like a banshee, grabbed my equipment, drove even faster to their house, ran in with my oxygen tank and my doppler, put my hands out, and caught the baby.

They had a neighbor there to help, because it was looking like the baby was going to arrive before I could, and the neighbor had the foresight to take some pictures. Afterward, when the extended family saw the pictures they said, "Wow, must have been really messy if the midwife had to wear her bathing suit so she could hose down afterwards." I always get a good chuckle out of that.

The truth is it isn't messy. People just think it is because they've seen so much red gelatin on TV. I double make the bed

with sterile sheets and plastic between the layers, and you'll never see a smidge of blood anywhere. I cannot speak for all midwives, but my team serves in many ways at a home birth other than simply being your birth attendants. We are the maids. We provide lots of doula services. We cook for you and do all the cleanup. We do the birth laundry. We take pictures and videos. We choreograph family and friends. We take care of kids and pets. We even water plants.

Working with a Midwife

There are a lot of great studies that show the wisdom and benefits of waiting to allow babies to come when they are ready.[104] Homebirth midwives generally attend far fewer births per month, which allows us to be much more relaxed and patient and to follow the process as opposed to trying to make things happen. I currently attend one or two births a month and my clients get a lot of attention. During the COVID-19 pandemic, many US homebirth midwives attended many more births than that per month, because many women saw hospitals as potential sites of contagion and chose home births instead. Since then, women are choosing to plan for a home birth in increasing numbers.

I can't speak to what each and every individual midwife does. I can only give you a broad understanding of what I provide for my clients. You can interview midwives in your area and see what standard of care they provide in their practice before you make your choice.

First Consultation

I give everyone who contacts me about attending their birth a free two-hour consultation. I do it because I want more information out there in the world about birth and empowerment. I want people to know about a safer way of giving birth, and a different approach to the entire experience. I want to educate people. I want to bring awareness to and lift the dialogue.

 I encourage partners to come to every prenatal visit. I have a lot of dads say, "What am I doing here?" Partners, you are the support system. It is really hard for the woman to remember and incorporate everything. You need to actively participate. Help with meal planning, shopping, cooking. Learn what's going on with her body so you can help with any problems she's having. Know the lingo. Be involved. She will love you more and more for every step you take in support of her and of your family.

Initial Visit

If, after that first consultation, the woman decides she wants to be my client (and vice versa), the next step is a two-hour initial visit. First, I draw the woman's blood to screen, which helps me assess her current health. Most doctors and many midwives screen for thyroid problems in early pregnancy. It's part of the initial lab work done for many women. It's an excellent idea to check for issues early on, because thyroid or hypothyroid is very common and must be addressed for a healthy, easy pregnancy.

After drawing the mother's blood, we go through a detailed personal medical history. I want to know about any allergies and medications used, any surgeries, injuries, accidents, illnesses, or other trauma. We

talk all about diet and health habits, weight information, and exercise. I ask all about the father. I want to know about his health and if he has conceived other children. I ask about the woman's menstrual and birth control histories. We discuss any previous pregnancies and births in great detail; they can help to inform me about how this pregnancy might go. We then talk about the present pregnancy in great detail. I spend considerable time going over the vitamins and nutrition that will best serve my client. I give each one of my clients a notebook filled with information about pregnancy, birth, and babies. It has all of the charts and forms that are going to be used for birth and the postpartum period, and we go over those as well. You can see why it takes two hours.

Physical Exam

During the third two-hour visit, I conduct an in-depth physical exam. I look in the eyes, ears, nose, and mouth and talk about oral hygiene and all the cool new stuff that's out there. I think it's kind of nice to get to know people before you get down and do a vaginal exam. All of my doctor's visits have been like, "How do you do? Lie down."

"Um, can we chat first?"

Nope. They have to get right down to it because they don't have time; they're seeing so many patients.

I palpate the lymph system and thyroid. I palpate the liver, spleen, uterus, and abdomen. I check over range of motion, muscle tone, skin tone, and spinal alignment. I check for edema (water retention leading to swelling in the hands, legs, feet, or face). I look for varicosities and ask about hemorrhoids.

I check blood pressure and pulse. I listen to their heart and lungs. I'll assess your reflexes. I perform a breast exam and teach all about breast cancer prevention and doing regular breast exams. I teach all the men about doing breast and testicular exams. I talk a lot about preventing cancer—in US society at large we are not talking enough about the cancer epidemic. I have even detected cancer in some of my patients who had been seeing OB/GYNs. Here again, the issue is that our doctors are incredibly overtaxed and simply don't have the time or resources to catch everything.

Then I do a speculum exam and a pap smear, if it's time for one. I always offer the woman an opportunity to look at her cervix. I use a mirror and flashlight. Most women are amazed by how beautiful their bodies are. I point out the os, where sperm goes in and blood comes out. It is tightly closed to keep the baby in there through the pregnancy, and it is the spot that opens up to 10 centimeters during birth.

At the physical appointment we also go over health habits to develop.

I then do a vaginal exam and assess the pelvis to make sure the pelvis is adequate for birth. Most women have much bigger than adequate pelvises, and there are no issues at all. I can also confirm that the reproductive system is normal and presenting appropriately for the baby's assumed gestation, and that there are no cysts tumors or abnormalities. It's comforting for my clients to know all these things are on track and her body is doing

what it is supposed to. In the rare instance where there are issues, the earlier we catch something, the better.

When I Advise an Ultrasound

Forty percent of my clients don't ever have an ultrasound at all. Ultrasounds have only been around for less than fifty years. There were never any ultrasounds before that ever, and our species reproduced just fine for thousands of years before they existed.

The American College of Obstetricians and Gynecologists (ACOG) recommends that prenatal ultrasounds be used only when medically necessary and that they be performed by trained healthcare professionals.[105] There are times when an ultrasound is called for and useful. I do require my clients to have an ultrasound in the following situations.

- If they are experiencing maternal bleeding.
- If the baby is not growing properly.
- If the size of the uterus doesn't match the dates.
- If it seems there is too much or too little amniotic fluid.
- If and when the mother reaches Week 42.

I find it useful to do an ultrasound when there is fetal malpresentation (the baby isn't in the optimal position for birth), to see if it will be possible to turn the baby. These are the circumstances where I require people in my care to have an ultrasound. Otherwise, I suggest forgoing them.

One of the reasons I am not in favor of ultrasounds is that I believe the process is uncomfortable for some babies. The ultrasound can create a field of pressure on baby's ears, akin to the sensation some people have when driving and someone rolls down a backseat window. I see babies during the ultrasound who are flinging themselves around, flailing, and putting their arms up. I've heard the technician say, "Oh look, the baby's waving." Babies in the womb don't know what waving is. They're not trying to say, "hello." I believe some babies are uncomfortable, and if they're waving, they're likely trying to get away or to make it stop.

Ongoing Prenatal Visits

After the first three two-hour visits that take place over three weeks, I see my clients for an hour once a month through the seventh month, then twice in the eighth month, and once a week in the ninth month until they are in labor, when I will be at their home.

During these ongoing visits I check my client for water retention and weight gain, and I test her urine. I'm looking for sugar, blood, ketones, and protein in the urine, which can be indicators for gestational diabetes, urinary tract infections, diabetic ketoacidosis (DKA), preeclampsia, or toxemia in pregnancy. I take her blood pressure and pulse, look for edema, and check her reflexes. I will palpate the uterus and baby, assess the baby's position and the amount of amniotic fluid present, and listen to fetal heart tones. Most importantly, we'll talk about how my client is feeling and how she is doing. I ask about her relationship, family, finances, work, etc. I listen.

It's so important that we build a strong relationship and that my clients trust me and can relax around me. This is true of every midwife. Spending so much time together really helps this process. We talk about what I do from start to finish and make adjustments as desired to fit her birth plan. I want to understand what she wants and to make sure that her birth experience will reflect that, to the best of my ability. Everyone is unique and will want things at their birth tailored to their needs, and they absolutely deserve that.

Childbirth Classes

I require that my clients take my childbirth classes starting at Week 30. The classes consist of seven two-hour sessions, and they are intentionally designed to put my clients in control of the process, to give them the information they need to let their minds relax throughout the birthing experience. You will find all the information from my classes in this book and *The Book of Birth Volume II*, but it also helps to access new information via different methods. Some people learn by reading, others by watching, listening, or doing. Find the medium that works for you and seek out good sources of information that align with your best method for learning.

Home Visit

Two to three weeks prior to my client's due date, I will visit them at their home. This visit helps to orient my team and me to their environment in advance of the birth. I also help them to prepare for the birth and postpartum period and answer any questions they may have.

The Big Event: Birth Equipment

I carry about 175 pounds of equipment with me to every birth—$15,000 worth of equipment. I carry IV fluids, drugs to stop hemorrhage, medication for violent vomiting, some pain medication, tools for resuscitation, and equipment for the baby. I bring several tanks of oxygen, a birth stool, a full homeopathic and herbal kit—I'm much more likely to use herbs or homeopathy before I resort to Western medicine, but the Western techniques that I can use as a registered nurse and midwife have lowered my transport-to-hospital rates dramatically.

I carry supplies to catheterize a laboring mother, to use if she is unable to pee. I can even put in an indwelling Foley catheter

(a device to help her pee without having to get up and go to the bathroom) if the mother is exhausted after the birth and needs to rest for 12–24 hours. I carry everything needed to anesthetize the area for the very rare episiotomy and to do any suturing necessary if there is a tear(s) during birth.

I carry everything needed to weigh and measure the baby, check their vitals, administer Vitamin K and eye drops, and perform all of the baby's aftercare.

Other equipment I bring includes a blood pressure cuff, stethoscope, doppler, everything to draw blood, oxygen masks for momma and baby, Ambu bag (infant resuscitation device), antibiotics, yoga blocks, a foldable stretcher, gauze, pads, gloves, scrub solutions, instruments, pressure cooker for sterilization of thirty-five instruments, footprint pads, file box with paperwork, etc.

My team and I set all of this up in a way that is very unobtrusive. All of my equipment stays in tackle boxes that we

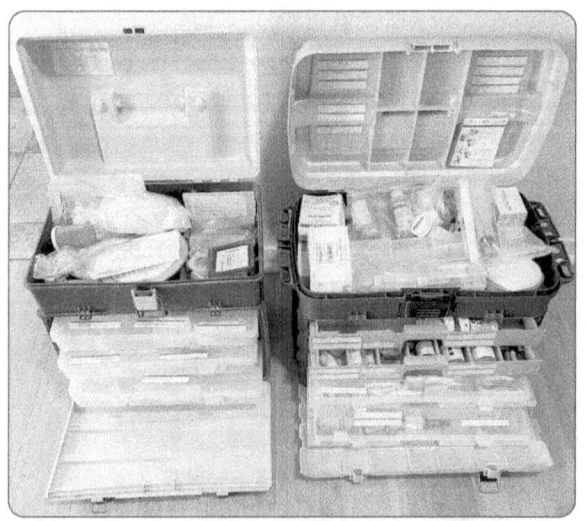

MariMikel's Equipment in Tackle Boxes

place against a wall in my client's home. I also have two cases with supplies that we keep in another room, out of the way until and if they are needed. We do this so the bedroom doesn't look like a medical minefield.

Birth is an intimate experience and I find that most women prefer the comfort of their partner. I am present for the birth, but I fade into the background until and unless I am needed. I provide the laboring woman with guidance about how her birth is going, helping her to gauge where she is in the process, and I make suggestions for things she might like to try. I get her consent for any intervention I recommend. My team and I are very present for her at the end and coach her through pushing as her baby enters the world. I'll go into much greater detail about this in The Labor and Birth Process chapter.

Complications and Transport to the Hospital

I want you to know that I have a plan for every single thing that could happen and the equipment to deal with it, and that includes knowing what I am not equipped to handle. If something comes up that I cannot handle, we immediately go to the hospital. Every midwife is trained to know when the situation is beyond their ability and always carries the health of the mother and the baby as her foremost concern.

If we do need to transfer to the hospital, I go with my clients and I stay there with them. I am their advocate. I run interference and interpret what the hospital staff is doing and saying to make sure they don't do anything that my client doesn't want (unless it is medically necessary). I stay

there until the baby is born and we either get to go back home right away or it may be that they stay in the hospital for a few days.

If you are still concerned and want more information about whether or not a home birth is safe, I encourage you to look at the complications section on page XX to see how I and many other midwives will approach any difficult or complicated situation.

Your Birth Story

I write a lengthy, accurate story about each birth to give to the family based on the copious notes I take during their birth experience. I document every aspect, what everyone is doing and saying, and provide them with a very accurate medical record and journal of the birth. These end up being five to ten pages long. I write these in legible handwriting. I have found so many of my clients cherish this documented birth story that they are able to read even years or decades later, and that they can share with their child if and when they want when they are older.

Postpartum Visits

I do think one of the reasons I don't see symptoms of serious postpartum depression in my clients (I don't want to say that no one has a hard time, it's just not life threatening) is that they have a loving, attentive care provider who wants to be sure that they are all right. I pay a lot of attention to them. I am there for them. I counsel and support them. I lift them up. And this is true for the vast majority of US homebirth midwives, who are generally amazing women with huge hearts full of love and compassion for their clients and brains full of wisdom and knowledge about how to facilitate normal physiologic births and how to identify and deal with birth complications when they arise. Statistics show that complications occur in only 13.6 percent of midwife-attended home births in the United States.[106] Compare this with the US hospital birth c-section rate of 31.8 percent, which is only one possible complication in birth.

My clients see me again for multiple postpartum visits in the days after birth (I go to their home or to the hospital if they are there) and have continual access to me via phone. I encourage them to call me with any questions or concerns at all. After two weeks, postpartum visits happen at my clinic.

Choosing a Care Provider

I know this has been an incredibly deep dive, but your ideal, perfect pregnancy and birth experience is the whole point of this book, and I want you to be informed about the care you choose for this experience. Hopefully I was able to dispel some of the myths and fairy tales you may have heard about hospital births, freestanding birth centers, and home births and to give you a better idea of what it's like to have a home birth or birth center birth with a modern midwife and what it's really like to have a birth in a modern hospital.

It is Your Choice

Now it's time for you to select someone to be your care provider, the person who will shepherd you through your pregnancy. If you haven't already, research the available options in your area. Find out if they take your insurance. Some midwives take insurance; some don't. I do not take insurance, but my fees work out to be approximately what you would pay out-of-pocket to meet a deductible and the percentage of service fees owed.

I want you to choose the practitioner who's best for *you*. I encourage you to look at midwives and think about whether it might be a good option for you, and I want you to have enough data to make an informed choice. There may be no midwives available in the area that you live in, in which case you will have to make another choice. In those instances, rely on your head and heart to make these decisions. Get the data and information about the person that you are interested in, and then go and visit them. Let your heart tell you if they are respectful, informative, and make you feel like you want to feel.

I'd like to take a moment to address surrogacy. A surrogate of pregnancy occurs when a woman carries a baby and gives birth for a couple who cannot do so themselves. Usually, the biological parents' genetic materials are in-vitro fertilized. The embryo is implanted in the surrogate mother's womb where it develops and then is born. At that point the biological parents take over parenting the new baby

I have assisted on several surrogate pregnancies. All of the women serving as surrogates were women who were married with children and were doing this as a kindness and also for financial compensation. It is an incredible gift and blessing to give this to a couple who cannot carry their own baby. But I think having a care provider who has more time for you through your pregnancy and birth, and who can give you the emotional and spiritual support that you need in this complicated situation, can be very valuable. While this is a gift and a blessing, it also is emotionally challenging to the surrogate mom. Pick a care provider who can be supportive.

If your idea of an ideal, perfect birth is one where you are in a hospital environment, attended on by professional strangers, and you like the ideas of blocking the pain and having the convenience of interventions, then that is what your ideal, perfect birth looks like, and I encourage you to keep reading with *absolutely no judgment from me.* I promise you I am not anti-hospital. I have learned so much from doctors and I have great respect for the work they do. I would love to offer the hospital practitioners some relief so that they can perform at peak levels instead of constantly being overworked and overwhelmed with patients. They are handling so much.

I know I can at times come across as very authoritative and opinionated, and the truth is, I am those things. Please understand that the foundational bedrock, though, is my absolute support of your desires and wishes. I truly want you to have *your* perfect, ideal birth. I ask that you consider the things that I feel strongly about, and simply discard them if they are not for you. But please do keep reading. I feel certain that no matter your path, you will find valuable insights and help in these pages. I do not want you to feel alienated if you are not choosing to work with or do not have the ability to work with a midwife.

Depending on where you live, hospital care may be your only option. It's difficult to achieve the depth of care you need and deserve through your pregnancy from mainstream practitioners because, again, they are overwhelmed. They must jam pack their schedules with patients to keep their practices afloat. Please keep this book by your side and let me be a guide when they cannot.

Questions to Ask a Potential Provider

Every doctor is different just as every midwife is different. There will be great ones and not so great ones. As a consumer, I want you to be conscientious. Don't just go with the first provider you find in your network. Conduct interviews. Get references. Gauge whether this is a good doctor or midwife to be with or not, the same as you should be doing with all your health care practitioners.

When you are figuring out the route for you, I think it is very helpful to go and meet with several midwives and hear what they have to say. Then take a tour of the local hospital and see what they have to tell you and what their labor and delivery rooms look and feel like. Interview OB/GYNs. Finally, visit some freestanding birth centers if they are available near you and see what they're like and what their ideas surrounding birth are. Without going and visiting you're not going to have all the information that you need to make this very important decision.

The hospital practitioners—nurses and doctors alike—simply do not have the time to get to know their patients as individuals. Many hospital-based nurse-midwives do try to develop relationships with their patients, so if you can find a certified nurse-midwife (CNM) who can serve as your primary care provider, you are likely to be much better cared for than if you choose an obstetrician. I also recommend birth and postpartum doulas if you choose to work with a doctor. We'll talk more about what they offer in The Second Trimester chapter.

When you are able to find someone who has enough time to give you something more than just medical care it helps a lot. This is easier said than done. We have a lot of people giving birth and not enough midwives to provide the kind of care that I provide. It is challenging for you to find someone, but I suggest that you look. They are out there, and the more we seek them, the more women will choose to become midwives, and the more available they will be.

Here are some questions you can ask to assess if a potential provider is right for you:

- What are your credentials, i.e., education?
- How long have you been in practice?
- How many births have you attended?
- What is your complication rate?
- What is your c-section rate?
- What is your epidural rate?
- What is your maternal/infant mortality and morbidity rate?
- Do you come for each birth or is it an on-call situation where you are there for example on Tuesdays, Wednesdays, and Saturdays?
- Do you work with other doctors or midwives? If so, will I meet them ahead of time? Will I have prenatal visits with them?

- For midwives: Where do you transport to in case of complications.
- For midwives: Do you stay with me when there is a complication and transport to the hospital?
- How many prenatal visits will I have with you and how long will they last?
- What does your postpartum care entail?
- For midwives: Do I come to you or do you come to me?
- For birth centers: What is a typical labor experience like here? Is it more like a home birth or more like a hospital birth experience? In what ways?
- Will there be shift changes during my labor and birth? Will I see different care providers and attendants during my labor?
- What do you charge?
- How are payments made and at what intervals?
- Does insurance or Medicaid cover any of this?
- How involved can my partner be?

Believe in the ability of the female body to propagate the species without the need for surgical intervention. If the doctor you're talking with has a c-section rate approaching or higher than the national average of nearly 32 percent, I advise you to keep looking unless you too want to be strongarmed into having a major abdominal surgery.

If you have had a previous c-section and are wanting a VBAC (vaginal birth after C-section) it is important to ask questions about this, too.

- Are you comfortable supporting me through a VBAC?

- What is your experience with VBACs—how many have you attended and what is your success rate?

- Do you allow induction or augmentation with VBACs if necessary, and is the facility (hospital or birth center) supportive of VBACs?

Assess your comfort level in talking with each provider you interview. Are they open to your questions? How do you feel when you are in the room with them?

Once you've made your selection, make your first appointment! Know that most OB/GYNs will not want to see you before ten to twelve weeks because of the risk of miscarriage. They'd rather start after the majority of that risk has passed and knowing that you likely have a viable pregnancy. They are also less likely at that point to have to deal with morning sickness, nausea, and the emotional upheaval of early pregnancy.

How to Find a Midwife

Not every midwife works the way that I do. If you decide you'd like to have a home birth, interview several midwives in your area, and ask for references and their statistics related to transport to the hospital, episiotomies, interventions, maternal and infant mortality, etc. Listen to what your intuition tells you about them. By doing this you have an excellent chance of finding a midwife who resonates with you.

To find a midwife in your area, it's always a good idea to use a search engine to look for "midwives near me." Many midwifery practices have their own websites and social media pages where you can learn more about their philosophy of care, services offered, and insurance coverage. There are a few directories available that may also help you to find midwives near you.

- Sistamidwife.com maintains a directory of Black doulas and midwives https://www.sistamidwifedirectory.com/home

- The Midwives Alliance of North America (MANA) has a directory of midwifery organizations and resources state by state which may help you find midwives near you. https://mana.org/about-midwives/state-by-state

- Birth Centers.org: This is a directory of freestanding birth centers in the United States. While not all birth centers are run by midwives, many are, and this can be a good resource if you're looking for a midwife-attended birth.

- La Leche League may also be a good resource for you to find midwives in your area.

- State midwifery groups can often be a good resource (e.g., Association of Texas Midwives (ATM), California Association of Licensed Midwives (CALM)).

Schedule a consultation with several midwives/practitioners if you can, and then select the practitioner you most resonate with.

What Will it Cost?

Children are expensive, regardless of how you have them. A recent study by the Brookings Institution estimates it takes $300,000 to raise a child to age 17 in the US.[107] Childbirth costs will vary depending on several factors, including your choice of providers and your insurance deductible and coverage. The study also found that the cost of raising a child varies significantly by income level, with higher-income families spending more on their children than lower-income families.

Insurance and Insurance Issues

Your personal finances and insurance may set you up to think you must travel in a certain lane in order to have the least expensive birth. I encourage you to understand what your deductible is and how much you will have to pay out of pocket. The difference in cost between midwifery care and a hospital birth may not be as vast as you'd think. If you'd like to have a midwife as your care provider, I'd also encourage you to engage in a conversation with your chosen midwife about what payment plans and/or insurance she takes. In my experience, midwives want to find a

HOW MUCH IT COSTS TO HAVE A BABY IN THE USA

This was my fourth baby and fortunately everything was cookie-cutter smooth, no high risks, no extra ultrasounds. It was a very smooth pregnancy and vaginal delivery. I paid a total of $1,823 for my OB and prenatal care. I paid $99 for genetic testing and an early gender reveal. The hospital bill for me was $7,400, but insurance covered $4,100 and I got a pay-in-full discount of 30 percent, so I only paid $2,288.

The hospital bill for my baby was $1,174 and other expenses for my baby were $1,239. I got an epidural and the bill for that was $1,680, but after insurance I only paid $211. I have very average insurance—definitely not the worst, but it's not winning any awards. So, in total I paid $6,834 out of pocket to have my baby.

—Addison Jarman, 2023

way to work with you in a way that is good for both of you.

Home birth is the least expensive option for giving birth, averaging $4650 in the US and costing 68 percent less than hospital birth.[108] Home birth is suitable for low-

	Average cost of childbirth in hospitals	Average out-of-pocket cost for health insurance plan members
Childbirth	$18,865	$2,854
Vaginal delivery	$14,768	$2,655
Cesarean	$26,280	$3,214

Source: Peterson-KFF Health System Tracker, 2022. Costs are based on large group health insurance plans.

Penelope: When I had my first child, the Affordable Care Act had not yet been passed. I was a freelancer without insurance, and pregnancy was considered a pre-existing condition, so I couldn't get health insurance. I assumed that midwifery care would be out of my financial reach, and I so wish that I hadn't.

I did contact the hospital ahead of time and negotiated with their finance department to give me a payment plan and a discount for their services. I was able to cut the stated costs nearly in half. It still cost me over $6,000 more than 15 years ago. I can only imagine it's more expensive now. Whatever your choice, be a great advocate for yourself.

risk pregnancies. A birth center is another option that is somewhere between home and hospital in terms of cost. A birth center allows for a quick discharge after birth and is usually covered by insurance. A hospital birth is often the most expensive option, especially without insurance.

I typically have two to four apprentices with me, and my fee is the same regardless of the number of attendants, the length of the birth, or the duration of birth services rendered (meaning, you can start seeing me as soon as you get pregnant or in your second trimester; the fee is the same). I currently charge on a sliding scale of $3,500–$6,500. I am absolutely worth $6,500, but I don't want to turn away the people who really want and deserve to have a different experience but have limited finances. I don't want people to be horribly stressed out about finances; I want them to have an amazing birth.

Many midwives, myself included, do not accept insurance (or conversely, most insurance plans don't support midwifery care), but some do, and most midwives will work with you on a monthly payment plan if the fees are too much all at once. Medicaid does cover some home births—

it's worth checking if you are covered this way! If your insurance won't pay, you can often work out a payment plan with a midwife, paying $350–$650 a month for ten months, which is very worth it to have a dramatically different birth experience than if you were in a hospital.

I am providing this information to show that the out-of-pocket cost of having a birth at home with a midwife may be quite similar to the cost of birthing at a hospital when you have insurance—and quite a bit less expensive if you do not.

If you don't have insurance and are planning a hospital birth, you can negotiate with the hospital directly to both reduce the cost of the service (they are often willing to do this if you have good credit and it means they don't have to deal with an insurance company) and to set up a payment plan.

Demystifying Pregnancy Dos and Don'ts

Myth: You Can't Have Sushi

You can have sushi and lox. Now, don't eat the sushi from the corner store in Waco, don't eat the sushi from places that don't specialize in it ... Make sure it's fresh and from a good source. Feel free to sit in front of the sushi chef at a fabulous restaurant and tell them, "I'm pregnant! Give me the freshest fish you have, please."

Myth: You Can't Get in a Hot Tub

Hot tubs are fine. It is getting overheated that is not okay. If the hot tub is at a reasonable temperature and you don't stay in it too long, it can be beneficially relaxing.

It's perfectly fine to get in the hot tub. As soon as you feel warm, get out and cool off a bit. The problem isn't the hot tub, it's overheating. It is much more common to become overheated working in the yard or attending an outdoor event in the summer. You can also become overheated by taking a shower or bath that is too hot. Always be careful in these situations, because overheating affects your baby's umbilical cord and can cause problems.

Myth: You Can't Have Soft Cheeses & Lunch Meats

This one is also untrue. You can have soft cheeses and lunch meats. Again, what's important is the sourcing and freshness.

With lunch meats, even with decent brands, if it's been delivered from an outside company to your grocery store it's likely been in the package too long, and that's the problem. However, you can go to a natural grocer (Whole Foods, Nature's Market, Natural Grocers, Sprouts, etc.) and get freshly sliced sandwich meat from their deli counter. Austin's Central Market makes beautiful roasted turkey breasts on the daily. If you go to Central Market or a

similar grocer and let them shave you off some turkey, you're going to be fine. The big key is that it has to be a reputable store with a very high turnover of products, so you are always getting fresh lunch meats that were cooked in the last 24 hours without the addition of preservatives.

Many high-end grocery stores, like Whole Foods, have world class cheeses. They carefully check out their cheese sources, and you don't really have to worry about their cheeses. The problems come when things aren't fresh. You simply have to be a conscientious consumer.

Myth: Don't Drink Any Alcohol, Ever

Some time ago, I asked a whole bunch of my doctor friends, "Where's the study that said a glass of wine would harm the baby?"

They told me, "There isn't one."

I then asked, "Why are you telling women that even a single glass of wine will damage their baby?"

They all said, "Well, you know women. If you tell them they can have one, they'll have ten."

I said, "Let me get this straight. You think women are so hysterical, indulgent, and uncontrollable that we have to lie to them to get them to do the right thing?" That was pretty much the end of our conversation.

Of course, women are fully capable of following the safety guidelines if they are properly explained. If you don't struggle with addiction, one glass of wine a week is just fine. Danish studies followed a cohort of women who consumed minimal amounts of alcohol (defined as less than nine drinks a week!) and found no adverse effects in their children over time.[109] Remember, with all things that may be questionable to you, the choice is yours and yours alone. Your body, your choice.

I think alcohol can occasionally be beneficial when used medicinally to combat stress (except for the people for whom it's not beneficial). If it helps you to unwind with a single glass of wine once a week, absolutely do that. If you don't face addiction issues, it's perfectly fine to drink alcohol in pregnancy, as long as you don't overdo it. The time to use alcohol is when you're stressed out, because stress is really harmful for babies, and really harmful for you. Alcohol suppresses stress hormones; it suppresses cortisol.[110]

If alcohol addiction is something that you struggle with, don't wrestle with that demon. Find another method of relaxation. If you do choose to use alcohol to help combat stress, I suggest at most two to four alcoholic beverages a month. I suggest doing it medicinally when you are really stressed. Stress hormones are, I believe, far worse for your growing baby.

Myth: Sex Will Hurt the Baby

Nope. Nope, nope, nope. Couples should absolutely have sex during pregnancy, as long as you are both 100 percent into it. It's good for your baby and good for mom. Every time you have sex it makes your uterus create more receptor sites for oxytocin to attach to, so you have an easier birth.[111] It produces more oxytocin in the pituitary to make the whole thing go better. It also produces endorphins, which are natural painkillers.

Anything shy of swinging from the chandeliers is fine, as long as you and your partner are both fine with it. You will not hurt the baby with normal sex, and it will help you physically, emotionally, and it will definitely help with your relationship. As you get further along in your pregnancy, you might need to be a bit gentler if you are typically more adventurous in the bedroom.

Use whatever positions feel good, although later in the pregnancy, when you've got a big belly, what feels good is not usually somebody on top of you. For a lot of women lying on their side with their partner behind them or on their hands and knees is comfortable and pleasurable. But really, anything that is good for you is *good*.

If your partner is unavailable, masturbation will help to achieve the same oxytocin activation. Have fun!

Many women notice a marked decrease in their sex drive when they are pregnant. If this is you, don't shame or judge yourself. It's important for the reasons I mentioned above, though, and for the health of your partnership (if you are in one), that you work to find ways to stimulate your sensuality and sexuality during your pregnancy.

Remember that you are not the only partner in your partnership, compromise is important, and having sex is one of the keys to having an easier birth. Notice when your sex drive is stimulated and work to stack those triggers so you can get in the mood.

MariMikel: Many years ago, I had 12 women in my care over an 18-month period who had no sex at all during their pregnancies, and nine of them had c-sections. Two had 48-hour labors, and one of them had a normal experience. It dawned on me that the sexual energy that gets the baby in there is the same energy that gets the baby out.

Communicate with your partner about what you find attractive right now. Maybe you need extra soothing foreplay in the form of a massage with warm oils and sexy music. Maybe you find intellectual conversation, talking about sensual times from your shared past, or sharing dreams about your future together to be quite stimulating. Be playful. Experiment.

It's also important that you maintain sexual hygiene to decrease the risk of vaginal infections. Both partners must stay clean, and if you are struggling with a yeast infection, bacterial vaginosis, or any other vaginal infection, I recommend you use condoms.

If you are bleeding or cramping, do not have sex. Instead, call your midwife immediately.

If you find vaginal dryness to be a problem, I recommend ASTROGLIDE, K–Y True Feel, and K–Y Ultragel.

Myth: You Can't Lie on Your Back

There is a huge myth that you cannot sleep on your back in pregnancy. I have seen many women who have been told that they can only sleep on their left side. It is ridiculous to imagine that you can only sleep on one side for nine months; it doesn't even make sense. Historically, women did not have a book or myth that told them to never sleep on their backs in pregnancy.

This myth does originate from a valid concern, though. When you get to be very big at the end of your pregnancy, if you are on your back for too long, the weight of the baby, uterus, and amniotic fluid can compress veins and arteries and decrease the oxygen that flows to the baby through the umbilical cord. When this kind of pressure occurs, every woman feels uncomfortable. It makes you feel like someone is sitting on your chest and you have trouble breathing. It is not a situation that is going to sneak by you, and you will move. Your body has systems in place to help you and your baby stay safe.

Another thing to consider is that everyone's belly protrudes differently. Some have a very prominent belly as early as 34 weeks. Alternatively, some women's bellies are not prominent because they have a deep torso and abdominal cavity and even a quite large baby can somewhat hide in there and they may not show much at all, even toward the end of the pregnancy. The woman who is huge at 34 weeks may need to stop sleeping on her back earlier than a woman who is not showing as much nearer to the end.

When it does not feel good to be on your back, simply move into a different position. I think if you are on your side for too long your hips and shoulders can start to hurt, and you may experience numbness in your hands. It is most sensible to move from side to back to side throughout the night and not stay in any one position for too long. The truth is, at the very end of your pregnancy, you won't want to spend much time on your back. Remember to trust your intuition.

Myth: Once a Cesarean, always a Cesarean

VBAC is an acronym for vaginal birth after cesarean. The US cesarean section rate has stayed stable at around 32 percent since 2011, meaning that around one-third of American women have a cesarean birth. Many women believe that once you have a c-section, you must have c-sections for subsequent births. There is a very small chance (0.5 percent in the US) of uterine rupture in a VBAC,[112] and this has been found to be prone to happen when the woman was administered heavy doses of Pitocin. The Pitocin increases the strength of the contractions so intensely that the former scar can tear open. Hospitals have stopped administering Pitocin in almost all VBACs, but in the last few years they have been occasionally using minimal amounts of Pitocin for VBACs and finding that if you give small enough amounts of Pitocin, you can achieve positive results without harm.

There are many benefits to VBACs, but one that is not discussed often is how important it is for the baby to be squeezed by the uterus, contractions, and pelvis during the birth. This squeezing is something like a full-body massage, and it does something beneficial to all of the parts of the baby—the brain, the body, and possibly the spirit. An astonishingly important element of the natural, vaginal birth is the flood of oxytocin that does not

happen in a planned c-section. In the US the VBAC rate is a paltry 14 percent. The overall attempted VBAC success rate is 70 percent,[113] which frankly means not enough women are attempting a VBAC. It can be done. My personal VBAC success rate is approximately 80 percent, which I believe is an excellent indicator that a VBAC is very possible.

While I am a huge proponent of VBACs, there are times when they should not be attempted, and a repeat c-section is the very best and safest plan:

- If in your previous c-section you had to have a vertical incision from your belly button straight down to your pubic bone, this is a contraindication to having a VBAC, because that type of scar ruptures much more frequently.

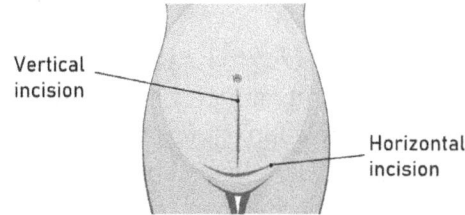

Types of Cesarean Incisions

- If you had a c-section after many hours of labor with a normal size baby and you were told that your pelvis was too small, a repeat c-section may be the best choice.

- If you develop high blood pressure, gestational diabetes, or placenta previa, these could all also be reasons to have another c-section.

- A twin or multiple birth stretches out the abdomen and uterus of the women much more intensely than a singleton and I think a VBAC would also be contraindicated in these instances.

If you are attempting a VBAC and labor does not progress, most care providers are going to be quicker to suggest a repeat c-section, and with good reason. Each situation needs to be examined uniquely by your care provider to assess the risks and safety.

If you are preparing for a VBAC, I strongly recommend you take evening primrose oil to help soften the scar tissue and create more elasticity, so it does not tear. I also strongly suggest that you use a belly support system from 30 weeks on or whenever the baby is head down after 30 weeks. This will help to take the pressure off the scar and equalize the pressure around your abdomen and back. Your insurance provider may cover this cost—they often do.

I suggest you also massage the scar tissue to help to break up any tense spots and to help it to be more supple and soft, so it stretches more easily. Use olive oil or Vitamin E oil to lubricate the area, then use two fingers and massage in small, 2- to 3-inch circles. Move from right to left circling clockwise. Then move left to right circling counterclockwise across the scar. Pay particular attention to any tense spots as more massage on those areas will help them to soften up. You might have to spend 15–20 seconds on those harder spots to feel the difference. This massage only takes a few minutes a few times a week throughout the pregnancy and it can make such a huge difference.

In terms of your emotional and mental readiness, focus on affirmations, visualizations, prayer, meditation and mindfulness, and anything that will help you feel confident, relaxed, and positive. It is very easy after you have had a cesarean to have unconscious and subconscious fears. There is a very deep part of you as a woman that may think you cannot do it, that your body does not work, and that you cannot trust the process. But these are not necessarily true. Our minds are so incredibly powerful, and we are so creative with our thoughts that it is critical to put out the thoughts that you want to have happen. "My body works." "This process was designed to work." "I trust that I can push out my baby through my vagina."

 Your partner will also impact this process. How they feel and what they say is going to affect you. This is an important point and you both must work together as a team and find the tools to combat any fears that may reside in either of you.

In order to not be afraid, you must also have a care provider who feels confident in VBAC delivery and is skilled and experienced. We've discussed the importance of finding a care provider who is supportive of your desire to attempt a VBAC. Make sure to have these discussions early in the pregnancy so you are supported.

Most of the time vaginal birth after cesarean works, and it is worth trying. If it ends up not working out, then interventions are available, and you may end up having another c-section. Don't let this possibility stop you from trying for a vaginal birth.

Truth: You shouldn't Wear Thong Underwear

This is advice that I absolutely agree with. Do not wear thong style underwear. It increases your chances of Group B Streptococcus (GBS or strep B), yeast, Gardnerella, and other vaginal infections because it rubs between your rectum and acts like a wick to move those bacteria toward your vagina. These infections can pose very serious potential complications, and avoiding thong-style underwear is something easy you can do to prevent problems. If all you own are thongs, put them away and get yourself some comfortable, larger, cotton panties. There are many beautiful, full-bottomed underwear out there. They don't have to be granny panties.

I will acknowledge there is research showing that hygiene is more important than the type of underwear you don, but in my experience too large a percentage of my thong-wearing clients develop vaginal infections for there not to be a correlation, and I think it is smarter to choose to not wear thong underwear.

Handling the Common Discomforts of Pregnancy

In this section I'll cover several of the common ailments and discomforts many women feel during pregnancy and what to do about them. This is information to help you if you are having any of these issues, but *always* feel free to call your midwife if anything is troubling you. I do recommend you keep track of any issues and be sure to let your midwife know if you are having any of these symptoms at your next prenatal appointment.

When to Call Your Midwife

I do want you to call your midwife[1] *immediately* if:

- There is water leaking from your vagina.
- There is any bleeding from your vagina (a little touch of pink or red is not necessarily abnormal, especially after sex, serious exercise, or a long day on your feet, but call anyway).
- You get sick, i.e., sinus infection, bladder infection (burning, stinging, or an urgency when peeing), stomach flu, respiratory infection symptoms, food poisoning.
- You take a bad fall.
- You experience severe emotional upset.
- You are in a car wreck.
- You experience regular contractions before 37 weeks that are getting longer, stronger, and closer together.
- You have a vaginal infection (indicated by itching, burning, and/or a fishy or foul odor).
- If you just need to talk (if you're working with a midwife or doula).

It is important to note that any physical pain that is getting worse and worse requires immediate attention and intervention. For example, if you have sharp pain in your lower abdomen, midline behind the pubic bone or in your vagina, this could be a bladder infection or your cervix opening. Do

---

[1] As a reminder, if your care provider is not a midwife, feel free to substitute "Care Provider" or "OB/GYN" here.

not suffer in silence! If you are struggling, call your provider and let them know what's going on. You deserve to be cared for.

Morning Sickness

For many women, mornings are difficult during the first trimester. There is a reason they call it morning sickness. Part of it is because you're nutritionally challenged. Feeling off in the morning can last until you are ten to fourteen weeks pregnant. Very rarely, but occasionally, it lasts longer than that, but if you follow my nutritional recommendations for what to eat and how frequently, it's more likely that won't be the case. I see less morning sickness in my clients because of what I recommend to them via the Sevenfold Approach.

If you do struggle with nausea, no matter what time of day, I have a few techniques for you to try:

Tiny Meals at Nighttime

First, make sure you're following my recommendations for nighttime eating on page 120.

Ginger

Many women find ginger lozenges, suckers, or candied ginger to be helpful in calming their stomachs.

Herbs/Acupuncture

Work with an acupuncturist and/or herbalist to alleviate your symptoms.

Cannabis/CBD

I have seen women who were greatly benefited with horrible pregnancy nausea by a little bit of cannabis or CBD. You have to weigh this for yourself and make your own educated choices. Refer to my earlier discussion of cannabis on page 57.

Prescription Medication

If you continue to struggle, find a doctor or nurse, and ask for a prescription for an anti-nausea medication. Typically, they will prescribe Zofran.

Headaches

The two most common causes of headaches during pregnancy are 1) dehydration from not drinking enough water and 2) low blood sugar from not eating enough. Another possible cause is that the volume of blood inside your body doubles in pregnancy to support the baby and to prepare for breastfeeding. Headaches can develop when this fluid stretches out the blood vessels in the brain. It may be uncomfortable, but this stretching of vessels will not harm you or the baby. Hormones can also be the cause of headaches in some women.

To alleviate most headaches, stay on top of your eating and drinking schedules. Your body needs fuel and hydration right now, and it will find an unpleasant way to tell you if you're slacking.

Migraines

Migraines are their own special beast and require quick remediation. If you're prone to migraines, I have a few strategies to help you out. The first is that you must stop consuming caffeine regularly. If you regularly consume caffeine, this method will not work. This is fantastic to do for your baby, too. See my approach for how to get off coffee without losing your sanity on page 62. Make sure you're drinking your four quarts of water a day absolutely faithfully. Then, if you get telltale signs that a migraine is coming on, follow these steps and hopefully it will shorten the duration of the migraine, or possibly keep it from coming on altogether.

1. The first thing you do is stop completely. I mean everything. If you're at work or grocery shopping or wherever, you go home. Leave work mid-meeting if you have to or abandon your grocery cart in the aisle and go home immediately.

   If you work from home, you stop working. You know it's going to incapacitate you anyway and you're not going to be able to do anything, so just call a halt to whatever you're doing.

2. Hang a sign on the front door that says, "Do Not Disturb Upon Pain of Death." You don't have to be that dramatic. You could just leave it at DO NOT DISTURB: MIGRAINE. Whatever you choose, have the sign ready to go ahead of time, because you have to move fast once the migraine is in motion.

3. Drink a quart of water while you accomplish the following steps.

4. Make a cup of coffee—keep freeze dried espresso in the freezer so you can just heat some water up and make it quickly.

5. Chug the coffee down with two or three 200 mg ibuprofen (two if you weigh less than 150 pounds, three if you weigh 151+ pounds), fill a plastic bag with ice, and go to your bedroom.

6. Darken the room. Unplug everything. Power your phone off. Lie down and put the ice on your head. Close your eyes. Visual stimulation makes it worse. You can wear an eye mask if you like.

7. Succumb to your desire to take a nap.

If the migraine gets you, you're done. But, if you move fast enough and make all of this happen before it gets you, it is very likely that the combination of caffeine, ibuprofen, ice, darkness, and quiet will encourage you to fall asleep for a short nap and when you wake up, you'll be fine. You'll absolutely ward off the migraine. However, if you're already drinking coffee every day, this won't have the same effect. If you suffer migraines, take steps now to get off any caffeine habit you may have.

Constipation

Constipation is a common occurrence in pregnancy and can be very uncomfortable. The most common causes of constipation are not drinking enough water, not eating enough food, eating the wrong foods, and not getting enough exercise. If you were very physically active prior to pregnancy and stop exercising (as I advise) in the first trimester, your body may get constipated as it adjusts. Pregnancy, especially early pregnancy, is constipating because your intestinal motility slows down. When you're very low ebb and can't really do as much, that can sometimes get you as well.

If you're not eating enough food, your body is going to hold on to whatever you're eating and try to wring a few more calories out of it.

Be careful of foods you know to clog you up. For me it's pizza. I do love it, but the flour is my downfall. I now am very enamored with the cauliflower crusts. I can't tell the difference and I just pile tons and tons of sauce and veggies on it and a tiny bit of mozzarella and parmesan and it's fantastic and not in the slightest bit constipating.

The vast majority of people simply eat too much white flour, and the conventionally grown gluten is exceptionally detrimental. Many people unknowingly have conditions that are linked directly to their consumption of gluten or US-grown grains.

There are so many alternatives out there now; it's really easy to substitute. You don't have to cut every scrap of gluten out of your diet, but experiment with having less. If you do cut it out entirely, you may experience flu-like symptoms (headache, weakness, chills, shakes) in the first week after eliminating it from your diet. To alleviate these symptoms, drink hot chicken or bone broth.

Eat fresh fruits, dried fruits, and bran. You can also take bran tablets. You will want to eat 100 percent whole grains as a preventative measure (whole wheat bread, brown rice, rye, etc.). Eat plenty of fresh, raw, and steamed vegetables. The fiber in these will help with your bowel movements.

Avoid an excess of dairy products (especially cheese), conventionally grown red meat, and processed foods that include so many empty calories and tons of sugar and salt, etc. Limit caffeine such as coffee, black tea, sodas, and chocolate, as these contribute to the problem with long term use.

Do not wait if you feel the urge to use the bathroom. Go immediately. Sometimes pulling your knees up to your chest and putting your feet on the seat or on a small stool in front of the toilet (Squatty Pottys are great) compresses your intestines and makes elimination easier.

Do not take laxatives during pregnancy. Laxatives can cause severe stomach cramps and occasionally cause miscarriage or early onset of labor. Don't do enemas or colonics during pregnancy either.

Do not take laxatives or do enemas or colonics during pregnancy.

If you have been constipated for two days or longer, use a glycerin suppository (available over the counter from any pharmacy) to lubricate and relieve the lower bowel. Once hard stools have been moved, the preventative measures described above will be more effective.

Glycerin suppositories are very effective for helping you to go. They're shaped like a bullet and about the size of two digits of your little finger, quite small. You will insert the suppository into the rectum. You have to relax enough to get up in there. If you just barely get it into your rectum, you will feel it and it will be uncomfortable. If you push it in about an inch it will effortlessly melt over about 10 to 20 minutes and lubricate the lower bowel, helping dry stool to pass gently. Wash your hands carefully after insertion or use a disposable glove.

Do not suffer through constipation for days. This is waste that needs to come out, so use the glycerin suppository. Don't be scared. It's not painful and it will bring you relief.

Herpes

The first trimester is a very stressful time for the body. It is undergoing some serious stress from the pressures of pregnancy and the physical and hormonal changes. I see an increase in herpes outbreaks at this time. Pay careful attention to the prodromal symptoms and do everything you can to mitigate them. I find that sometimes a cool cloth (not cold) can sometimes slow down or stop the outbreak. You must slow down and reduce stress as a preventative measure. For more information, you can visit the detailed explanation of how to deal with herpes on page 90.

Pregnancy Brain

In early pregnancy you may be more forgetful and possibly clumsier than you normally are. This affects some women more than others.[114] We call this pregnancy brain, and it is a real thing. I believe it is because so much of your vital life force is going to the creation of this dynamic new being that it takes *everything*, and there's just not enough left for you to be sharp and snappy.

If you don't already, you may find it useful to implement the use of a project management system or planner, so you don't forget as much. Schedule alarms to remind yourself to check it until you are used to working with it. Some free, web-based project/task management systems include Asana, Trello, and Habitica.

MariMikel: I remember for one of my pregnancies I received a reminder call at 10:00 a.m. for an appointment later that day at 2:00 p.m. I said, "Oh, thank you so much for letting me know. Yes, I'll be there."

At three o'clock, the office called to ask me if I remembered the conversation we'd had that morning about my two o'clock appointment. I said, "Well, that does sound vaguely familiar." It was pretty shocking to have forgotten so completely so rapidly.

Aleah: I went on a trip with some girlfriends when I was in the early stages of pregnancy with my first baby. We were sightseeing in a park and were all chatting happily. I tried to tell them what I was feeling about how beautiful the park was. I said "This is really just one of the most beautiful places I have ever been, the trees are beautiful, the flowers are blooming and the ... the ... well, you know that thing in the sky that shines... oh jeez, what is it called?" We all laughed hysterically as they reminded me that yes, that big ball of light in the sky was called the sun.

Well, it was definitely funny, but also completely disconcerting to me at the same time. I was someone who was proud of my brain. I had accomplished a master's degree and I used my brain a lot for all that my work entailed. This feeling was so foreign! How could I have forgotten the word sun? The pregnancy brain was in full effect and I knew it would not always last (which it didn't) but it is real and can be discombobulating.

One of the things that you need to remember is that all of this is going to go away. You are going to return to your sharp and savvy self. But give in to it for now and act accordingly.

Uterine Cramping and Spotting

In the first trimester, cramping and spotting can happen, especially around the time of your missed period. In the first two months, you can have a kind of constant feeling of an impending period and that is completely normal.

When you experience cramping and spotting in pregnancy it is always very scary as these are associated with miscarriage, but they do not always mean that you are miscarrying at all. I had cramping and spotting in every one of my pregnancies. If you are spotting, call your midwife. This is an appropriate time to schedule an ultrasound for reassurance.

Bleeding

Women can continue to have periods throughout their pregnancies. Once, I found what I thought was a large tumor in my abdomen. I went to the doctor because I knew that couldn't be okay. They did an ultrasound and said, "Well, ma'am, your tumor is fourteen weeks old and has arms and legs and is waving at you."

I said, "No, no, no. I have very heavy, normal periods, and I just had my period a week ago."

"Ma'am, would you like to look at your smiling, waving baby? Because this is not a tumor, this is a pregnancy, and you are fourteen weeks along."

This is how women can go to term not realizing they're pregnant and have unexpected births. Some women have periods throughout their pregnancies. Sometimes the hormones of pregnancy and the hormones of menstruation fight for dominance and you can have periods while you are pregnant until finally the hormones of pregnancy win out and you no longer menstruate while pregnant. There are even people who have had periods through their entire pregnancy, although this is rare. The baby implants in one little spot in your uterus and the whole rest of the uterine lining that can potentially slough off while not affecting the baby at all.

The body is so amazing.

So, that was my shortest pregnancy ever; I had the baby five and a half months later. It was an eye opener for me. You can have periods while you're pregnant. You can also skip a period and think you are further along than you truly are.

Leg Cramps

Leg cramps are very common in pregnancy. Three Ultra-Mins tablets a day will help tremendously to prevent these.

If you're in the midst of a cramp, flex your foot backward toward the shin and hold it. You must train yourself as quickly as possible to not point your toes. Flex your foot back only. Massage sometimes makes it worse and can sometimes help.

Breathe.

Pain from Ligament Stretching

Pain from round ligament stretching is very common up to about Week 24. It's a very sharp pain on either side of your torso, down low. It is particularly intense if you twist suddenly. Avoid this motion. The Ultra-mins you are taking contain manganese, which softens the ligaments and enables them to stretch more easily as a preventative measure. Evening primrose oil also helps immensely. I'll talk more about ligament stretching in the Second Trimester chapter, as most women commonly feel it then.

Varicose Veins

Varicose veins can occur in different parts of your body. The most common place is on the legs. The vein becomes softened and forms a bulging area that can be seen and sometimes even sticks out. They are often bluish purplish in color and can be minimal to very serious. You can also have varicosities in your labia. Hemorrhoids are varicose veins of the rectum.

Varicosities are often genetic. If your mother, grandmother, or sister has problems with varicose veins there is more of a chance that you will, too. Prevention is critical. Once you've got them, they are likely to get worse, and it's difficult to get rid of them while you are pregnant. A lot of varicosities go away after you give birth if you work to keep them under control during the pregnancy.

Prevention

- Take 800 IU mixed tocopherol E and 2,000 mg of Ester C a day. This is included in my vitamin recommendations, so if you've started those, you're already on top of this.

- Drink 4 quarts of water a day.

- Eat less wheat and gluten.

- Exercise—strong muscles will support the blood vessels and keep them from relaxing and enlarging. Some walking is good, but it sometimes will make the condition worse. Swimming is ideal because there is no impact, you are horizontal for the exercise, and it is cooling. Exercise before you become pregnant and again when you start feeling better, usually in the second trimester.

- If you have had varicose veins in a previous pregnancy or non-pregnant state, you must put support hose on early in the pregnancy before they start getting bad.

Treatment

- Take two **white oak bark capsules** twice a day.

- Add one more **Vitamin E** to your supplement regimen per day, for a total of 1200 units.

- Wear **support hose**. This is not optional. Wearing support hose can help a lot. Depending on the degree of your varicose veins you will need the medium grade or strongest grade of support hose. The light ones will not work. You must put them on in the morning before you get out of bed and wear them every day. It is critical that you keep the veins compressed so they can't balloon out.

- Lie on your back on something comfortable and put your legs at a

45-degree angle up against a wall. This will help the blood to flow and take the pressure off the vessels. Stay in that position for 5–10 minutes per day.

If you find a red spot, swollen spot, or hard spot in one of your varicose veins you must call your midwife or doctor immediately! It could be a thrombus (blood clot) that if allowed to progress could be life threatening.

Acne

Acne is often related to nutrition or hormones. A lot of people are sensitive to wheat, dairy, sugar, and processed foods, and when they cut back on these, their acne clears up. Many women break out with acne when they get pregnant, and that may be hormonally related. When people take the vitamins and supplements that I recommend (especially the mixed tocopherol Vitamin E and omega-3s), I don't see them break out as much. Be sure to wash your face before bed every night and wash your pillowcases frequently. It can also help to get a silk or satin pillowcase. Clean your makeup brushes regularly and replace your makeup every six months.

Also, while it may seem counterintuitive, using a good quality face oil can help, even if you have acne-prone skin. Make sure you get something that is made for acne-prone skin and is safe to use in pregnancy. There are all types of products out there and it is important to be a conscientious and informed consumer of all your skincare and beauty products. The INCI beauty app may help here.

Sometimes you may be eating perfectly and taking great care of your skin, but with the hormones coursing through you, you may still get acne. It will pass eventually.

Nosebleeds

Your capillaries are fragile in pregnancy. The Vitamins E and C you're taking will help mitigate nosebleeds. If you do experience them, sniffing salt water will help. Use two teaspoons sea salt per one quart of warm water. Cup it in your palm, bring it to your nose, and inhale deeply. It will run out of your mouth. I recommend standing over a sink, or in the shower or tub, for this.

You can also use a cotton-tipped applicator to apply Vitamin E or petroleum jelly directly to the insides of your nostrils. Poke a hole in a Vitamin E capsule and squeeze the oil onto the applicator. Then "paint" the inside of both nasal cavities as far back as you can get. Be thorough. This acts as a barrier to prevent further chafing and irritation and helps the blood vessels to be stronger.

Bleeding Gums

Sometimes brushing with salt and baking soda will toughen gums. Mix a tablespoon of salt with a tablespoon of baking soda and add enough coconut oil to form a paste. Often if your gums are bleeding, you need to be getting more of Vitamins C and E. Also, make sure you're flossing faithfully, once a day at least, because the biggest cause of bleeding gums is not flossing, it's the bacteria that can build up under and around the gums. Flossing will help to disrupt the proliferation of bacteria. Brush, floss, and use mouthwash daily. Consider using a water flosser. They can really help to toughen gum tissue and make your gums less fragile.

Dizziness

Because your body is getting softer in preparation for the birth, your blood can pool in your legs and make you feel dizzy when you stand up too quickly or stand without moving your legs for too long, especially if you have low blood pressure. You need to always talk with your healthcare practitioner about your blood pressure—ask questions like "What is it?" and "Is that high? Low? Mid-range?" Also ask, "What does that mean?"

It is important that you move your legs around before you stand up to get your muscles activated. While still sitting, slightly bounce from one leg to the other. Also move them gently if you must stand for any length of time. Do not lock your knees in place while you are standing.

If you feel faint it is super important that you lie down and get flat wherever you are. You cannot stand in the grocery store and think, *Wow I feel really weird I wonder if I'm going to faint?* By the time you get through this little discussion with yourself, you will be on the ground with worried people gathered around you. Fainting is your body's way of getting you horizontal, so if you start to feel really funny you have to get horizontal no matter where you are (yes, even in the grocery store), so you avoid the risk that comes with falling. A little embarrassment is much better than passing out or hurting your baby.

Yeast or Bacterial Infections

You may experience yeast or bacterial infection symptoms in the first trimester, but most women will experience these types of symptoms in the second trimester, after Week 12. I'll cover this in more detail in the Second Trimester chapter.

Symptoms

Some symptoms of yeast or bacterial infections can include vaginal itching and burning and/or irritation of the labia. With a yeast infection you can also see an increased discharge that can look like cottage cheese or lots of white discharge. Bacterial infection can also cause a weird discharge and may have a funky odor. Sometimes sensitivity during or after sex can indicate these types of infections as well.

Miscarriage

This may be an anxiety-inducing or triggering topic for you to think about, and please feel free to skip ahead to the next topic if that's the case. It is my sincere hope that you will never need to refer to this section, but many women do, and it's so important to acknowledge and talk about this subject.

The first thing to say about miscarriage is that it is incredibly normal and incredibly common. Some studies have suggested that upwards of one in three pregnancies ends in miscarriage.[115] A lot of those happen before people even know they're pregnant. It is so important at the very beginning of any discussion about miscarriage to say that they are almost never caused by something you have done, and I want to suggest that in many cases it may even be happening for good reasons that we just can't know about … the body has decided there is something not quite right in the fetal development and rejects it. YOU DID NOTHING WRONG and while you may wrestle with grief, please do not also saddle yourself with guilt. If you experience a miscarriage, know that it is *not your fault*.

When women have serious bleeding or serious cramping in the first trimester—or anytime during pregnancy—that is the time to go in and have an ultrasound. That's when it's medically indicated. Whenever there's a question about whether everything is okay or not, I tell people to go in and check.

If the ultrasound reveals a heartbeat, I advise my clients to lie down and not move around. Don't do too much. Don't have sex. Don't exercise. Don't go to work. Just stay down. What's likely happening is that an edge of the placenta has pulled up a little bit, and you're getting some bleeding and cramping as a result. The cramping is from the blood that's under the edge of the placenta, and the bleeding is a little bit that's actually getting out of the uterus and vagina.

If we don't find a heartbeat then I talk as gently as I can, because the baby is gone. If you experience this, I want you to know your feelings are normal. It is 100 percent okay to be terribly upset. It is also 100 percent okay if you are not.

There is so much guilt and so much shame around miscarriage. I had four miscarriages and six babies, and I can remember my family saying, "Don't talk about it; it will make people sad. It will make people afraid." When I learned how incredibly common miscarriages are, I realized this was harmful advice. I thought having a miscarriage meant there was something wrong with me, and I believed I had done something terrible or else everything would be okay. These are old, uninformed

thoughts, and all of it is just nonsense. I'm going to say it again, because it's just so important: If you experience a miscarriage, you will feel a lot of strong emotions. Please don't let guilt or shame be among them.

If you experience a miscarriage, you will feel a lot of strong emotions. Please don't let guilt or shame be among them.

Most miscarriages occur between 6–12 weeks and begin with either cramping or spotting. Even though miscarriages are common, they can be quite traumatic. There are two ways of handling a miscarriage. You can allow it to happen naturally at home or you can go into the hospital for surgical help. If you have a family practice doctor and you are faced with a situation where the pregnancy is not viable and you need to release the placenta and sac, there are doctors who can prescribe medications that you can take at home to help you to safely pass the tissue. If it doesn't happen at home naturally, the hospital is where you need to be. Sometimes the hospital is the first place to be. If you just feel like that's the thing for you, then that's the thing to do.

As a midwife, I have helped hundreds and hundreds of women through their miscarriages. I have been there for them as they went through the process. I've spoken with them for many minutes to hours at a time and I've never charged for this service.

Sometimes it takes your body knowing consciously everything is not okay for it to let go physically. In my own experience, my body held on, spotting and cramping and giving me all kinds of weirdness until I had an ultrasound and saw there was no little embryo, that the placental sac was empty. Then, as I intellectually realized this was not a successful pregnancy, my body was able to let go. It was able to surrender and proceed with the miscarriage.

I had a woman in my care recently who I sent in for an ultrasound because I was concerned about the size of her uterus, and we found there was no heartbeat. The baby apparently stopped developing at around seven weeks. As I am writing this, it has been 2-1/2 weeks since she found out, and she wants to wait it out. She doesn't really want to go in and have surgery, she wants it to happen naturally. We're doing acupuncture and Chinese herbs to try to move it along in a natural way. Most of the time a miscarriage will occur naturally, and you can stay at home, but sometimes it's complicated.

This lack of support or acknowledgment of miscarriages represents an error in our thinking and in our societal norms. We need to be more supportive. The women in my care often don't even think they can take time off work to have their miscarriage, or they feel they have to go back to work immediately. This is because we're not discussing the fact that miscarriage is fairly common, and you have got to let your body go through the process and heal. I suggest taking at least three days off.

When to Go to the Hospital

It's more than possible to allow the process to happen naturally at home. If you start running a fever or bleeding heavily you should go into the hospital immediately.

Bleeding heavily in this context means soaking a sanitary pad every thirty minutes to an hour. If you soak one or two, that's probably okay, especially if you're in the throes of the actual miscarriage, but more than that can be a sign to go in and get some help.

If you are anxious about the bleeding and you don't have anybody to talk to, go into the hospital. Err on the side of caution always. It's much better to go in and be told, "You're okay, you can go home," than to not go in and not be okay.

If you go to the hospital and are bleeding heavily, they will no doubt suggest a dilation & curettage (D&C) to remove the placenta and clean out the decidual tissue to help you stop bleeding.

Miscarriage at Home

I have experienced four miscarriages, and I experienced three of them naturally, at home. For one of them I was bleeding significantly and had a D&C at the hospital to stop the bleeding. Of paramount importance is your health, but it is often possible and perhaps preferable to experience a natural miscarriage at home.

For my clients who want to take this natural approach, we discuss their options and what to expect, and, if they want me to, I support them through the process.

What to Do

I recommend that you put cheesecloth over the toilet bowl and then place the toilet seat down to secure it. With this in place, when you are on the toilet blood can go through the cheesecloth, but anything solid will be stopped so it can be examined. You have to see that the little placenta came out. You have to open up the clot and see if there is tissue within that clot. You want to identify the little embryonic sac. It's usually the size of a silver dollar. The placenta looks like tissue and it's kind of a bluish/purplish/reddish color and there's usually membrane attached to it. Clots are very common at this stage and often people think that they are the placenta. Clots look like liver, are very solid, are a deep, dark red, and are not the same as the placental sac, which may or may not contain an embryo.

My clients send me pictures and I can identify whether what comes out is the placenta or not, or they can save it for me to see when I see them next. People are so grateful and appreciative. They just need somebody to be available who's knowledgeable and compassionate.

There are a few things you can try to help the process complete. Acupuncture and herbs (at the direction of a naturopath or herbalist) can be very effective. Sex (with a condom for cleanliness! This is essential for not getting an infection) can cause contractions to stimulate completion of the process. Brisk walking can help (but stay close to home).

Watch for infection. You must take your temperature daily to make sure you're not running a fever and your midwife should do occasional bloodwork to check your white blood cell count.

When you find that tissue you can bury that little person and give their body back to the Great Mother Earth or have a ceremony befitting your own spiritual beliefs. You don't have to do that, of course, but you may find it helpful in the grieving process.

More time has passed since I first wrote about the woman I mentioned a few pages ago who wanted to let her miscarriage happen naturally, at home. She tried everything—herbs, acupuncture—but after three weeks the placental sac still hadn't passed. She and her husband had a wonderful trip to Europe coming up and I advised them to make an appointment at the hospital to expedite the process, so she would have time to heal and still be able to go on their trip, hopefully to make it a healing journey for their spirits.

Four weeks is my cutoff. If the placenta hasn't passed in that length of time infection can occur or it could lead to some difficulties or problems with the lining of the uterus that could affect subsequent pregnancies. So, after four weeks if the embryo still has not passed, it really is time to go to the hospital.

Emotional Aftermath

Know that this is a death in your family, and it is normal and natural to grieve the loss of your baby. People said the most horrible and stupid things to me when I miscarried. They said, "Oh, well, thank God it happened so early. It's like it never even happened." But in my mind, I'd already birthed my baby and named them and imagined them grown up and through college and I'd visualized her amazing life. I grieved desperately for the little teensy baby who never had a chance to develop, and I felt anger for the people who discounted my pain. Mostly they just didn't want to hear about it. When they asked how I was doing, they wanted me to reassure them that I was fine so they could feel good. I recommend you not make room for those kinds of people in your life.

It was difficult to get all the support I needed. That said, there are many more resources available to modern women than there were when I was struggling with the emotional aftermath of my miscarriages. If you are struggling with this, I urge you to call on your support network. I have listed additional resources to help you through your grief in Appendix D.

I also felt like my miscarriages were portentous. I think the little spirits that choose us as parents sometimes skip like stones over a river. They'll dive in and go, "Oops, not the right time," and dive right back out. Once, I was trying to get pregnant and I did, then miscarried. I didn't realize how critical it is to not get pregnant again immediately after a miscarriage and got pregnant again two weeks after the miscarriage. I miscarried again. It was awful, and I was just horrified. But soon after, I found out I had a terrible tumor on my shoulder and had to undergo major surgery. Had I still been pregnant, I would have been 20 weeks along when I had a 15-hour surgery to remove the tumor. If the baby had survived ... it may not have been very good for them.

> I think the little spirits that choose us as parents sometimes skip like stones over a river.

So, I think she landed and left, and landed and left, and then within three months after the surgery I got pregnant again. I intuitively knew it was the same little spirit who had been trying to come in but arrived and realized, "Oh, there's a problem here. This is not the right time. I'm out of here," and then I dragged her back in, and she realized, "Hey, this is still not okay," and dashed out again. I found the tumor, handled it, and then she landed, and we've lived happily ever after since then. I've introduced you to this beautiful spirit already; her name is Aleah.

I think it's super important to keep encouraging intuition. We do not encourage intuition enough in our medicalized approach. Our society considers it to be like witchcraft or ancient superstition and it's not. Intuition is a very powerful, very real, dynamic part of a woman's ways of knowing, and it's not respected in this culture. Our patriarchal approach denies us this avenue. Listen for, pay attention to, and learn to rely on your intuition. It is a gift that can be developed. It is a gift from the divine.

Often people are wondering how they can replace what they've lost when they miscarry, and you simply can't. You can't replace what you've lost. You can add to your life, but there is no replacing your baby, and it is important to give your heart and your mind time to grieve and let go of the lost potential. Surrender to the present moment.

Breathe.

When to Try Again

 A woman should have two normal periods after the miscarriage is completed in order for the lining of the uterus to build back up properly before trying again. Until that time, your partner has got to use condoms; you must use barrier birth control methods. Don't fool around without them. Semen are present in pre-ejaculatory fluids. I've known many people who got pregnant immediately after miscarrying. Your fertility is enhanced a bit after miscarriage. It's like your body wants to get right back on it. If you do get pregnant again too quickly, the lining of the uterus may not be adequate to support the pregnancy in the very beginning and you could miscarry again, which is what happened to me. Please don't give yourself that heartache.

Natural Remedies for When You are Sick

Beyond common complications in pregnancy, there also exists the possibility you'll succumb to a virus or infection. Take a holistic approach to your health. Western medicine has its place and antibiotics are also an option when you are ill. I especially recommend antibiotics if strep A bacteria is found in the throat, for ear infections that do not respond to garlic and mullein, for bladder infections that do not respond to natural measures, for breast infection (mastitis), and for serious sinus infections, to name a few.

Preventative Measures

I want to encourage us to all do better as a society to not spread illness. So often I hear from my clients when they are experiencing the first signs of illness, "I have allergies." I feel some of this is ignorance and sometimes it's because our personal situations force us to engage in less-than-ideal situations, like sending sick kids to school or going to work when you're sick because your sick days have been exhausted. The fact is we are getting each other ill by these practices and we must stop! If you must go out when you are feeling poorly, please wear a mask to slow the spread of contagious illnesses. They do work, and what you think are allergies may be a contagious cold.

Wash Your Hands

The first and best line of defense to stop the spread of germs is proper hand washing. Many germs live for up to 48 hours on hard surfaces. Wash hands often and well. Hopefully we all learned how to wash our hands the right way in the 2020 pandemic, but as a reminder: Wash hands for at least 20 seconds, scrubbing in between fingers, on top of your hands, and your wrists in addition to your palms. Use soap and hot water. If you have older children, make sure they wash their hands several times a day, especially before eating, after using the bathroom, and when returning from public places.

Don't Sleep in a Bed with Sick People

One of the ways we continue to spread illness is by sleeping with sick people. I strongly recommend that you do not sleep in the same room or bed with anyone who is sick, including your closest family members. There are certain viruses that, if contracted by the mother at particularly vulnerable points in her pregnancy, can cause very severe damage to the developing baby. It is better to err on the side of caution than to continue sleeping with a partner who is ill and may expose you to the same illness. Protect yourself and your unborn baby.

Additional Best Practices

Here are a few more best practices for you to put in place:

- Wipe down doorknobs regularly.
- Ask how people you will come in contact with for an extended time are feeling and avoid those who admit they're not feeling their best or have really bad allergies.

- Make it a practice for all who enter your home to remove their shoes upon arrival. Our shoes are in contact with all kinds of germs and pathogens and there's no need to track them throughout your home.

Steps to Take When You Feel an Illness Coming On

In this section you'll find my recommendations for what to do when you begin to feel sick or suspect you have been exposed to an illness. This is where the Natural Medicine Chest you've been building up comes into play. If you have any questions about these remedies, you can refer back to my explanation in the Conscious Conception chapter of this book. All of my recommendations are natural and safe to use in pregnancy (even if the package says to consult your doctor if you are pregnant before using); I have been recommending them for decades. They are safe and they work.

Anytime you are feeling like you may be getting sick, take the steps on this list. You might be coming down with a respiratory infection, sinus infection, breast infection (mastitis), cold or flu, bladder infection, cough, sore throat, stomach virus etc. Whatever it is, you can greatly diminish or stop the threatening illness altogether if you take it seriously as soon as you feel off. The key is to start immediately.

- **Stop all activity and go to bed.** Do not go to work, clean your house, be on your feet, shop, etc. Your body needs the energy you would expend on these tasks, so it can fight off the illness. If you slow down right away, it will likely take only a few days instead of possibly a few weeks for you to knock out whatever's ailing you. If you go out of the house, you can spread the infection to others. If you must go out, wear a mask to protect others and slow the spread.

- **Significantly limit your intake of wheat, red meat, dairy or sugar.**[116] These are very mucous producing and hard to digest. They also create large amounts of metabolic waste that forces your body to expend energy on something other than fighting the infection.[117]

- **Avoid processed and refined foods.**

- **Eat as much organic food as possible:** Extra fresh fruits and vegetables and healthy proteins and fats.

- **Increase your Vitamin C intake from 2000 mg to 3000 mg per day.** Taking 500 mg every four hours is a good way to do it. An effervescent

Ester-C drink is also a beneficial way to get the extra Vitamin C you need, as are supplements.

- **Stay hydrated**—Drink 4 quarts of water per day (at least!). If you have a fever, you need more fluids, at least 1 extra quart per day.

- **Eat lots of fresh garlic** and/or you can take it in capsule form.

- Boost your immune system with "**The Remedy Shot**" (see below)

- **Sleep alone** to decrease the risk of spread.

The recommendations for viral illness versus bacterial illness are different. A bacterial illness would be something like a sinus infection, toothache, bladder, or breast infection (mastitis), strep throat, a boil, or a severely infected cut/abrasion.

Viral infections that can be treated with some of these natural remedies include the flu, colds, coughs, RSV (Respiratory syncytial virus), and other respiratory and stomach viruses.

The Remedy Shot

This remedy is very effective for all illnesses and infections EXCEPT stomach viruses and food poisoning.

Timing

If you have been **exposed to an illness**, do this twice a day. If you have not gotten sick after 48 hours, you can stop.

If you feel like you **might be coming down** with something, start this protocol immediately and do it every 6 hours. If you are feeling better after 36 hours, you can stop.

If **you are sick** do the remedy every 4-6 hours (it is not necessary to get up in the night) for three to five days.

Instructions for Preparation

- Use a small glass (like a shot glass) and put 1-2 oz of strong juice in it. Grapefruit, orange, grape, black cherry, or pomegranate are great options.

- Add 1 dropper full of echinacea tincture and 1 dropper full of astragalus (shake each bottle well before use and squeeze on the dropper a few times to flush the liquid in the dropper out before filling and putting it in the glass so it is fully mixed).

- Add Colloidal Silver liquid (follow label on bottle for correct amount).

- Add 10 drops of grapefruit seed extract (GSE) and then stir the entire mixture very well. If you don't stir it, the GSE falls to the bottom and stays there.

- If you have a bacterial illness, slowly add 6 drops of oil of oregano in the middle of the glass so as not to touch the rim. The oil will float on the surface of the liquid. When you drink the remedy shot, shoot it back so the oil does not touch your lips, because it is very strong and can be uncomfortable.

Following are additional recommendations for specific illnesses.

Fever/Pain

Fever is a natural response by the body's immune system to heat up and destroy bacteria and viruses. It is appropriate to let your body gently bake for a little while before you suppress fever but if you have a fever over 102F, that is high enough that you should work to suppress it right away. Fevers are very dehydrating, so you must take in extra and frequent fluids.

Acetaminophen (e.g., Tylenol) is an amazing fever reducer but it's not very good for pain. Ibuprofen (e.g., Advil) on the other hand is excellent for pain because it is an anti-inflammatory and reduces the swelling and inflammation in infected areas of the body. Inflammation causes most of the unpleasant and painful symptoms during illnesses. The inflammation is caused by your immune system's reaction to the virus and/or bacteria, not necessarily the virus and bacteria themselves.

There are warnings on ibuprofen that it is not to be taken in pregnancy. The issue is that 2 ibuprofen given every 4 hours for more than 3 days can cause a platelet lowering effect from minimal to major which can affect your blood clotting factor. There is some research that has shown that, taken in the Third trimester for more than 24 hours, ibuprofen may be correlated with lower birth weights and serious lung issues. I suggest you only use ibuprofen in the case of serious pain, headaches, or body aches, and that you do so for a short duration.

Recommendations

For pain, I suggest two 200 mg ibuprofen every four hours (faithfully!) for **no more than 24 hours/6 doses at a time**. It is important to keep the ibuprofen levels up during this time and not miss a dose in those 24 hours. This is definitely at a low enough dose so it won't cause any problems but will help you considerably.

For fever, take two 200 mg acetaminophen every four hours.

For fever and pain, you can take acetaminophen and ibuprofen in conjunction. Start with two 200 mg acetaminophen, two hours later take two 200 mg ibuprofen, wait two hours, and repeat for no more than 24 hours.

Respiratory Infection

In my experience almost everyone who is developing a respiratory illness of any sort says they have allergies. The problem is that you cannot tell the difference between allergies and illness in the first day or so. You have to err on the side of caution and start acting as if it's an illness, and it will become pretty obvious if it was just an allergic moment. If you wait to treat it and find out it is an illness, you'll have missed the opportunity to beat it back. In order to effectively stop or lessen an illness you have to catch it in the very beginning.

It will not do you any harm to start any of these recommendations if it does end up being allergies but if it is not and you wasted days, the chances of you being able to lessen the symptoms are reduced dramatically. It's important to stay on top of respiratory infections because if you develop a serious cough, it is possible to cough severely enough to detach the placenta and lose the baby.

- Elderberry syrup as directed for illness on the package.

- Sniff salt water and xylitol.

- This flushes the sinus and nasal passages (a neti pot is a daily hygiene ritual for cleaning out your nose but does not reach your sinuses). Dissolve 2 level teaspoons of xylitol and 2 level teaspoons of sea salt in a quart of warm water. Once you have your mixture prepared in a large, wide bowl, stand over the sink with the mixture in front of you so you don't make a mess. Alternatively, you could do this in the shower. Cup your hands and sniff the salt water as hard as you can up into your nose and through your sinuses, it will come out your mouth. It will force all the bad viruses, bacteria, allergens, and mucus out while cleaning the passageways and providing a barrier from infection. Do this 2–4 times a day depending on how bad the symptoms are.

- Sleep in a slightly elevated position; lying flat makes it harder to breathe.

- Boil a large pot of water then turn off the heat and move the pot to a cool spot on the stove. Then add 5–10 drops of both eucalyptus and tea tree oils into the pot (you want it to be strong smelling). Stand over it with a towel over your head and cover the pot so the aromatic steam rises into your face where you are inhaling it through your nose and mouth. *Be so careful not to touch the pot and burn yourself.

- You can suppress a minor cough with tea and honey and a very small amount of whiskey added to it.

- You can suppress a serious cough with Robitussin DM. You might find yourself spotting after very serious coughing. This is fairly unlikely, but it is best to get a serious cough under control quickly.

- Significantly minimize your intake of any mucus-producing foods to help reduce and thin mucus.

Flu

Oscillococcinum is the go-to homeopathic remedy for the flu or flu-like symptoms. It has been used for more than fifty years and is the most commonly used remedy in France.[118] Take it at the first sign of illness to lessen the duration and severity of fevers, aches and pains, headaches, chills, and low energy. This remedy comes in a small tube; place the contents of the tube under your tongue and allow it to dissolve. Repeat every six hours, up to three times a day.

Stomach Viruses

- If you are throwing up do not eat or drink anything until you have not thrown up for 2 hours (anything you put in will come back up and if you throw up too much you can dangerously lower your electrolytes).

- Darken the room and make it cool, and completely reduce all stimuli (no TV, phone, or computer).

- Put an ice-cold cloth on your throat. This slows the firing of the vagus nerve and lessens the urge to vomit. It's a great trick! Keep a bowl of ice water by your bed so you can continue to cool the cloth when needed.

- After two hours without vomiting, try tiny amounts of ice chips very slowly until you are able to keep those down for one to two hours.

- Next you can try coconut water to replace some of your lost electrolytes.

- If you keep the coconut water down, try real ginger ale next. You want ginger ale with real ginger in it, available at most large grocery or health food stores. Occasionally it is called ginger beer but is not alcoholic. Ginger is a stomach soother. The carbonation in the ginger ale can also be very soothing to your unhappy stomach.

- When you have kept the ginger ale down for at least an hour, then take 1 dose of Pepto-Bismol. It's not natural, but it is very effective. Do not be alarmed if it turns your stool black.

- The rest of the day try liquids like chicken, vegetable, or miso broth as well as sugarless fizzy water like Topo Chico or Perrier.

- When you are ready for solids, first try one of the following: mashed potatoes, oatmeal, apple sauce, or very well-cooked vegetable soup.

Bladder Infection

- Increase your water intake. Bladder infections are often caused by being behind on drinking water.

- Take cranberry extract with D-Mannose in pill form.

- Drink unsweetened cranberry juice.

- Always use the bathroom after sex for prevention. The bacteria in the vagina are pushed into the urethra during intercourse and can cause infection if not flushed out by urination.

You can take phenazopyridine (marketed under the brands AZO or Pyridium). It is a bladder anesthetic. This drug only helps with symptoms and will take away the worst of the pain but will not do anything to help with the infection. If your bladder infection is bad enough to use this, you need to be on antibiotics. This product will turn your urine bright red.

Cough, Cold, or Sore Throat

- Gargle with warm salt water and xylitol 3–4 times a day.

- Sniff warm salt water and xylitol (see respiratory infections for directions).

- Blow nose frequently for cold symptoms, this will help reduce the viral and/or bacterial colonies in the nose.

- Use zinc lozenges.

- Take a blow dryer and hold it up to your face blowing crosswise (do not blow directly into face). Take 15 deep breaths through your nose and then

15 deep breaths through your mouth. Dry, hot air over 107 degrees kills bacteria and viruses on contact.

- Take elderberry syrup as directed for illness on the package. If you have a bacterial infection there is no need to take elderberry syrup.

- If your sore throat does not get better with these natural remedies after two or three days, you absolutely must go and do a throat culture to see if you have strep. Strep throat can absolutely be deadly if untreated, and you must take antibiotics if you have it.[119]

Allergies

Allergies can turn into sinus infections very quickly so follow these steps faithfully to prevent them from getting that far.

- Gargle with warm salt water and xylitol 3–4 times a day.

- Use a neti pot daily to clean out your nose.

- Clean all the air filters in your house at least once a month if not more often, depending on how bad your allergies are.

- Clean your house very thoroughly. Wet mop all hard floors, clean all mini blinds, ceiling fans, AC and air purifier vents, and shelves with a damp rag, then again with a dry one so you are not just stirring up the dust but actually capturing it. Wash or dry clean all curtains.

- If you have carpet, it is imperative to have it professionally cleaned once a year (or more if you have very severe allergies). It is also a great idea to remove old carpets and replace them with hardwood, bamboo flooring, tile, laminate, or vinyl to help eliminate allergens that reside in carpet fibers. You can then use area rugs, which can be washed or cleaned more regularly.

- If you have persistent allergies, it could be because of mold in your air conditioning ducts. A professional duct cleaning company is imperative in this case; they can determine if you do have black mold or other types of mold spores and then take care of it for you.

- Get a room air filtration system for your bedroom. You will at least sleep allergen-free. I recommend Blueair systems, but there are many wonderful systems.

Ear Infection/Pain

Garlic and mullein oil drops can help alleviate this pain. Place a few drops of the warmed oil in ear canal and insert a cotton ball.

Use Astragalus as directed on the package for immune support as a preventative measure along with our proven vitamin regime and a diet that contains lots of fresh veggies, fruits, nuts, and seeds, yogurt, and lean chicken, turkey, and fish.

Asthma

Albuterol inhalers are perfectly fine. Albuterol is safe in pregnancy, so don't be worried about having to use an albuterol inhaler for asthma while you are pregnant. Sometimes asthma is benefited by pregnancy and sometimes it's exacerbated. Follow the recommendations for allergies, above.

I do not recommend the use of steroid inhalers during pregnancy. Try alternatives if you are habituated to steroid inhalers. They are not a great idea during pregnancy, as the steroid can get to the baby.

What if It Doesn't Work?

These natural techniques are remarkably effective a lot of the time. But if it has been a few days and you have not significantly turned the corner toward wellness, it is very possible you're dealing with a bacterial infection and need to go to the doctor to get antibiotics. While antibiotics are overprescribed, they are at times necessary. It's not useful to keep trying to do alternative healing techniques when you are getting sicker. Antibiotics can be lifesaving when they are needed, and you should take advantage of them for bacterial infections like strep throat, bladder infections, bad ear infections, toothache, and mastitis.

10-12 Week Genetic Screening

Genetic screening is usually performed during Weeks 10–12. It's done by collecting a small amount of the mother's blood. The screening identifies changes or abnormalities in the baby's gene profile to confirm or rule out possible genetic conditions. It is only very recently in terms of how long women have been giving birth that we have had the know-how to conduct genetic screening and have implemented it on a wide scale.

Genetic screening is a personal choice. There are certainly plenty of mainstream medical practitioners who are going to insist that genetic screening should be done on every single fetus. I do not believe that this is true. I believe if your risks are small and you're not going to do anything with the information besides worry, then relax and everything will be revealed at the appropriate time when the baby is born. On the other hand, if you know that you could not carry a baby that had a problem or if the problem were terminal to the baby and you would make other choices, then genetic screening is a really good idea.

Consider that if the results of the genetic testing do indicate something is wrong with your baby, this information can rob you of your possible joy and harm your relationship with your unborn child. It can transform your relationship with your baby into a relationship with a diagnosis. It's difficult to be thinking about the uplifting part of having a baby join your family when you're consumed with thinking about the downsides.

What I have seen too often is when someone finds out there's something wrong with their baby, all they can do is agonize over that one thing for the rest of the pregnancy. It can serve to negate the unconditional joy and imagination of the limitless potential of the new person coming into this world.

Years ago, I had a client who had an ultrasound at about 20 weeks in her pregnancy. The ultrasound showed a very bad condition with her baby. I remember thinking at the time, *Oh my God, we have caught this, and every single person needs to have this screening to find out if there is something like this so they can prepare for it.* I think that's a natural human response. The woman's entire pregnancy was taken up with going to a hospital four hours away to meet with specialists who could potentially help with this very serious situation and to prepare for it.

The baby was born via c-section, and the situation was very severe. Doctors at the hospital started performing surgeries immediately. I think the baby had eight surgeries in total. But what I remember the most is that the baby never smiled in the eight months that they lived. They had a lot of pain, and I thought to myself, *If we'd forgone that screening and not known about this condition, she would have had that baby at home. The baby would have died peacefully in her arms without ever having been tortured.*

That baby did die. There wasn't any fixing what was wrong with them. If they had been at home for the birth and it had been fixable, we would have been able to get to the hospital in time. We would have gone immediately, and the doctors would have done something immediately, but this baby wouldn't have survived at all without instantaneous intervention. I've asked myself, *Was that the right thing?*

I have seen that when women were told there was something wrong with their babies they did not even want to look at their babies when they were born. They wanted to look at the baby's arm or foot or whatever body part the defect was

associated with. They had spent their time in pregnancy bonding with the anomaly instead of with the person inside of them, and this created a barrier between them.

I have had circumstances where an anatomy scan showed there was something wrong, but when the baby was born there wasn't anything wrong with them at all.

When the baby comes out the mother goes through this incredible bonding dynamic. Her heart opens and oxytocin levels rise to orgasmic levels. Transformation occurs and she calls out, "My baby, my baby." She is in love. It doesn't matter that there's something not quite right with her baby physically.

After a little bit I might say, "Honey, I think there might be a little problem with their foot."

She might say, "Oh, okay," or glance up at me and say, "I'll look at that in a minute." She's madly in love with her baby. She didn't bond with the problem in her baby's foot, she bonded with her child, and together nothing will keep them from handling those issues that may have come with the baby.

I've come to believe it can be better not to know. I believe that anything challenging is a challenge that can be handled after the birth, after you've met and fallen in love with your baby.

Some may feel they have to plan for a serious problem with the baby or even a minor problem with the baby, but consider it may be better to plan for no problems and have the emotional and spiritual lightness that not knowing brings. Trust there will be plenty of time to think about what to do and to handle it *if* the time ever comes. Again, this is a personal choice.

You may feel differently, and the choice is yours to make. If you are interested in genetic screening, talk with your care provider about your options.

Pets

Dogs and cats are totally aware that something is up when you become pregnant. Their noses are so much more sensitive than ours. I'll talk more about how to prepare these family members for your coming baby in The Third Trimester chapter. For now, I just have one bit of advice if you have cats.

Cats

Cats are absolutely wonderful and fabulous. You do not have to get rid of your cat to have a baby.[120] Follow a few safety guidelines while you are pregnant, though. Keep your cat indoors. Wear gloves when you change the litter box.

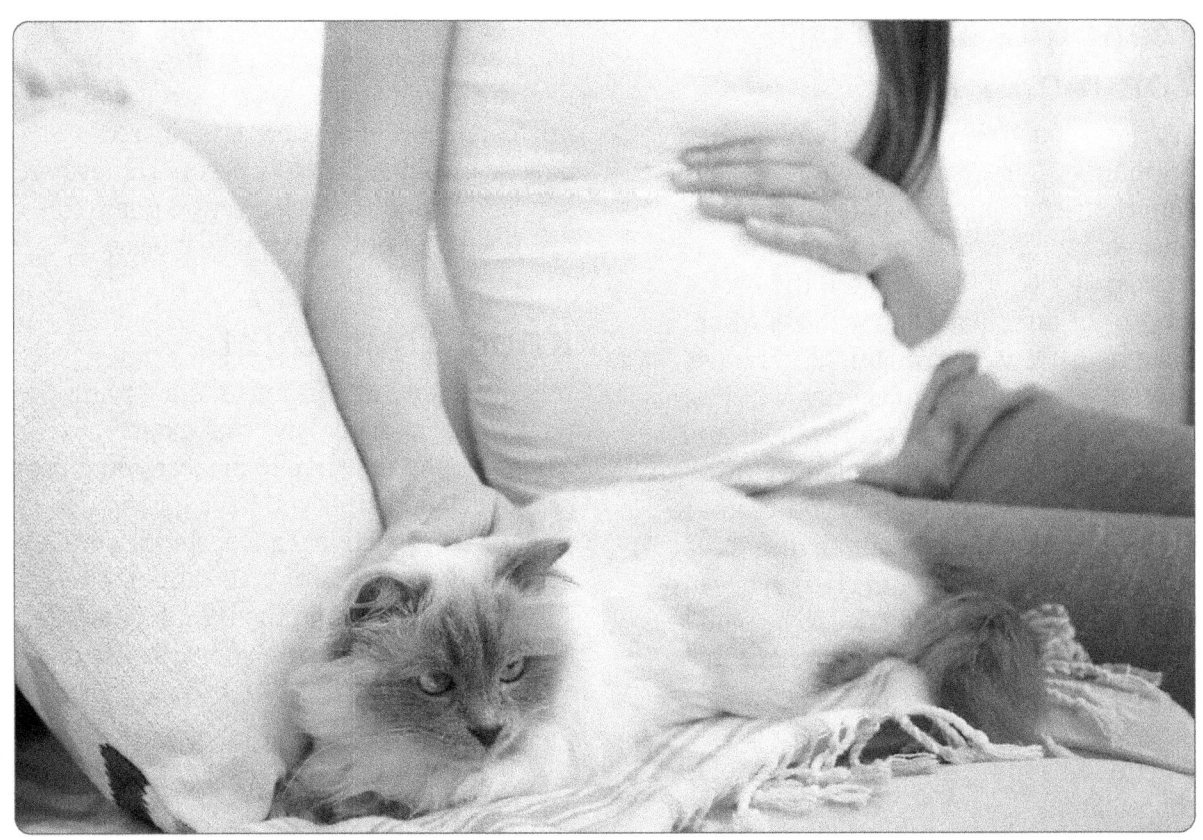

Take a Few Precautions and Your Cat is Going to Be Just Fine

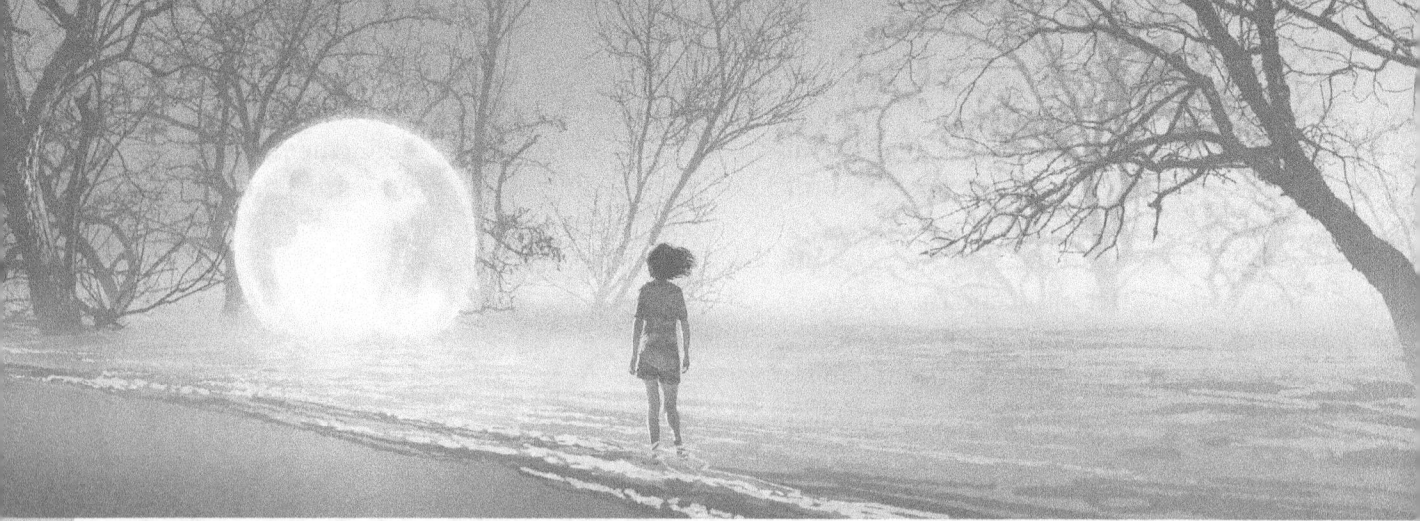

Rest

Feeling Low Ebb is Common

Try not to push yourself too hard in the beginning of pregnancy. Avoid remodeling your house or taking on big work projects. Give yourself permission to be more relaxed. It's very likely that in the first months of pregnancy you will feel what I like to call *low ebb*. You might not have a ton of get-up-and-go energy. You'll likely swing between being ravenous and wanting to take naps. As you move through these early days, remember, you've got to pace yourself and space out anything that requires an expenditure of energy, because there's almost always a price to be paid until you reach the halcyon days of the second trimester.

The brilliant thing to do when you feel low ebb is *absolutely nothing*. Your body is telling you it's time to slow way down. *Listen to it.* Magical things are happening inside of you.

Your baby requires a tremendous amount of your body's energy. Any energy or nutrients you expend on exercise aren't going to the baby, so rest and give that energy to the new life inside of you. Take heart if you are feeling low ebb. There is an incredible change coming. It usually occurs somewhere between 10 and 16 weeks. You're going to feel great. But until then, take it easy.

Know Your Rights

It is incredibly important to understand your rights and any laws that exist wherever you may live to protect you during pregnancy and after you have given birth, so you can proactively advocate for your needs and the needs of your family. There is recent legislation in the US, for example, that I want to make sure you're aware of.

Extended Parental Leave

First, in recent years many states have expanded their extended parental leave (EPL) from two months to twelve months. Check to see if you live in one of the (currently) 37 states that have legislated this for their constituents, and know that if you do, your workplace may be legally required to provide this.

Each state's EPL policy has its own eligibility requirements, benefit levels, and other provisions. For example, some states require employees to have worked for a certain period of time before being eligible for leave, while others do not. Some states also offer different levels of benefits to birth parents, non-birth parents, and adoptive parents. To find out more about your rights under your state's EPL policy, you can visit the website of your state's labor department or contact your employer's human resources department.

Pregnant Workers Fairness Act

The Pregnant Workers Fairness Act (PWFA) prohibits employers from discriminating against pregnant workers on the basis of pregnancy, childbirth, or related medical conditions and requires employers to provide reasonable accommodations to pregnant workers. This applies to discrimination in hiring, firing, pay, promotions, and other terms and conditions of employment. The PWFA applies to private and public sector employers with 15 or more employees. It includes protection for conditions like morning sickness, gestational diabetes, fatigue, and pregnancy-related high blood pressure.

Under the PWFA, you may be entitled to:

- More frequent breaks
- Lighter duty assignments
- Temporary alternative assignments
- Modified work schedules
- Assistance with lifting or carrying heavy objects

- Provision of a stool or chair
- Restrooms that are more accessible

PWFA also expands access to family leave for pregnant workers and new parents. The PWFA requires employers with 50 or more employees to provide up to 12 weeks of unpaid leave to employees for pregnancy, childbirth, or related medical conditions. The leave can be taken all at once or intermittently, and it can be used for any purpose related to the pregnancy, childbirth, or related medical conditions.

The PWFA does not require employers to provide paid family leave, but it does make it easier for employees to take unpaid leave without fear of losing their jobs or their income. The PWFA also provides protections for employees who take unpaid leave, such as prohibiting employers from discriminating against them or retaliating against them for taking leave.

Every workplace is different. Some are more supportive than others. Knowing your rights as a pregnant worker puts you in the best position to advocate for yourself during your pregnancy.

Babymoon Vacation

The first trimester of your pregnancy is definitely not the time to take a chance on a vacation. I have known far too many first-trimester women who went on vacation anyway, felt horrible, and could not do any of the fun stuff they had planned. If you get pregnant and have a vacation already planned during your first trimester, I strongly suggest that you reschedule it, if at all possible, for your second trimester.

Start Preparing for Your Maternity Leave

One of the things I'd like you to start planning for now is your maternity leave. Do not plan on working through the end of pregnancy. I want you to stop working at least two weeks before your due date if that is at all feasible for your family. In my practice, I see a higher percentage of complications in women who work up to the very end of their pregnancies. When you stop two weeks before the end it is *wonderful*, and you will be relaxed and really ready for your baby when they arrive.

Those weeks allow you the space to shift away from your professional life and make room for you to step into the mother you are about to become. Don't get me wrong, I am a working woman and I understand how important that can be. The vast majority of your life you can spend a lot of your energy on your career. But when your baby is about to arrive, it's better if you can make the space and shift your energy to being fully present for this new little human about to enter your world with the power of a meteor impacting a planet.

Plan ahead of time to take more time off than you think you'll need. People think that 12 weeks will be enough and it's just not. Twelve weeks is the normal amount of postpartum maternity leave you get in the United States. If you do as I suggest and take off two weeks prior to being due, this may mean you are only getting nine to ten weeks after the baby arrives. Many European countries offer mothers one to two years of paid maternity leave, and the fathers also get many months or up to a year of paid leave. This is as it should be everywhere, but alas is not our experience here in the good ole' U S of A. Unless you're going to go to hell in a handbasket financially speaking, it's just a terrible idea to take only twelve weeks off. No baby is really ready to be away from their mom that much and moms are also not ready to be away from their baby. I think it just messes with you, hormonally. I mean, when the baby arrives the whole body, spirit, psyche—all of that—is just geared toward being a mom and raising kids and having them survive, and so there are alarm bells that go off in your limbic system with separation. You will benefit from more time with your baby. Plan now to take as much time as you can.

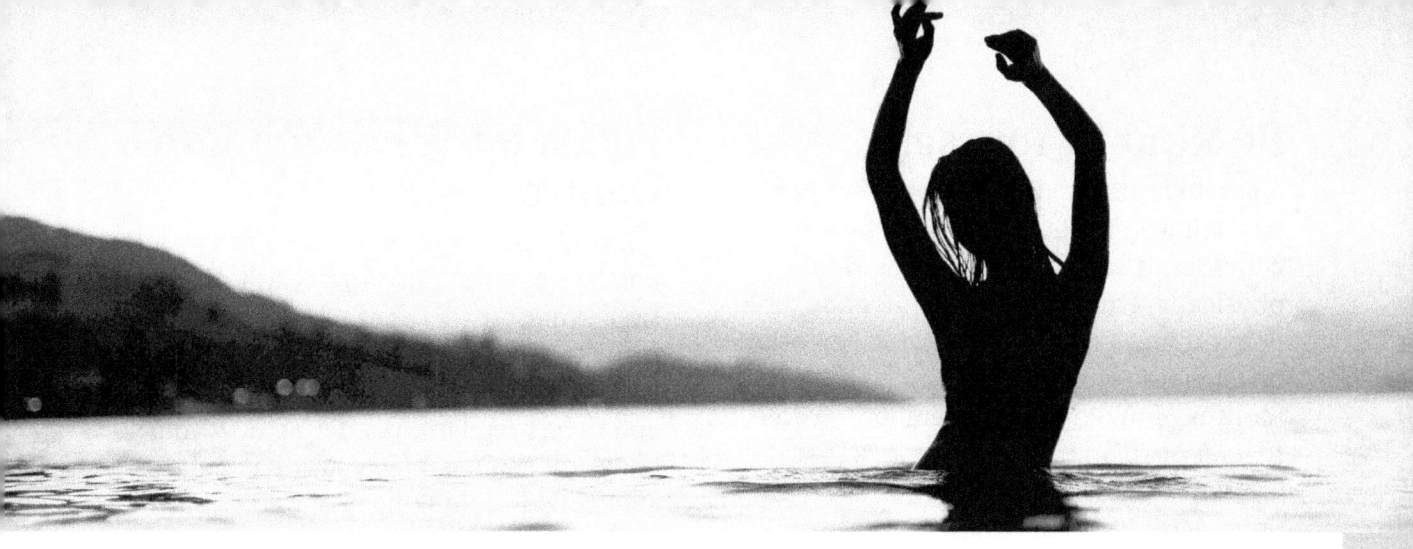

Joy

Creating a Positive Birth Experience

Taking care of your physical health during your pregnancy is crucial, and experiencing joy can contribute to a healthier pregnancy. Furthermore, joy and positivity during pregnancy can set the stage for a positive birth experience. When you approach childbirth with joy, optimism, and confidence, you are more likely to have a smoother and more positive birthing experience. Your emotional state and mindset during labor and delivery can impact the progression of labor, your perception of pain, and your overall satisfaction with the birth.

As I've mentioned before, joy is the inverse of stress. It releases stress and can serve as a shield against stressors and negative thoughts. Exercise is perhaps the best way to shed residual stress from your body. However, I've told you I don't want you exercising in this first trimester. Thankfully there are other ways to let go of stress, and most of them include accessing joy. Revisit my suggestions in the Conscious Conception section on Joy (see page 105) and incorporate joyful activities in your daily life.

Bonding with Your Baby

Joyful emotions and positive experiences during pregnancy can enhance the bond between you and your baby. When you feel joy, your body releases hormones and develops neurotransmitters that promote positive emotions and can positively impact the developing baby's well-being. Your joyful experiences and emotional states can create a nurturing environment for the baby's development and lay the foundation for a strong emotional connection even before birth. Babies are keenly sensitive to their environment and the emotional energy surrounding them both in and out of the womb, so build up your joy receptors and your inclination to feel joyful *now*.

Be Kind to Yourself

A great way to be kind to yourself in the first trimester is to prioritize self-care activities. It can be a challenging time physically, emotionally, and mentally, and doing things that feel good can be greatly beneficial to enhancing joy in those early months of pregnancy. Remember to listen to your body and choose activities that are comfortable and safe for you during pregnancy. If you have any concerns or questions, consult with your healthcare provider for personalized advice.

Engage in an activity that nourishes and rejuvenates your emotional well. This could include:

- Taking a warm bath with soothing essential oils, relaxing music, and candles lit to enhance the mood.

- Reading an uplifting book and escaping from the day-to-day realities of the world around you. One of my favorites is *All Creatures Great and Small* by James Herriot.

- Mindfulness or meditation practices.

- Going for a walk through a natural environment and enjoying the beauty the world has to offer.

- Making time for a hobby you love.

MINDFULNESS EXERCISE

Put one hand on your heart and the other on your belly. Breath slowly for five breaths and notice the sensations. Repeat this process as many times as you like. Smile and notice the sensations in your face and body. What happens to your thoughts?

Focus on What You Can Control

Remember to focus on what you can control and let go of the things you can't. In the first trimester there are a lot of changes to come to terms with—you are beginning the journey of discovering what it feels like for you to be pregnant, pondering how your body will change, how you will change as a person, and thinking about how your life will change as you become a parent. This is true even if you have other children. Every pregnancy is different.

It can be helpful to focus your energy on the things you can control, like eating well, staying hydrated, resting, and creating as much joy in your life as you can.

Some women experience discomforts in early pregnancy (nausea, cramping from the early growth of the uterus, hormonal ups and downs, emotional upsets, etc.) and it can be a stressful time. Focusing your energy and efforts on the principal elements of the Sevenfold Approach is a great way to concentrate on the tangible things you do have control over instead of letting your mind wander to stressful things that are out of your control.

Connect With Nature

Connecting with nature during pregnancy is a wonderful way to promote relaxation, reduce stress, and enjoy the beauty of the natural world. Here are some safe ideas to connect with nature while pregnant:

- **Gentle nature walks.** Take leisurely walks in nearby parks, gardens, or nature trails. Choose well-maintained paths that are not too strenuous and ensure they are safe and accessible for you while pregnant.

- **Picnics in the park.** Pack a healthy picnic lunch and head to a nearby park or garden. Find a comfortable spot to relax, enjoy the fresh air, and soak in the natural surroundings while you eat.

- **Outdoor yoga or gentle stretching.** Find a quiet outdoor space where you can practice a short prenatal yoga session or gentle stretching. This allows you to connect with nature while promoting relaxation, flexibility, and your overall health and well-being. Remember, nothing too strenuous at this stage!

- **Gardening or plant care.** Engage in light gardening activities or caring for houseplants. Planting flowers or tending to houseplants connects you with nature and the joy of watching things grow. It can be a perfect pairing as your own pregnancy begins to grow and blossom.

- **Sunrise or sunset appreciation.** If you are getting enough sleep, it can be beautiful to wake up early to watch the sunrise. Alternatively, find a serene location to enjoy a breathtaking sunset. Take a moment to appreciate the natural beauty and the changing colors of the sky.

> **NOTICING EXERCISE**
>
> Take off your shoes and socks and walk on the grass or earth. Pay attention to the sensations you feel and notice the connection between your body and the earth beneath you.

Spend Time with Your People

Spending time with your loved ones who support and care for you during early pregnancy can bring immense joy and uplift your spirits in the moment while laying down a healthy foundation of support that you can rely on during this journey of pregnancy, birth, and parenting. Focus your energy on cultivating healthy and supportive relationships. Surround yourself with friends who lift you up and encourage you. Prioritize spending quality time with people you feel good around. Nurture these relationships by actively listening, offering support, and reciprocating their love and kindness. Remember, a strong social support network is a vital aspect of self-care and can contribute significantly to your overall well-being and happiness during pregnancy and beyond.

As I mentioned before, have lots of lovely sex with your partner or pleasure yourself.

Pregnancy can be a time of mixed emotions, including excitement, anxiety, and vulnerability. Being around people who love and support you provides a safe space to share your feelings—your joys, challenges, and concerns. They can provide a listening ear, offer comfort, empathy, understanding, and encouragement, helping you navigate the emotional ups and downs of early pregnancy. Surround yourself with people who support your choices, offer you their love, and lift you up. Laughter, engaging conversations, and shared activities can help stimulate the release of endorphins, the "feel-good" hormones that are so beneficial during pregnancy, while simultaneously promoting relaxation and shifting your focus away from stressors.

Having these types of people in your inner circle also allows them to actively join you in celebrating the milestones of early pregnancy. You will feel more comfortable in sharing the news of your pregnancy, hearing the baby's heartbeat for the first time, or having them come with you to early prenatal appointments when you've nurtured these intimate relationships.

Your friends' and family's enthusiasm can amplify the joy and excitement you feel during these special moments. You can discuss the physical changes, preparations for baby, and anticipate together. Sharing experiences, advice, and stories can deepen your bond and create a sense of togetherness.

Family and friends who support you can also provide practical help during this time. Whether it's helping with household chores, offering rides to appointments, babysitting older kids if you have them, or providing emotional reassurance, their assistance can alleviate stress and allow you to focus on taking care of yourself and your growing baby.

The first trimester can be such a pivotal and transformational period in your life. Spending time with loved ones during early pregnancy allows you to create memories you'll cherish when your life is full of diapers and sippy cups, and you have less time for such endeavors. Whether it's going on outings, enjoying meals together, or simply having meaningful conversations, these shared experiences become part of your pregnancy journey and contribute to the joy and connection you feel.

Surround yourself with people who believe in you and your ability to navigate pregnancy and parenthood for a boost to your own self-confidence. Their support and reassurance can help to remind you that you are not alone.

By actively working to experience joy and doing things that bring you happiness, you can reduce your stress levels and create a more harmonious and peaceful environment for you and your baby. There are so many fun and uplifting activities you can enjoy with your family or friends. Here are some ideas:

- **Dinner Party**
- **Girls' Night**
- **Dates** with your partner or a friend or family member.
- **Dance Party**
- **Outdoor Picnic:** Organize a picnic in a nearby park or garden. Bring delicious food, snacks, and drinks to enjoy together while soaking up the fresh air and sunshine.
- **Movie Marathon:** Plan a movie marathon with your favorite films

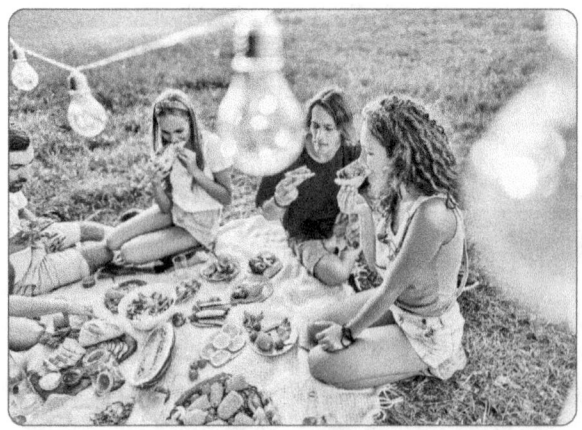

Outdoor Picnic

or a theme-based movie night. Get cozy with blankets and popcorn while enjoying a series of movies that uplift and entertain you.

- **Arts and Crafts:** Engage in creative activities like painting, drawing, pottery, or DIY crafts. You can collaborate on a project together or have individual creative sessions.

- **Cooking or Baking Party:** Gather in the kitchen and cook or bake together. Choose a recipe that everyone can contribute to and enjoy the process of preparing and sharing a delicious meal or treats.

- **Scavenger Hunt:** Organize a scavenger hunt, either indoors or outdoors, with clues and hidden treasures. Divide into teams and enjoy the adventure and excitement of searching for clues and solving puzzles.

- **Game Night:** Have a game night with board games, card games, or video games. Engage in friendly competition, laughter, and bonding over shared experiences.

- **Karaoke Night:** Sing your hearts out with a karaoke night. Set up a karaoke machine or use online karaoke platforms and take turns performing your favorite songs. Enjoy the laughter and camaraderie.

- **Music Exploration:** Go to a concert or explore a new playlist together to dive into music you already love or new music you haven't ever been exposed to.

- **Outdoor Adventures:** Plan outdoor activities like short hikes, canoeing, or a trip to the lake or beach. Engage in adventurous activities that allow you to enjoy nature and each other's company.

- **Volunteer Work:** Find a local community service project or charity event that you can participate in together. Giving back to the community as a group can be incredibly fulfilling and uplifting.

- **Storytelling or Book Club:** Have a storytelling session where each person takes turns sharing a favorite story or memory. Alternatively, start a book club and read and discuss uplifting and inspiring books together.

The most important aspect of these activities is the opportunity to connect, share laughter, and create positive memories with your loved ones. Adapt the activities based on your own preferences and the interests of your family or friends and enjoy the time you spend together. Don't forget to take pictures!

Remember, it's important to surround yourself with people who uplift you and respect your choices, especially if you are

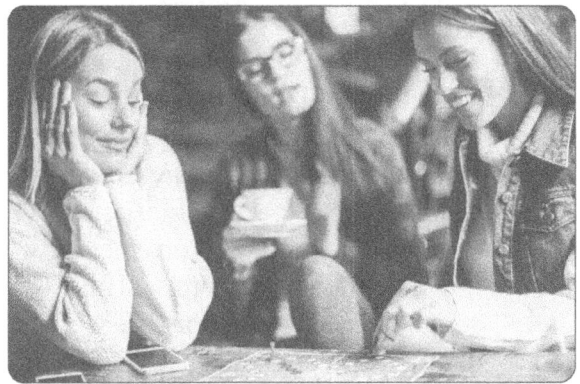
Game Night

choosing to use a midwife and have a home birth. Their love, care, and presence can be instrumental in enhancing your overall well-being and joy during early pregnancy.

Pamper Yourself

Anything you can do to relax and let go of stress is very beneficial for you and the baby. Massage is particularly beneficial because it is not only relaxing, but it is important for your cardiovascular, lymph, and immune systems. If you can, schedule regular massages throughout your pregnancy. If this is a splurge for you, save it for the final trimester. You will want to make sure that whoever works on you will be providing a *prenatal* massage and will have the proper prenatal massage table and/or support pillows to make lying down comfortable for you and safe for your baby.

If you are new to massage, I want you to know that you are free to communicate with your message therapist to convey what you like or don't like, and to let them know if the pressure is too strong or not strong enough. Don't hesitate to express your preferences! This should be enjoyable for you. Speak up and let your needs be known.

Sing, Dance, and Listen to Music

Incorporating singing, dancing, and listening to music during early pregnancy can be a joyful and beneficial experience for both you and your baby. Here are some ideas to explore.

- **Sing to Your Baby:** Singing is a beautiful way to bond with your baby and stimulate their auditory development. Choose soothing lullabies or songs that bring you joy and sing to your baby throughout the day. It doesn't matter if you think you have a "good" voice; what matters are the loving connections and the positive vibrations your voice creates.

- **Take Prenatal Singing or Music Classes:** Consider joining prenatal singing or music classes specifically designed for expecting mothers. These classes often involve gentle movements, vocal exercises, and songs tailored to support the well-being of you and your baby. They provide another an opportunity to

Don't Hesitate

Mary Oliver

If you suddenly and unexpectedly feel joy, don't hesitate. Give in to it. There are plenty of lives and whole towns destroyed or about to be. We are not wise, and not very often kind. And much can never be redeemed. Still, life has some possibility left. Perhaps this is its way of fighting back, that sometimes something happens better than all the riches or power in the world. It could be anything, but very likely you notice it in the instant when love begins. Anyway, that's often the case. Anway, whatever it is, don't be afraid of its plenty. Joy is not made to be a crumb.

connect with other pregnant women and create a supportive community.

- **Dance and Move:** Engage in gentle and safe dance movements to uplift your spirits and promote physical well-being during pregnancy. You can explore gentle forms of dance like ecstatic dance, belly dancing, or even freestyle movements in your own living room. Allow the music to guide your body, embracing the joy and freedom of movement.

- **Create a Pregnancy Playlist:** Curate a playlist of songs that inspire joy and uplift your mood. Include songs that hold special meaning for you or that evoke happy memories. Play your pregnancy playlist during quiet moments of reflection, while engaging in self-care activities, or simply to add a joyful atmosphere to your daily routine.

- **Listen to Music for Relaxation and Meditation:** Incorporate soothing and calming music into your relaxation and meditation practices. Choose instrumental pieces, nature sounds, or guided meditation tracks that promote deep relaxation and reduce stress. Set aside time each day to listen to this music, allowing yourself to unwind and connect with your baby.

- **Attend Musical Performances:** If you enjoy live music, consider attending musical performances or concerts that align with your interests and comfort level. Look for soothing and uplifting genres, such as classical, acoustic, gentle rock, or indie music. Ensure ahead of time that the venue and environment are safe and comfortable for you.

- **Create a Musical Bond:** Encourage your partner or family members to participate in musical activities with you. Sing or play music together, dance as a family, or simply enjoy listening to music collectively. This creates a shared experience and strengthens the bond between you, your baby, and your loved ones.

- Enjoy the power of music to uplift your mood, strengthen connections, and create a joyful atmosphere during early pregnancy.

Gratitude Practice

In these early days of your pregnancy, I would like you to start the practice of using gratitude to help you adopt a joyful mindset. If you started reading this book after you conceived, you may have missed my explanation of this practice. You'll find it on page 113 in the Conscious Conception chapter.

Noticing what we are grateful for brings our awareness to all the abundance and wonder in our lives. Practicing gratitude is also a powerful way to enhance joy and cultivate a positive mindset.

Here are some ideas for incorporating gratitude into your daily life:

- **Deepen Your Gratitude Journaling Practice:** As you continue your practice of recording things you are grateful for, work to be more specific in your detail. Rather than just saying you are grateful for Naomi, maybe write "I am grateful for Naomi's constant willingness to jump in and help out. She really brings me a lot of relief" or "I am just so grateful for the way Alex never passes me without gently touching me and letting me know of his love."

This practice helps shift your focus toward the positive aspects of your life and fosters a sense of gratitude. If you are struggling emotionally, go bigger and aim for one thing for each year you've been alive. This practice will help you to adopt a mindset of joy.

- **Gratitude Letters or Notes:** Write a letter or note expressing gratitude to someone who had a positive impact on your life. They could be a friend, family member, mentor, or colleague. Share your appreciation for anything they did that made a difference to you. Deliver the letters personally or send them via mail or email. This practice not only uplifts others but also enhances your own joy and connection with them.

- **Gratitude Rituals:** Incorporate gratitude rituals into your daily routine. For example, start your day by expressing gratitude for three things before getting out of bed or create a gratitude jar where you write down moments of gratitude and place them inside. At the end of each week or month, take time to reflect on the contents of the jar and feel the joy that arises from recalling those moments.

- **Mindful Gratitude Practice:** During meditation or quiet reflection, focus your attention on gratitude. Bring to mind things you are grateful for and allow the feeling of gratitude to fill your heart and mind. Engage your senses by visualizing and savoring the experience of gratitude. This practice deepens your connection with gratitude and enhances the sense of joy it brings.

- **Gratitude Walks:** Take mindful walks in nature or around your neighborhood, and as you walk, consciously direct your attention to the things you are grateful for. Notice the beauty of nature, the warmth of the sun, the gentle breeze, or the sounds around you. Allow yourself to appreciate the abundance and wonder of the world. This practice promotes a sense of awe and joy.

- **Gratitude Sharing:** Incorporate gratitude sharing into your conversations with friends, family, or colleagues. During social interactions, take turns expressing something you are grateful for. Or, if making it a group activity feels weird, just make sure you express your gratitude when you notice it. "I'm so grateful you got this report to me on time. It makes my life easier. Thank you." Or "I just love hanging out with you. I'm so grateful for our friendship." This practice creates a positive and uplifting atmosphere, deepens connections, and amplifies joy.

Penelope: When my firstborn was three and presented typical, overwhelming, three-year-old challenges, I signed up for a parenting program to help me. It had the added bonus of providing me with a built-in community of parents in the same boat I was in.

One of the first things the instructor did was pair us off and give us a series of questions to answer every day in an email to one another. My partner and I still exchange daily emails answering these questions. It has become the cornerstone of my day. I answer the questions, and then I'm ready to go. The questions are:

What filled your cup yesterday?

This is noticing the glimmers of good in your life.

What will you do to fill your cup today?

This is actively anticipating and working toward having a great day filled with glimmers of goodness.

What five things are you grateful for right now?

This cultivates an attitude of gratitude.

How are you feeling right now?

This is where you can get real and avoid toxic positivity, which is when you cover up or suppress negative emotions and pretend everything is fine when it really isn't.

What are you joyfully anticipating?

Anticipation is half of happiness. Anticipating a joyful event can make it even more fulfilling when it actually takes place. Joyful anticipation for me has ranged from looking forward to a European vacation, moving to a new state, seeing a friend, or a delicious lunch. I often use this space to visualize and manifest.

What is your intention for the day?

This is a short statement. I might say something like "peace and productivity" or "progress and laughter" or, on a harder day, "one moment at a time."

What have you learned?

Sometimes this question provokes a profound and interesting response. Sometimes it's more like, "Did you know there's an arrow on the dash pointing to which side of the car the fuel tank is on?"

Even if you're not comfortable sharing these with a friend, you can answer them daily for yourself. I really like the accountability of sharing. When one of us fails to do the template for a few days, the other of us will kick us back into gear. This practice helps me to manage my emotions, makes sure I'm checking in with myself, provides a support system (my partner and I often are each other's cheerleaders and counselors) and sets my mental state first thing in the morning, so I can stay positive throughout the challenges of parenting life.

- **Gratitude in Challenging Times:** In challenging situations, intentionally seek out aspects to be grateful for. Shift your focus from what is lacking to what you still have. It could be the support of loved ones, personal strengths, or lessons learned from adversity. Finding gratitude in difficult times can help cultivate resilience and open the door to joy even amidst hardship.

- **Gratitude Reminders:** Place visual reminders of gratitude in your environment. Use sticky notes, quotes, or images that evoke a sense of gratitude and place them where you'll see them frequently, such as on a mirror, desk, or refrigerator. These reminders serve as prompts to pause, reflect, and experience gratitude throughout your day.

Remember, the key to cultivating gratitude is consistency and intention. Choose practices that resonate with you and make them a regular part of your life. Over time, practicing gratitude will become a habit, and you'll notice an increased sense of joy and appreciation for the abundance in your life.

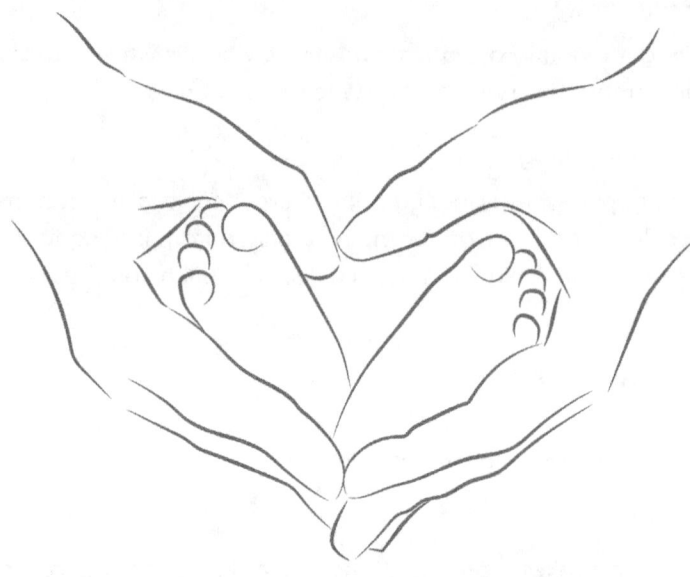

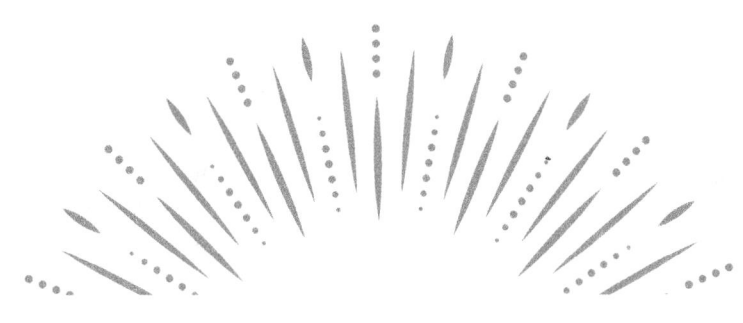

THE SECOND TRIMESTER

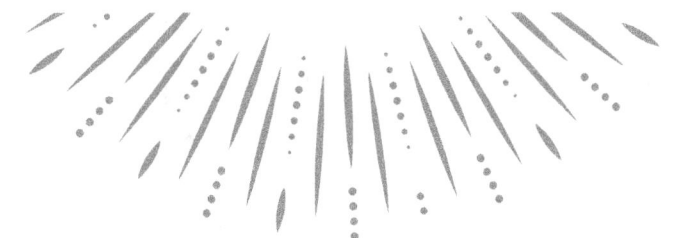

Introduction

Welcome to Your Halcyon Days!

There is an enchanting myth about the origin of the term *halcyon days* that is full of love and loss and ultimately beneficence and rebirth, and you can look it up if you like, or you can just know that I use the term as it's come to mean: halcyon days are marked by prosperity, success, abundance, peace, and calm. In your second trimester, you'll feel good, better than you have in months, and you can eat and move more and resume so many activities that may have been a struggle in early pregnancy. This is a beautiful time.

The difficulties of early pregnancy are behind you, the discomforts that can come in late pregnancy are months away, and during this time you get to enjoy the calm and peace that comes with all the progesterone flowing through your body. Chances are you've been able to hear the baby's heartbeat by 10–12 weeks, and that can also be very comforting. You can settle in and deeply enjoy this part of your pregnancy.

 Partners, when you are prepared emotionally, physically, and psychically, when you step into present, conscious being, you lift your woman up with the power of your energy and life force. When it comes time, you will be able to support her flagging energy in the depths of labor with your own, and she will be lifted by the gift of your support when she feels depleted. Don't underestimate the effort this will take. Prepare for labor as assiduously as your partner does. Eat well, rest well, move your body, and take care of your mental, emotional, and spiritual health in advance of this life-altering event. The time to prepare is now.

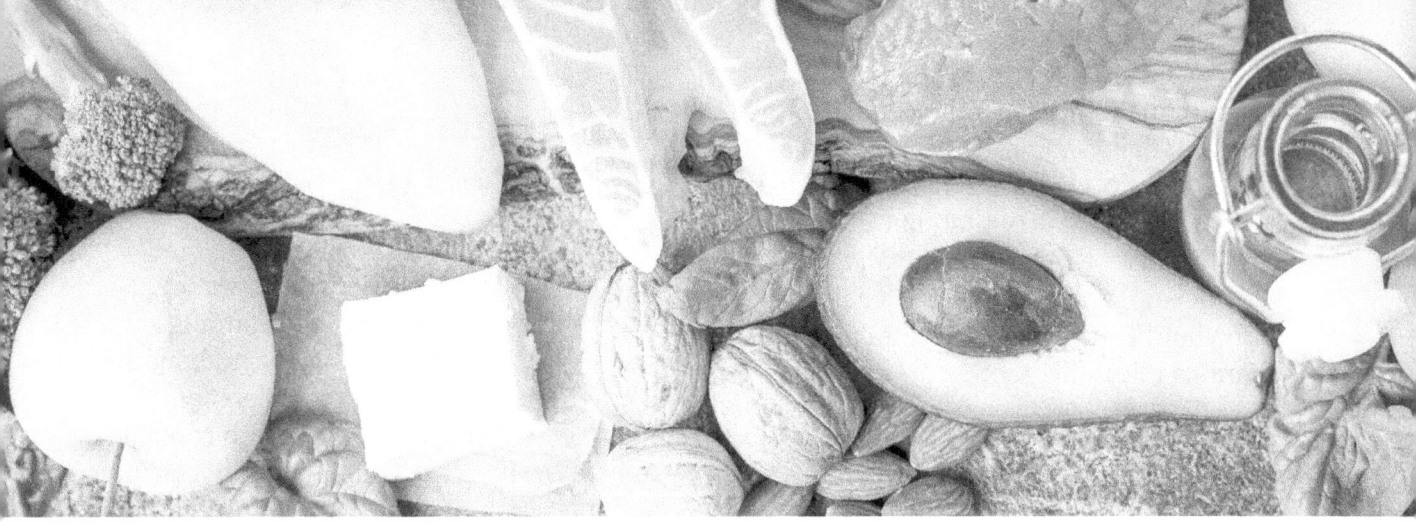

Nourishment

Weight Gain Window

It is very important for most women to gain an average of at least a half a pound a week over the course of their pregnancy. Give your baby plenty of the right kind of food to encourage a healthy and thriving life for both of you. I truly believe supporting your nutritional needs is one of the most important things to help your baby to be optimally healthy. The key to gaining is to eat regularly and often, but many newly pregnant women struggle with this. Gain as much as possible through healthy eating in the first six months. If you struggled to gain weight early on, there is a great window for weight gain between 18–28 weeks.

If you were to call me wanting a home birth halfway through your pregnancy and you hadn't gained at all, I would think it's possible you should have your baby in the hospital rather than at home. I've had a few stillbirths in my practice, and about 60–70 percent of them were in women who did not gain nearly enough weight in pregnancy. I think these stillborn babies were simply not strong enough to survive.

By the same token, it is not a good idea to be seriously overweight and pregnant. The problems are aggravated, especially with high blood pressure. Work with your midwife to understand what

You'll likely be ravenous in this phase of your pregnancy, but gaining too much a month in the third trimester is how you end up with big babies that are difficult to get out. Gain the weight that you can *now*.

If You're Struggling to Gain

If you feel like you're eating everything you possibly can, and still aren't gaining weight, my suggestion is to start taking a weight-on powder. You can find them online, in health food stores, and in some grocery stores. Athletes use this to help put on weight to reach competition requirements. Find one with as many calories per scoop as you can possibly get. Opt for one with high-quality fats and maybe a little protein. Avoid powders loaded with carbs/sugar.

You can mix it into any milk you like or add it to your daily smoothie. This is an easy way to add 1,000 calories a day. Real food is what you should try first, but if you need help to add on the fat that you and your baby need, then implement this daily along with your healthy meals. Keep taking your vitamins faithfully, too!

If You're Still Struggling with Nausea

Many people don't gain at all in the first trimester—some even lose weight—and almost inevitably those are the women who are seriously throwing up, can't eat anything, and are miserable and feel horrible through the first trimester. If you are one of the few who is still experiencing intractable nausea and vomiting at this stage, the prescription medication Zofran can offer significant relief.

Satisfying Your Sweet Tooth

Sweet treats do bring us joy, but they can bring too many calories from sugar. You can find several great recipes that satisfy the sweet tooth without being overly sugar laden in Appendix B. You might try:

- Angel food cake with fruit
- Avocado pudding
- Chia seed pudding
- Tapioca and fruit
- Halved dates pitted and stuffed with nut butter and sea salt, cashews, or almonds

Supplements
Add an Ultra-Mins to Prevent Muscle Cramps

At about Week 16 you may start getting leg cramps because the baby is pulling so much calcium out of your body. Add another Ultra-Mins tablet to your supplement regimen at bedtime at 16 weeks to combat or prevent this. The combination of calcium and magnesium in the Ultra-Mins will help prevent this from happening to you. It will help you to sleep better as well as preventing muscle cramps.

At about Week 16 you may start getting leg cramps because the baby is pulling so much calcium out of your body.

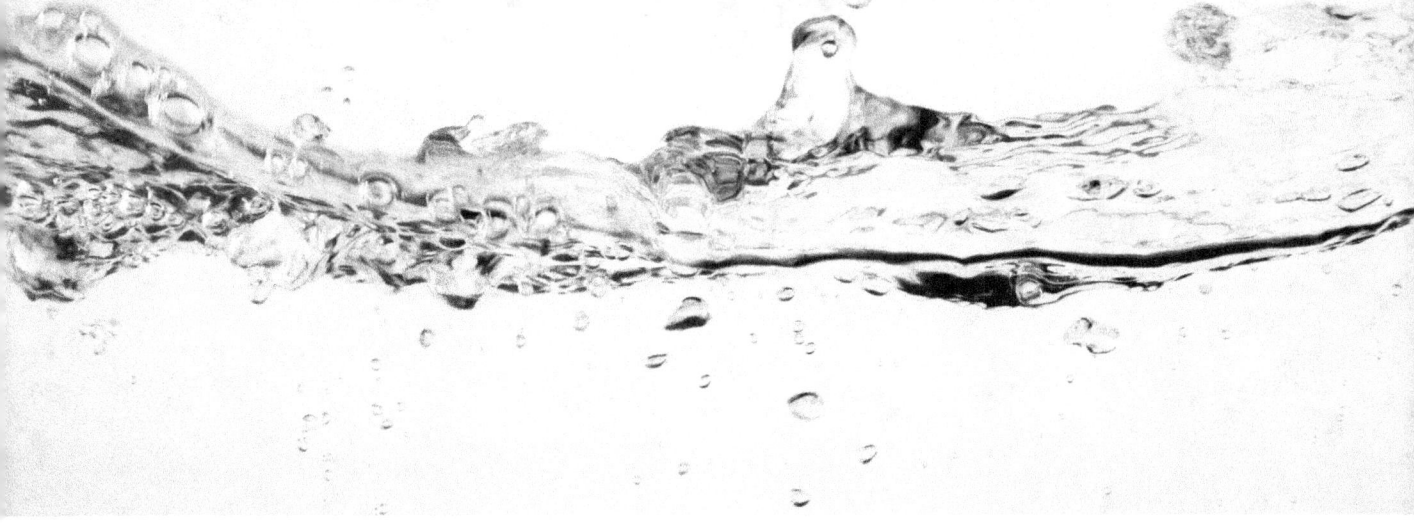

Hydration

 My recommendation for hydration remains constant. You must absolutely be drinking one gallon of water every day. Pregnant or not (your partner needs to do this, too!) That's 4 quarts or 16 cups. Cups are smaller than you think. Drink one 8-ounce cup of water every waking hour of your day. Set an alarm on your phone or smartwatch if it helps. You may find it easier to drink 16 ounces (2 cups) every two hours. That's fine, too. Keep this habit up for life.

Alternative Methods of Hydration

It's totally fine to hydrate yourself with liquids other than plain water. What's not fine is to load those drinks up with sugar. Stay away from powders you add to your water; they're almost always loaded with sugar or chemicals. The less sugar you consume, the more your body will be okay with consuming less sugar. Laboratory studies have shown that sugar is an addictive substance that creates dependence.[121]

Great alternatives to plain water include:

- Coconut Water
  - Coconut water is one of the highest sources of potassium out there. It's much better for you than a banana, providing potassium and other sources of electrolytes.

- Lime/Lemon Water
  - Just squeeze a little juice from a lime and/or lemon into your water.

- Fruit Waters
  - Chop strawberries and chill them in your water for a bit prior to drinking.
  - Gently macerate blueberries and/or raspberries and let them diffuse in water.
  - Be sure to eat the pulp when you get to it.

- Decaffeinated Herbal Teas
  - Mint tea
  - Nettle tea
  - Alfalfa tea
  - Hibiscus tea
  - Ginger tea
  - Pregnancy tea

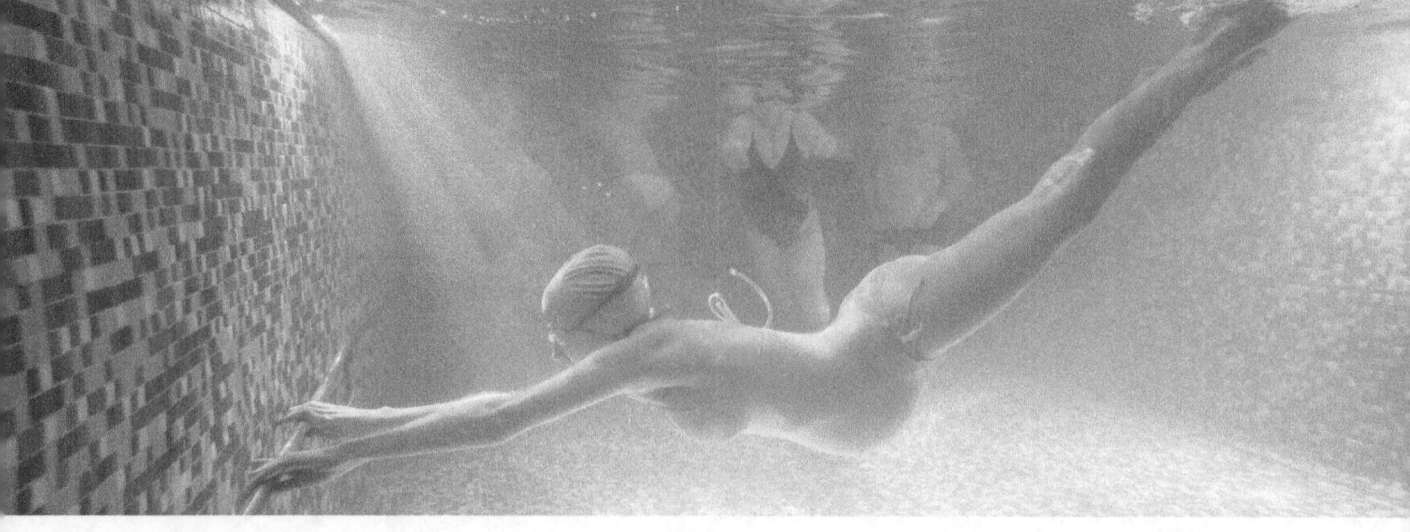

Movement

I suggest you start exercising as soon as you start feeling good, usually between 12 and 16 weeks. Steroids are shooting around in your body during pregnancy to facilitate this teensy embryo growing to be a baby weighing several pounds at nine months. So, you can build muscle in pregnancy like never before or never again in your adult life. Take advantage of this natural boon!

One of the reasons I want you to have really good upper body strength is for pushing. First time mothers especially tend to have longer labors. I recently helped a momma with a tough birth. She had 17 hours of pant-blow breathing through difficult contractions and then three hours of pushing. Birth can be an Olympic marathon. I say this not to scare you, but to prepare you. I want you to get in excellent shape again now, like you were during your conscious conception.

Go back to your cross training: walking, swimming, yoga, and weight work. If you started reading this book after you became pregnant and skipped the Conscious

Conception chapter, go to page 64 to see my recommendations for your exercise routine.

Considerations for Exercising While Pregnant

Yoga

Once you are pregnant, make sure you are doing prenatal yoga positions only! Many positions done in regular yoga classes

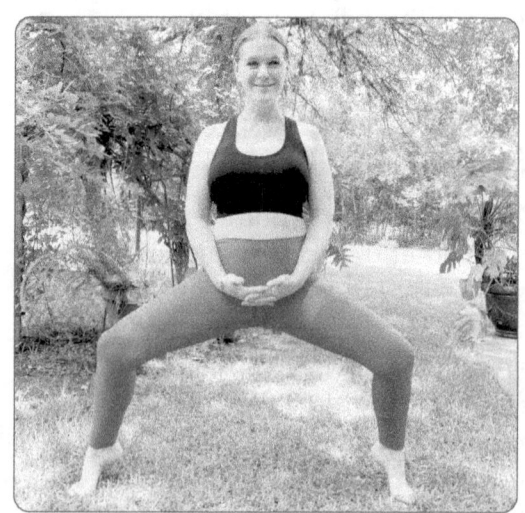

Prenatal Yoga is Excellent in the Second and Third Trimesters

involve inversions that could possibly tangle the baby in the cord. Prenatal yoga can also stretch out muscles and ligaments in the pelvis to help you push your baby out more easily.

Swimming

When swimming, avoid flip turns between laps. There is a possibility of the baby becoming entangled in the cord or turning breech with this motion.

Impact Exercise

Continue to avoid anything that causes an impact like jumping on a trampoline, skiing, horseback riding, jogging, and bicycling because of risk of injury due to a fall or collision. A stationary bike is fine; it's not the motion of cycling that's a problem, it's the risk of losing your balance and falling from a moving bicycle or getting hit by a car.

I don't think you should run—in fact, I don't want you to be running in pregnancy at all. Honestly, if you're a runner, you might want to reconsider whether you still want to be a runner after you have your baby. Every part of your body is going to change. Your uterus becomes unhinged from its moorings a tiny bit, your breasts certainly change, all your body will have been stretched out by the pregnancy, and running can be too hard on many women after they've given birth. You can power walk while pumping your arms and burn a similar number of calories and work more muscle groups than jogging.[122]

Do work yourself back up into a regular exercise routine as soon as you possibly can.

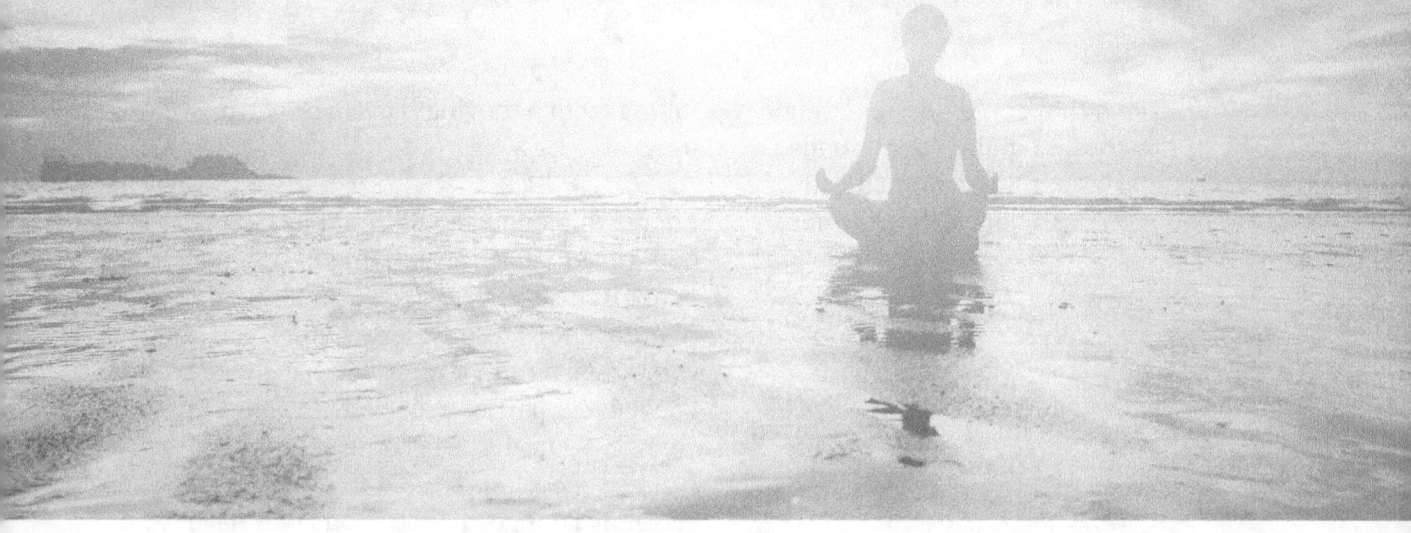

Emotional/Spiritual

Bolster Your Body Image

It's hard to accept all the changes your body is going through, hard to not think, *I'm getting fat.*

No! You're not getting fat, you're pregnant! When else will you ever be encouraged to gain 20–40 pounds in nine months in your life? This only happens when you're pregnant. Enjoy it!

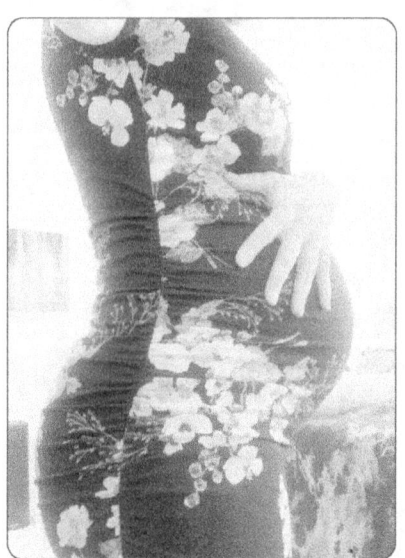

Second Trimester Baby Bump

You've got to do your best not to fret about weight gain. It can be a difficult psychological adjustment to go from being very slender to not being slender. But you do want to gain weight, and you must do so by eating healthy food. Food is life for your baby.

Reassure yourself that you're not getting fat. You're nourishing your baby, helping them grow, and showering them with nutrients. In return all the fat you've built up is going to turn into breastmilk and continue to nourish your baby after birth, melting right off you.

Reassure yourself that you're not getting fat, you're nourishing your baby.

If you do face negative voices in your head, notice when they are there and counter their negativity with the truth. What society has taught us about body image

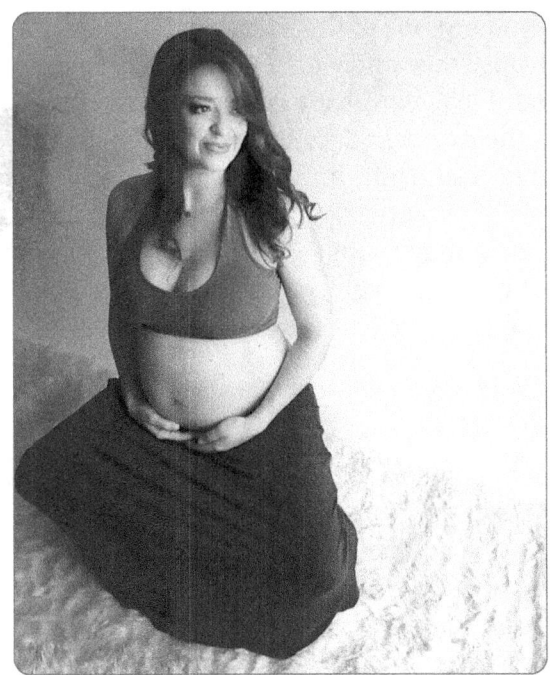

Aleah in the Second Trimester

Connect with Your Baby

It can be more difficult for women to connect spiritually and emotionally with their developing baby in the first trimester than it is later in pregnancy. In those first few months, women cannot feel it or see any hint of pregnancy besides some enlarged breasts and emotional volatility. Most of the effects feel negative: fatigue, nausea, etc. But when your baby starts moving in the second trimester and you start to develop the baby bump, your baby becomes more real to you. As a midwife and as a woman with many friends who have given birth, I have seen so many people that seemed so over-the-moon in love with their unborn baby.

sneaks into our brains. These voices tell us things like, *Oh my God, I'm getting fat. Oh my God, my butt's getting bigger* ... and we feel the accompanying emotional messages of *No one will love me if I'm big* and other lies.

To counter this lying voice, you must repeat the truth to yourself. *I look great! I feel so healthy. I am doing so well. I am radiant. I am glowing with happiness. My baby is going to be so healthy. This baby is going to suck all that extra weight right off me. My body is doing something miraculous. I am beautiful.* Repeat these messages until you believe them because they are true.

Partners, every single day is a great day to remind your pregnant mother-to-be how incredibly radiant and gorgeous she is, and how much you treasure her for the transformation she is undergoing for your family.

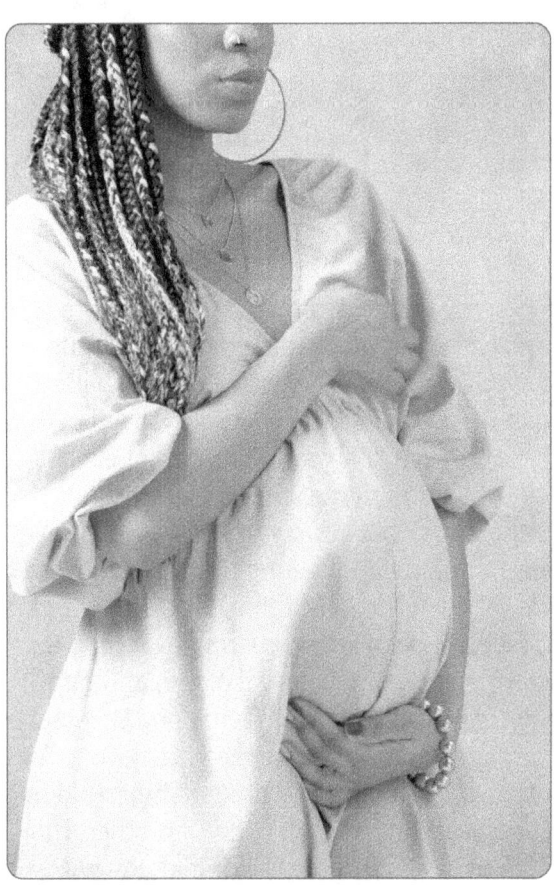

The Baby Bump Becomes Real This Trimester

I struggled a little bit. I loved my unborn babies, but I wasn't head over heels and over the moon in love with them, and this concerned me. I have since talked to so many hundreds of women who have had similar feelings and concerns about these feelings or lack thereof that I had a realization. Some women I believe are protected from the possibility of a devastating loss by a little tiny bit of emotional distance.

Pregnancy is a sacred time, a period when the divine energy of creation flows through you, connecting you to the miracle of life itself.

—Eckhart Tolle

When my baby was born and put up into my arms, I felt my heart open like a lotus flower. I could hardly draw a breath with the rush of oxytocin and love that flooded over me, and as the baby and I looked at each other I could tell that this was happening to the baby, too. I know the baby must have been thinking and feeling the same things I was—because they do think and feel—and it must have been so interesting to be in a dark warm place, somewhat all alone, and one day things really start moving and the gentle massages that have become part of your life intensify for hours and hours. Then suddenly a *big squeeze*, the bright light, and then there is mom in all her glory gazing at you with eyes of love.

If you are one of the women who struggles at this stage and worries about whether you'll love your baby enough, know that as the oxytocin does its job, you, too, will have your heart unfold like a lotus flower of love. If you are choosing a medicated birth, Pitocin may change this experience initially, but trust that your love for your baby will be deep and true just the same.

Develop Your Intuition

Some people are more aware of intuition and access it more easily than others. For those of you who don't feel a great connection to your intuitive self, I want to encourage you to develop that way of knowing a bit more. Here are a few ideas for you to try:

- Pay attention to your gut feelings. When you have a gut feeling about something, take note of it; don't dismiss it as "just a feeling." Instead, try to explore it and see where it leads you.

- Be mindful of your emotions. Your emotions can also provide valuable information about your intuition. If you're feeling anxious or stressed about something, it may be because your intuition is telling you something is wrong.

- Don't be afraid to trust your instincts when you have a strong feeling about something. This doesn't mean you shouldn't listen to intellectual reasoning by any stretch, but it does mean you should be open to listening to your intuitive feelings.

- Get out of your comfort zone. One of the best ways to develop your intuition is to push yourself into unfamiliar territory and try new things. In a new situation your intuition is more likely to kick in.

- Meditation can help you to quiet your mind and supports you becoming more aware of your intuition. There are many different types of meditation, so try several to find one that works for you. Some might not resonate at all, while others may significantly help you.

- Journaling can also help you to track your intuition and see how it develops over time. When you have a gut feeling about something, write it down. This can help you to see if your intuition is accurate.

- Talk to people you trust about your intuition. They may be able to offer you insights you hadn't previously considered.

- There are apps and games that can help you to develop your intuitive skills. You can search for "intuition games" in your app store or look for the Magic Intuition or Intuitive Life games.

Affirmations

This is a good time to revisit your affirmations and consider changing them. Maybe now you're starting to think more about the future with your new child, or maybe you have some affirming to do about the upcoming three months.

Sample Affirmations for Pregnancy

- I am continuing to fully nourish myself and my baby and to prepare for the work of labor.

- My body is gorgeous. Seriously gorgeous.

- Labor is a normal, natural process that my body innately knows how to do.

- I welcome the support of my tribe.

- I can handle the discomforts of pregnancy with ease.

- The universe loves me and supports me and my baby.

- This baby is a welcome and wonderful addition to our family and our relationship will be phenomenal.

Noticing

The second trimester is a great time to tune in and listen to yourself. Take the occasional moment each day to check in with your emotional self, your spiritual self, your mental self, and to ask your body where it's at and what it needs. You may hear responses you did not expect.

Writing in your journal for a few minutes—or making voice/video recordings on your phone for those who prefer talking their thoughts out—is a great way to practice noticing at the end of the day. You can spend as little or as much time as you like. This practice is just for you. You don't have to share these thoughts with anyone, and you can even delete or get rid of them afterward as a symbolic cleansing of those thoughts or feelings from your mind. Take a few moments for yourself every day to notice and reflect on your current state of being.

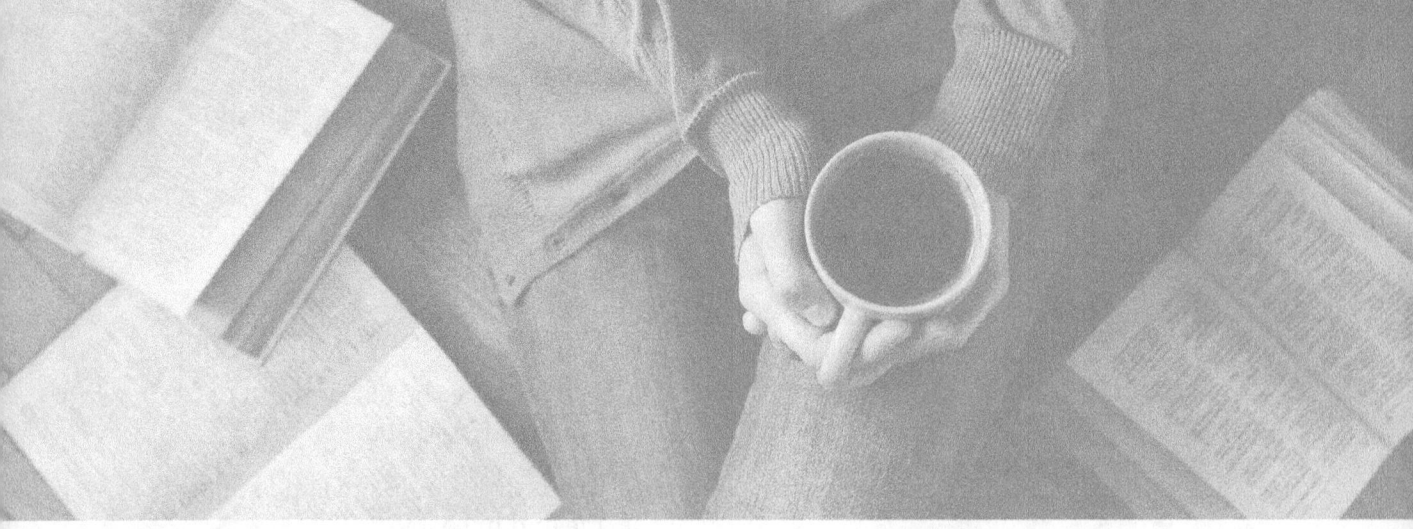

Knowledge

When you start feeling better in the second trimester it's the perfect time to learn more about what's going on in your body, your baby's development, what's coming with the birth process, and to cultivate your ideas about how you'd like your birth experience to be. Many women are simply too low ebb to study or read much in the first trimester. The second trimester is the right time to read and learn as much as you can. Please do not rely on TikTok or Instagram for your education. There is some great advice to be found there, but there can also be damaging information. Vet your sources.

READING ON A BUDGET

For those of you on tight budgets, I've got a few ideas to make your dollars stretch (or stay in your pocket!)

Your local public library, one of our nation's greatest institutions, is a wonderful resource. Librarians love to help. They can set you up with an account and show you how to access ebooks and audiobooks through their website—so after your initial visit you won't even have to go to the library to check those out and return them. You can reserve physical books that others may be currently reading or check books out immediately from the shelves. You can use their computers and internet service. You can chill out on a bean bag chair or at a desk. Libraries often host classes and workshops. And all of this is absolutely free of charge to you in the US. It's so brilliant.

Chirp and BookBub are sister companies that offer deals on audiobooks and ebooks, respectively. You can visit their website (chirp.com or bookbub.com), sign up for free, tell them what kinds of books you are interested in reading, and they will send you a daily email with books in the categories you specified that are deeply discounted for you to buy if you like. They are excellent curators, and only offer books that have passed their quality inspection.

Friends who have had babies in recent years and are past their pregnancy and infant years may have libraries of their own that they're happy to lend or pass on to you. It doesn't hurt to ask.

I suggest you complete reading this book and also read *The Book of Birth Volume II: Your Postpartum Journey through the Fourth Trimester* during your second or third trimester, so you are forearmed with the knowledge you need to carry you through the coming months. Also, for the record, my editor assures me that audiobooks totally count as reading.

What's Going on in My Body?

Your baby is getting bigger and bigger, and you may become noticeably pregnant. The difficulties of early pregnancy are behind you and the struggles of late pregnancy are in the distant-seeming future.

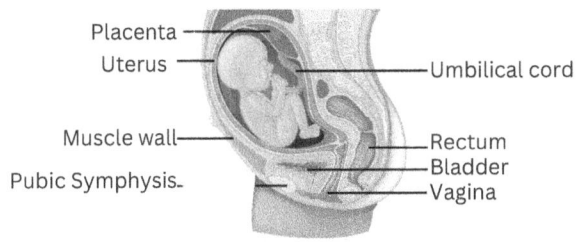

Anatomy of Pregnant Mother and Baby at Five Months

At five months, the mucus plug has developed and is blocking the cervical canal. The baby weighs about three quarters of a pound (12 ounces), is 6 inches long from head to heel, and the placenta is attached to the uterine wall.

Uterine Contractions

Your uterus continues to contract regularly, as it has since implantation. Most women cannot feel the sensations of the contractions until much later in pregnancy, but many women can feel the hardening of the uterus with their hands on their abdomen. From about 16–18 weeks on, the uterus forms into a hard ball when it contracts. Many women think it's the baby doing something. I've heard them say, "Oh, look, the baby's in the shape of a ball!" Well, the baby doesn't form the shape of a ball, but the uterus sure does. When you've had a few babies, you might start noticing your uterus much earlier on and you may notice the movement of the baby much earlier, but again, there are no real sensations of the baby until later in the pregnancy.

Ligament Stretching

The uterus is held in position in the pregnant and non-pregnant state by sets of two different ligaments, the round and the broad. The round ligaments are toward the front on either side and attach the uterus to the pubic bone. The broad ligaments are in the back part of the uterus and attach the uterus to the sacrum.

When you are not pregnant the **broad ligaments** don't have a large function, but you likely notice them during your period when you have a backache. In pregnancy, the broad ligaments work to hold the uterus and baby up and keep them from falling forward out of the abdomen. If the woman does not have decent stomach muscles, the broad ligaments will do the job of holding her uterus in place as it grows.

When you are not pregnant, your **round ligaments** hold your uterus within the pelvic cavity, so it is protected from blows and accidents. In pregnancy the uterus goes from being the size of a plum that weighs 6–8 ounces when you are not pregnant to the size of a cantaloupe that weighs 4-½ pounds right after the birth. The round ligaments stretch in pregnancy to accommodate this growth. They go from being about 4 inches long to sometimes over 10 inches long. Luckily, the human body softens dramatically to allow these changes to occur. However, the stretching of these ligaments as they lengthen can cause sharp pains on either side of the abdomen. Sharp pains on the sides of your abdomen are almost always round ligament pain. Taking evening primrose oil as I described on page 125 will help with this pain.

Placental Growth

The placenta is made up of the maternal side and the fetal side. The maternal side does all the work of oxygenating the baby, getting nutrients to the baby, and removing waste products and carbon dioxide. Your baby does not poop during pregnancy; they drink and breathe amniotic fluid about six to nine times per minute. They pee into the amniotic fluid and the placenta filters out any impurities. The umbilical cord has three vessels: two arteries and one large vein. It attaches to the baby on one side and the placenta on the other. There are two sacs surrounding the baby; the inner sac is the *amnion*, and the outer sac is the *chorion*. The amnion is the sac the baby is in contact with.

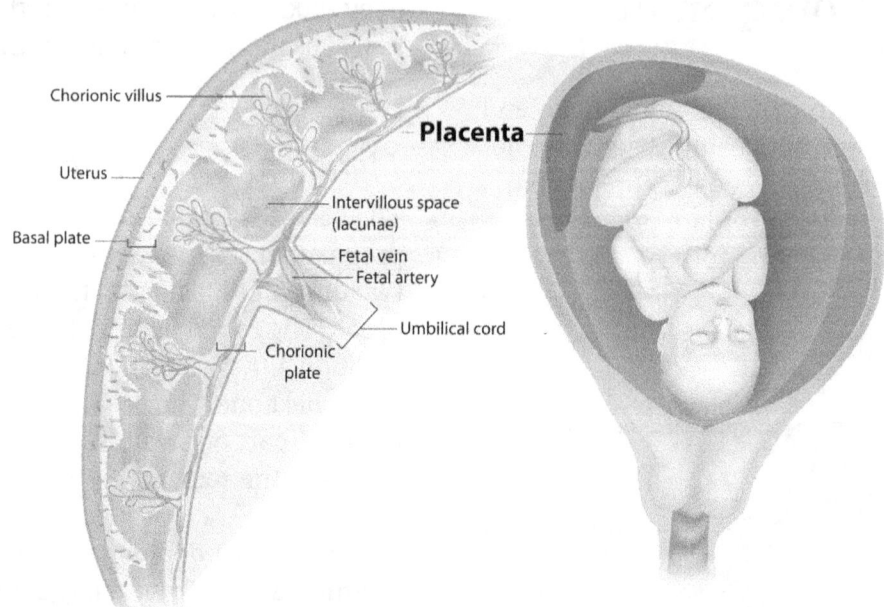

The Placenta

My team and I give our parents a tour of the placenta after the birth if they so desire. We wash it off first. Many people are very interested in seeing the apartment their baby's been living in. The women I help have placentas that are so incredibly beautiful. Even when they give birth at Week 42, their placentas are healthy and in great shape because they follow my Sevenfold Approach.

The placenta usually implants to the back of the uterus. Occasionally the placenta will attach to the front, which can sometimes make it difficult to hear the fetal heart tones, but it is usually not a problem otherwise. The reason this placement makes it difficult to hear the baby's heartbeat is because the placental sac is larger than the baby in the early weeks of development, and it echoes the mother's heartbeat, covering up the infant's heart tones.

Baby's Movements

Most women feel the baby begin to move at Weeks 18–22, with Week 20 being the most common. It can be a lot later if the placenta is attached to the front of the uterus. Women who have had babies before can sometimes feel fetal movement as early as Week 15.

Oftentimes a pregnant woman is feeling the movement of the baby, but it feels so much like gas in their intestines that it's hard to tell which is which. I'm always amused when women early in their pregnancy say, "I'm feeling lots of movement" and when I ask where they are feeling it, they point to their upper abdomen. I have to gently remind them that the baby's not up there. Then there are the women who say, "I'm not feeling the baby move yet, but I'm having lots of gas" and when I ask them where they are feeling it, they point right to their uterus. I get the joy of telling them that while these sensations feel very similar to gas, what they are actually feeling are the gentle, early movements of their baby.

Pelvic Floor

The tissue between the rectum, anus, and vagina is called the perineum. The following illustration shows the location of the pelvic floor muscle. Some people know this as the "Kegel" muscle or associate it with "Kegel exercises." Dr. Kegel named the female perineum after himself ... I always have had a little trouble with that. I prefer the term *pelvic floor muscles*. The pelvic floor muscle is the figure-eight-shaped muscle that goes around the vagina and around the rectum. It is used to stop urine mid-stream or to hold it in. It is also the muscle that stretches during birth.

Here's a diagram showing you where these muscles are located in the female reproductive system.

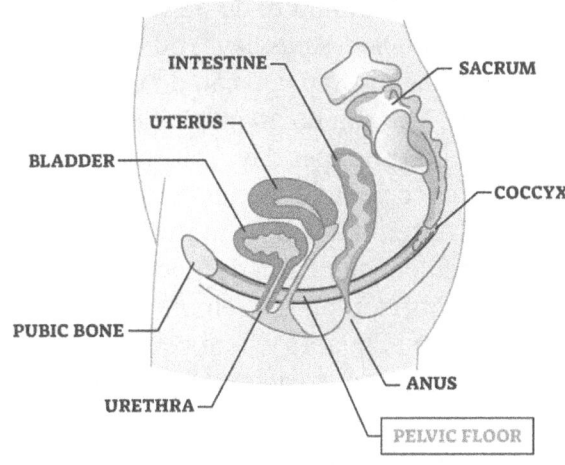

Location of the Pelvic Floor Muscles

And this diagram shows the muscles as if we were looking at them facing the vagina.

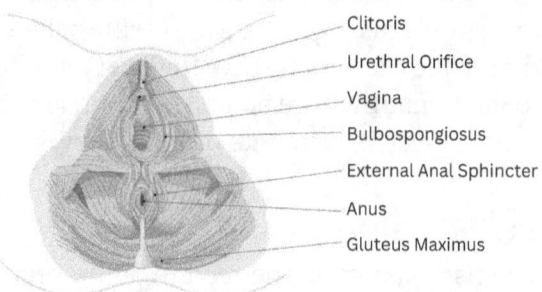

- Clitoris
- Urethral Orifice
- Vagina
- Bulbospongiosus
- External Anal Sphincter
- Anus
- Gluteus Maximus

Pelvic Floor Muscles

As mentioned previously, you begin to have contractions the moment the embryo implants into the uterus. These contractions are often called Braxton Hicks contractions. I have a hard time with this as well, because this is yet another man who named a woman's process after himself. Women, let's leave these men out of our bodies and call them what they are, which is *contractions*, plain and simple as that.

Pelvic Floor Exercises

Some of the most important things you can do to strengthen your pelvic floor are to walk every day and to do pelvic floor exercises 200 times per day. You can do them quickly, and you can do them anywhere. You can do 20 pelvic floor exercises 10 times per day. You can put up little notes to yourself with "PFE" written on them to remind you to do these. Great places include your car's dashboard, the bathroom mirror, on the remote control … These are all places where you can do 20 PFEs while you're doing something else like stopped at a traffic light, doing the dishes, brushing your teeth, etc. You can also set multiple reminders on your phone.

Or you could do them at the top of the hour when you're getting your cup of water to drink. (Habit stacking is a great idea!)

What to Do

The way you do these exercises is to contract your pelvic floor as hard as you can, hold it for a second, and then release. You can do these anywhere.

Where are My Pelvic Floor Muscles?

If you don't know which muscle you're supposed to be contracting, one way to learn it is to stop peeing midstream. The muscles you use to squeeze off your urine when you're peeing or keep yourself from passing gas are the exact same muscles you want to strengthen. Now, this is not something you want to continue to do once you've located the muscle, as it could reduce the long-term effectiveness of emptying of your bladder, and that's not a good thing. So just use this trick once or twice to figure out where exactly your pelvic floor muscle is.

Another method is to put your finger into your vagina and feel what's happening there when you squeeze. You should feel the vaginal muscles gripping your finger. Once you can control these muscles and really grip and feel that clamping down, you know you've got it, and you can continue to strengthen and tone your muscles from there.

This practice will also help you to strengthen and thicken the perineum. If that tissue is thin, it will likely tear a bit during the birth, but if it is thick, it will be more likely to stretch beautifully and go right back to normal soon after the birth.

Developing strong perineal and pelvic floor muscles will greatly reduce the risk of uterine prolapse and bladder incontinence as you age. The following illustration shows you what can happen when you don't have good muscle tone. The whole uterus can prolapse and fall into the vagina and make you super uncomfortable. This is why I want you to stay down for two weeks after giving birth!

Finding Out Your Baby's Gender

That old wives' tale about you presenting as wider when you are having a girl and more pointed out in the front for a boy is total nonsense, and you should ignore that completely. I think a lot of people are just more psychic than they realize and they're getting vibes that are correct.

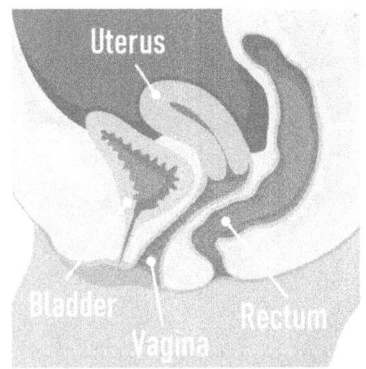

Normal Anatomy

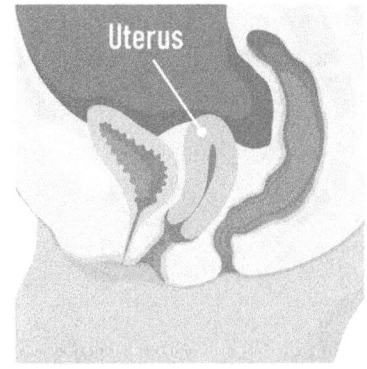

Stage 1 – the uterus is in the upper half of the vagina

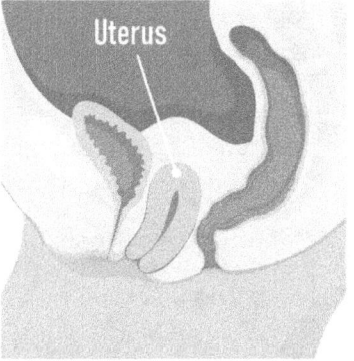

Stage 2 – the uterus has descended nearly to the opening of the vagina

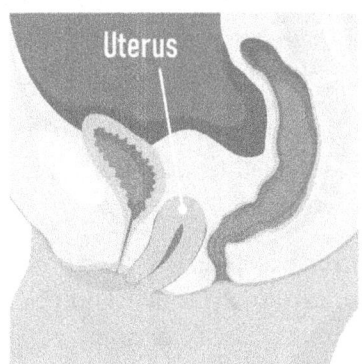

Stage 3 – the uterus protrudes out of the vagina

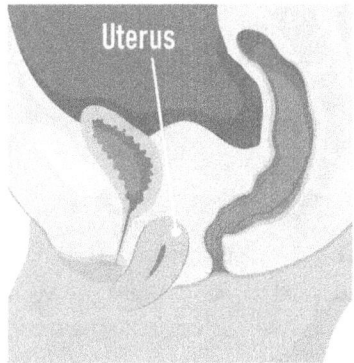

Stage 4 – the uterus is completely out of the vagina.

Stages of Uterine Prolapse

Robbie: I intuitively knew with absolute certainty that my first baby was a girl, so during that pregnancy, I only bought girls' clothing. With an equally strong intuition, I knew that my second was a boy, so I only bought boys' clothes. I never had an ultrasound to confirm my intuitive knowledge, and my intuition was right both times!

Aleah: Something that always stuck with me deeply were MariMikel's words about finding out the gender of your baby. She said, "When you don't find out ahead of time, it's the biggest surprise you're ever going to get; it's the biggest surprise of your life."

It made me think of Christmas and the anticipation of opening a gift and not knowing what it was going to be, and this was going to be the most amazing Christmas gift ever. I felt very deeply that I didn't want to find out in advance. That's totally a personal decision. For me it felt so special having that wonder, that excitement of not knowing. I love surprises, so this was perfect for me.

I will never forget the moment my baby was born and placed up on my belly, the joy and awe of birth that already exists was compounded by that moment when one of us asked, "Is it a boy or a girl?"

My husband Frankie said, "I don't know."

I said, "Look, look!"

He did and when he said, "It's a girl," I just cried with joy. I would have been incredibly happy with a boy or a girl, but that moment is forever deeply etched in my soul and something I will never forget and truly cherish always.

I do want to add that you might check out the Chinese gender calendar. You can search for that term online and easily find a free one. It's just a fun little thing to do, but I have found that it is surprisingly accurate. I don't know anybody who's had an incorrect prediction. I don't know how it works but they have been doing this kind of thing for a very long time. It is cool, especially if you are wanting to not find out but maybe have an idea of what your baby might be.

I really wanted the gender of my baby to be a surprise, but my husband really wanted to find out if we were having a boy or a girl, so I told him about the Chinese gender calendar. It accurately predicted that we'd have a girl.

With our second baby it also predicted she was going to be a girl. We did end up finding out her gender through an ultrasound at about Week 20. My husband said he just couldn't handle the suspense the second time around. We had a lot of pink hand-me-downs, and if it was a boy, he wanted us to start getting things that would be more gender neutral. I decided that would be okay. I'd had my surprise and we would find out the gender of our second baby so he could have the comfort of that knowledge throughout the pregnancy. Regardless of whether your find out the gender in advance, the Chinese gender calendar is pretty cool.

Penelope: I'd never heard of the Chinese gender calendar before, but I did check it out and tried it for the one child for whom I was certain of their conception date and found that it accurately predicted his gender! It seems to be based on a lunar calendar and relies on the mother's lunar age and the baby's conception date.

I did find out the gender of my first two babies, and having had a boy and a girl already it was easy to let the third baby's gender be a surprise to us. When baby number three practically fell out of me I didn't even remember that I didn't know their gender. We were so focused on getting them skin-to-skin, warm, and making sure that they were breathing that it was several minutes before I remembered to ask if they were a boy or a girl. My husband looked and the midwife confirmed we'd had a girl.

Because we didn't know their gender, we had a lot of fun picking out names for boys and girls and we spent a few days with our precious newborn getting to know her before deciding on her name. Having done it both ways, I think there are benefits to either approach. There are a lot of gender-neutral color choices (if you care about that) so you can easily take the *surprise-me* approach for your first baby.

Know that ultrasounds can be incorrect in assessing gender, especially when based on an exam done prior to Week 18. For a definitive answer, you can get a blood test at any point after Week 18.

Cord Blood Banking

I am a huge proponent of cord blood banking and I think this is a good time for you to be learning about it, thinking about it, and planning for it if you decide to do it. I think that banking your child's cord blood is an awesome idea. It is an insurance policy for your family. When you store the stem cells that are in the cord blood at the time of the baby's birth, they can be used to help with an amazing number of awful things.

Why do it?

There are 16 types of cancer that medical professionals use stem cells for as the number one way to heal, and more diseases are found every year that stem cells help treat.[123] Advances in use are rapidly accelerating.[124] Scientists are very close to being able to cure spinal cord injury with stem cell therapy.[125] They also are within a few years of being able to create the insulin-producing cells of the pancreas through stem cell therapy.[126] When a person suffers burns or deformation in something like a bad fire or a car wreck, they can now create noses and ears and lips from stem cells that are bioidentical to the person who the stem cells are from, and because of that they will never be rejected by the injured person's body.[127]

Your baby's blood can also help other family members. Cord blood is a match for siblings at a rate of 50–70 percent. Parents are a 25–50 percent match and grandparents are a 25 percent match, so it's not just your new baby you are creating an insurance policy for.

There was a little girl who had leukemia and the treatment had been unsuccessful so far. She was going to die. The parents learned about stem cells and the father had his vasectomy reversed. They became pregnant, had the baby, and banked her cord blood. That baby's cord blood was a match for her older sister, and they were able to cure her sister's leukemia with stem cell therapy.

Another mother in my care had complications in labor, and after many hours I transported her to the hospital. After another 12 hours laboring in the hospital, the baby was born with some brain swelling. They were able to use the stem cells that they collected at the time of the birth to help with the damage that can occur from brain swelling.

How Does it Work?

The birth happens and the baby goes up into your arms. As soon as I confirm the baby is breathing well and is nice and pink, then we go to the cord. I clean the cord and insert a big needle into the cord close to the vagina—there's no feeling in the cord; it's like hair or fingernails. It has absolutely no nerve endings for hot, cold, or pain, so this does not hurt at all. The blood drains out of the cord, and I

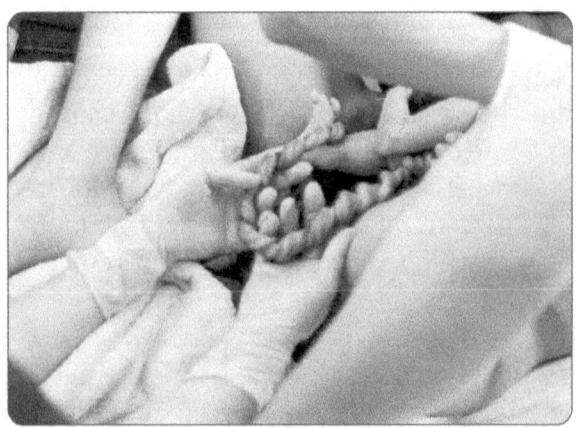

Umbilical cord

capture it in a little bag. This blood would normally drain back into the placenta, form a clot, and be eliminated by your body with the birth of the placenta, so cord blood banking is not taking from baby or momma's resources.

How Much Does It Cost?

At the time of this writing, most reputable cord banks charge several thousand dollars for retrieval and decades of storage. It is an expensive outlay if you do it all at once, but many reputable cord blood banks offer payment plans. There are several companies I recommend, listed in Appendix E.

Many Americans pay thousands and thousands of dollars every year for insurance they rarely use. Think of this as a highly personalized insurance policy against a lot of terrible things that can happen to people, and I believe it's worth the investment.

In my practice, it is my client's responsibility to make arrangements with their preferred cord blood bank and to get the collection kit and have it ready. It is their responsibility to include the kit with the supplies I ask them to have on hand for the birth, and it is my responsibility from there. My team will fill out the paperwork, complete the kit for my clients, and arrange for the couriers to come and pick it up. I'll make sure everything is taken care of, but my clients need to arrange for and pay for the services ahead of time, which is why we're talking about this in the Second Trimester. Talk with your midwife about their methodology for cord blood banking collection and follow their guidelines if this is of interest to you.

Private versus Public Stem Cell Banks

Private blood banking ensures that the stem cells and tissue that you bank are available to your child and your family only.

Public cord banking is another option if you choose not to bank the stem cells for your family. This provides a donation of stem cells to further scientific research into new therapies and help people who may not have privately banked. There is usually no charge for public banking.

You will need to research which hospitals in your area offer this or arrange with your midwife to handle the donation. If this is of interest to you, you can find additional resources in Appendix E.

Regardless of whether you choose private or public cord blood banking, both provide immense benefits.

Handling the Complications and Common Discomforts of Pregnancy

In this section I'm going to revisit a few previous topics and broach some new ones in light of where you are in your pregnancy. You may or may not be experiencing these symptoms. If it stresses you out to read about these topics, I suggest you scan the list below to familiarize yourself with what they are, so you can return to this section if you need to. If this is you, skip ahead to page 248 to learn about Other Helpful Practitioners you may want to rely on during your pregnancy, labor, and birth.

In this section we'll cover:

- Anemia
- Back Pain
- Congestion
- Cramping and Spotting
- Fatigue
- Gestational Diabetes
- Hemorrhoids
- Herpes
- Indigestion
- Ligament Stretching Pain
- Pregnancy Brain
- Varicose or Spider Veins
- Yeast and Bacterial Infections, Gonorrhea, and Chlamydia

Anemia

At about Week 20 the baby starts siphoning iron from momma. Babies must store all the iron they're going to need from birth until they are eating solid foods (around 5 months of age) while they are in utero; there is no iron in breast milk. You may experience anemia when this happens. Know that this is normal and natural, but it can be very debilitating. This is one of the reasons I recommend you take Ultra-Mins, which have an absorbable source of iron in them as a preventative measure, but sometimes it's not enough and you have to supplement more.

Anemia stems from either your body not making enough red blood cells or not absorbing enough iron. Absorption of Iron is improved with Vitamin C consumption. Iron comes in two forms in our food: heme and non-heme.[128] Beef, chicken, pork, lamb, fish, and shellfish provide more bioavailable iron (heme) than vegetables.

The iron in vegetables is less bioavailable to us (non-heme), and how the vegetables are raised is important in terms of their actual mineral content. Minerals are in the soil and are then absorbed by the vegetables. If we are eating conventionally grown produce, we are eating foods grown in depleted soil, and mounting evidence shows they are simply not as nutritious as in times past.[129]

Anemia can be harmful to both mother and baby. If your hematocrit level is below 32 and/or your hemoglobin is below 11, you should take supplements to raise your iron count. Here are a few recommendations you can select from to help you (I am not recommending you do all of these). As always, consult your midwife for personal guidance.

- **Ultra-Mins**—Take three a day faithfully.

- **Ideal Iron**—Manufactured by Thompson's. Take two tablets two or three times a day on an empty stomach with Vitamin C.

- **Yellow Dock**—Herbal capsules. Take two capsules two or three times a day.

- **Organic Desiccated Liver Tablets**— Take three per day.

- **Mint-flavored Liquid Chlorophyll**— Take 2 tablespoons twice a day. Mix with 8 ounces of water or juice if you prefer.

- **Fe cell salt**—Fe is the atomic symbol for iron, and this is a homeopathic remedy—use as directed on the package.

- **Floradix Liquid Iron**—one tablespoon two times a day.

If you take iron supplements, **don't** take them at the same time that you take **Vitamin E** as it can be an iron absorption blocker.

Definitely take them with 500 mg Ester-C because that will help you to absorb the iron from your gut.

If your bloodwork shows you're low in iron or you are anemic, you can focus on including more iron-rich foods in your diet.

- Protein: beef, chicken, pork, lamb, fish, and shellfish
- Dried peaches are best—but they can't be sulfured (which preserves their pretty color; they taste just the same when they're darker.)
- Apricots (unsulfured)
- Raisins (unsulfured)
- Dark leafy greens, spinach
- Dry beans and peas
- Nuts
- Seeds
- Nut butter
- Tempeh
- Tofu
- Beets/beet powder
- Raw oysters—Check these out carefully; make sure they're fresh. Don't eat them if they are gaping open, dry, or if they smell or taste different from how you expect. Oysters are one of the highest sources of absorbable iron out there. I recommend Pacific Northwest oysters and Atlantic northeast oysters. They are from colder waters, and I think are safer to ingest in pregnancy. I live in Texas, and I do eat and love gulf oysters, but I only eat them when the waters are colder,

in the winter. A good rule of thumb is to only eat from these warmer waters in months that have an "R" in their names. Avoid May, June, July, and August.

- Blackstrap molasses

If you are vegetarian, you might also try whole grain or enriched cereals, brown rice, pasta, and butternut squash. You can also obtain more iron by cooking in a cast iron skillet.

Back Pain

Inactivity and poor posture are the root causes of back pain. Women too often relax their stomach muscles, sway their back, tilt their tail bone up/pubic bone down, lock their knees, and balance by leaning back from the waist up. This leads to back pain.

Remedies

You want to lift your pubic bone, engage your stomach muscles, and tuck your tailbone. Stand up straight. Shoulders back. Walk that way! It's critically important. Walking is one of the things that helps your back the most, but you must control the angle of your pelvis. Use mirrors to check your posture.

Sit properly! Slouching promotes poor positioning for your baby and a more painful labor for you if the baby stays that

SECOND TRIMESTER

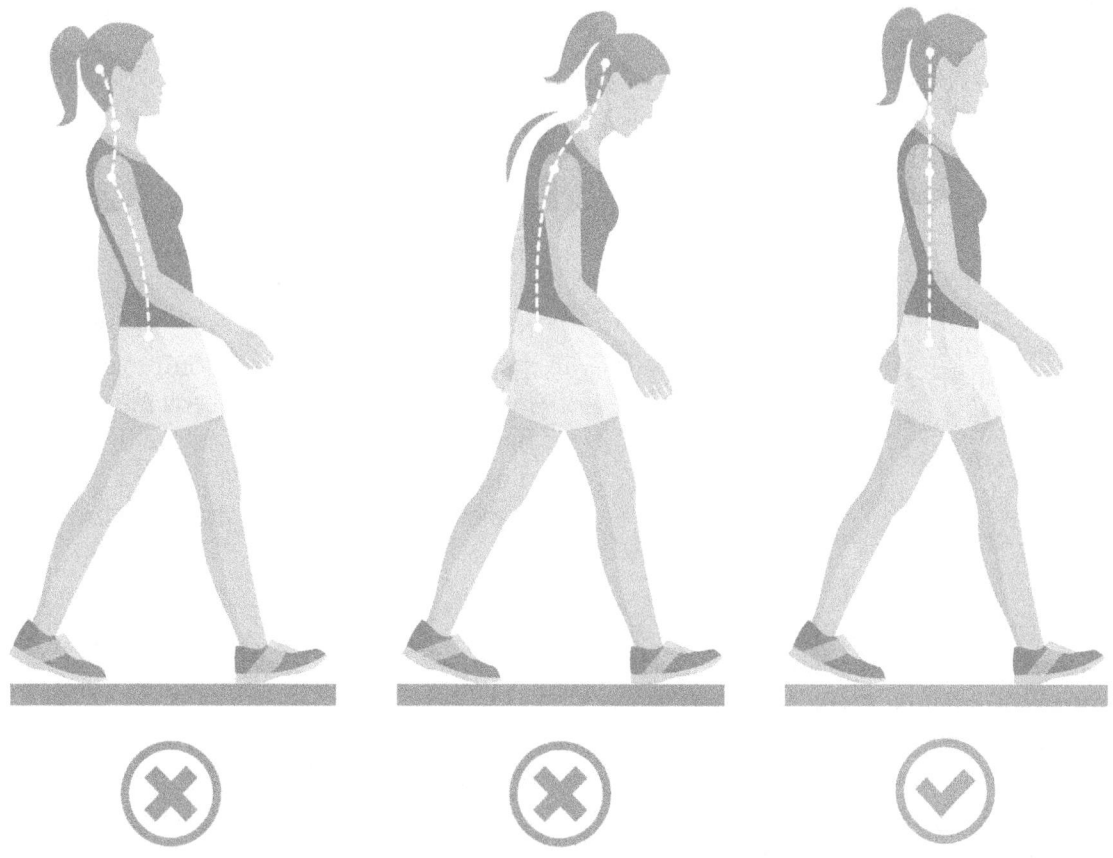

Incorrect and Correct Walking Posture

way. Don't slump while you're sitting; keep your spine straight and your shoulders back. Activate your core and stomach muscles. This will encourage optimal positioning for your baby.

If you are struggling with back pain, chiropractic care is essential, massage is recommended, and acupuncture is valuable.

Congestion

There are folds in the nose called turbinates that moisturize and filter the air you breathe as it comes in through your nose. These folds have a lot of blood vessels in them and because the blood fluid volume of a pregnant woman increases so much, there is an unpleasantry that can happen in pregnancy: Whenever you lie down, your nose may become congested, and there is not much to do about this aside from positioning. You could elevate the head of the bed just enough to help provide relief, or get a wedge-shaped pillow designed for this.

Note that I strongly discourage you from using nasal drops or sprays to open your nose. Once you start using these, your body will come to rely on them as a crutch and may not produce as much lubrication naturally.

Cramping and Spotting

After the first three months, cramping is less normal and should always be an indication to call your midwife. Any time you feel cramping, you should reduce physical activity, do not have sex, and possibly drink a glass of wine to stop the uterus from contracting. Alcohol, in small amounts, is an excellent and safe way to slow uterine activity down when it is concerning you. It is a smooth muscle relaxant, and your uterus is a smooth muscle.

Worrisome cramping usually takes place behind the pubic bone in the middle of the low abdomen and upper vagina. If cramping is occurring on either side instead, know that it's probably coming from your round ligaments and is not as worrisome. Much of the time, this cramping is caused by a lack of water. Dehydration concentrates the oxytocin in your bloodstream, causing these cramps. You can also have cramping from your intestines if you are constipated.

Remedy

Call your midwife and follow her advice. Get off your feet and lie down. Rest. Drink more water.

Fatigue

There are several causes of routine fatigue that are very common in pregnancy.

Not enough **movement**. You are building up stamina for birth. If you don't exercise, you lose energy. Inactivity breeds fatigue. You have been more inactive in the first three months and now must start the gradual climb to being in great shape for the birth.

Inactivity breeds fatigue.

Nutrition. Vitamin C, Vitamin B, the whole regimen ... Everyone who takes the vitamins and supplements I recommend reports feeling better and having more energy and less fatigue after starting. I notice that if I miss a few days, I really do feel that my energy is depleted.

Sleep. You must be striving for eight hours a night. See my recommendations for sleep hygiene in the Rest section in the Conscious Conception chapter (page 99). Allow yourself to take naps when you feel the need. Try not to nap past 2:30 p.m. or it may interfere with your nighttime sleep.

Hydration. When you are hydrated, your body is able to more easily perform its functions and provide you with extra energy.[130] I have noticed this feels very true when my own hydration flags.

Gestational Diabetes

The Mayo Clinic defines gestational diabetes as "diabetes diagnosed for the first time during pregnancy (gestation). Like other types of diabetes, gestational diabetes affects how your cells use sugar (glucose). Gestational diabetes (GD) is a condition where your blood sugar is elevated past the point your body can respond to it, and that can affect your pregnancy and your baby's health."[131]

While it's not always the case, a large percentage of GD is due to poor diet. If you have a genetic predisposition to gestational diabetes, you might need to be more careful. Most people don't realize that during pregnancy they simply can't eat as many carbs as they are accustomed to.

Carbs are everywhere in our standard American diet (SAD). Rice, pasta, bread, potatoes, sweet potatoes, carrots, cereals, and all the processed foods, candies, and

sweet treats ... they're all carbs. All fruits and vegetables are carbs as well, but they're not the problem. The human pancreas was not designed to metabolize that much sugar. The grains and starches consumed in the SAD overload our insulin response. This kind of diet pushes us firmly toward a propensity for developing GD in pregnancy. I've been astonished at how many people can turn GD around completely with diet.

Most people would rather say "I can't" or "I could never do that" than make lasting changes. Sometimes a partner will present an obstacle as well. On top of that, you have to guard against the culture that promotes sugary foods over nutritious foods. Avoid making impulse purchases. Marketers try to tempt you with these products. Avoid: purchasing from end caps (end of aisle product displays) and point-of-sale displays, drive-through up-sells, and midafternoon media that often has advertisements for sugary foods to take advantage of the fact that people's blood sugar often dips during those hours.

Watch the volume of simple carbs and sugars you consume. Watch ingredient labels for hidden sugars. It's important to get *some* carbs; no diet should exclude carbs completely, at least not in pregnancy. Please eat as many vegetables as you like! Track your carbs for a week to see what your average daily consumption is and note what kind of carbs you're eating. Check with your midwife to see if that's a healthy amount for you.

At 28 weeks, I screen to see if a woman is at risk for developing GD. If I see sugar in a woman's urine during the pregnancy, this is also an indication of a risk for developing

GD. If women are at risk, the first thing I advise them to do is to monitor their carbs and start eating fewer simple carbs, more protein, and more vegetables. I also suggest that they buy a glucose monitor and check their fasting blood sugar levels when they wake up in the morning and then occasionally after they eat. Tracking this data allows you to work with your care provider to make better decisions about whether the situation is a problem. I also ask my clients to educate themselves about the diabetic diet and the outcomes if they allow this to go unchecked. All of these are great ways to monitor and address a potentially worrisome situation.

If you do develop GD, know that your proclivity to develop Type II diabetes is increased postpartum and later in life as you age.

Hemorrhoids

The Mayo Clinic describes hemorrhoids as "swollen veins in your anus and lower rectum, similar to varicose veins. Hemorrhoids can develop inside the rectum (internal hemorrhoids) or under the skin around the anus (external hemorrhoids)."[132] Most women feel them as small lumps around the anus or may see a little blood when they wipe after a bowel movement.

Prevention

Like varicosities, hemorrhoids often run in the family. If you are prone to them, do your best to not get constipated. Drink four quarts of water a day. Remember, an excess of wheat, red meat, dairy, and sugar are all constipating. Eat these in minimal to moderate amounts. If you are having a flare up, don't eat them at all.

Avoid sitting for long periods.

Be careful when squatting. It can increase the chance of hemorrhoids. When practicing squatting, tighten your perineum and rectum while you squat, and don't bear down while in that pose.

If you are not able to have a bowel movement, use a glycerin suppository. It will usually make you go to the bathroom within thirty minutes and will keep the hemorrhoid from becoming worse. Do not sit on the toilet any longer than you absolutely must (no reading or cell phone use!).

Wipe with Tucks medicated pads whenever you have a bowel movement. Wiping with toilet paper will abrade the exposed mucus membrane. You do want to push the hemorrhoids back into the rectum with a good oil or Vitamin E. You must keep them lubricated. Wash your hands thoroughly after doing this or use medical gloves.

Treatment

Keep hemorrhoid cream on the hemorrhoids after you wipe. Push the hemorrhoids back into the rectum, if possible. Wash your hands carefully before and after you treat your hemorrhoids.

Make a poultice of grated raw, starchy potato, and apply to the area for a minimum of twenty minutes (baker or Russet-style potatoes work the best, red potatoes do not work as well). This method dehydrates the tissues and reduces the fluid in hemorrhoids, helping to decrease inflammation and size. This works. If you're in pain, I urge you to try it. It may sound weird, but trust me, this will really help.

Soak a cotton ball in witch hazel and put it in the freezer. Once very cold, apply to the hemorrhoid for fifteen minutes.

With both the potato and witch hazel, you'll want to apply the remedy, put on a sanitary pad, and lie down. Stay still for 15–30 minutes so the remedy has time to work.

White Oak bark: this is an amazing herb. You can buy it in capsule form and take one or two twice a day depending on how bad your hemorrhoids are. It helps to firm up the rectal vessels.

If you do have severe hemorrhoids, you'll want to support your rectum. You can put a few sanitary pads against it to provide that support and hold them there with panties that are tight enough to keep them in place.

Herpes

Many women have fewer herpes outbreaks in their second trimester. It is a much easier time for you and your body, but still watch for those prodromal symptoms and take the mitigating actions if they flare up. See page 90.

Indigestion

One of the leading causes of indigestion (aka heartburn) is the softening of the cardiac sphincter, which is the sphincter between the stomach and esophagus, and the stomach herniating into the esophagus, which causes the stomach acid to be pushed up into the esophagus.

In pregnancy, everything softens. The uterus pushing up on the stomach makes this condition worse. One way to stop this problem is to physically push the stomach

back down through the sphincter. A knowledgeable practitioner should perform this. I do this for my clients and show partners who feel comfortable how to do it, so it can be done at home as needed. You might ask your provider if they can help you with this. Here are other remedies and preventative measures you can employ:

- Eat frequent, small meals or a large meal slowly, over two hours.

- Always thoroughly chew your food.

- Limit your consumption of spicy foods, fermented foods, citrus, tomato-based products, carbonated beverages (including carbonated water), vinegar, and hot sauces.

- Take papaya enzymes before eating.

- I recommend Tums brand calcium tablets for relief; get the natural kind. Calcium carbonate is a natural substance and isn't a drug. But if you just try to treat indigestion by taking lots and lots of Tums, you run the risk of calcifying your placenta by having too much calcium carbonate in your diet. I'm talking several times every day. Resist the urge to do that. You need to discover what is causing your indigestion and take action at the root of the problem, as opposed to suppressing the symptoms.

- Don't eat after 6:30 p.m. after the first trimester (unless you are experiencing nausea. If you are experiencing nausea, eating before bed and during the night is crucial.).

- The stomach produces several major digestive enzymes. They each digest a particular type of food. When you chew your food, salivary enzymes in your mouth tell your stomach what food is coming and what enzymes to excrete to aid in digesting those foods. If you drink a large amount of liquid with food, you interfere with these enzymes in your mouth and your stomach doesn't produce these prep enzymes as efficiently, which can hinder your digestion. To avoid this, drink minimal to moderate amounts with meals. This isn't the time for chugging.

- Cold drinks consumed immediately after eating can cool the stomach temperature, also slowing digestion and adding to a feeling of sluggishness. Consider room temperature drinks instead, or better yet, don't drink during meals.

- You can buy digestive enzyme complexes in supplement form, and those can be very helpful sometimes. They'll have papain, bromine, amylase, and protease, which can really make a difference. Some of these also have wonderful herbs in them.

- Stop drinking fluids one hour before bedtime.

- Sleep at a slight incline. Use two pillows to raise the head of the bed, get an incline pillow, or elevate your adjustable base to achieve this.

- Acupressure: If you're in the throes of it, place your thumb and index finger on either side of the large vertebrae at the base of your neck, massage firmly (but not too hard) in a circle for a few seconds, move down to the next vertebrae and repeat. Do this for three or four vertebrae, go back to the top, and repeat. Your heartburn should diminish in 20–60 seconds.

Ligament Stretching Pain

You might feel sharp pains in your lower abdomen from time to time as one or the other or both round ligaments stretch.

One of the reasons I suggest you take evening primrose oil is that it helps to soften the round ligaments and can help them to stretch without discomfort. Doing the ab work to strengthen your abdominal muscles can also help. Be careful not to bend or twist too rapidly or forcefully as it can tear the attachment of the round ligament to the uterus and can be painful for days. If you are getting bigger more rapidly, wear a belly support system earlier as it will help to take the pressure off your round ligaments and distribute it to the back. As I mentioned before, your insurance company may cover this expense; it pays to check. Ligament pain is usually harmless and goes away on its own after childbirth.

Here are some additional tips for helping with ligament pain in pregnancy:

- Get plenty of **rest**, especially during the second and third trimesters.

- **Gentle exercises**, such as yoga, can help to strengthen the muscles in your pelvis and abdomen.

- Applying **heat** to the affected area can help to relieve pain and inflammation. Use a hot water bottle or warm compress. You can also fill a long sock with rice, tie it off, and microwave it for a minute. If it's not warm enough, heat in 30-second increments until it is.

- Applying **ice** to the affected area can also help to relieve pain and inflammation. You can use an ice pack or frozen peas wrapped in a towel.

- **Massage** can help to relax the muscles and relieve pain. Ask your partner or a prenatal massage therapist to massage the affected area.

- **Arnica** cream or pellets: Frequent applications of arnica cream applied directly to the sore spot will help the pain to go away faster. You can also take arnica pellets orally (as directed on the bottle) for 24 hours.

If you are experiencing severe ligament pain, talk to your midwife about it. They may recommend medication or other treatment options. I have suggested that women with a serious round ligament tear take two ibuprofen every four hours for 24 hours **only**. This is a very small amount of ibuprofen over a very short amount of time, and it will not hurt your baby. This will reduce the inflammation and allow the tear to heal much more quickly. During this time, it is critical that you stay down and not move. Allow the healing process to be effective. Remember that when you are hurting, the tear is being exacerbated, and when you're pain free it is healing.

Pregnancy Brain

Pregnancy brain usually gets better in the second trimester. You have more vitality, the baby is not growing quite as dramatically, and—while it's still an issue—you should find it less of a problem right now.

Varicose or Spider Veins

Your midwife should screen for this issue in your family because it's hereditary.

If varicose veins do run in your family, take one capsule of white oak bark in either the morning or evening to firm up the vascular system. This is a preventative measure.

The combination of Vitamins E and C (as recommended in my regimen) supports the circulatory system and creates a stronger cardiovascular system in the baby and in you, helping to prevent and treat varicosities.

If you experience serious varicosities, quit using the evening primrose oil supplement and take one or two white oak bark capsules in the morning and evening depending on how bad it is.

Gluten also seems to be a very big factor here. If you haven't already, cut it way down or out altogether. If you find you have flu-like symptoms when you cut out gluten, know that this is normal and due to your body's withdrawal from the substance. Drink some hot bone broth or chicken broth when you feel the symptoms of headache, foggy brain, fatigue, and/or shakiness or chills. The symptoms usually subside within minutes of ingesting the broth.

If you have varicose or spider veins, wear compression socks and/or support hose. Put them on to compress the legs before you get out of bed in the morning to prevent expansion of the vessels. They need to be strong enough to compress. It's awful to have to do this in the summer, but it's better than getting a bad varicosity/blood clot that could potentially harm you. Keep your legs compressed at all times unless you're in the shower or in bed.

Vaginal Infections

I'm going to address these conditions somewhat together as their treatments are very similar.

Yeast Infections

A yeast infection is a fungal infection that can occur in the vagina, mouth, and other parts of the body. The most common type of yeast infection is a vaginal yeast infection, which is also known as vulvovaginal candidiasis.

Yeast is a normal inhabitant of the vagina, but sometimes during pregnancy the pH of the vagina changes and if the balance of bacteria and yeast in the vagina is disrupted, the yeast can grow out of control and cause an infection. The most common cause of yeast infections is eating too much sugar. Remember, all carbs turn into sugars in the body and can exacerbate yeast symptoms. (Yeast loves sugar.) Yeast infections also can often follow antibiotic use.

Symptoms

Yeast infections can cause vaginal itching and burning as well as irritation of the labia. You may also see an increased discharge that can look like cottage cheese or lots of white discharge. Sometimes sensitivity during or after sex can indicate yeast as

well. I see lots of yeast infections with no adverse symptoms—this does not mean it doesn't need to be treated. It can still infect your baby's mouth after the birth causing thrush, and potentially getting thrush into your nipples, which can cause severe pain when you breastfeed your baby.

Bacterial Infections

A vaginal bacterial infection is an infection that occurs when the balance of bacteria in the vagina is disrupted. This can happen for several reasons, including taking antibiotics, having a weakened immune system, having a new sexual partner, as well as being pregnant. Douching on a regular basis can also be a factor. Douching should only be used to handle moments that are out of balance, to try to heal things without having to resort to antibiotics.

I also think serious stress can throw the vaginal flora off, and it can put your whole body off-kilter. Your immune system takes a nosedive under serious stress because your body's too busy working on adrenaline, cortisol, and epinephrine to handle everything it should. Work to eliminate stressors as much as you can; it may be the most impactful thing you can do for your health in every aspect of life, and especially in pregnancy.

Bacteria are normal components of the vagina, but there are bacteria that are not supposed to be there. There are a number of different types of vaginal bacterial infections, including:

- **Bacterial vaginosis (BV)**—the most common type of vaginal bacterial infection. It is caused by an overgrowth of Gardnerella vaginalis, a type of bacteria that is naturally present in the vagina. BV can cause symptoms such as a thin, grayish-white discharge with a fishy odor, itching, and burning.

- **Trichomoniasis**—a sexually transmitted infection (STI) that is caused by a parasite called Trichomonas vaginalis. It can cause symptoms such as frothy, yellow-green discharge, itching, and burning.

- **Chlamydia**—an STI that is caused by a bacteria called Chlamydia trachomatis. It can cause symptoms such as a clear or white discharge, burning when you urinate, and pain in the lower abdomen, although many Chlamydia infections can be symptomless.

- **Gonorrhea**—an STI that is caused by a bacteria called Neisseria gonorrhoeae. It can cause symptoms such as a yellow or green discharge, burning when you urinate, and pain in the lower abdomen.

Chlamydia and Gonorrhea are both STI's that can cause blindness in the baby, and it is a legal requirement that pregnant woman be screened for both by all care providers during pregnancy.

- **Group B Streptococcus (GBS)** or more commonly strep B, is a type of bacteria that is commonly found in the vagina and rectum of about 25 percent of healthy women. It is usually harmless, but it can sometimes cause infections in newborns. GBS can be transmitted to the baby during childbirth and very rarely in pregnancy.

If a baby is infected with GBS, they may develop early-onset GBS infection (EOGBS), which occurs within the first six days of life. EOGBS can cause serious complications, such as sepsis, pneumonia, and meningitis. Late-onset GBS infection (LOGBS) occurs in babies between 7 days and 6 weeks of age. LOGBS is less common than EOGBS, but it can still be serious. There is a simple test that can be done during pregnancy to screen for GBS. We will talk more about GBS/strep B in the Third Trimester chapter. Most strep B infections have no symptoms.

Prevention of Vaginal Infections

Diet is a big factor when considering prevention of yeast infections. Simple carbohydrates such as sugar, fruit, honey, maple syrup, agave nectar, fructose and glucose provide yeast infections with a fuel source. Foods made with yeast or containing yeast may also promote yeast growth (beer, bread, pizza). The less gluten, dairy, bread, pasta, potatoes, rice, sugar, and alcohol you consume, the lower your chance of yeast infections.[133]

I have found more strep B infections in women who wear thongs than those who do not. Thongs rub between the rectum and the vagina, potentially inoculating the vagina with strep B. There are few if any symptoms of strep B, but I take a culture toward the end of the pregnancy to identify any of these abnormal organisms. If you own thong underwear, I suggest you put them away and get full-bottomed, cotton underwear. If you must wear pantyhose, cut the crotch out of them.

The use of condoms is the best way to prevent the transmission of STIs. If you think you may have any vaginal infection it is also a great idea to use condoms so as not to pass any of these things back and forth between you and your partner. This is not only important for treatment but for prevention as well.

Treatment

The typical treatment for yeast infections is an over-the-counter vaginal suppository. My experience strongly suggests that these are not very effective, as most women's diets push them toward this imbalance, and the yeast returns shortly after completion of the medication. There are all kinds of natural ways to handle this problem. The method I suggest (instructions to follow) washes the yeast colony out of the vagina, changes the pH, and creates a less hospitable environment for the yeast to proliferate. Additionally, it creates a more hospitable environment for the good bacteria of the vagina, which normally keep the yeast in check. This method is also appropriate for any of the other conditions I listed at the beginning of this section.

Most douche apparatuses you buy are one-time use devices that use a very small volume of fluid. What I find to be effective is to use a hot water bottle with a douche apparatus. You can find these at most drugstores. This device has an enema tip as well as a douche tip. It can be used as a cold or hot water bottle or for enemas, and for the douching regimen I'm about to share with you. There is a clamp that attaches onto the tubing so you can pinch it off and stop the flow.

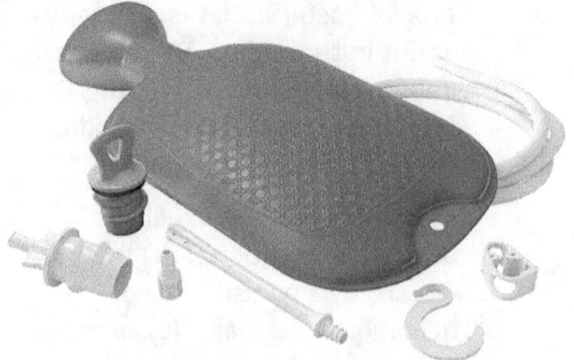

Hot Water Bottle with Douche Apparatus

I recommend that you use the ingredients listed below. Use one ingredient each day, and then repeat the sequence, for a total of eight days of douching.

- **Days 1 and 5:** Put 2 tablespoons of apple cider vinegar or white vinegar in the hot water bottle and fill it with warm water. This changes the pH of your vagina to one inhospitable to yeast.

- **Days 2 and 6:** Put 10 drops of tea tree oil in the hot water bottle and fill it with warm water. This is an excellent fungicide.

- **Days 3 and 7:** Put 2 teaspoons of boric acid crystals or powder (available online or at your pharmacy) and dissolve it in a little bit of hot water before adding it to the hot water bottle, then fill the bottle with warm water. Boric acid powder in this miniscule amount is perfectly safe to wash out the vagina. Boric acid powder often has a warning on the label that says it's not for internal use, and this means for God's sakes, *don't eat it*, but the active ingredient is in many of the over-the-counter natural remedies for yeast and bacterial vaginal infections, and it is perfectly safe. This is an extremely effective treatment for yeast.

- **Days 4 and 8:** Add ½ cup of natural plain yogurt with live acidophilus from the health food store (e.g., White Mountain—don't trust the mainstream grocery brands) to the bag, then fill with warm water. It may help to use a funnel to facilitate this process. The acidophilus in the yogurt replaces beneficial bacteria that normally keeps yeast in check.

How to Douche

I do not recommend douching as part of your regular hygiene—the vagina has its own ways of balancing the flora, and regular, daily douching in pregnancy for extended periods has been linked with preterm delivery.[134] However, douching very occasionally to manage these issues is perfectly safe in pregnancy, and it is the only thing I have found in my 50 years of practice that really seems to work for yeast infections in pregnancy. The only times I suggest douching is when you have yeast or bacterial symptoms, visible yeast upon speculum or vaginal exam, or if you see thick or curdy white discharge on your partner after sex. Here is what you do.

1. Lie down in an empty bathtub.

2. Let the water run through the tubing to remove all the air before you insert the tip into the vagina.

3. Insert the douche tip gently, as far back into the vagina as it will comfortably go. It is important that you put the douche tip far enough in

or the douching will not be effective. Typically, this will be about 3–5 inches but it depends on the length of your vagina. Some are long, some short. Usually very tall women have longer vaginas and vice versa.

4. Rotate the douche tip in a circular motion around the cervix while the fluid completely empties from the bag. It should not hurt.

5. Use the whole amount until the bag is empty, then remove the tubing from your vagina. Allow the mixture to get up around the back of the cervix where the yeast colonies live and let it slowly wash out the vagina.

Continue to douche for the full eight-day regimen. Symptoms should subside after three days, but don't stop the treatment! After you have finished the treatment, you may need to continue to douche once every two or three weeks with one of the mixtures (you can alternate between the four) to keep the yeast at bay. It can come back, especially if you don't change your diet, so keep after it by occasionally douching. After the birth, the yeast often disappear, but pregnancy exacerbates yeast colonies quite significantly for some women.

Severe Yeast or Bacterial Infections

If the above treatment does not control your yeast, or if you have a bacterial infection, you may have to douche twice a day for eight days alternating the four mixtures mentioned above with the herbal mixture I describe in this section, i.e.: Day 1: Mixture 1 in the morning, herbs in the afternoon. Day 2: Mixture 2 in the morning, herbs in the afternoon, and so on.

In order to prepare the herbal mixture, you will need to purchase 2–3 ounces each of echinacea leaf, eucalyptus leaf, comfrey leaf and ½ ounce of myrrh powder. Keep the herbs stored separately, preferably in glass and in a cool, dark place to preserve the properties of each. You may need to order these online.

Herbal Mixture

In a glass or ceramic container pour 1 quart of boiling water over ¼ cup of each herb and 1 tablespoon of myrrh powder. Let it steep for 30—40 minutes, until just lukewarm. Strain the mixture in a large mesh strainer or colander lined with cheesecloth (the herbs can fall through the colander's holes if you don't use the cheesecloth). Once cooled, pour the strained tea into the hot water bottle and douche.

Additional Remedies

- Take oral acidophilus from the refrigerated section of your health food store. You'll want to choose one that has many different strains of lactobacillus. Taking one tablet or capsule a day for ten days helps to replace the good bacteria of your gut and vagina. Be sure to store it in your refrigerator.

- Putting a whole, uncut, peeled clove of garlic in the vagina between each douching session day and night is an excellent treatment in addition to the douching. Make sure there are no knicks or cuts in the garlic flesh or it may cause a burning sensation. Leave it in no longer than 8 hours.

- There is a product called Yeast Guard, which is a homeopathic suppository you can insert in the vagina after douching in the morning. Some people have found this to be effective as well.

- In difficult cases, putting a gelatin capsule (you can buy empty ones at the health food store) filled with boric acid crystals or powder into the vagina after douching in the morning can be very helpful.

If none of this works, you are welcome to try one of the over-the-counter yeast preparations such as Monistat or Gyne-Lotrimin. As previously mentioned, I have not found these things to be very effective or I would certainly suggest you do something easier than this douching regimen. These medicines do not seem to work during pregnancy, and they are relatively expensive. If you are opposed to the treatments described above, feel free to try these medications first.

Other Helpful Practitioners

I tend to think of Western medicine as reactive, and alternative or natural medicines as preventative. You will benefit from pursuing preventative, alternative health care to help you reach optimal health during your pregnancy. In an ideal world, you would be seeing an acupuncturist once a month, a chiropractor every two to four weeks, and a naturopath every six to twelve months. Employ other practitioners at your discretion. Always tell any practitioner you work with that you are pregnant. This goes for your regular providers too, like your dentist.

Acupuncturist

Acupuncture is a form of traditional Chinese medicine that involves inserting thin needles into specific points on the body. These points are believed to be connected to energy pathways (meridians) that run throughout the body. By inserting needles into these points, acupuncturists restore the flow of energy and promote healing. Acupuncture has been used for centuries to treat a variety of health conditions, including pain, nausea, anxiety, depression, and infertility.[135]

Acupuncture is a great practice to engage in during pregnancy and before birth, and it's something that I think everyone should do as part of their self-care. Acupuncture is about improving the energy flow in your body. If there are blockages, excesses, or insufficiencies of energy in your body in places, a talented acupuncturist can harmonize or unblock these channels, which can make your body function better

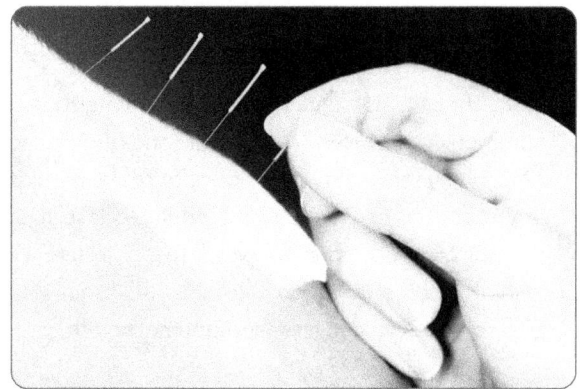

Acupuncture Needles

and ultimately help you to have an easier pregnancy, labor, and birth.

Chiropractic Care

Chiropractic work is also good to get ahead of time. You want your body to be properly aligned and to have nerve endings optimized, so all of the messages transition optimally, and chiropractic care does that. It can also help to alleviate back pain and other pains in the body, such as hips or joint pain.

SECOND TRIMESTER

CHIROPRACTIC CARE IN PREGNANCY

I have been in practice since 1990. My wife Jennifer and I have four kids who were all born at home. I have helped countless pregnant women during my career in addition to caring for my wife through four pregnancies. Jennifer and I met MariMikel in 1997 when pregnant with our second child. Following MariMikel's Sevenfold Approach to an Ideal, Perfect Conception, Pregnancy, and Birth in combination with chiropractic care was the reason for our healthy pregnancies and successful home births.

Chiropractic care is an essential part of a healthy pregnancy, labor, and delivery. From the moment the egg and sperm meet, and cells begin to divide. The first organs to form are the brain, spinal cord, and nerves, which make up the nervous system. These form first because the nervous system is the master system that regulates and controls all functions in the body.

As the skull and spine develop, they become the armor protecting the nervous system. Your spinal cord begins at the base of your brain, and it runs through the center of your spine with the nerves exiting between the bones of your spine. The nervous system controls and coordinates the function of every cell, tissue, gland, and organ in the body.

(continued on page 250)

CHIROPRACTIC CARE IN PREGNANCY *(continued)*

Your health is dependent on uninterrupted communication between your brain and body. At no time in your life is this not important and essential. Stressors that cause the spinal bones to lose their normal alignment and motion cause interference with the communication between the brain and body and can lead to less-than-optimal health.

There are three types of stress our bodies are constantly managing and adapting to, physical, chemical, and emotional stress. Physical stressors include accidents, injuries, repetitive motions, poor posture when sitting, standing, and sleeping. Chemical stressors include air and water pollution, food additives, pesticides and chemicals, drugs, and alcohol. Emotional stressors include trauma, loss, major life changes, conflicts, worry and uncertainty. These stressors are things we cannot avoid in our daily lives. We can minimize and manage them to some degree, but it is essential that we improve how our bodies respond and adapt by maintaining a healthier spine and nervous system.

Chiropractic care is a great way to help improve the health of your spine and nervous system and your body's ability to adapt to these constant stressors. Chiropractors look for misaligned bones in the spine that interfere with the nerves and make adjustments that restore proper motion and alignment to the spine. This reduces stress on the nervous system, allowing for better uninterrupted communication between the brain and the body. This in turn helps the body to better adapt and manage the effects of the stressors.

Most women seek chiropractic care during pregnancy for back pain. Back pain is common during pregnancy due to the increased physical stress on the spine from the substantial changes that occur during pregnancy. As pregnancy progresses into the second and third trimester, the weight of the baby pulls the spine forward causing a shift in the center of gravity. This puts a greater load on the spine and can lead to muscle tension, joint pain, and discomfort.

Many women are surprised to find out they have pre-existing alignment problems in the spine that they were unaware of until there was the additional physical stress from carrying a baby. Exercise such as walking, swimming, weight training, and yoga are great types of exercise and an important part of a healthy pregnancy but are also physical stresses not well suited for a poorly aligned spine during pregnancy. Chiropractic adjustments can help alleviate pain and discomfort in the back, hips, and pelvis, helping women to stay active more comfortably during pregnancy. This is a much better approach to the management of pain during pregnancy than using over the counter medications and other prescriptions drugs which would be additional chemical stressors on mother and child.

It is also important to understand that physical stress on the spine only begins with pregnancy. Once the baby is born there is a lot of time spent breastfeeding, looking down, bending, lifting, carrying car seats, bags, and strollers. As your child grows, they become heavier, harder to lift and less cooperative. Women who begin chiropractic care during pregnancy often continue with care after delivery to help them with the most physically demanding time in their life. Most chiropractic practices are filled with moms and dads with young kids because of the physical demands this time in your life places on your spine.

A misaligned pelvis can cause complications during pregnancy, labor, and delivery. Pelvic misalignments alter the size of the pelvic opening which makes up the birth canal. Chiropractic adjustments can help to restore proper alignment of the pelvis, reducing the

CHIROPRACTIC CARE IN PREGNANCY (*continued*)

risk of complications, such as breech presentations, prolonged labor, and back pain during labor. Improved pelvic alignment can help optimize fetal positioning by reducing tension in the surrounding muscles and ligaments. Research has shown that chiropractic care during pregnancy can reduce the need for a cesarean delivery.[136] By improving pelvic alignment and optimizing fetal positioning, chiropractic care can help to facilitate a natural vaginal birth.

Chiropractic care can help to alleviate stress on the nervous system and promote overall well-being for both the mother and the developing baby. A healthy nervous system can improve immune function, digestion, and sleep, which are all essential for a healthy pregnancy. For your body to optimally utilize the health benefits of good nutrition, vitamins, exercise, sleep, and hydration you must have a healthy, well-functioning nervous system.

If you are pregnant and considering chiropractic care, consult with a qualified chiropractor who has experience working with pregnant women. Chiropractic care is safe for both mother and child during pregnancy. It should be an important part of every woman's prenatal and postpartum care. You can start care at any stage of pregnancy, but it is best to start early to prevent potential complications with pregnancy, labor, and delivery.

—David R. Wagner, DC

Naturopath

A naturopath is a healthcare professional who practices naturopathic medicine, which is a system of healthcare that emphasizes the use of natural remedies to promote health and healing. Naturopaths use a variety of therapies, including herbs, diet, exercise, and lifestyle counseling. The goal of naturopathic medicine is to help the body heal itself. Naturopaths believe the body has the ability to heal itself if it is given the right support. They use natural remedies to help the body's natural healing processes. Herbology is the study and use of herbs for medicinal purposes and is a branch of naturopathic medicine.

Naturopathic medicine is not a replacement for conventional medicine. Naturopaths often work alongside conventional doctors to provide a more comprehensive approach to healthcare.

Here are some of the benefits of seeing a naturopath:

- They can help you find natural ways to improve your health.
- They can help you make lifestyle changes that will improve your health.
- They can help you manage chronic conditions.
- They can provide you with care that complements conventional medicine.

If you are considering seeing a naturopath, it is important to do your research. Find a naturopath who is licensed and has experience in treating the condition in which you are interested. It's a good idea to visit with a naturopath in advance of labor to get remedies tailored to your personal conditions.

Abdominal Massage Therapist

In the Conscious Conception chapter of this book, I mentioned that abdominal massage can be incredibly beneficial. Abdominal massage is a gentle massage technique that is often used during pregnancy. It can help to relieve a variety of pregnancy-related discomforts, including back pain, constipation, leg cramps, round ligament pain, stress, and anxiety.

Abdominal massage can also help to improve circulation to the uterus and placenta, which can help to deliver nutrients to the baby. This practice can help to release tension in your muscles and tissues. Abdominal massage is generally safe for pregnant women, but it is important to talk to your provider before getting a massage. There are some conditions that may make abdominal massage contraindicated, such as placenta previa or preterm labor.

If you are considering getting an abdominal massage during pregnancy, it is important to find a qualified massage therapist who has experience working with pregnant women. The therapist should use gentle, circular movements and avoid applying too much pressure.

Counselor

A counselor or therapist is a mental health professional who provides guidance and support to people who are struggling with emotional, behavioral, or mental health problems. They can help people to understand their problems, develop coping skills, and make positive changes in their lives. Counselors and therapists use a variety of techniques, including talk therapy, cognitive-behavioral therapy, and group therapy to name a few. They may also provide medication management or referrals to other healthcare providers.

It is so important to be healthy in every aspect of your mental, emotional, spiritual, and physical lives, to take a holistic approach. A great counselor can help you step through trauma so your life isn't so burdened by hurts from the past and you can release thoughts, habits, and emotions that are no longer serving your greatest and highest purpose. They can also help you to be a better parent by helping you to release your own parental issues, and they can help immensely in your relationships and with communication skills.

If you don't heal what hurt you, you'll bleed on people who didn't cut you.

—Anonymous

Dentist

Being pregnant makes it more likely you'll develop cavities. You can pass the bacteria that cause cavities to your baby during pregnancy and after birth, which can cause problems for your baby later in life.[137] So, I encourage all of my clients to go to the dentist during pregnancy and have their

Aleah: There's an old wives' tale that you lose a tooth for every baby. I had heard this before ever becoming pregnant, but never in my wildest dreams did I think that would become a reality for me. I had a rude awakening when, two months after my first baby was born, I started feeling a soreness in one of my teeth.

I had perfect teeth (not even one cavity) until my mid-20s when I had my wisdom teeth removed. Their removal gave the rest of my teeth room to space out, and even with my normal brushing and flossing routine (which, I will admit, was not completely, 100 percent up to par) I ended up with six cavities. Three of those progressed to the point that I needed root canals for them within two years of having my wisdom teeth removed.

I hated that experience and was determined not to repeat it. I became an avid, twice-a-day brusher and flosser. I take really good care of my teeth, so feeling any kind of issue with them sent me into fear mode.

After feeling that sore spot, I immediately made an appointment with the dentist. I didn't have anyone to take care of my baby, so I took my eight-week-old into the office with me. Thank goodness she was tiny and slept through the appointment in her car seat while they examined me. Sure enough, they told me that one of the other teeth that had gotten a cavity after my wisdom teeth came out now needed a root canal.

I was lucky not to actually lose a tooth, but it was so shocking and, of course, cost a pretty penny. Root canals are incredibly expensive, even with insurance. The point of this story is even if you have perfect teeth to begin with and take all of the supplements in support of your pregnancy, this can still happen. Take extra care to stay on top of or up the ante on your hygiene routine. This is just another key example of why taking such good care of yourself during pregnancy helps to prevent issues postpartum.

teeth cleaned. When you do this in the second trimester, you're past the point where your gag reflex is stronger, and it's better than having dental work done in the first trimester. There is an old wives' tale about losing a tooth for every baby, and I know that this is rooted in a common experience. It's super important to have your teeth checked, your gums examined, and to get your teeth cleaned. If it's been a long while, you can safely have dental X-rays taken. Your dentist will shield you and it will be fine. Your midwife may have to sign off on this for the dentist to be willing to work on you while you're pregnant.

Doula

According to DONA International, a doula is "a trained professional who provides continuous physical, emotional and informational support to their client before, during and shortly after childbirth to help them achieve the healthiest, most satisfying experience possible." A doula serves to assist the laboring mother and often helps in the initial postpartum period. They can be an excellent source of support. Many midwives provide doula services, so if you are choosing to work with a midwife, a doula may be superfluous. Check with your midwife to

Penelope: I hired a doula for my first birth when I was a single mom. I can't recommend this highly enough. My doula helped me to solidify my birth plan. She helped me to understand more of what I was in for with a hospital birth. She was a constant present and presence at the end of my pregnancy, throughout my labor, and we are dear friends to this day more than a decade later.

My doula kept me company in early labor while I binge watched shows. She helped me to chart contractions, she helped me to get through contractions, she drove me to the hospital and stayed by my side through a grueling labor. A short time after what had been a traumatic experience for me, she gifted me with my birth story as told to my new baby. The story helped me to reframe my experience and to see it in a more positive light. I was someone who was facing labor as a single mother, and she became my trusted birth partner.

Robbie: I so wish that I had hired a doula to be with me and my husband during our first birth, which ended in an unnecessary cesarean that perhaps could have been prevented if a doula had been with us. I did have a doula for my second birth, which was a home VBAC. I was in early (latent) labor for the first two days, until active labor finally kicked in on Day Three. During those first days, my midwives would come to check on me, shake their heads, tell me that I was still only 4 cm dilated, and go home to care for their kids. Yet my doula, Rima Star, was my constant companion. Without her ongoing reassurance and support, I might have given up and gone to the hospital, and I'm so glad that she was there, because birthing a 10-pound baby in my own bed in my own home was the most empowering experience of my life!

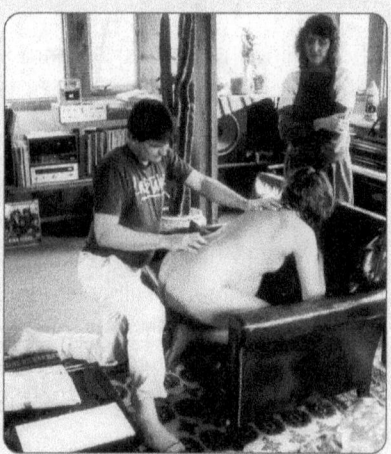

One of Robbie's Midwives Delivering the News

see if she provides these services. If you're working with an OB/GYN, a doula may be exactly the support you need for your ideal, perfect birth. Now is a great time to start investigating whether you'd like to hire a doula. Dona.org is a wonderful resource for learning more and locating a trained doula. DoulaMatch.net also allows you to search for doulas in your area. Sista Midwife Productions has a directory of Black doulas and midwives (www.sistamidwifedirectory.com/).

Doulas are exceptionally helpful, especially if you are electing to have or end up transitioning to a hospital birth. If you haven't already hired someone to serve in this role and want to, now is the time.

Homeopath

A homeopath practices exclusively in the realm of homeopathy. Homeopathy, or Homeopathic Medicine, is a medical system based on the belief that the body can cure itself. Those who practice it use tiny amounts of natural substances, like plants and minerals, to stimulate the healing process. Homeopathy is holistic because it treats the whole person, rather than focusing on a diseased part, symptom out of context, or a labeled sickness. Homeopathy is natural because its remedies are produced according to the US FDA-recognized Homeopathic Pharmacopoeia from natural sources. So much of homeopathy is based on emotional as well as physical components; it's important to establish this relationship before you need care.

Massage Therapist

A massage therapist is a healthcare professional who uses their hands to manipulate the soft tissues of the body to improve health and well-being. They use a variety of techniques, including kneading, rubbing, and tapping, to help relieve pain, improve circulation, and reduce stress. Massage therapy is a complementary and alternative medicine (CAM) therapy that has been used for centuries to treat a variety of health conditions.

Massage is an intensely relaxing experience and can release deep tension and pain in your body. I recommend that every woman get a massage every month. During pregnancy, be sure to find someone who specializes in prenatal massage.

Repatterning Practitioner

I have recently tried repatterning and it is so cool. These practitioners are intuitive, and this process can feel quite magical, albeit draining. Repatterning practitioners are professionals who specialize in helping people change their unwanted patterns of thinking, feeling, and behaving.

Repatterning practitioners can help people with a wide range of issues, including:

- Anxiety and depression
- Phobias and fears
- Eating disorders
- Weight loss
- Pain
- Relationships
- Careers
- Self-esteem and confidence issues
- Sports performance
- Personal growth and development

They use a variety of techniques, including hypnotherapy, NLP, and EMDR, to help people identify and release the root causes of their problems and create new, more positive patterns. Some practitioners work in person and some offer phone consultations so you can work with practitioners who live elsewhere in the world.

Educate Yourself

This is a great time to start learning about different styles of parenting and different ways to successfully raise your children. Read everything you can about their brain development, their emotional development, and their social development. See Appendix F for my favorite recommendations.

This is also an excellent time to take a First Aid/CPR class if you haven't already been certified.

Penelope: My sister turned me on to a repatterning practitioner. She couldn't really describe what the session was about. She used words like "guided meditations" and "wild energy floes" and "sparkling lights" when she talked about it. At first it sounded like hocus pocus, and honestly, she's a little more gullible than I am. But she was convinced repatterning could help me and bought me a session with her practitioner, who lives several states away and provides consultations by phone..

I scheduled the session and wow! What an interesting, fascinating experience it was, unlike anything else I'd ever experienced. Plus, it was immediately effective in helping me shed years of emotional issues I'd carried surrounding my relationship with my mother. I've since done a few more sessions and each one is a very different, very spiritual, very cool experience. My sister was right; they are difficult to describe, and maybe intimate enough that they shouldn't be.

I loved it so much I encouraged my best friend to try it when she was struggling. She called me after it was done and said, "I don't know what that was, but I am never going to counseling again. I'm just doing this."

Many of my friends love their counseling sessions and counselors have helped them so much. Personally, as someone who has long conversations in her head already, that was never the case for me. I always felt like counseling was expensive and carried no return. I don't need a counselor to feel heard. I need concrete help with specific issues. For me, repatterning is the magic bullet that counseling never was. Your mileage may vary. Try different approaches until you find what works for you.

Continue to read on in this book past where you are currently at in your pregnancy, so you can mentally begin to prepare for your birth experience. Reread the Third Trimester and The Birth Process chapters of this book as you enter your Third Trimester and refer to them whenever you like as you approach your birth experience. I also recommend that you read *The Book of Birth Volume II: Your Postpartum Journey through the Fourth Trimester* during your second trimester, so you can begin to prepare yourself mentally and physically for life with your newborn.

Don't forget the Sprout pregnancy app to keep up with the baby's development and the changes happening week by week.

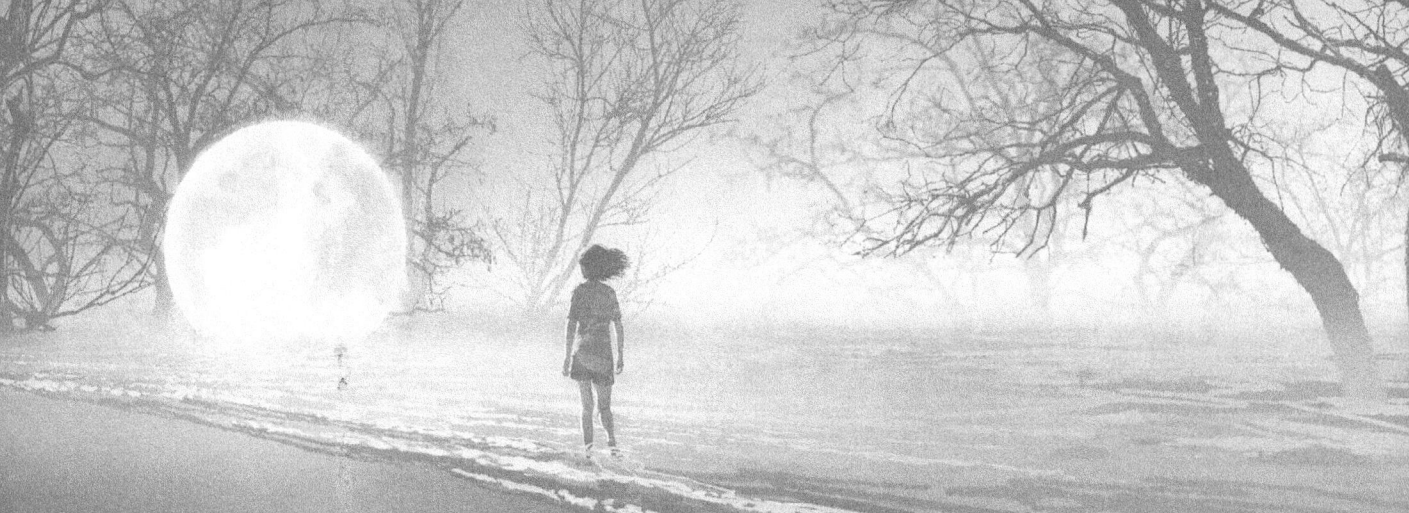

Rest

Most people don't sleep enough. They watch way too much TV and engage in too much phone or screen time. They might have children who go to bed at 8:00 p.m. and they want a few hours to themselves before they go to bed, so they get maybe six hours and feel absolutely fatigued all the time. You must be striving for at least eight hours a night. Take naps. *Rest*.

When you get closer to the birth in the third trimester, your body will begin to practice for labor, and it may wake you up in the middle of the night. Many women find their sleep becomes more and more interrupted in the weeks leading up to birth. Take advantage of the ease you feel in the second trimester and rest deeply as much as you can.

As your belly starts getting bigger and you're lying on your side, put a pillow to serve as a wedge under your abdomen to counteract gravity. On your side, your uterus will hang toward the bed and pull everything on your high side down. If you support the abdomen with even just a small pillow, you will sleep much more comfortably.

Find a balance between rest and pushing yourself. When you are resting, REST. Pregnancy is exhausting. What it takes to create a human being is beyond our ability to truly understand; what it takes to create the baby physiologically is beyond our ken. It takes so much out of women, way more than we give credence to, it's harder than society thinks. You have full permission to give over to your need to rest.

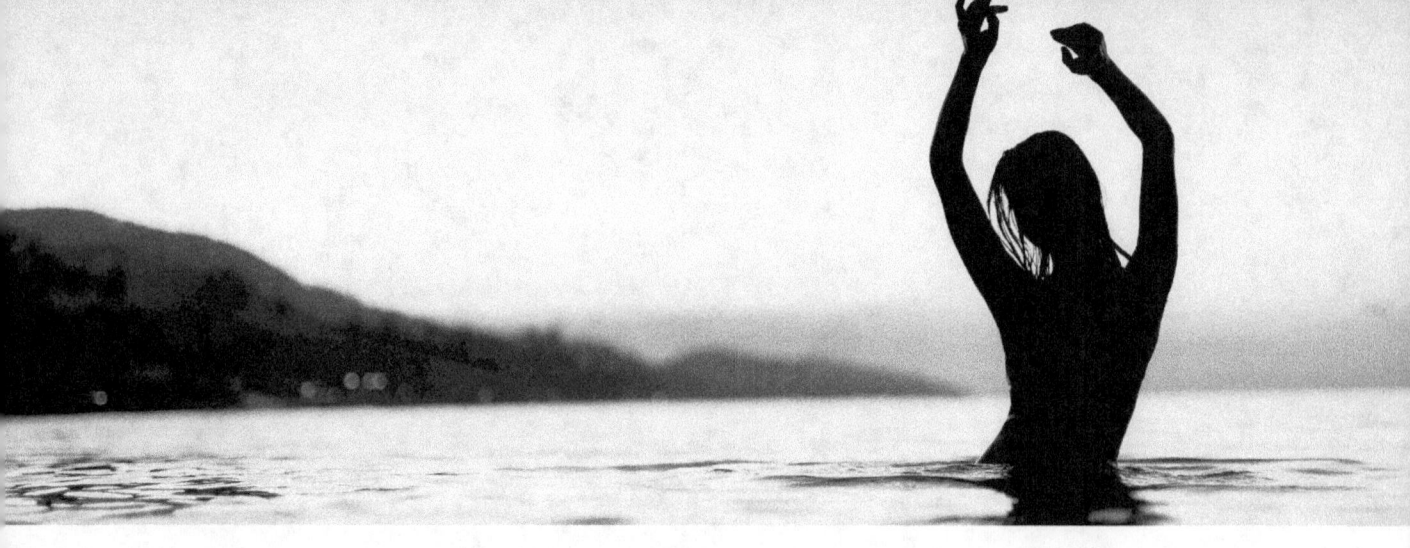

Joy

Cultivating joy during pregnancy sets the foundation for a positive transition into parenthood. When you fill your pregnant life with joyful experiences you are setting yourself up for a sense of fulfillment, connection, and well-being in parenting. Joy also acts as a source of resilience and strength during the postpartum period, helping you navigate the challenges of caring for a newborn.

Self-Care in the Second Trimester

During the second trimester of pregnancy, when many women experience increased energy and decreased discomfort compared to the first trimester, self-care activities can be wonderful ways to amplify your joy quotient. Here are some additional ideas for self-care during this phase of your pregnancy.

Prenatal Massage

If you didn't get one in your first trimester (or even if you did), treat yourself to a prenatal massage performed by a certified prenatal massage therapist. Prenatal massages are specifically tailored to the needs of pregnant women and can help alleviate muscle tension, reduce swelling, and promote relaxation.

Manicure and Pedicure

Book a manicure and pedicure session at a salon that offers pregnancy-safe services and products. Tell them you are pregnant when you call. Enjoy having your nails trimmed, shaped, and polished, and indulge in a soothing hand and foot massage.

Facial or Skincare Routine

Pamper your skin with a facial or develop a pregnancy-safe skincare routine. Opt for facials that use gentle, natural products and avoid treatments with harsh chemicals. Alternatively, establish a simple and nourishing skincare routine at home, including cleansing, moisturizing, and using gentle products suitable for pregnancy.

Hydrotherapy

Consider exploring hydrotherapy options, such as visiting a spa with a warm water pool or tub for gentle water-based relaxation.

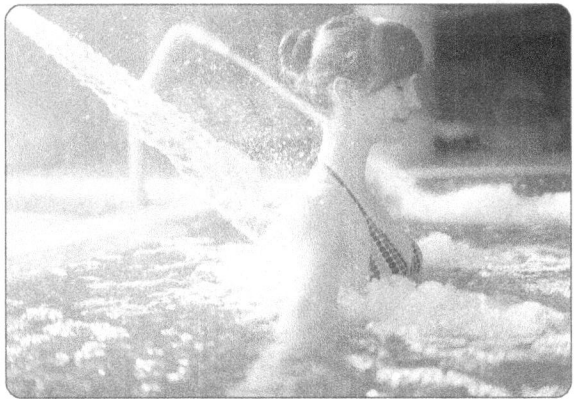

Hydrotherapy

Stretch Your Pampering Dollars

Spa treatments can be expensive. If your budget is stretched, there are still plenty of ways to incorporate self-care practices into your life without spending a lot of money. Here are some alternatives:

Create a Home Spa

Transform your own space into a relaxing sanctuary. Take a warm bath with essential oils or bath salts, play soothing music, dim the lights, and light candles to create a serene atmosphere. You can give yourself a facial using homemade masks or practice self-massage techniques.

Treat yourself to DIY manicures and pedicures. Take the time to trim and shape your nails, apply nail polish, and give your hands and feet a gentle massage.

Discount stores like TJ Maxx and Marshall's usually have great products for home spas at great prices. You can also find affordable products at drugstores and online.

Stretching and Prenatal Yoga

Engage in stretching exercises or practice prenatal yoga at home. There are numerous free prenatal yoga classes available online or through smartphone apps. Make sure the classes you select are specifically prenatal yoga. Yoga not only helps improve flexibility and strength but also promotes relaxation and mindfulness. Try different classes until you find a prenatal yoga instructor you love.

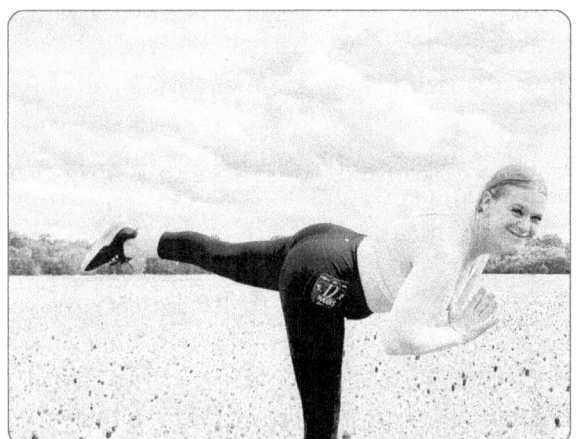

Getting Back into Yoga in the Second Trimester

Massage

 Partners, learn some basic massage techniques to release tension and promote relaxation in your pregnant woman. Look for tutorials or videos online to learn different techniques.

Women, you can also learn self-massage techniques. You can use your hands, foam rollers, or tennis balls to target areas of muscle tightness.

Meditation and Mindfulness

Continue to dedicate time to practice meditation or mindfulness techniques that help you relax and connect with your body and baby. Use guided meditation apps or online resources specifically designed for pregnancy to support your relaxation journey. If you need a refresher, refer to the Joy section of the Conscious Conception chapter (page 111).

Remember, self-care is not limited to expensive treatments or products. It is about intentionally taking care of yourself and prioritizing your well-being. With creativity and resourcefulness, you can find numerous ways to incorporate self-care practices into your life that are accessible and affordable.

Tailor your self-care routine to your individual needs and preferences and embrace this time as an opportunity to nurture yourself and your growing baby. Keep in mind, it's essential to prioritize your safety and comfort during self-care activities. If you have concerns, always feel free to consult with your midwife before trying new treatments or products.

Connect with Nature

Connecting with nature during pregnancy is a wonderful way to promote relaxation, reduce stress, and enjoy the beauty of the natural world. Here are some safe ideas to connect with nature while pregnant that can be particularly enjoyable in the second trimester during your halcyon days.

Remember to always prioritize your safety and comfort. Stay hydrated, dress appropriately for the weather, always wear

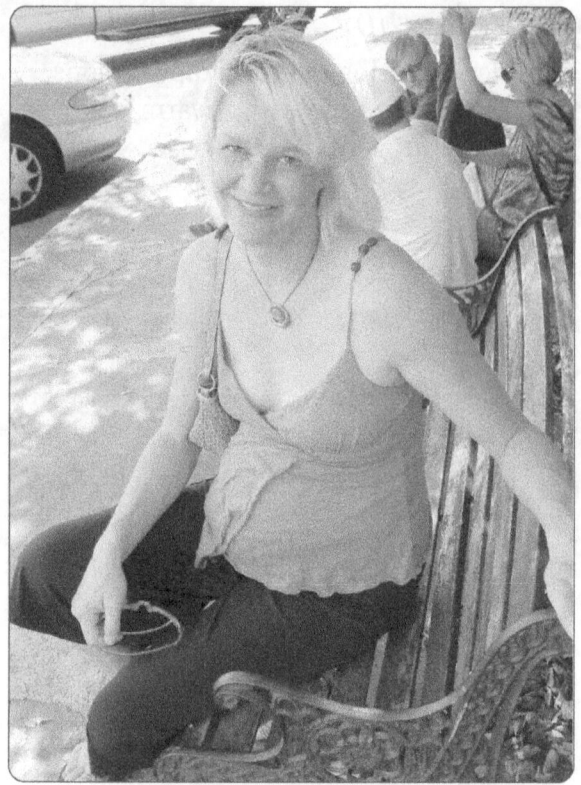

Penelope Enjoying a Day Trip to a Quaint Town in the Second Trimester

sunscreen when outside, and listen to your body's signals. It is also always a good idea to consult with your midwife about any specific concerns or limitations related to your pregnancy.

Nature Hikes

Make sure to select trails that are suitable for your fitness level and pregnancy stage. Look for well-maintained paths with gentle slopes and terrain that is not too challenging or strenuous.

Listen to your body and hike at a pace that feels comfortable for you. Take breaks whenever needed and allow yourself time to rest, stay nourished, and consistently hydrate. Eat a hearty breakfast and/or lunch before you go, and pack nutritious snacks and plenty of water to keep your energy levels up during the excursion. Pay attention to any signs of fatigue or discomfort and adjust your pace accordingly.

Choose loose, breathable clothing that allows for easy movement and layer appropriately for changing weather conditions. Wear supportive and comfortable footwear that provides good traction on uneven terrain. Remember to pay attention to your posture while hiking, engage your core muscles and maintain an upright posture to support your changing body. Take shorter steps and use trekking poles if needed for stability. Lightly engage your perineal and rectal muscles as you walk or hike. Have some intention in your crotch.

Make sure to protect yourself from the sun—apply sunscreen, wear a wide-brimmed hat, sunglasses, and lightweight, breathable clothing to shield yourself from excessive sun exposure.

It is also important to be mindful of your surroundings and potential hazards or wildlife. Avoid steep ledges, slippery surfaces, or areas with overgrown vegetation. Respect the environment by not disturbing plants or wildlife. Carry essential items: Pack a small backpack with essentials such as a fully charged cell phone, a map or trail guide, a basic first-aid kit, insect repellent, and any necessary medications you may require during your hike. Always hike with a buddy.

Watch out for poison oak/ivy. Be careful to look before you sit or put your hands down. If you don't know what they look like, it's easy to look up online.

Nature Photography

Embrace your creative side and take up nature photography. Grab your camera or smartphone and capture the beauty of the natural world around you. Even simple walks can become an opportunity to appreciate the small details of nature. You might want to save some of your favorites to put in your pregnancy journal.

Nature Inspired Arts and Crafts

Engage in artistic activities that draw inspiration from nature. Botanical crafts like pressed flower art, creating natural dyes, botanical jewelry making, or making prints of flowers, leaves or other plants onto paper or fabric can be really satisfying to your creative self. Sketching, painting, or drawing while outdoors is very stimulating. Make candles or wreaths—bonus points if you do it outside.

Camping or Glamping

Plan a camping trip to experience a few nights in nature. Set up a tent (or rent a glamping yurt!), cook and eat meals outdoors, and engage in activities like hiking, swimming, stargazing, or simply enjoying a campfire. This is so rejuvenating.

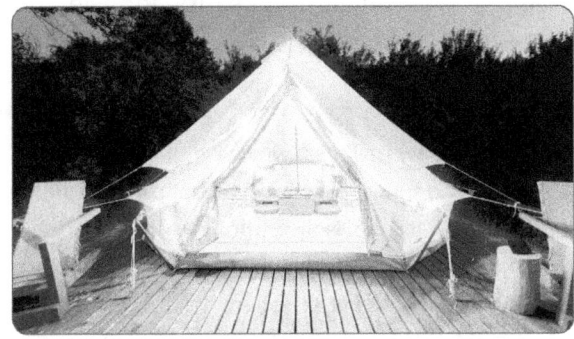

Glamping Setup

Outdoor Sports and Water Activities

If it's safe and appropriate for your pregnancy, consider activities like swimming or gentle water exercises in natural bodies of water such as lakes or gentle rivers. Ensure you follow any safety guidelines and consult with your midwife as needed. If your pregnancy allows and you have a safe place to engage, consider participating in outdoor activities like kayaking, canoeing, or paddleboarding. These activities allow you to not only connect with nature but also engage in physical exercise. Don't forget to use SwimEar a few times a week when you're swimming.

Nature-Inspired Journaling

It can be fun to seek out creative activities that draw inspiration from nature while also supporting your self-care rituals. For nature journaling, it's as simple as sitting outside and journaling about your thoughts and experiences in nature.

Sunrise or Sunset Appreciation

Wake up early to witness a beautiful sunrise or find a serene location to enjoy a breathtaking sunset. Take a moment to appreciate the natural beauty and the changing colors of the sky.

> Spend a few minutes watching the sky, the clouds, or a sunrise or sunset. Watch how the light changes in the sky. Notice what you smell in the air and how the air feels against your skin. What do you hear? Reflect on how you felt when you started and how you feel after doing this exercise.

Build Your Support Network

This is a great time to reach out to find other like-minded pregnant women in your area and to find additional layers of support within your network. This can be so invaluable. You can forge new relationships through local meetups or other online groups. If you don't see a meetup that appeals to you, make one!

When it comes to being a conscious consumer, there's no better resource out there than moms who are a few steps ahead of you and who can help inform you about the products and services that really helped them, and which were a waste of resources. It's so fantastic to have a tribe of women going through what you are going through. They can empathize like no one else and may have wonderful advice for you when you're struggling. Likewise, your ability to offer emotional support to them is rewarding for you.

Birth Plan

A birth plan is your written visualization of your ideal, perfect birth. Think about what you want for your birth and write it down. It's as easy as that. This might include specific music to be played, a poem or prayer to be read, a song to be sung, the person you want to cut the cord, weigh the baby, wash the baby's hair, and/or dress the baby. You might want specific essential oils in a diffuser or a special scented candle to be lit (only for a home birth).

It should also include a description of your ideal, perfect birth. If you're working with a midwife, you'll likely develop a vision together as she gets to know you. It helps you and your birth team to understand your desires and what they should be working toward. Your birth plan might include that you want a natural labor without intervention unless it's medically necessary for the health of the mother and/or baby and so you don't want medication to be offered. Or it might say that medication should be supplied only if and when you, the mother, request it. It might state a preference for pain relief medication. The only important thing is that it accurately and specifically states your wishes and desires.

You'll want to understand the services your provider will attend to. At the births I attend, my team and I are happy to do whatever you want. We often act as doulas, maids, and coaches. If you want us to stand on one foot and whistle, we will! Your practitioner may be different, and you may want to enlist the aid of a doula to help you through your labor. If you do, specify her role in the birth plan as well.

You may not yet know what you want. That is okay too. You might explore what others have done and see what resonates with you. If you're looking for inspiration, you can find some great ideas just by using a search engine to see what others have done.

What to Put in Your Birth Plan

State your desires. You might start with something like, "I want to be calm and peaceful and be able to be with my partner at home."

You might start by freewriting what you want your birth experience to be like and then craft a plan once you see that dream outlined. You might include things like:

- I want to be able to be in the water.

- I want specific music playing in the background.

- I'd like a specific candle to be burned or a specific essential oil to be used in a diffuser. (Electric candles are okay in a hospital.)

- I do not want to be offered unnecessary medication or intervention.

- I do want an epidural, but only after I've reached 6 cm of cervical dilation, so the epidural won't slow down my labor.

- I want an epidural as soon as possible after I get to the hospital. It will only slow my labor by about 30 minutes.

- I want it to be very quiet when the baby is born so they can hear my voice.

- I'd like to say a specific prayer over the baby when they arrive.

- I'd like to say specific prayers together at every stage of birth: when the midwife arrives, when I start pushing, and when our baby arrives.

- I'd like a specific poem to be read when our baby arrives.

- I'd like a specific scripture to be read when our baby arrives.

- I'd like our baby to go straight to my belly after birth before the cord is cut.

- I want to delay cord clamping until it quits pulsing, and the placenta has been born.

- I want a specific person to cut the cord.

- I don't want our baby to be given formula/I only want my baby to have breastmilk (Note that if you are at a hospital and your baby needs supplementation, they often have access to breast milk and can supplement with that if requested instead of formula.)

In each of these instances where the word "specific" is used, go ahead and specify what you want—which playlist, which scent of candle, which scriptures, which prayers, which person, etc.

I heard once that art is decoration for your walls, and music is decoration for time. Isn't that lovely? When you are building your playlist for the birth, consider making two of them. Make one playlist with music you love or songs that are meaningful to you for earlier in your labor. Play it during your pregnancy, too. When you hear these songs years later, they will bring you back to these moments of the miraculous joy of new life and your part in all of creation.

Make a second playlist with music better suited to the depths of labor. I recommend slow tracks with deep, arhythmic bell tones, like mediation music or music for *savasana* in yoga classes. More rhythmic music can be off from the rhythm of your labor as contractions intensify, and so these soothing tones are often better for the later stages of labor.

Put your arhythmic playlist on when you practice your breathing with your partner in the third trimester. That way, when you play them in labor, it will serve as an additional Pavlovian signal to your subconscious that you are in a safe place and your body knows what to do. It will help you get to *the zone*, and it will help you to relax and initiate breathing through the tougher contractions.

Placenta prints are another great idea to plan for. For my clients who request it, I use a piece of nice art paper to make a print of their placentas; these turn out beautifully and often resemble the Tree of Life.

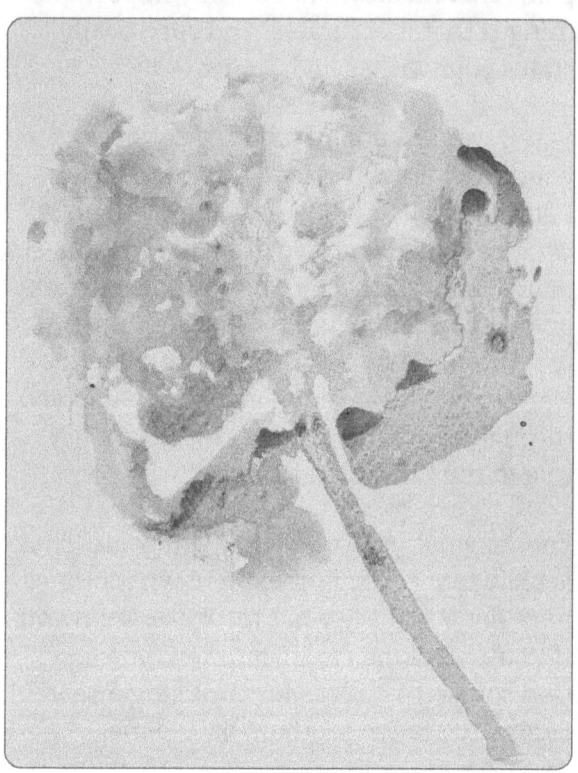

Placenta Print

Another option is placental encapsulation. This service dehydrates and powders your placenta, then places it in a capsule for mom to ingest after the birth to help with the uterus going back to shape, the milk coming in, and the hormonal balance/postpartum mood stabilization. You'll find more information about these in *The Book of Birth Volume II: Your Postpartum Journey through the Fourth Trimester.*

Some of these things are obvious and what you have agreed upon with your midwife, but it's still good to put them in your birth plan. If you start out at home and need to be transported to the hospital, it is useful to give a copy to the nurses so they can understand what you're going for. They may react to it with varying degrees of respect, but as more hospitals get more and more help from the midwifery community, this practice of having a birth plan will become more expected and supported, or so I hope and believe.

If you are planning a hospital birth, it's also an excellent idea to have everything you desire stated in your plan so that the nurses can familiarize themselves with it during your labor.

Surrender

It is a great idea to create a birth plan. I love birth plans and get all kinds of elaborate multi-faceted birth plans from my clients. I think it is great to set goals. If you set goals, you are more likely to strategize and prioritize, be disciplined to implement behaviors that support your efforts, and ultimately to achieve your desired outcome. Birth plans are fantastic expressions of goals.

It is equally important to understand that not all goals can be achieved. In my life all kinds of things didn't work out the way I thought or hoped they would. Two of my planned home births ended up in the hospital. I was right where I was supposed to be, but it was not what I had envisioned, wanted, or was happy about.

I talk frequently about surrendering, and this is why. I had to surrender in those moments. You set goals, make plans, and shoot for your highest and most ideal birth experience, but then you must relax and trust that how your birth unfolds is exactly how it is supposed to. It is perfect. You do the work throughout your pregnancy, and in labor you let go, relax, and trust.

When the time comes, allow yourself to go with the flow and to be flexible. If your wise advisors tell you things need to change, trust that they have your and your baby's best interest in mind, and if they are deviating from your plan, it is to try to preserve the health of you and your baby. So, plan for what you want but then relax into the situation because ultimately whatever happens is what you and the divine have put together for your greater good, though it may be hard to see that in the moment.

There is a certain power to our imagination. It is a form of projecting our expectations into the universe. I think it can shift energy toward what you want to happen. Expect to be surrounded by abundance, love, peace, and all of that, and you will find a lot of abundance and love and peace in your life. If you expect people to be horrible and birth to be frightening, you'll likely find the world is exactly as you expect.

Build Up Your Emotional and Spiritual Health

During these halcyon days, while you are feeling strong and good, I want you to build up your emotional and spiritual health. Affirmations, visualization, prayer, and meditation—all of these are ways to do this.

I think it's just as important as any other part of what you are doing for yourself and your baby's health. Once you've crafted your birth plan, spend time visualizing your labor and birth proceeding exactly as you desire.

Avoid Negativity

Avoid negativity. You have got to protect yourself. Now that you are visibly pregnant, you will be shocked by the number of people who want to tell you horror stories—strangers, friends, and family included. I'm going to remind you now, as soon as someone starts telling you a birth story you need to say, "Is this a happy story?" If it's not, tell them you don't want to hear it.

People might think you're joking. Make it clear you aren't. Be firm about this. If they launch into it anyway, say, "I'm not kidding." You do not need that negative energy or those negative visualizations in your life. Their story has absolutely nothing to do with you. This is particularly hard when it's a family member. Stand strong! You have to learn to stand up to your family at some point. You are becoming a momma bear, a protectress, and to become that, you must first protect yourself.

 Partners, when you're in a social situation, step in and be the guardian against these stories on behalf of your pregnant woman. It takes energy to ward off negativity, and you can serve as your pregnant woman's shield, letting her devote more of her precious energy to your baby.

Work to protect yourself against the negativity in the world at large. Avoid watching the news. There's not much

you can do about the conflicts overseas; there's not much you can do about the latest disaster in Europe or here in the US. There's not much you can do about climate change ... except to vote and get everybody you know to vote. So, be a good citizen, but avoid bumming yourself out with the news of the world.

If you previously had a habit of watching the news a lot, it's easier to replace that habit with a new one than it is to simply stop it. When you regularly tune in to the news, instead search out a light comedy or find a great YouTube channel about a calming hobby you enjoy. Better yet, spend that time working on your hobby, or reading a great book. Refer to the reading list in Appendix F. There are so many options for healthier, more positive distraction.

Sun Your Belly

Put your belly in the sun! Take your clothes off or pull your shirt up off your belly and get out there with bright, full sun on your back and on your belly. Your baby will see so many colors: they'll see orange, red, coral,

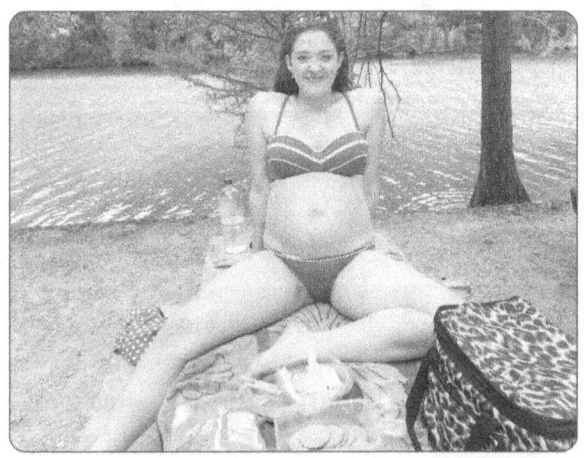

Aleah Sunning Her Belly, Enjoying Nature, and Staying Hydrated and Fully Nourished

salmon, pinks, and all kinds of beautiful warm colors and interesting shapes. Our ancestors were out in the sun with bare skin and now we simply aren't very often. Babies are stuck in the dark underneath all our clothing. Get out in the sun and stimulate your baby's senses!

Babymoon Vacation

This is the ideal time to go somewhere and do something fun. Get away for a little bit. Renew and refresh your relationship. Stop work and have a big fun time. People think they're going to resume life as usual and vacations as usual with a new baby, but most are shocked at how much work a new baby is and how little they feel like they can do in terms of a vacation with a new baby in the first three to four months. In the middle of the pregnancy, however, most women feel great and have a lot of energy. This is a wonderful time to take a little break with your beloved and your family before the baby comes, and your life becomes overtaken by them for a little while.

Take it All In

This time is for many the most relaxing and enjoyable part of pregnancy, and it will be over before you know it. Be present and mindful and immerse yourself in the moment. Take it all in. These are your halcyon days to enjoy.

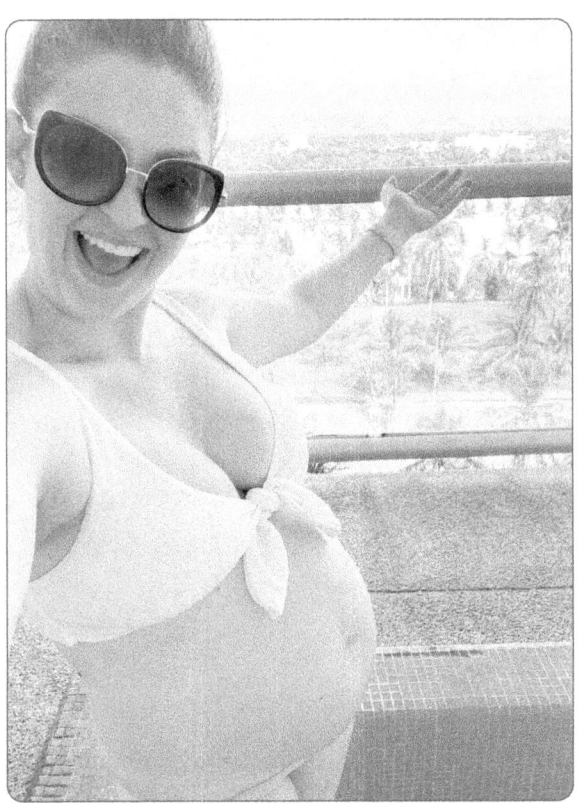

Aleah's Babymoon Vacation in Mexico

"When you moved, I felt squeezed with a wild infatuation and protectiveness. We are one. Nothing, not even death, can change that."

—Suzanne Finnamore,
"The Zygote Chronicles"

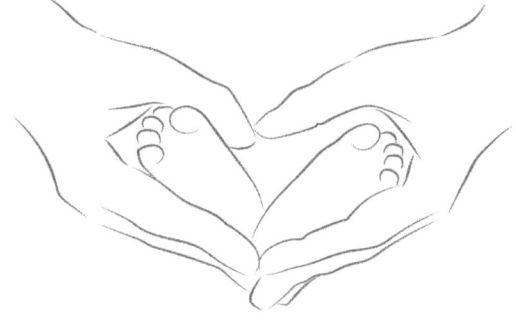

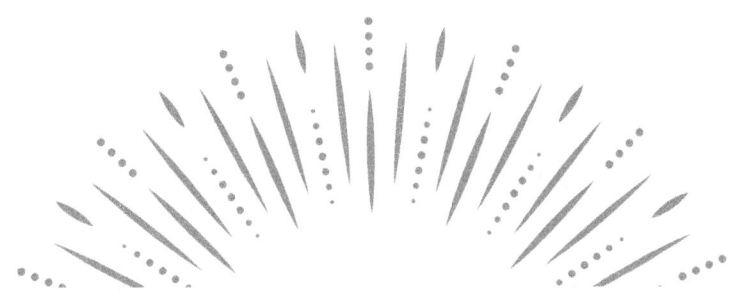

THIRD TRIMESTER

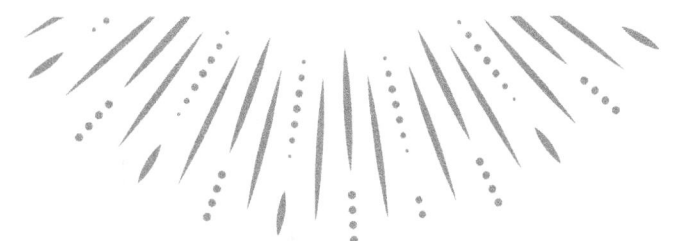

Introduction

These final weeks may seem interminable, but *you are so close now.* More and more of your everyday thoughts are likely going to how your baby is almost here, how you can't wait to meet them, and wondering what your birth experience will be like. These final few months have their own challenges and joys, and at the end of it all, you get to meet your beautiful baby!

When you eat fantastically, take all the vitamins I recommend, drink your gallon of water every day, exercise to increase your strength and stamina, focus on joyful interactions, get plenty of sleep, and generally take such great care of yourself, the placenta is more likely to stay gorgeous and your baby can safely stay in the womb longer, continuing to develop and to put on more fat. Each additional week in the womb produces quite dramatic developmental changes in your baby.

When you are not taking all those vitamins, drinking the proper fluids, exercising, and generally taking care of yourself, your placenta may not be as healthy.[138]

This is one reason why some women may give birth earlier. Their placenta just gives out because it does not have enough left to sustain the baby, and the body decides the baby will do better on the outside by getting breast milk. It can also be genetic to give birth at 37–38 weeks—some women's babies simply gestate faster than others.

Now is the time to stay focused and really continue to implement all of the Sevenfold Approach to your pregnancy, so you have a much better chance of having a wonderful birth experience and a super healthy baby.

There will come a day when you are 70 percent likely to have your baby the next day, then 80 percent, then 90 percent, and then a day when it is 100 percent certain that you will have your baby the next day. The only problem is, you do not get to know when that countdown begins, so it is so important at the end that you act as if every day could be the last day before your baby comes.

Go to bed on time, drink your water, and keep your health and nutrition at the forefront. If you skip a day and eat the wrong foods, stay up late, neglect to move your body, and then go into labor, you may regret the choices you made. Stay constant. Your baby may be healthier, and your labor may be easier for it.

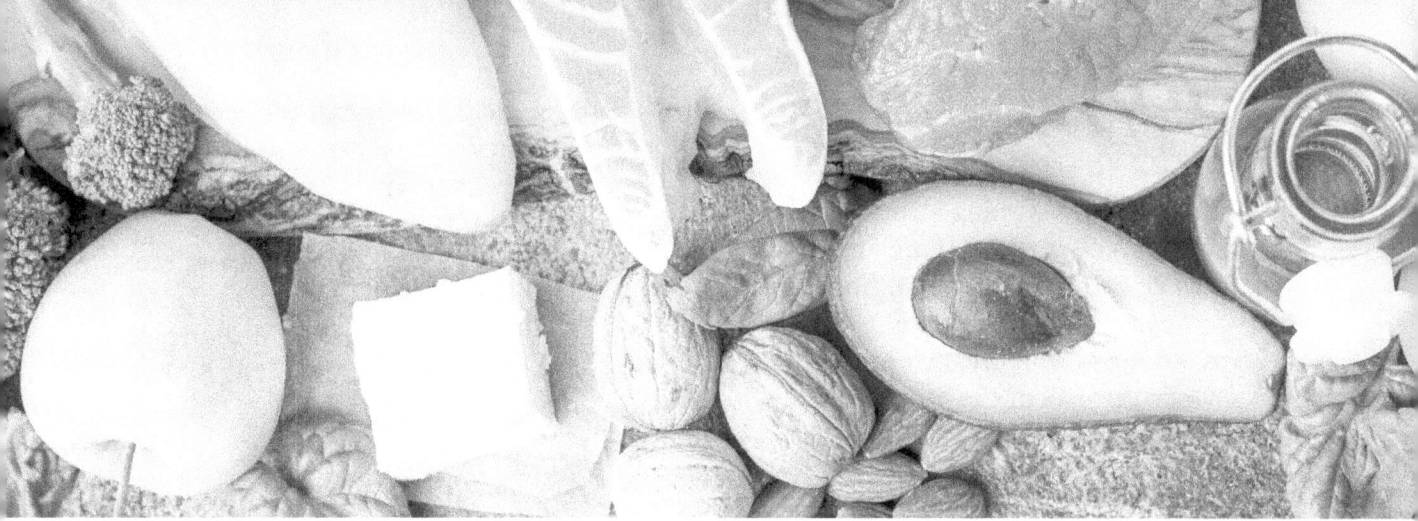

Nourishment

You need to keep eating fantastically, and very regularly. There is no milk present in the first few days of your baby's life, just small, increasing amounts of colostrum. Your baby is designed to live off their fat stores for the first few days. They lose a significant amount of weight in the first three days while they are working hard to bring the milk in. The more fat they have on them when they come out, the better they will withstand the first few days, and they will be much less likely to develop jaundice or be seriously fussy and unhappy, because they'll be hardier. You must keep eating, so your baby can build up these stores of fat and thrive when they are out of the womb.

When your baby puts on 6–10 ounces of fat, it does not make it any harder to give birth. All the difficulty of giving birth is getting the head and shoulders out; fat is just not a big deal. This doesn't mean you want to gain ten pounds in the last month, because that kind of late weight gain can make you much more likely to have a 10-pound baby rather than a 7–8-pound baby.

You have to keep eating healthy food frequently. It should feel like you are eating all the time. Graze. Eat tons of vegetables, chicken, fish, salad, and plenty of fruit, Include good quality grains in your diet (barley, millet, quinoa, and brown rice)—but not too much. One cup of cooked beans and one cup of cooked rice is about 400 calories. You must be careful what you eat, so you won't gain so much that you have a huge baby. In order to do that, you have to eat all the time, but don't go heavy on simple carbs, fats, or high-calorie items.

Cheese is an American downfall, and cheese, bread, and pasta are an incredible combination for too much weight gain. It's often what we want to eat, but we must choose to eat less of it.

Supplements

Continue the regimen of supplements you've been taking. See my recommendations on pages 50–51.

Borage Oil, Evening Primrose Oil, or Black Currant Oil

The Vitamin E and evening primrose oil are fantastic sources of GLA (gamma linoleic acid), which helps your body to produce all of the important pregnancy hormones—relaxin, estrogen, and progesterone—that make you softer. All of the body parts related to getting the baby out, the uterus, the vagina, the perineum, the lower uterine segment, and so forth, will be softer and you will be less likely to tear. Your cervix will also soften, so it can more easily dilate and efface in preparation for birth. These supplements come in gel caps. They are a bit expensive, but well worth it.

When not enough softening or *ripening* has taken place, I suggest you take evening primrose oil or black currant oil. I suggest you take 2 capsules three times a day, beginning four to eight weeks before your due date. I ask that every woman who has had a previous long and difficult labor, or who had a c-section and is attempting a VBAC, take these. Check with your midwife before implementing this suggestion yourself.

After you give birth, these supplements are also very helpful for PMS when your cycle resumes. You can take 1–3 capsules every day (depending on the severity of your symptoms), starting when you ovulate and continuing until your period starts.

Herbal Blend for Birth Preparation

There are many beneficial herbs that have been used for eons in other countries and in the Americas to support the birth process.

Using these herbs in the last few weeks of your pregnancy to increase your hormone levels helps your cervix to become more effaced, dilated, and softer by the time you go into labor. You'll want to search for "birth prep herbs" online or work with your midwife to understand her preferred blend. My clients use Dr. Christopher's birth prep blend.

The herbal blends typically include spikenard, squawvine, red raspberry leaf, nettles, as well as blue and black cohosh, and they are wonderful to help you have an easier pregnancy, birth, and postpartum period. Squawvine and spikenard are labor builders, blue and black cohosh are uterine tonics, and nettles are blood builders.

While I have not seen these herbs stimulate an early labor, some women do go into labor early. **If your cervix is dilating early or if you are having lots of contractions, do not take these herbs.** You also do not want to take them after 3 p.m. because you may be kept up with contractions.

- **Week 34:** Take 1 capsule a day in the morning.

- **Week 35:** Take 1 capsule in the morning and 1 capsule in the early afternoon.

- **Week 36:** Take 1 capsule in the morning, 1 capsule at lunch, and 1 capsule around 3:00.

- **Week 37:** Take 2 capsules in the morning and 2 capsules around 1:00.

- **Week 38:** Take 2 capsules in the morning, 2 capsules at noon, and 1 capsule at 3:00.

- **Week 39 and until you go into labor:** Take 2 capsules in the morning, 2 capsules at noon, and 2 capsules at 3:00.

Very rarely, a woman may be quite sensitive to these herbs. If they make you feel nauseated, I don't want you to continue to take them. Try them with food and on a few different occasions before you make your decision. I also suggest not taking them if you have high blood pressure or other high-risk situations (and consult your midwife or physician as well).

As long as you are building up carefully like this, you should be fine. Anytime you take these herbs, you want to remember to take them earlier. Skip them altogether if you forget, because they could make you have contractions at night and not allow you to sleep well. Sleeping is so key at the end of your pregnancy and can already be difficult to achieve given that you are so big and likely unable to get comfortable, so you do not want to mess with your sleep any more than it already is.

Preparation for Postpartum Nutrition

Once you give birth, you must eat faithfully, on a schedule. At 7:00 a.m. you eat a small snack, then have a nice big breakfast at 8:30, a lovely snack at 11:00, a great lunch at 12:30, a nice snack at 3:30, dinner at 6:00 and then eat a good tiny meal before bed at 9:00 or 9:30. That's a lot of food to be thinking about for two full weeks while you stay in bed, so I suggest you prepare by making menus together and preparing and freezing meals in your third trimester, at about 37 weeks. I'll remind you later.

Avoid gas-producing foods in your menu as they can stimulate colic, which makes your baby so uncomfortable, and gassy or colicky babies let the world know it for hours and hours. Gas-producing foods include:

- Brassicas: Brussels sprouts, broccoli, cauliflower, cabbage, and kale.

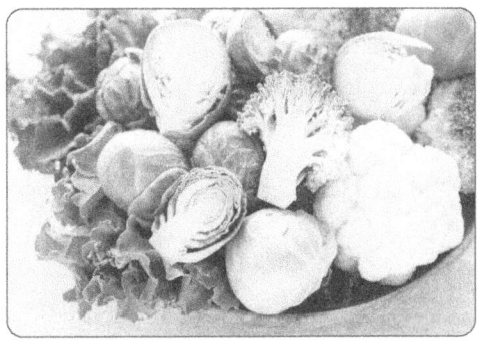

Brassicas

- Legumes: all kinds of beans, peanuts, split peas, lentils, hummus, etc.

- Soy and tempeh: all forms of tofu, including soy milk.

- Large amounts of starchy carbs like rice and pasta

In addition, some moms and/or babies have a hard time with very heavy foods with a lot of oil or fats, meals high in dairy like lasagna or mac 'n' cheese. If you think your baby may be gassy or developing colic, examining what you are eating can be helpful so you can eliminate those food culprits. (Although, food is not always the issue when it comes to colic. I'll talk more about colic in *The Book of Birth Volume II: Your Postpartum Journey through the Fourth Trimester.*)

 Your partner will likely be the one cooking, and it is so helpful to have two weeks of breakfasts, lunches, dinners, and snacks already written down and planned for. Do your shopping, make food a few weeks in advance of your due range and freeze it, make snack packs with cheese cubes, fruits, veggies, and nuts, and store them in the fridge—all in preparation for a time when everyone will be too tired to cook. I suggest you start this food preparation at around 37 weeks; I'll share more with you later in this chapter when I cover what to do then. That is also a good time to start signups for a meal train; there is more information about this in the *Joy>Baby Shower Ideas* section of this chapter (page 370).

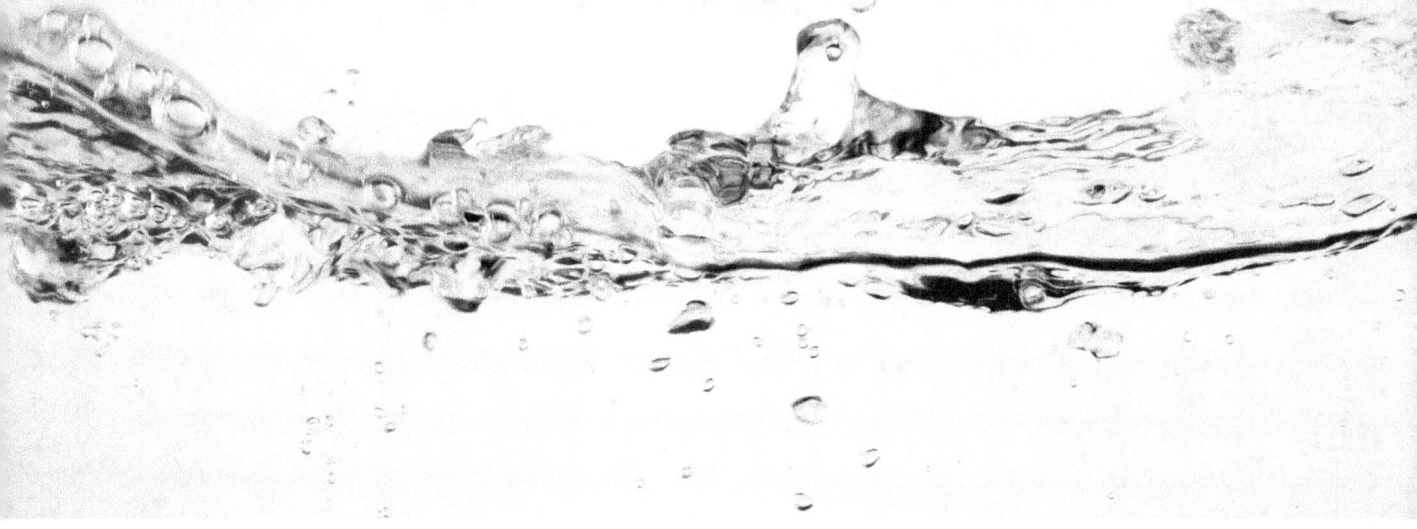

Hydration

Stay hydrated. Continue to drink four quarts of water a day, faithfully.

Continue to drink red raspberry leaf and pregnancy teas.

Buy coconut water now in preparation for the birth. Coconut water is very high in potassium and electrolytes. It is very easily digested and good for nausea or when you just can't eat.

Some people like coconut water and some don't. Try different varieties to find the brand you like; they do taste different. Costco carries an organic, no-sugar variety at a great price. It may be that one brand disgusts you, but you find you like another one. It's such a great option for birth that I encourage you to experiment until you find one you like. It is perfect for while you are in labor, so stock up ahead of time. I suggest you buy a case—which is typically 10–15 bottles. Organic is ideal, but if you cannot find it, make sure you are buying coconut water with no sugar added. Check the labels every time to ensure the only ingredient is coconut water. Even some of my favorite brands have changed ingredients and added sugars, so be diligent and read the labels on all your foods.

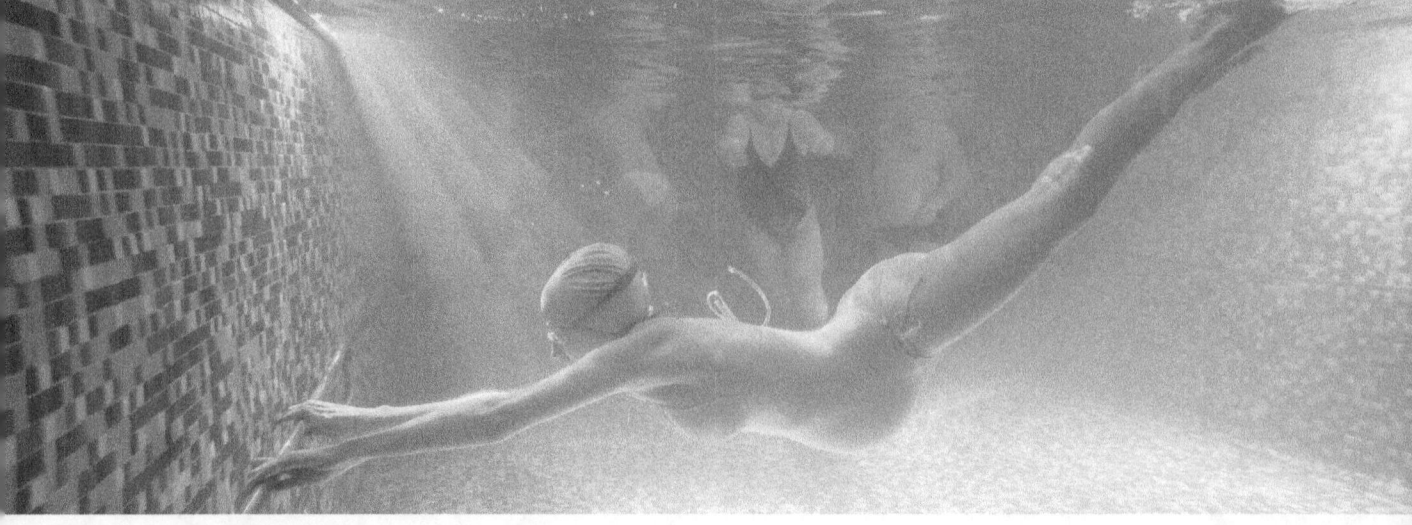

Movement

I hope you will keep exercising, and we'll talk more about that in a bit, but I want you to know up front that this section also includes really important breathing techniques and exercises for you to use in labor. I want you to take these very seriously. They need to become a part of your routine as you prepare for birth. They may not feel natural at first, which is why practice is so important. You want them to become second nature, so you can fall back on them in labor. They can really, really help you.

Make sure to listen to your body. If it is telling you to rest a lot and you feel like you need to sleep twelve hours and take a two-hour nap during the day, then do that, but until you reach the final weeks of your pregnancy, during the day, while you are awake, make sure to also exercise. This is the key to keeping your stamina up, so you feel good and have lots of vitality at the end of your pregnancy and for the birth and postpartum period.

Exercise

Before I tell you anything else, I need to say this: **Do not exercise** if you are experiencing any of the following:

- lots of warm-up labor,
- contracting and cramping,
- swelling in your feet and/or legs,
- or pubic bone pain.

Please be in regular contact with your midwife if you are experiencing these symptoms.

If these symptoms do not describe you, then now is the time to get yourself in the best condition you possibly can, because you could be facing a heroic task in the days to come. It is so important that you are in good shape for the birth. Birth is a physically demanding event, and good muscle tone, flexibility, and excellent stamina are crucial to be able to get through the birth and still have energy left over for bonding. The endorphins and oxytocin that are released through exercise are much needed to create adequate contractions and help to get you through the birth process.

Birth is an athletic event. Pregnant women expend approximately twice as many calories as a non-pregnant adult—even when they aren't doing anything.[139] Pregnancy, labor, and the birth process will likely be among the most strenuous experiences of your life.

In popular media, natural labor is often rendered as a brutal and unrelenting onslaught. It is painful, at times, but it is so different from how it is often portrayed. In natural labor your body gifts you with an absolute storm of beneficial hormonal activity that will help to carry you and power you through the experience, and it will grant you the space to find your breath, rest, and prepare for the next contraction.

Exercise, exercise, exercise, but don't overdo it. This isn't the time to be heading out on three- or four-mile hikes but do absolutely get in several shorter walks of 20–40 minutes every week. Don't waste yourself. Don't get so fixated on getting ready for when the baby comes out that you use up all of your reserve energy before the

---

> Don't get so fixated on getting ready for when the baby comes out that you use up all of your reserve energy before the big event even begins.

---

big event even begins. Too often I have had to transport women to the hospital because they have gone into labor absolutely depleted of their energy. They cleaned too much, took on too much, worked too much, and tried too hard. The key at this stage is to exercise, but in moderation.

I'll say it again: The best way to be prepared for birth is to exercise and be strong. It is the key to an easy birth. About 8 percent of my clients end up being transported to the hospital, and I would estimate about 60 percent of those women did not get in adequate shape for the birth during their pregnancies. So, keep up your workouts, because more muscle tone and stamina will help in labor, and exercise stimulates your body to produce more hormones like oxytocin as well as endorphins that will help you to have an easier birth. They also can help you to sleep.

You want to encourage your body to produce a lot of endorphins as they will help you to feel less pain in labor. Endorphins are produced in high amounts during exercise, sex, trauma, and in very high amounts during birth. So, prepare yourself by exercising regularly and having *as much sex as you can.* I suggest you continue doing cardio, swimming, walking, low impact aerobics, rowing, elliptical training, Pilates, or ride a stationary bicycle.

Swimming

Swimming is one of the things I suggest the most at the end of your pregnancy. It is excellent for keeping the baby in a head-down position. When you swim, it puts you in that belly-down position, which helps the baby rotate into an occiput anterior position—exactly what you want. So, any position that gets you down on your hands and knees—working in the garden, certain yoga positions, etc.—will help the baby find their way to the right position for birth.

Swimming also keeps you cool at a time when most women find themselves continually overwarm, and it will help you to build upper body strength and muscle. Water provides a lovely, weightless environment at a time when you are generally feeling so heavy. Swimming also sucks the water retention weight off your hands, feet, and body when you swim.

Swimming can become a spiritual practice as well, a meditative time where you can think about your baby and give them energy. Practice your visualizations or repeat your affirmations in your head as you swim. I love to pray and commune with the divine while I swim. Consider using this time to deepen your own spiritual practice, whatever that may be.

I recommend you do the breaststroke to help build upper body strength in front, i.e., your pectorals, which you will need in the months to come as you carry your baby in the heavy car seat, and all the accoutrements that you will need. The breaststroke also moves your body in such a way that the baby is encouraged to move into an anterior position. But any stroke where the front of your body is facing down will be beneficial.

Walking

Walking is important because it builds your lower body muscles (glutes, legs,

thighs, and calves), as well as your stomach and lower back muscles, all of which are important during birth. Both swimming and walking build stamina. As you near the end of your third trimester you will want to limit how far you walk, so you are never too far from home.

Squatting

First-time moms often are often encouraged to squat to push and to stand in between contractions, which is quite a workout. I suggest you start squatting ahead of time and practice getting comfortable being in a squatting position and standing repeatedly, so you are prepared in advance.

 During labor, your partner should help you up and down in between contractions, so partners, you should be doing these squats with your pregnant momma-to-be *now*. Help her up and down for a few minutes and you'll begin to understand what you are in for. Know that in labor this could go on for hours.

Getting the baby into the correct anterior position is really, really important. It just makes everything easier. Getting the baby's head into the pelvis in a good way is also important. Squatting brings the baby's head down into the pelvis and flexes their head, so their chin is on their chest. This is ideal. When the chin is on the chest, a much smaller diameter is presented to the birth canal and it's much easier to deliver. The head acts as a wedge against the cervix to help open it, and the squatting can help to get the head flexed, tucked, and engaging properly in the pelvis and against the cervix. Gravity helps, too. Squatting is an exceptionally beneficial position for the baby in labor, but it's not one that we employ often in our day-to-day life the way our ancestors did, so practice!

How to Squat

If you are alone, put your back up against the wall, feet on the floor. If you can't get your heels all the way down yet, use yoga blocks or a rolled-up towel under them for support. Open your knees way apart, so that your knees are wider than your pelvis and pointed at 2 o'clock and 10 o'clock, because that opens you up. Now squat. Hang out there for a count of three and come back up

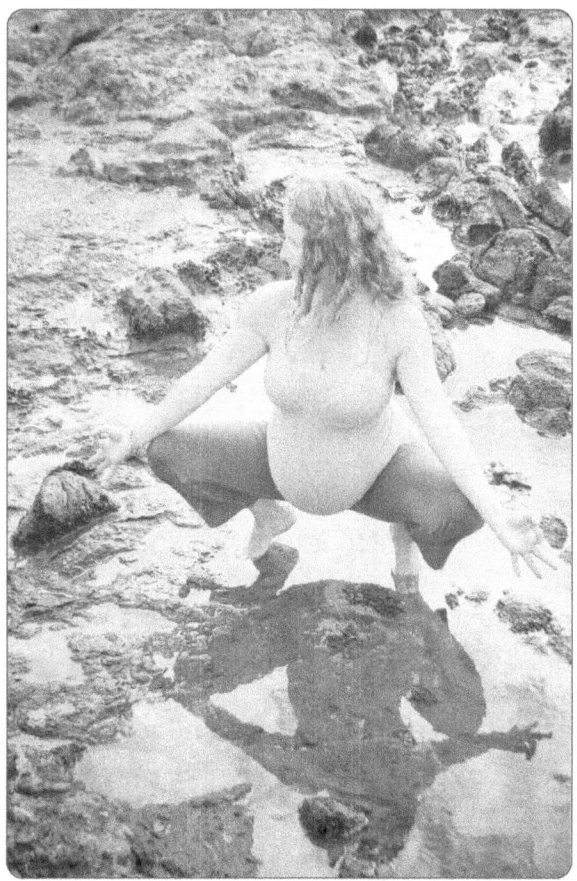

Pregnant Woman Squatting

while keeping your back straight. Gradually increase the time you spend in the squatting position. Use your legs, not your back, when coming out of a squat.

 I highly suggest you work with your partner and do these together. Have your partner sit on the bed, legs wide apart. Stand in between their legs with your back to your partner. You're going to be calling the shots in labor, so practice that now.

Here's what to do: Pretend a contraction is coming on. In one smooth sequence, say, "Contraction begins, one, two, three," then immediately take a deep cleansing breath as your partner's hands guide you into the squat. He should support you enough that you are not carrying all of your own weight. Practice one of your breathing techniques for a few seconds (don't worry, we'll get to these shortly). As the practice session ends, you'll take another deep cleansing breath and say, "One, two, three, up!" and rise with your partner's assistance.

Please practice this in advance. Work with your partner to build up these muscles. Squatting will save first-time mothers a tremendous amount of time in labor.

Weight Work

I also suggest using weights to work out. Heaving around my giant babies after birth threw my back and neck muscles out at times because I didn't have enough muscle. Build muscle! Often you have your baby in a heavy car seat on one arm, and your purse and a diaper bag with all the baby accessories on the other arm—it can just be so challenging. Using weights will help your body to prepare.

Upper body strength is difficult to develop naturally when you are not doing a lot of carrying. Carrying water, food, firewood, and their children in times past helped women to have strong upper body muscle tone. In our modern world, with its conveniences and our newly sedentary lifestyles, most of us don't do these things. Many of us are lacking in upper body strength. A lot of research has shown that building upper body strength can help you now, as well as significantly later in your life, to improve bone density and bone health.[140]

Continue Abs Work

Preparing your stomach muscles is also very important. When you are pushing you use your stomach muscles to help squeeze the baby down and out, so you want those to be strong. Continue your daily ab routine (see page 131).

Prenatal Yoga

Prenatal yoga is another great activity at this stage. It is beneficial in calming you, centering you, and connecting you to your baby. It builds flexibility and stamina.

Research has shown that ancient people naturally got into many interesting positions—reaching high to pick a piece of fruit or dig behind a plant to reach a root—that required stretching and balancing, which our modern, convenient environment simply does not require.[141] I believe good balance is so important to keep both our bodies as well as our brains

active. Certain yoga poses have you upright and balancing on one foot or the other. It really does wonderful things for your brain. There are studies that suggest that balance training can be an effective way to improve memory and spatial cognition in healthy adults.[142]

Different poses stimulate your body in different ways. I think you have to really work to stretch out the muscles you build by swimming and walking and lifting weights—these tighten you up—and yoga is an excellent way to stretch you out and make you more flexible, especially in your legs. You want to practice those particular positions that open your hips and stretch your leg muscles as they will be helpful during labor, which means less work for both you and your baby.

When to Stop

At the very end of your pregnancy, you have to give up exercising. You'll want to, too. At 38–40 Weeks it will be all you can do to lounge around in some lovely water. A 40-minute walk won't feel good by this point because you're soft; everything in your body softens to get ready for the birth, and it doesn't just soften the vagina and the cervix. It softens everything. You may notice that your feet spread out from the softening, and you may gain half a shoe size or more. You may find it uncomfortable to simply walk across a room. Relax now. Rest now. You have a big event on the horizon, and a life-long marathon after that. Do not exhaust yourself before it begins.

Breathe.

Rise Carefully

Sometimes if you've been sitting for a really long time, especially if you have low blood pressure, it's important to wake your muscles up *before* you stand up. Jiggle your thighs, clench, and release your buttocks, wiggle your whole body a bit and then move your legs to get your blood pumping.

Late in one of my pregnancies I sat in a movie for two hours and then the lights came up and everybody stood up and walked off, and I stood right up and walked off with them, but when I got to the aisle, I thought, *Oh no, I'm going down.* I knew I was going to faint, so I immediately laid down on the floor instead of risking a fall. It caused a little commotion; people wondered if they should call EMS. I told them I was fine, just pregnant and needed a moment, which was true. Wiggling your legs will firm up the relaxed muscles and keep your blood up in your head. All this is to say, jiggle and wiggle before you get up, and if you do feel like you're going to faint, it's better to control how you get to the ground and go down carefully and of your own accord before that happens.

There is an old wives' tale that women often faint in pregnancy, and it is so true. Pregnant women faint for a multitude of reasons, one being hypoglycemia. If you don't eat frequently enough it can really get you, and hard. Another is the muscles soften and aren't as efficient at keeping the blood in your head, so the blood flows out of your head and into your extremities and you faint. Both of these potential problems are preventable by eating frequently and engaging your leg muscles before standing as just mentioned.

Breathing Techniques & Relaxation Exercises
No Single Way

There are lots of different techniques for handling the sensations of labor. I am a firm believer in partner-coached childbirth, and I am a trained Lamaze instructor. I'm sure many of you have heard of Bradley and Lamaze, but each of these is only one way to handle the sensations of labor. There are as many ways to give birth as there are women to do it. Look around, check with the other mothers you know and see what they liked. Experiment.

One of the biggest things I can recommend to you at this point is that you read lots of books, take classes, or watch YouTube videos about how to handle the pain of labor. There are so many ideas and theories and if you are open to extending yourself to look into those possibilities you will have many options to choose from.

A midwife is a woman who understands the rhythmic flow of life, who listens to the whispers of a woman's body and soul, and who holds the space for miracles to unfold.

—Dr. Michel Odent

The more options you have to respond to the sensations of labor, the better prepared you feel, and the more relaxed you will be. And just like surrendering, relaxation is key to a shorter, easier, less difficult time during the birth process.

Any way that you can get more oxygen to the baby is good. The less oxygen you have, the more it hurts and the more stress and anxiety you and your baby will feel. Breathing techniques are used by about 85 percent of my clients during the birth process. A lot of them deep breathe through most of their early to mid-stage labor and then pant-blow in later stages. Any of these will help to oxygenate the baby.

Some of my clients use visualization or self-hypnosis to help deal with fear in advance of the birth experience and to access other methods and tools for handling the challenges of natural labor.

I have worked with plenty of people who don't use breathing techniques in labor. They moan, they roar, they do other types of vocalizations—singing and such. There are lots of ways to approach labor, and you have *complete permission* to do everything and anything that you want during your labor. I do want you to learn these breathing techniques, so you have these tools if you need them.

I will also say that while it can feel good to vocalize your experience, if you are moaning by four centimeters, you'll be screaming by nine. In my experience this is stressful for the baby and everyone else in the room. These babies tend to come

out with an elevated heart rate and seem freaked out. Many women choose another method when they learn this.

How Often to Practice

 Practice is so crucial for both you and your partner. One of the things I find about some folks attempting these techniques is that they can be kind of lackadaisical about it, just going through the motions. That level of effort will not help you when you are facing intense and painful sensations in labor. If you really work on this and practice intentionally and enthusiastically during pregnancy, it will be more automatic during labor. That's important because while you are in labor, it is not the time to learn new skills.

All told, I'm asking for less than 15 minutes a week for you both to practice this, but I want you to be fully present for those few minutes. You only have to practice for three minutes each session (one minute per breathing technique), two to four times a week. If you have had babies before and have used breathing methods successfully before, practice them twice a week, but if you haven't, do it four times a week or every other day.

Partner's Role

 Partners, if your woman loses her rhythm due to the intensity of a contraction, you will want to get on *her* track, following her rhythm, and then guide her back to where she was. You cannot breathe five times slower than her; that won't help. You must first match where she is and then help

guide her back to the proper rhythm. And if your woman needs someone to breathe with her for 15 hours during her labor, that person will be *you!*

The best reason to practice is that when you do so together, it gives you a sliver of potent time as a couple, face-to-face, focusing on this little baby, this labor, and this birth. These can be tender, quiet moments where you are not focused on all of the other minutiae of life. These are magical minutes. You will be opening your hearts to this process, and to a still place to focus and let the baby communicate with you and you with them.

Be eye to eye and take a few moments to focus on your baby, sending your lifeforce to the baby, thinking about the baby and how you will handle the sensations of labor.

You have the opportunity to connect your energies together during this process. Partners, lay your hands on your lovely mother-to-be. Give your vital life force and love to this incredible woman. You can send your strength to her in this process, and if you practice these techniques, they will likely work so much better during labor.

Breathing Exercises

I'm going to describe each of the breathing exercises to the best of my ability with words, below, but you may also find it helpful to see and hear them demonstrated. If you'd like to see me demonstrate these techniques, you can find recordings of these techniques on my Instagram page @marimikelthemidwife, saved in my posts and stories.

Deep Cleansing Breath to Kick Things Off and Wrap Things Up

The first thing you do at the beginning and ending of every practice is to take a deep, cleansing breath. It is in through the nose and out through the mouth, and it is very vigorous and very quick.

This deep, cleansing breath is very important—it serves as a signal to everyone in the room during your labor that a new contraction is beginning or that the contraction you were just experiencing has ended. It is your stop and start and bookends each contraction. When you practice, make sure you do this at the start and stop of the session and relax on the exhale.

Focus

Next, you want to pick a focal point for your eyes. It can be your partner's eyes or a fixed point on the wall. It really doesn't matter what you look at, just find a place for your eyes to rest. Your inner vision will ideally be focused inwardly on your uterus, your cervix, on the baby moving down on the cervix, the uterus pulling up on the cervix to open it, the thinning of the cervix, and everything that goes along with your body physically ripening. I want you to be able to visualize all this in your mind's eye to aid your body in this process during labor.

A lovely project is to draw and color a circular mandala that you can use in labor to rest your eyes. This provides a focal point that is centering, opening, and expanding.

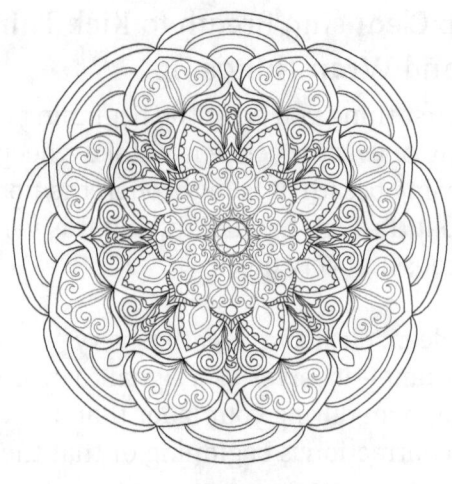

Mandal

As you practice the different techniques listed below, I want you to visualize white light coming in with every breath that you take in. You know, it is no accident that the intake of breath is called "inspiration." There are many sacred traditions that teach that your breath is a connection to God. The Hindus believe that there are two manifestations of God in the physical form. *Prana* is your breath, and *prahbā* is light. When you are breathing in, I want you to feel that you are breathing in all the love in the world, all the peace, joy, prosperity, love, tenderness, and forgiveness. I want all good coming in. And as you exhale, release all fear, tension, pain, upset, worry, and all negativity. It is a beautiful circle of white light welcomed in, with darkness pushed out—a *yin-yang*, if you will.

Deep Breathing

Deep breathing needs to be fairly vigorous. It is in through the nose, out through the mouth, six to nine times per minute somewhat slowly (for one minute), beginning and ending with your cleansing breath.

Connect the inhale to the exhale. It is very important that there are no gaps between the inhale and exhale, absolutely no holding of your breath in between. It is also equally important to equalize the inhale and the exhale; if one is shorter or longer than the other, it can cause you to hyperventilate because your carbon dioxide and oxygen balance can be thrown off. If this happens, you will not feel good—you will feel dizzy, and your hands and lips will tingle and feel numb—so it is very important for you to make sure your inhale and exhale are of roughly equal lengths. It may help you to do a slow count in your head as you breathe.

Relax on the exhale. Every time you exhale, let your shoulders go, feel your back and neck let go, feel your belly let go, feel your vagina let go, feel your legs let go. With every exhale you deepen the level of relaxation, releasing more and more of your body's tension.

After one minute, end with another deep, cleansing breath.

The Pant

The pant starts with a cleansing breath and continues with a series of quick *hee-hee-hee-hee-hee-hee-hees* (for one minute) and ends with a cleansing breath. These *hees* are each very, very quick inhales and exhales. I do about 20–30 in ten seconds. Take about half a breath of air in first, then pant on top of it. You have to put your tongue on the back of your bottom teeth and make a *hee* sound, which forces your lips into a smile. Think of the way you see animals panting when they are hot, happy, or stressed. I have seen a number of animals give birth, and they all panted in labor. So, I think this is a natural way to handle the discomfort and intensity of the sensations of labor.

You want to equalize the inhale and exhale. If you start to run out of air you can let it out and then just pull more back in, but keep your rhythm equalized. No matter what you are doing, stay on that path of equalized breath and keep the same rhythm, letting carbon dioxide out in a few *hee-hees* and pulling oxygen back with the next few *hee-hees*.

The Pant-Blow

Last but not least is the pant blow. Start with a deep, cleansing breath, then *inhale* three quick *hees*, and exhale a *whoo* equal in length to the three *hees*. *Hee-hee-hee whoo, hee-hee-hee whoo, hee-hee-hee whoo.* Do this for one minute, then end with your cleansing breath. If you do make the exhale too short or too long, again, you will unbalance the intake and output and you can hyperventilate and feel bad; it has got to be equal. Remember, you are breathing in and out with each *hee*.

Practice faithfully, and these three techniques will be yours to draw on when labor gets intense.

Practice Relaxation

 I want you to continue to practice relaxing. It is not an easy task to deeply relax in our modern society. This culture is not really supportive of relaxing and letting go, having a comfortable moment where all of your muscles go limp. And we certainly do not generally know how to go limp to our partner's touch. When your partner touches you, your body's natural reaction is to physically respond to them rather than to go limp.

At this point I want to teach you something different, so you can let go of muscles that are tense during labor and go limp at your partner's touch. This technique will not take you much more than three to four minutes. If you do it a few times a week, it will be valuable time spent connecting to each other, and you can achieve much more heightened states of relaxation, which will be so helpful during labor and birth, as well as life.

Women can really tense up during labor and there is nothing worse than having someone say "relax." Instead, let's learn what's called touch relaxation. I am sure you have heard of Pavlov's dog, who developed a conditioned response to salivate at the sound of the bell. Similarly, I'd like you to become conditioned to go limp at your partner's touch.

Here's what you will do together:

Women, lie down and put your arms down to your sides.

Partners, gently stroke her arm. This is how you will begin and end each session. Next, gently squeeze her arm muscles.

Women, when you feel that gentle squeeze, let go of all tension in that muscle and go completely limp.

Partners, once you have relaxed the arm muscles, pick up her hand and give her arm a little shake to see if that muscle is relaxed. Make sure to always be gentle and never tickle. If her arm rises up to meet you, it's a sign she is not yet fully relaxed. Don't drop her arm when you're finished. Lay it down gently.

Then, go over to the next arm and repeat this process. Stroke, gentle squeeze, lift, gentle shake, and gentle release. Once you've achieved relaxation, stroke the arm again.

Move to the legs. Stroke one leg, give it a small squeeze as a reminder to relax, and then put your hand under the thigh (try not to go under the knee—the popliteal artery is under there and you can cut off the circulation). It should feel relaxed and floppy. If the leg rises up to meet you, then she is not yet relaxed. Repeat the squeezes until she achieves relaxation. End with a stroke.

Repeat this on the other leg: Stroke, gently squeeze, lift and gently shake, then gently release.

Now put your hands on her head. I want you to feel the energy in your body and your hands. I want you to feel that energy flowing from you to her. One of the things

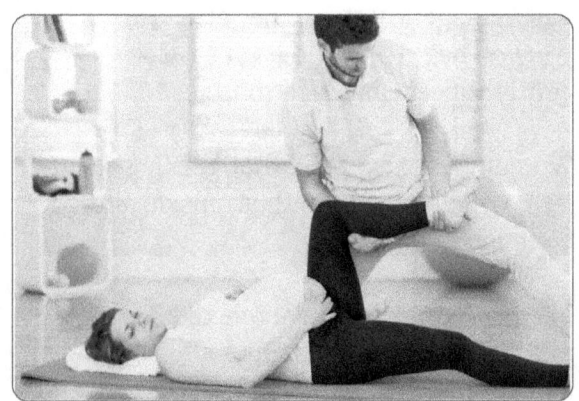

Practicing Relaxation

you can do to help your woman in labor is to transfer your energy to her. This may feel a little strange at first, but with practice you can visualize the energy moving through you to her.

In that moment, think about your vitality flowing into her. Then, massage her forehead a bit, massage her temple a little bit, get your hands down below her shoulders and massage the back of the shoulders; we all carry so much tension right in there. And then move up into the neck, into the space where her neck meets her head. Feel that the head can freely move and be completely relaxed. Stroke her cheeks and forehead gently and visualize and feel all of your love flowing into her. By this time, her whole body should be very relaxed.

When you put your hands on your loved one and you feel your life force and vitality flowing from your hands and arms into her, you can spiritually and energetically lift them up and through a tough moment. This is what the laying-on of hands is all about. It works, and it is so powerful. Spiritual healing and the healing power of touch is just phenomenal.

Often in labor partners feel they do not know what to do to help. The truth is you are feeling these labor pains and they are not. You are in many ways alone. You have people there to support you, number one should be your partner, but it is still quite a solitary experience, all things considered. If you practice this in advance, when labor comes and you are feeling tense and having a hard time relaxing into the intense sensations of the contractions, your partner can help you. They can give your arm a gentle squeeze, or your leg, or the muscles of your shoulders or neck, and your body will more naturally respond by relaxing to their touch instead of tensing up more. This is a great trick to use in labor and a mutually beneficial way for your partner to support you and feel they are actually doing something to help when you are riding those waves of labor pains.

Take a few extra minutes to do this practice in tandem with your breathing practice. These moments together where you are able to meet each other in the closeness of this experience, thinking about your coming baby and birth, and the joy that you have created together will make a world of difference in your labor.

Women, if I could sum all of this up in one word, that word is *surrender*. Surrender to the higher power at work, open your heart to the spiritual power all around you and allow it to flow into you.

Surrender to the pain, don't fight it—just surrender to it and let it flow.

Robbie: During the three days of labor for my at-home VBAC, I kept trying to *do something* about the pain. I tried chanting with it, singing with it, dancing with it. Then, during very active labor toward the end of the third day, I dove face-down onto my bed and let go. I said to the pain, "Take me, I'm yours." And suddenly, I became one with the pain and then there was no pain. I had entered into a state of total relaxation and ecstasy that midwives often call "laborland," which MariMikel calls "the zone." I stayed in that state for a very long time, just flowing with the contractions without even feeling them. That's how I learned the true meaning of what MariMikel calls "surrender."

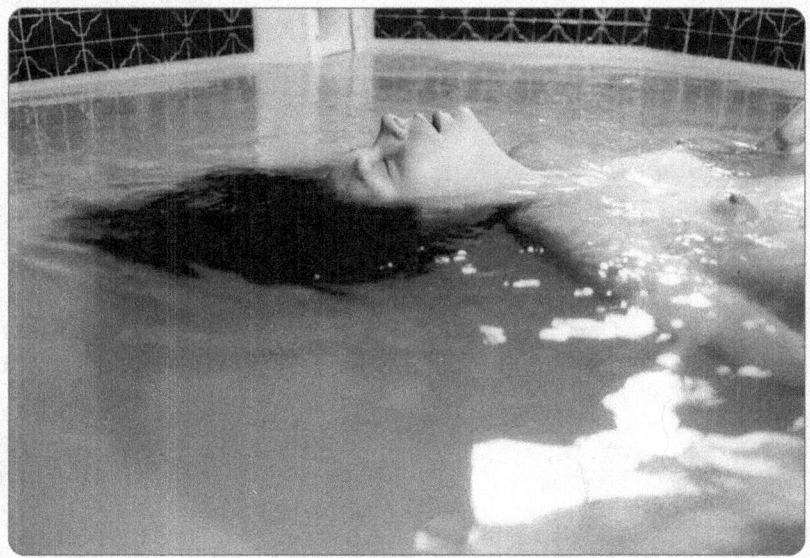

Robbie Surrendering during Labor

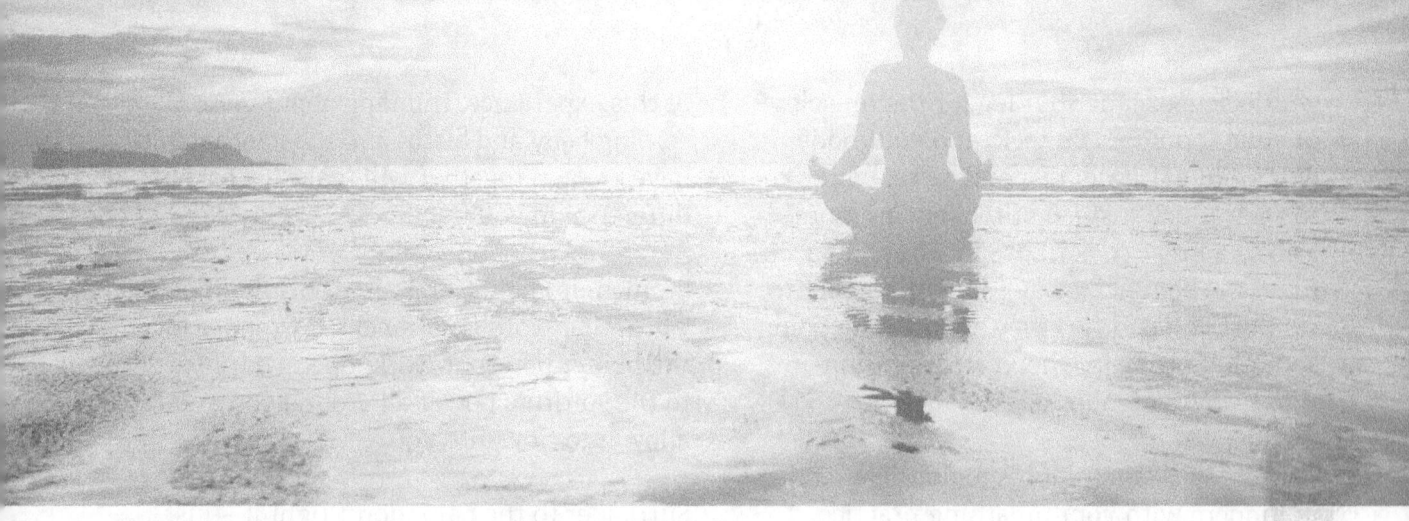

Emotional/Spiritual

Fear and Spirituality

There are reasons why there is so much fear surrounding birth. In pre-modern times 2–3 percent of all women and babies died in childbirth.[143] They didn't have the ability to diagnose or handle common complications that arose and the four most common causes of death in those times were blood pressure issues, hemorrhage, infections, and stalled birth. Now we have ways to monitor and compensate for these issues and, as long as you are under the supervision of a competent birth care provider, you will be taken care of.

But these issues do exist and that's why it's important to have someone by your side. You can't read a few books and expect to be able to handle a birth alone at home without support or competent medical supervision and care. Do not try any aspect of this alone.

One of the biggest complications with labor is when there is unsolved emotional work in the momma. Labor is sensitive to turmoil. If you have family members or friends who are drama prone, you owe it to your baby to break free from those emotional ties and relationships for now. You also owe it to yourself and your family to get the help you need to heal that trauma.

As I've told you, part of the problem with the OB/GYN community or with midwives in hospitals is that they're all just so taxed with an overwhelming workload. If I were attending 20 births a month, there is no way I would have time to check in with my patients, to make sure they had someone to talk with to guide them through combatting those fears, to ask if they had opened themselves up to the divinity of the universe, and if they were praying.

Some women have cut themselves off from spirituality. I have had clients who've said they don't believe in a higher power. I believe that it believes in them, and I've asked them if we can talk about it. Often, I've found they've had a bad experience with a church or have been fed overly restrictive beliefs. When we talk, they come to understand that spirituality is not religion and religion is not spirituality ...

except when it is. The bottom line is, if you can find a path to any sort of spiritual connection in your life, it will really help, especially during labor and birth.

Components of a Holistically Safe Birth

There are several factors that will aid you in your pursuit of your ideal, perfect birth. Many of these I am sure you have already incorporated into your pregnancy.

You need the *knowledge and learning* about what you're going through to calm the fears of your mind. This allows you to prepare the mind and understand what to do.

You need the emotional preparation of *stress relief and relaxation,* communion with nature, and resting.

You need the *spiritual connection* to open your heart and calm the fears of your soul. Prayer is also wonderful for labor preparation. Open your heart to God, the Goddess, the spirit, the Universe, whatever you believe in. Almost all women reach out to something during birth; they reach a point where they are hoping that their God/dess is there to help them. I believe that the spirit is available to you, to flow through you and lift you up when you cannot handle it anymore.

You need *loving community* around and in support of you, so you have people to talk to and work through and calm the fears of your heart. Especially if you have experienced trauma around birth before, it's very important to have this network of support around you. If you are a single mom, call on your besties to support your pregnancy and birth experience!

You need a *knowledgeable and attentive care provider* in support of you to monitor things like blood pressure and glucose levels, cervical readiness, and presentation, etc. to prevent or overcome any issues.

Remember, your thoughts are powerful, and you are manifesting your reality. A lot of this is done on the unconscious and subconscious levels, but the more you can bring your conscious mind to bear, the more you can affect your unconscious and subconscious and therefore what manifests in your life. If you expect the worst, I think it subtly pushes things toward that happening.

Expect the best. You are very powerful.

Visualizations are another wonderful thing to do. You can lie down, close your eyes, relax, and visualize your ideal, perfect birth. When do you go into labor? How does it feel? What is the experience like?

> *It's 4:00 a.m. and I wake to strong contractions, but I am able to doze in between them. The sun comes up and I rise with it; the contractions are strong, and they hurt a little, but I handle them with ease, breathing with each. I progress perfectly over the next few hours and by mid-morning I am already six centimeters dilated.*

Get creative and strive to see this montage in your mind's eye. Imagine your perfect birth but remember to be realistic. You do not want to visualize a painless childbirth. For one, it is not likely to happen, and two, if it were to happen, well, that is how babies are born in strange or public places, and you don't want your baby falling out in the produce section at your local grocery store or in the elevator lobby.

Penelope: When I was very young, my mother loved to take me and my sister to McDonald's for breakfast. Our local McDonald's often ran contests for prizes. On the sly, my mother would swipe a ballot pad or two, bring them home, and have my sister and I fill out hundreds of entries. We were young enough we didn't realize this is known as "stuffing the ballot box."

To our delight, we won a trip to Disneyland and a family beach vacation with this method.

Here's where it gets interesting. I grew up believing I was someone who won things. Nowadays, as I am putting my ballot into the box for a giveaway or drawing, I visualize a hand plucking it back out of the hundreds or thousands of entries. I always say, "They're going to draw my name," or "I'm going to win," and it's not because I stuffed the ballot box (I don't.). It's because I believe it.

I recently attended a conference with a friend and, as we were filling out ballots for a giveaway, she said, "I never win anything."

I said, "I do." It shocked her. She'd never heard that from anyone before in her life.

Throughout that day, whenever we were together with others, she would tell them that I was going to win the drawing. She put so much good juju out there for me.

Guess who won the contest? Yup, it was me.

This does not always work, of course. But I have won many, many prizes from giveaways of this nature and I firmly believe that I am aided by all the people who tell the Universe, "I never win anything."

Change your mind; change your life.

I once watched an amazing video captured by store cameras where a woman in England was in the frozen food aisle and she suddenly said "Oh! Oh dear! Oh my

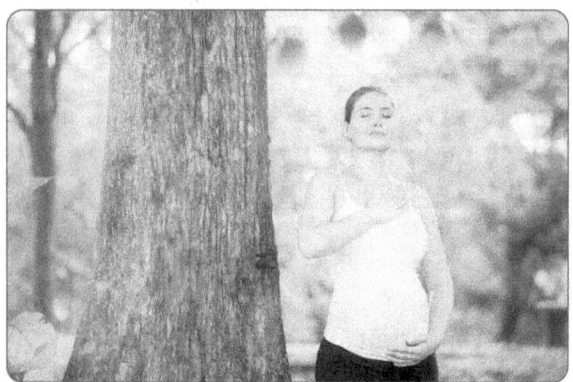

Taking Time to Visualize, Connect, and Bond in Nature

God!" and the baby was born right there on the floor! This is part of why your body is designed to feel some of the sensations of pregnancy, labor and births—so you know something is happening, and you won't have your baby someplace other than the place of your choice.

Meditation and mindfulness practice are also helpful to center yourself and feel at one with the universal creative force. I believe these are another form of prayer.

All of these components have their place in the process. Labor will do what it does. It's mainly a matter of hanging on and going into the zone. These components are the ones you can control; these components are what you can influence. As your due range grows near, put your time and attention to these activities rather than worrying about when your labor will start or what could go wrong.

Intuition

I talk so much about resting, relaxing, and listening to your body. Continue to practice listening to your intuition for guidance as you navigate this last part of the course. Use your deepening connection to yourself, your baby, and the divine to open your heart. Do what you need to do to take care of yourself and be prepared for the upcoming labor and birth. Allow your intuition to guide you, so you rest when you need to rest, eat when you need to eat, drink when you need to hydrate. Do not overload yourself and work too hard. Give yourself the space to focus on your emotional and spiritual self, have fun, and create joyful moments.

Affirmations and Visualizations

Affirmations and visualizations have changed my life and I think they are an amazing aid for pregnancy and birth. They can help you to get what you want out of life, and to have a safe, healthy, and connected pregnancy and birth process. Research has shown repeating affirmations for just a few weeks can have startlingly positive effects on your self-esteem and ability to perform well.[144]

Combatting Fear

Now I know I have said this before, but I think it helps to be reminded of these things at each stage of your pregnancy journey. Thoughts become things. When you feel fear about your coming experience, know that you can think differently. Your fear is not reality at all; it is a product of your thoughts and beliefs. You can say your affirmations and visualize a safe and thriving future where your fears have not materialized, erasing those particular fears. If you have fears or concerns about the birth or parenting, pregnancy, or the baby's health (which are all normal and common feelings), it is a great idea to face them head-on by creating affirmations around them. Fears left unchallenged can bubble up when you least need them to.

Nearly everything we think about ourselves is a learned response. Most learned responses come from our parents, but they also come from family, friends, society, culture, education, etc.—all of these things build our character and belief systems. Journaling can help us uncover these unconscious responses and identify things about ourselves we want to let go of (like fear) or improve. If there is something you are not happy with or do not like, you can actually change it by repeatedly programming yourself with a new message. It does help to write the new message down. Affirmations are most effective when you write them several times.

At the end of pregnancy, it is crucial that you are in the very best state possible emotionally and physically. But this is also when you may start to feel fear as you grow bigger and bigger, and the baby's delivery starts to become real. Think thoughts that provide a lot of resonant energy, some kind of charge; these tell you there's fear to work through.

Maybe the affirmation you need to design is to remind you that you can handle whatever childbirth throws at you, that your body was designed to do this and can do it easily. You are the current endpoint of an unbroken line of women who have successfully given birth back into the misty dawn of time and raised their babies well enough to have their own babies. You are carrying on this hundreds-of-thousands-of-years-long tradition.

> *I am strong. My body gives birth easily. This ancestral knowledge is deep in my bones.*

If one of your fears is that your perineum might tear or need to have an episiotomy, you can create an affirmation around it.

> *My perineum stretches perfectly and easily for my baby to come out without tearing.*

What a nice thought! Give it a try. It really, really works.

If you are afraid of the pain of giving birth, try:

> *The pain of labor does not make me afraid, and I handle it very well.*

It may be about motherhood. Maybe you're afraid that you will become someone alien to yourself, that you'll replicate the mistakes of your own parents, that you'll be neglectful, or just not good at the job. You might in that case choose an affirmation like:

> *I am a kind and empathetic mother. My baby can trust me and rely on me to be an excellent, nurturing guide.*

> *I am an informed and nurturing parent. I can model a new way of being for myself and my child.*

> *I am a conscious and loving mother, and my child can rely on me to break the chains of generational trauma.*

Here are some examples of affirmations you might choose to adopt now that can help address these types of fears about your body, your health, your baby, pain, labor and/or birth and/or motherhood. Feel free to use one of these or write your own.

- *I love myself, every part of my mind, body, and spirit.*
- *My body is beautiful, and I fully accept the changing body I am in.*
- *My body is nurturing my baby and me and doing the beautiful work it needs to do in pregnancy.*
- *I am connected to my growing baby inside.*
- *I am strong. My body gives birth easily.*
- *I am resilient and I can handle whatever childbirth throws at me. My body was designed to do this and can do it easily.*
- *I give birth calmly and joyfully, in an environment that is comfortable, with people I love who will support me through the natural sensations of labor.*
- *My baby and I are supported and nourished by the healthy actions I take for us.*
- *I am a being of light and love and a channel for the divine.*
- *My baby is developing beautifully, and I am the healthiest I have ever been.*

- *I welcome the sensations of labor and birth. They mean that I will meet my baby soon.*
- *I welcome the beauty and challenges motherhood will bring into my life.*

I suggest writing each of your chosen affirmations ten times a day for the last six to eight weeks of your pregnancy, but you can start to do them as early as you like. Doing this will actually help your brain to think differently and ease those fears. Reach out to friends, family, or a therapist when you need more support or someone to talk to. Sharing your feelings and concerns with others can provide comfort and perspective.

Noticing

The third trimester is the time to notice these last changes in your body and the changes that are coming to prepare you for labor. If you train yourself and practice paying attention, you will feel more and more of what's going on and notice the changes that are bringing you closer to the birth. This awareness will help you immensely as labor approaches. This is a fantastic time for daily body scans. Notice what you are feeling as you envision the light filling each area of your body. See page 138.

Whom to Invite to the Birth

Much of what I write in this section is intended for women who are planning a natural, unmedicated labor, regardless of where you plan to give birth. If you are choosing a medicated birth or must schedule a c-section, tailor my recommendations to your scenario.

Energy in the Birthing Room

Inviting someone to your birth is a real gift. Wherever you give birth is a sacred space. Everyone who attends the birth will bring their energy to the process. Good energy is so important. Inviting someone to your baby's birth is not something you do to help someone else heal; it is crucial you protect the emotional and spiritual space around yourself and your baby. I believe the energy at the birth can affect the baby and even imprint on them. You do not want scared, sad, or mad people around you, or—if you're having an at-home birth—people who do not agree with home birth or midwives; it is just not a good idea. Anxious people will have an effect on the process, no matter how quiet they are. There can be a palpable tension in the birthing space, emanating from these people's fears, and that fearful energy can so often be felt by the mother and baby. It is a delicate and sensitive time. Be careful whom you invite.

Until recently (evolutionarily speaking) women *never* experienced birth around strangers. Giving birth was a very intimate experience with the people around you who loved you. Your mother, your grandmothers, your aunts, all the wise women of your tribe who had given birth surrounded you and cheered you on. You had their wisdom behind you to help you through the process. Now a woman who plans for an unmedicated home birth and adopts this ancient practice of bringing in the matriarchs and women of her family might find herself surrounded by people who have not had that same experience and may not be fully on board with it.

When people are confronted with a different way of doing things, especially things that are as primal and life changing as giving birth, they can feel attacked. It is easy for others to fall into the trap of thinking that you are inherently criticizing them because you are choosing to give birth differently than they did. They may cling to a desire for you to have your birth the way they had their birth(s) in order to validate their experience, and that can be tough on your relationship. They may bring a lot of judgment, fear, and anxiety to the birthing room. This is something to consider when you are making your choices about whom to invite to join you while you labor and give birth.

I want to remind you that birth is on the continuum of sexual experiences, and it may be one of the most profound experiences you will have in your life. I suggest not inviting anyone to the birth that you wouldn't feel comfortable having sex in front of. I'm pretty certain this is a very short list. I tell people that birth is a sexual experience because a lot of the energy is centered on your sexual self. The oxytocin level is so high that it approximates the oxytocin levels in sex.

Birth is an intimate act of full vulnerability, and it needs to be undertaken in an environment of deep trust. I work to do my job, promote safety first, promote spirituality and the rights and needs of the mom, dad, and baby, but after that I feel I need to be in the background, and quiet at the birth. You want people who can be discreet and unobtrusive. You may have friends or family who are in that category and those who are not. If they are going to focus the energy and attention on themselves, they are probably not the best people to invite. You need to not be distracted by anyone else's strong energy at

your baby's birth, especially while you are in labor.

I walk into my clients' homes smiling and happy and so thrilled to be there. I am confident and have wonderful positive energy and that is important. You want that quality in all the people you invite to the birth. Family and close friends can be so wonderful to have with you. I fondly remember one birth I attended at an ashram where a woman had more than 40 people with her. Most were not present until she started pushing, but once she started pushing, she wanted all the people she lived with to be there. There were probably 10 people in the birth room and all the rest were right outside the open doors and windows. As the baby started crowning, they all started quietly "Om"-ing, and it was such a magical experience to be a part of. The energy was absolutely levitating.

How Many People to Invite

Birth is not a spectator sport and wanting to see the birth is not a good enough reason for someone to be there. It is not something you want to be observed while you're doing it. Most women are working as hard as they've ever worked, maybe as hard as they ever will work, to navigate this challenging process, and having people watch you while you struggle to find your way with pain and the fears and joys that come along with it is tough. You are incredibly vulnerable in labor.

The people in the room with you should have no agenda other than supporting you in your labor and birthing process. The more people you have there, the harder it is to reach the zone. I mentioned a fabulous experience at the ashram, but I have also transported

Aleah: I knew how important it would be for me to have the right people at each of the births of my two daughters. This came from what MariMikel teaches, as well as from listening to my intuitive self. It was important to me to have people there who I loved, who loved and supported me, and who would not be anxious or fearful.

I am extremely close with my older sister and had been at the births of both of my nieces. I knew I wanted and needed her to be by my side. I am also best friends with my sister-in-law and had attended her births. I felt so strongly that both my sisters needed to be there with me, and knew they would be loving, calm, encouraging guides for me through the process.

I am also incredibly lucky in my life to have a group of girlfriends I have known since childhood, for over 20 years, and I am still so close with them. They are not just friends but truly like sisters. Barring international travel with their own newborn during my first birth, I was able to have almost all of them at my side. I ended up having my partner, two midwives (including my mom), two apprentices, and five sisters in attendance. This may sound like a lot (and could be too many for some people), but it was exactly what I needed, and their presence surrounded me with the tangible, loving, levitating energy I was seeking for my labor and birth. It was a magical moment that I was able to share with most of the closest people in my life, and an experience I will cherish always.

women to hospitals in order to extricate them from the presence of a toxic person in the birthing room. I have seen babies simply refuse to come out in the presence of undue stress in the mother. If you are having a home birth, you want to make sure those present are confident, happy about your choice of a home birth, happy about your choice of a midwife, respectful of your decisions, and do not try to push you to make any choices *they* want you to make. They need to be there to help and support you with no further agenda. Consider carefully. You do not have to invite someone just because they expect to be invited. You have permission not to. Give yourself permission to make this experience about you and do what you need to do to feel as safe, comfortable, and supported as possible.

At a home birth, I ask one of your invited attendants to hold one leg at the time of the birth while your partner holds the other, because you need both of your legs to be fully supported. Having two people who can do that is pretty important. I usually have two apprentices at my side, and I can't always station one of them at the woman's leg, so I find it is helpful if to have approximately six people at the birth. The mom, her partner, the midwife, two apprentice midwives, and another friend, family member, or doula. Talk with your midwife to see what she recommends.

All this to say, you do need help, and it can be so helpful to have your friends or family at your side. In my practice, we work to help keep them busy and involved, and they can be such a blessing. But choose wisely.

Harmonious and Private

I've seen people announce they're coming for the birth (these are often mothers of mothers-to-be), show up without consent, and stay for two weeks waiting for that baby, tapping their feet, exuding stress. The baby just won't come out while in their presence. As soon as they leave, the baby comes. I have seen it time and time again. Women need to feel safe in order to give birth. Full stop.

In ancient tribal times, sex and birth weren't done in complete privacy, but rather in a kind of *offered* privacy. The rest of the tribe was present, but they turned their backs. It's not like the couple would leave their safe sheltered tribe to go out into the jungle to have sex where they could possibly be eaten by a jaguar or bitten by a venomous snake ... In modern times, we have forgotten the art of allowing people to feel private in front of us, allowing people to feel unwatched, unobserved, and unscrutinized while we are in the same room with them. But it's vital that those in the room provide this safety for the laboring woman. This is what we as midwives strive to achieve in the birthing room as well.

Inviting Your Mother

I ask a lot of questions when my client wants her own mother to be present at the birth. Many mothers of pregnant woman are quite helpful to have in the birthing room. But when you consider that most of them were both born and gave birth in a hospital, there's a fear factor there that has everything to do with their perception of normal. You don't need to introduce the energy of fear to your birthing room. It's not conducive to reaching the zone. A lot of communication that happens is nonverbal and this fear energy *will be communicated.* I often ask my clients if their mother is a giver or a taker. If their mother is a taker,

it may be better to not invite them until after the baby is born and the momma has recovered some from the rigors of labor and birth. If your mother can be generous and kind, take a back seat, shower you with love, accept your choices, and—most

During pregnancy, some baby cells migrate into the mother's bloodstream and then return to the child. It's called "*mother-fetal microchimerism.*"

For 41 weeks, the cells mix and circulate back and forth, and, after the baby is born, many of these cells remain in the mother's body, leaving a permanent imprint in the tissues, bones, brain and skin of the baby to mother, and they often remain there for decades. Every other child a mother has we'll leave a similar imprint on her body. Even if a pregnancy doesn't end, or if you have an abortion, these cells still migrate into the bloodstream. Research has shown that if a mother's heart is injured, fetal cells will rush to the injury site, and transform into different types of cells that specialize in repairing the heart.

The child helps the mother repair, while the mother builds the child.

This is often the reason why some diseases fade away during pregnancy.

It's amazing how the mother's body protects the baby at all costs, and the baby protects and rebuilds the mother in return, so they can safely develop and survive.

Let's think about pregnancy cravings for a moment. What did the mother need, that the child make her wish?

The studies also showed the presence of fetal cells in her mother's brain 18 years after birth. How wonderful is this?

—Nargis Kizalbash

importantly—you want her there, by all means invite her.

Watch Birth Videos

It helps for parents-to-be and those you are inviting to attend your birth to see videos of births and to become used to seeing birth as a natural and healthy event instead of as traumatizing. This culture has certainly fed us more than our fair share of anxiety-producing images about birth. One of the things I have to tell you is you will not see red gelatin. Every birth on TV the baby has this red jelly-like stuff all over them. In truth, in most births the baby comes out clean, having been washed in the salt water of the womb before they arrive.

If you have never seen a vaginal birth before, you should prepare yourself for what's coming by watching some birth videos on YouTube. You'll want to see some easy births, and you'll want to see some hard births. Repetition will help you get over the shock factor.

Almost everyone who sees a birth the first time gets this look of abject horror on their face and goes, "Oh my God! Oh my God! Oh my God!" The next time they see a birth they go, "Oh wow," but their reaction is not quite as horrified. The next one they see might say, "Oh look, the baby's crowning," and then the next one they see they have a big smile, and they say, "Look the baby's almost here; Oh my God!" But this last "Oh my God" is different from the first exclamations; it is said in awe instead of shock.

Repetitive viewing takes the charge off of the visual intensity of birth. You and anyone you're going to invite to your birth have to desensitize yourselves ahead of time. I think that people faint because they're not expecting what happens in birth to happen. If they've had a chance to see some birth videos, to see some different ways of doing things, then they can realize that there are a lot of approaches. Some women are quiet, some women are not, and all of that is within the realm of normal.

A lot of the blood people associate with birth is from episiotomies, which do bleed. A lot of people freak out at the sight of blood, so if you can show them a healthy birth and show them it's not really that bloody when there is no episiotomy, they can become used to what's going to happen, which is a good thing.

I attended a birth where the mother did the pant-blow for 17 hours and then pushed for three more. It was super hard. Super, super hard, and when the baby finally came out everybody was pretty wasted. The dad did great because he had watched some videos and he said, "Thank God I watched videos, otherwise I would have completely flipped out."

Watch videos in the last month of your pregnancy and encourage those you're inviting to your birth to do so as well. You can simply search YouTube for "midwife home birth videos" so you can watch at your leisure in the comfort of your own home.

Sibling Preparation

If you have an older child or children, it is important to prepare them for the birth of their sibling and their new paradigm to come. I encourage parents of older children to bring them along to prenatal appointments in the third trimester.

It is your decision whether or not you'd like your older child(ren) in the birthing room. This is a personal decision. Some mommas may need more privacy than that. If you invite them, designate someone, a known family member or friend, to take care of them. If you need to be transported to the hospital it is imperative that the designated person remain home with your older child(ren).

You should work to prepare your older child(ren) for what will happen at the time of the birth, the arrival of the new baby, and what's expected of them.

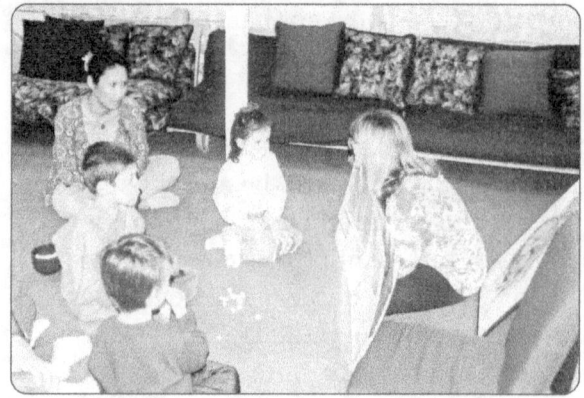

MariMikel Leading Sibling Preparation Classes

Here are a few ideas for helping older child(ren) to adjust:

- Read books together about becoming a big brother or sister.

- Have older kids participate in decorating the nursery or picking out baby's first outfit.

- Have conversations about the change to come for the family. Prepare kids in advance for how much attention the new baby will need from mommy and daddy because babies are needy, they mostly nurse, sleep and pee or poop. It can be fun to talk about how much babies poop and pee—kids just love talking about this stuff. Be sure to reassure them that they are not being replaced. "Even though mom will be very busy with the baby, we will still be together and have time for you and me."

- Make plans for your partner to provide support with the baby after your two-week lying-in period so you can have some one-on-one time with your other children, even just reading a book, doing a puzzle, or cuddling before bedtime. These

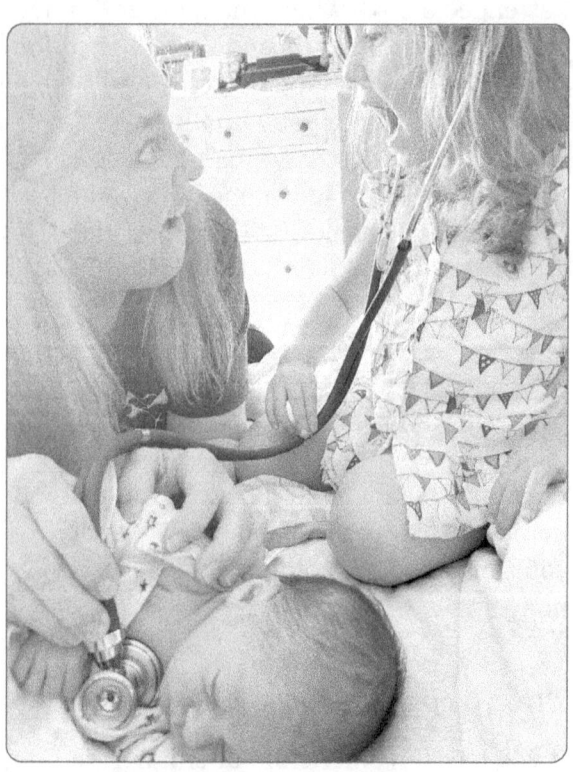

MariMikel Conducting a Postpartum Exam with a Sibling Present

> **Robbie:** My first child, a daughter named Peyton, always slept in our big family bed with my husband and me, at first because it was just so much easier to breastfeed her during the night, and later because we were all just so used to sleeping together. When our second child, a boy named Jason, was born around four years later, started sleeping in our big bed between my husband and me, I took the big low coffee table out of our living room and put it at the end of our bed with a nice, soft pallet on top of it. I also put those little felt sticky stars that glow in the dark on the ceiling above Peyton's new little bed. And there she slept happily until she was six years old, at which point she decided to sleep in her own room. Jason did the same at exactly the same age, and that was the end of our "family bed."

activities and time with your older children will help them to feel connected to you, safe, and less likely to be resentful of the baby getting most of your attention in those first weeks and months.

Co-Sleeping and the Family Bed

If you have a family bed, I suggest having a pallet in the room for the older child when the new baby arrives, as sleeping in the bed with the baby can be dangerous. If you do need them to sleep in the bed with you, have them sleep on the other side of one of the parents and not next to the baby. It's best to make this adjustment to a pallet before the baby arrives to lessen the association of rejection from the bed with the baby's arrival. You can get them excited about a transition to a "big" bed of their own and reassure them that after the new baby is more developed, they can rejoin the family bed if they like.

Friend and Extended Family Preparation

I believe it is vitally important that in the first few days with your newborn the only people in your world are you, your partner, and your child(ren). The first few days are such a crucial time for bonding with the immediate family, and if you have a multitude of visitors, you will be distracted from your most important job. Your baby will need you to give the full attention of your heart and spirit to your relationship, welcoming them to the family. The first few days are sacred. Your baby will need the constancy of your love and attention in these early days. I suggest preparing your friends and family for this. Let them know you will not have many visitors in the first three days, but after that you cannot wait to have them there. I will talk much more about this in *Volume II*.

Reserve visitation rights in those first few days to people of the utmost importance in your life and severely limit the number of these visits, if not foregoing them altogether. Your extended family and friends will have a lifetime to get to know your new, sweet baby. They can wait a few more days.

If you do invite people to visit you in these first few days, make the visits short and limit them as much as you can. I highly suggest you do not have three different two-to three-hour visits. It may feel like you want to see these people, or you know they will not understand asking them to wait (like your parents), but these visits can be so very overwhelming, taxing, and can seriously interrupt the bonding process. Carefully plan what is right for you and your family and make sure you advocate what is best for you and the new baby.

Alternatively, it may be that you have a difficult birth, or a long and exhausting pre-labor, and you call on someone to come and help you a few hours after the birth. Sometimes you and your partner may absolutely have to sleep after the birth for a few hours and it's nice to know that there's someone you can call on at the drop of a hat who will come and help cook, clean, and take care of other things while you and your partner rest and focus on the baby, healing, and bonding. Identify the people you would trust to step in this way and ask them now if they are willing to serve in this role, if necessary, when the time comes.

An Advocate

With a home birth, if complications arise, your midwife may need to transport you to the hospital ASAP, and you cannot have the people around you freaking out. People in the room must be able to be calm and respond effectively to the situation. Keep this in mind when you are deciding whom to invite to the birth.

You may find that some people you thought would be wonderful end up not behaving as you'd expected, or don't have your best interest in mind. You may need them to leave. Work out ahead of time who will take charge of protecting your sacred environment and who will escort anyone out of the room who isn't adhering to the baby and mother's best interests. It's best if the partner can be taking care of mom and baby; find another helper from your

birthing team who can serve to shepherd no-longer desired guests from the birthing environment. It doesn't matter if you're in the hospital or at home. This is too sacred a moment for people to not behave themselves or to try to take over and be in control of a situation that is not theirs to control.

Boundaries and Difficult Situations

The time to have difficult conversations and to set boundaries with those who may have expectations that differ from yours is *now*. You must have these conversations before you go into labor. I have counseled many women whose mothers, for example, expected to be present for the birth, expected to be able to live text the birth milestones to their friends ("Okay, she's at six centimeters! ... Okay, seven centimeters now! ... Oh, my goodness, she's pushing!"), and expected to have the role that mothers whose daughters have hospital births often play. If you want them to do this, that's great, let them. But if you do not, it is crucial you communicate this beforehand, so they know your wants, needs, and your expectations of them during your birth.

Some mothers of mothers-to-be may feel like not getting to play this role isn't fair to them. Well, it's not about them. It's about you. Hold this boundary firmly. You deserve to have the best possible birth experience for you and your baby.

I'll say it again. Birth is not a spectator sport. You do not need an audience. You need assistants and assistance.

Parents often still see their adult children as just children, and it is very hard for them to let that go. At some point you have got to stand up for yourself. I find it's very helpful to start by reminding them that they want what's best for you. I recommend saying something like, "I know you love me more than anything, and you want what's best for me, and so I know you'll understand when I tell you that I'm going to decide who is in the birthing room, and I'm sorry, but it doesn't include you. I need to do what makes me feel most comfortable in this situation. I love you, and I appreciate you so much. I know you're going to understand that this is what I need. Your support means so much to me. I can't wait to see you and have your help after our baby is here." Your parents weren't present for the conception; it's okay if they're not there for the birth.

A lot of mothers of pregnant women won't view their desire to be at the birth as selfish, but as supportive. They may or may not be accurate in their perception. Only you know if your mom is truly supportive in word and deed. If she is not, I suggest you let her know that she's not welcome at the birth (use the technique in the paragraph above) and then quickly turn the conversation to when you *will* want her company and when you *will* let her know about your joyous bundle. Promise her she can meet your baby so soon after the birth, but that you are keeping the birthing room quiet and intimate.

Going Radio Silent

Another scenario involves family members who are used to being in very close contact with you. When parents-to-be don't have these conversations in advance, family members who are usually in close contact can really freak out. They're usually already a little weirded out by the fact that you're giving birth outside of a hospital—if this is your plan.

If you are someone who is in contact with your family via text or phone all the time, when you go into labor and that communication drops off, they may worry. Some *really* worry. I have known adult women whose mothers have called the police to report a missing person if they were out of contact with their daughter for more than several hours.

You should address this ahead of time. "I know this may be difficult for you, but this isn't about what you think and what you want, this is about me right now. I need you to know ahead of time that you may not hear from me during my labor because I will be focusing all my energy on my baby. It is so important that I am not spending energy worrying about anyone else's thoughts or feelings. I do not want you to worry if I do not reach out or respond to messages or calls. I promise you'll be one of the first people we call, and I will let you know as soon as we are ready to communicate about the birth and have you come over, but I need you to trust me. I promise we'll contact you if anything gets dicey, but I don't expect it to. You have to believe that when I go into labor, no news is good news ... until our baby arrives, and I promise you'll be the first person we call."

People who are used to knowing everything about you can grow really concerned when the birth plan isn't explained ahead of time. I once had a family who was not prepared and not invited to the birth. When their daughter didn't respond to their messages, they called 911 and told the dispatcher that something horrible was happening. The ambulance arrived, and the EMTs checked on the situation, saw that everything was under control, and left.

But it goes to show that this is an emotionally charged time, and some people get a little crazed if they haven't heard the updates they mistakenly expected to or if they think it's taking too long. Please be sure to prepare your loving family in advance so they know what to expect, for your sake and theirs.

Continue to Avoid Negativity

I don't want you to use up all of your reserve energy before your labor even starts. This applies to mental energy, too. Know that with every passing day it becomes more and more likely that the next day will be the day that your baby arrives. It WILL happen. Don't allow yourself to become sucked into a never-ending loop of negative *what if* thoughts. Focus on your positive affirmations and trust the process.

Partners, Help Now

 Partners, here are ways you can actively support your pregnant woman.

You can bolster her spirit.

- "I'm so grateful for everything you've done this year." (Give her examples.)

- "I know it has to be wild going through so many changes, but I want you to know, you're incredibly beautiful to me."

- "I'm so excited for how we're going to grow together as parents. I'm so excited to see you be a mom."

You can help her rest.

- "What can I do today to help us get ready for the baby?"

- "I'm taking our older kids to the park for a few hours today so you can get a nap."

You can support her nutritional needs.

- "What are you hungry for right now? What can I make you?"

- "I made your breakfast smoothie for you."

You can help her prepare for birth.

- "Are you ready to do our breathing exercises?"

- "Let's practice squatting."

- "I want to help you. Let's do a relaxation exercise."

- "I can't imagine what you're feeling. You seem like you have it all together, but is there anything you're anxious about? I'm here for you. I can just listen."

Maybe you feel weird taking suggestions right out of a book. Here's the thing. It doesn't matter where you get your ideas. What matters most right now is that your woman feels supported, and that means checking in with her many times a day, in many ways. She doesn't care where you get your inspiration, and it will mean the world to her that you take the time to sprinkle her with love and affection. What she is doing is so hard. Help her.

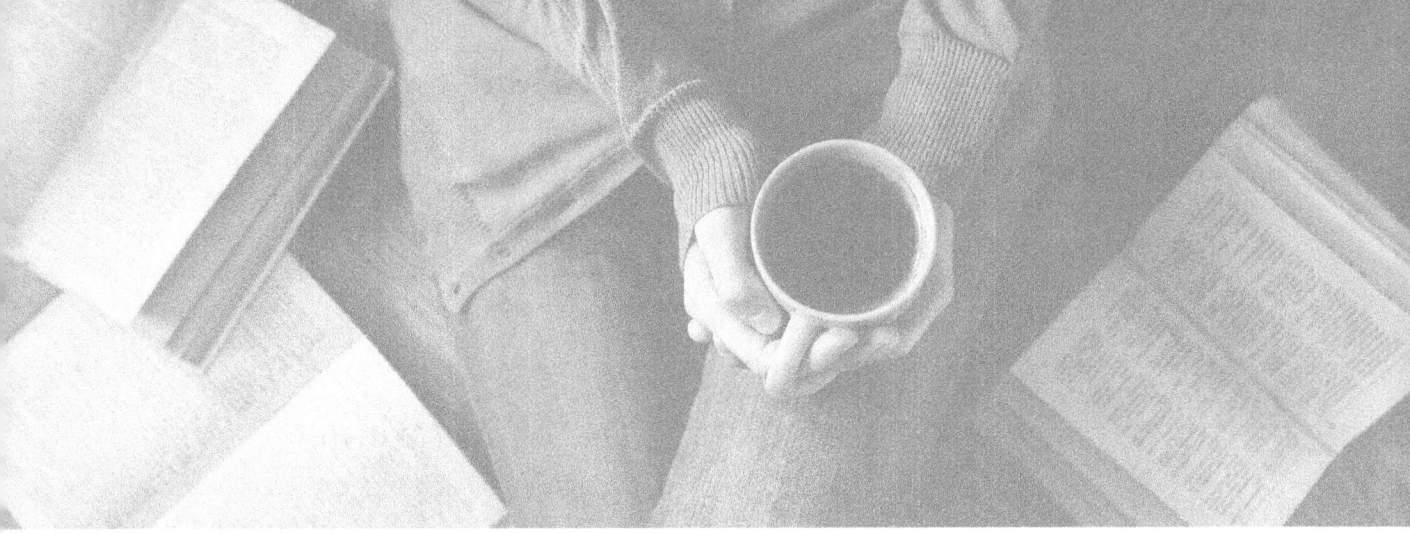

Knowledge

The time to catch up on your reading is *now*.

I don't say this to scare you, but there are some women who have a period while pregnant or skip a period altogether, and this can result in your due date calculation being as much as a month off. I want you to prepare early, so if you are among those whose due date was miscalculated, you're still ready for what's coming. Read ahead, take childbirth classes, and prepare in advance.

What's Going on in My Body?

Ripening and Softening

Your body is growing, ripening, and softening for birth. You're likely having more contractions and the beginnings of cervical effacement and dilation. As you reach the final weeks of your pregnancy, the baby may come down in the pelvis. This is sometimes called *lightening* or *dropping*; I refer to it as *engagement*. This doesn't happen to everyone prior to labor, but it does for many. You may feel a difference when the baby comes down into the pelvis— or not. There is more pressure on your bladder, and you'll have to pee a whole lot more. Your pubic bone may bother you when the baby's head is down against it. You may suddenly find you can breathe more easily. You may experience less indigestion, because the baby has moved down, and your stomach is not being as pushed up into your esophagus as it was before.

Most of the discomforts of pregnancy in the third trimester are due to the increasing size of the baby and the simultaneous softening of the mother's body. There is not as much resistance in your muscles, tendons, skin, and tissues to hold things as they get heavier and heavier.

Sometimes at this point this softening can cause more visual disturbances in your eyesight and more trouble with gag reflexes and swallowing. Your feet are softening as well, so not only do they spread and possibly your shoes do not fit, but you may also experience some foot soreness. Walking for exercise may become challenging (whereas swimming will provide relief).

Preparing to Breastfeed

Your breasts are getting bigger, and toward the end of your pregnancy you may start seeing colostrum produced in small to moderate to large amounts. Colostrum is your baby's first food; it's what is present in your body prior to your milk coming in. It looks like yellowish liquid, and it often forms crusty spots on the nipples. It has sugars, protein, and fats in it, and can be a breeding ground for bacteria. If you do have this production of colostrum prior to birth, you want to pay particular attention to keeping your nipples and those little areas of indentation on the nipple very clean.

Also, by the time they give birth, most women have as much as half again the amount of blood circulating in their bloodstream as they had before pregnancy. This happens in part so you can lose blood with the birth and not be negatively affected, and in part to prepare your body for breastfeeding. Milk is made from blood! I'll tell you more about that in *Volume II*.

Your Baby is Growing

Your baby is getting bigger, too. Up to 28 weeks the baby is usually three pounds or less, but by Week 32 most babies are around 4 to 4-½ pounds, and just get bigger every day from there. This puts a lot of pressure on the pubic bone, the bladder, and the cervix, and sometimes sex feels different because there's more going on in the pelvis than before.

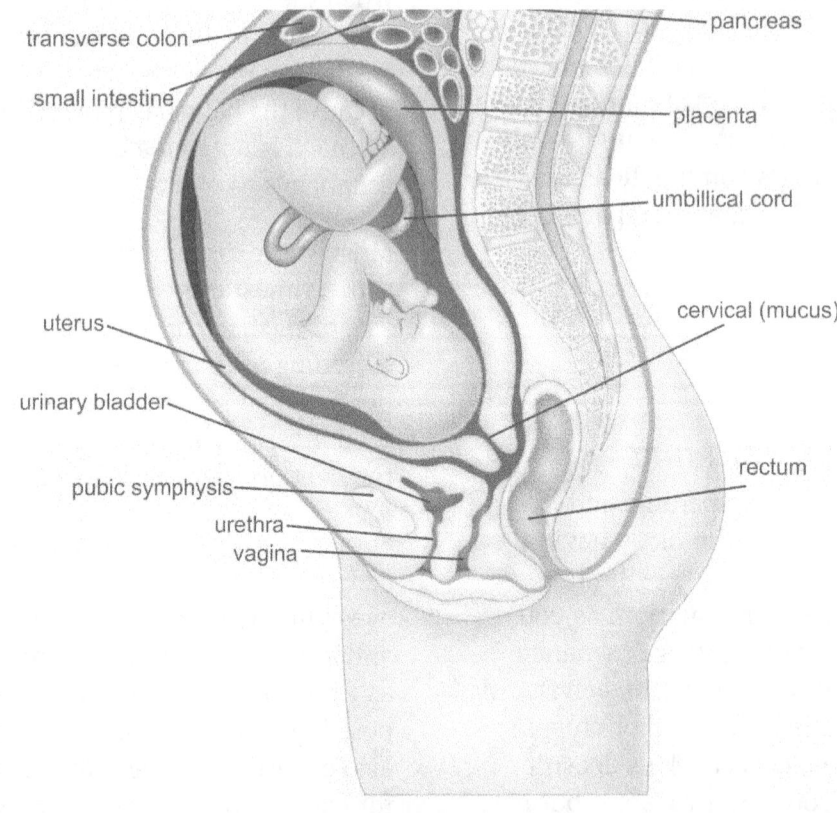

transverse colon
small intestine
pancreas
placenta
umbillical cord
uterus
urinary bladder
cervical (mucus)
pubic symphysis
urethra
vagina
rectum

Full-Term Baby in Utero

Why am I Peeing so Much?

The bladder is right behind the pubic bone and the uterus sits on top of the bladder. This applies pressure to the bladder, which makes you feel like you need to urinate. As your baby grows, the uterus pushes against your bladder, and this is why you have less and less capacity to hold your urine and must go to the bathroom more frequently. Your poor bladder, which previously had plenty of space, is overcome by the uterus and no longer has the same room it had prior to you becoming pregnant.

This changes as the uterus rises in the abdominal cavity in the second trimester and then gets worse again at the end of the pregnancy when the baby's head (typically) presses against it. In the following illustration you can clearly see why you may suddenly find you're visiting the restroom more and more often.

Handling the Common Discomforts and Complications of the Third Trimester

High Blood Pressure

I recommend herbs to my clients with high blood pressure in the last three to four weeks of their pregnancy. Talk with your midwife about taking these if this applies to you. I advise my clients to take them and then try to take a nap, because usually—especially the first time—there's a really good chance they'll make you feel sleepy. My advice is to take a dropper full of skullcap tincture and a dropper full of passionflower tincture. You can put it in a few ounces of water or juice and shoot it back. I suggest taking this before eating your big meal at midday. Always work with your midwife when taking herbs.

Don't Cross Your Legs When Sitting

Many chiropractors say that to prevent back and hip problems in pregnancy, refrain from sitting cross-legged from Week 32 on.

Another tip is to lighten the weight in your handbag to help reduce any pulling on your shoulders.

Swelling

The number one cause of swelling I've seen is excess salt in your diet. It's overwhelmingly at fault—I'd estimate 95 percent of the time. Big culprits are Indian food, Asian food, sometimes Mexican food, barbecue, chips, bacon … Avoid salty snacks. Read the label on processed foods you consume and avoid foods high in sodium.

To prevent swelling or make it go down, you want to drink a lot of water, use compression socks, elevate your feet, and rest. Get a handle on it and then manage it going forward. You can also lay on the floor with your legs up against a wall to encourage blood flow.

If you get really swollen, use liquid chlorophyll. It works as a blood builder and body purifier. It helps with excessive body odor too. It's a colon cleanser (though it will color your poop slightly green). Take 2 tablespoons five times a day to get the diuretic effect. I suggest you mix 10 tablespoons in 1 quart of spearmint tea with honey. Keep it in the fridge and drink 20 percent of the quart five times a day. It is an amazing and safe diuretic.

Take your rings off at night before bed. You can get a little too much salt in during the day, and your hands can swell while you're asleep to the point where you can't remove your ring. If that happens, I suggest you go to the ER, have the ring cut off, and then it can be repaired. Prevent this by not wearing your rings at night. If your hands get too swollen, you won't be able to wear your rings during the day either. At this point many women put their wedding ring on a chain around their neck. You can wear it on your finger again after the birth.

Herpes

Compared to the second trimester, herpes outbreaks tend to happen more frequently in the third trimester. It's very stressful for your body to be this pregnant and have the baby taking so much out of you. Oftentimes you're a lot hotter physically, there's more blood coursing through your veins, there's more friction because the labia can be swollen, and your legs and feet may swell as well. There's a lot to deal with.

Some doctors recommend taking Valtrex at the end of the pregnancy for a whole month before (and until) you go into labor to prevent herpes. I think eating carefully, taking care of yourself, resting, and maintaining your healthy living is a better plan than taking drugs. You have to make your own choice here, but it's not what I recommend to my clients. Try an alternative way. If you have a prescription for Valtrex, keep it handy, and if you start to develop an outbreak while already implementing the rest of the mitigating actions, start taking it then. Again, consult your care provider.

If you have a really serious case of herpes and have frequent outbreaks, taking Valtrex during the end of your pregnancy is probably a good idea. Most of my clients that have herpes have very infrequent outbreaks during pregnancy even though they have had herpes for a long time. In these cases, I think it's safe to do other management techniques. But if you have a real problem with it and experience frequent outbreaks, take the Valtrex.

Glucose Screening

At 28–32 Weeks, glucose screening is a wonderful idea to make sure that a woman does not have or is not developing gestational diabetes (GD). Untreated GD can damage the mother's vascular system, including the placenta, and create a very big baby due to the presence of large amounts of sugar in the mother's bloodstream. The way doctors traditionally test you is by doing a glucose tolerance test. This is where they take a fasting blood glucose measurement, have you drink an orange- or cola-flavored sugar drink with 100 grams of sugar in it, and then check your glucose levels one and two hours later. Most of my clients do not eat a lot of sugar in general, and this large influx of sugar can be dangerous, very unpleasant, and overwhelming. Years ago, I decided it's not a healthy way to check for GD.

The way I test for GD is to have my clients come to the clinic at Week 28. I take a drop of blood from their finger and check their fasting blood sugar on a machine in my office. They then eat a good, big breakfast with protein, fats, complex carbs, and a small amount of simple carbs, for example, an omelet with toast and jelly or breakfast tacos with a small glass of juice. Two hours after they finish eating, they return for a second blood sugar test. This is an excellent way to screen women who are healthy, eat well, and have not exhibited any symptoms of GD, such as spilling sugar in their urine. If the numbers resulting from this test are concerning, I have the mother work very hard to reduce the amount of carbs (sugars) in her diet and then we retest one week later. If that is also abnormal, I send them to the lab for a glucose tolerance test. Your provider will work with you to respond to a GD diagnosis. I'll tell you more about how I handle this later.

Pregnancy/Mommy Brain

Pregnancy brain is a real thing. So, you're entitled to some leeway. You get a bunch of get-out-of-jail-free cards when it comes to running behind or being forgetful. It becomes much more serious in the third trimester. Again, your body is working very, very hard to maintain the pregnancy, the growth of the baby, and all of your metabolic needs. If you nourish yourself emotionally, spiritually, and physically, and get enough rest, it will help a little bit, but you still might want to write everything down and check your list regularly to prevent serious things from being forgotten.

 Partners, you need to be prepared for this as a possibility and be as supportive as you can. It's hard to not be your sharpest self.

Wanting Your Partner to Understand What You're Going Through

 I was on a podcast recently where the host told me she wanted to buy her husband a 50-pound pregnancy outfit. She wanted him to wear it throughout the day and lift weights in it like she did, drive the car, hold their older child all day and night, and sleep in it like she had to. She wanted to know if it would be worth the money; would it help him understand what she was going through?

Doing something like that would certainly bring awareness, but the fact is, it's not the same experience at all. Your partner isn't designed to give birth and you are. Women actually make it look easy, and it's not. There's so much more going on, so much more that you're feeling and experiencing than just extra weight. Everything about your body and brain is changing. His

Penelope: I often find myself in a room and have absolutely no idea why I am there, other than knowing I was supposed to do something or get something there. I heard somewhere that when you pass through a doorframe, the brain erases the short-term memory. Since then, when I have one of those momnesia moments, I go back to the last door frame I walked through. Most of the time I instantly recollect what I was doing, and the second time I go back to get or do whatever it is I was doing or getting, my brain does a better job of holding onto its objective. Maybe this will help you with those momnesia moments, too.

understanding has to come from empathy. You are being remade just as you are making your baby. His understanding has to come from compassion, awareness, and communication, all those things. You need to listen to each other and hear what each other is saying, because you'll never recreate for him what it feels like to be pregnant.

Partners, it will be helpful if you can adopt a mindset of service. I had one father tell me that he realized, as he was up super early in the morning getting food ready for the day for himself and his pregnant wife, this was his future. While his wife's body was literally occupied, his body also needed to change, to act in support of his growing family. His body was also not his own. He had shifted into a place of service. He saw his service to his wife during pregnancy as preparation for serving her and the baby once the baby arrived. He embraced and welcomed that role. I think this is a beautiful attitude. Too often it is only our mothers who set aside so much of themselves in service of the family. If everyone were to do it, we would all retain a greater portion of our sense of self because the load would be more equally shared.

How Big Will My Baby Be?

An 8-½-pound baby is normal. Fifty percent of my clients' babies are 7–9 pounds, 25 percent are 9+ pounds, and only 25 percent of the babies weigh less than 7 pounds. I have found that babies often weigh close to what their fathers weighed at birth, though nutritional support throughout your pregnancy also plays a tremendous role in ensuring a healthy birth weight. How much weight

you gain does affect the size of the baby. As I've mentioned, if you gain a lot of weight (especially at the end) you are more likely to have a bigger baby.

28-32 Weeks

Belly Support

It's a great idea to get a belly support system at about 28–30 weeks depending on how big you are. I highly recommend that you go to a maternity and baby store and try several on, because they're all different. Find the one that's most comfortable for you and will accommodate your growing belly. You are going to get a lot bigger before this is over. It will help you to sit better and will support your abdomen, keeping it from pulling on your back muscles and helping to avoid back pain, which will in turn allow you to rest more deeply. It also helps to keep from separating your pubic symphysis. Wear it loosely enough so it is supportive, not constricting. This is not a girdle; Do not use it to constrict, it should be a gentle, helping hand. You can use this after the birth as well to help your uterus return to its normal position.

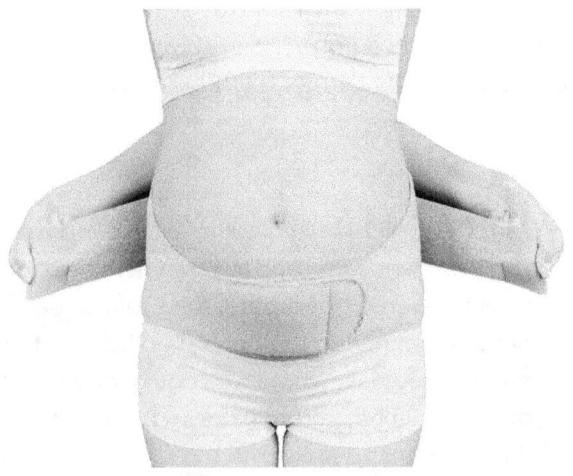

Belly Support System

Many insurance companies will now pay for a belly support band. Check to see if your insurance plan will, as this can save you some money. You might also check to see if they will pay for a breast pump at this time and purchase one concurrently to save on paperwork.

Childbirth Classes

Childbirth classes can really enhance your understanding of the birth experience. Before I required my clients take my childbirth classes, I found many of them foundered and were really scared during labor and birth, and many had zero idea of what to do for their baby and themselves after birth. Knowledge is power, and that power is incredibly helpful in the birthing room as well as throughout the journey of parenting.

I suggest you start childbirth classes at 28–32 weeks. Earlier than that, and there is a good chance you won't remember the information. Later than that may not leave you with enough time to learn, absorb, and implement the information.

If you have the option, I suggest taking classes in the morning, when your brain is fresh and you're more likely to retain the information. Take notes to reinforce important parts. Your midwife may recommend classes in your area or may provide her own classes. Here is a summary of what my birthing classes cover, so you have an idea of the breadth of information that birthing classes can provide:

- **Breathing Exercises and Relaxation Techniques**
- **Anatomy and Physiology**

- **Stages and Phases of Labor and Birth**
- **Preparing for the Birth**—gathering supplies, packing for the birth, sterilization for home birth, preparing home, family, kids, pets, and work.
- **About Birth**—recognizing labor, what it feels like, what it is, when to call the midwife, what to do as you go into labor, when you're in labor, the partner's role in labor, midwife's approach to the birth sans a birth plan; complications, what to do if any of the following occur.
  - Your waters break early.
  - Labor won't start.
  - There is meconium staining.
  - Labor isn't progressing.
  - Baby's heart tones drop.
  - There is bleeding in labor.
  - The placenta won't come out.
  - The woman tears seriously.
  - The woman's blood pressure is too high.
  - The baby isn't breathing.
  - The baby inhales meconium or amniotic fluid.
  - When a transfer to the hospital would occur.

It helps the parent to know that their midwife has a plan for all these possibilities.

- **Postpartum for Mom**—bonding, birth of placenta, initiating breastfeeding, and staying down for two full weeks.
- **Postpartum for Baby**—breastfeeding and baby care for the first 24 hours and the following days and weeks including diapering, sleeping, early infant wellness, weird but normal things with your baby,

what to look for that is not normal, as well as preventing thrush, colic, and jaundice.

- **Raising Kids**—education, discipline, creating cooperative children, creating communicative children, creating spiritual children, family planning, sexuality, infant nutrition, extended weaning, extended breastfeeding, when to start solids, staying out of the pediatrician's office and when to go, immunization, circumcision, and keeping the relationship alive.

- Exposure therapy via watching **videos of live births**.

- **Sudden Childbirth**—a guide for partners on what to do if the baby comes before your midwife does.

- **Review** of the most important information from all of the preceding classes.

I have been teaching childbirth classes for more than 45 years and have included the most important information that is essential to improve my clients' comfort and informed choice. If someone comes up to you in a labor that is not progressing well and says, "Well I think the baby got in there a little asynclitic, and probably was not very well molded, and the cervix was not ripe or effaced or engaged, and possibly the mid-pelvis is a little snug," you do not want to have to figure out what that means while you are in labor. It helps so much to have a baseline, so you're comfortable with what's happening, and it's not a big scary unknown. If you have only had hospital births and are now having a home birth, you still need classes to prepare you for it. It is really different.

Talk with your midwife at your next appointment about childbirth classes and do yourself the favor of signing up for them.

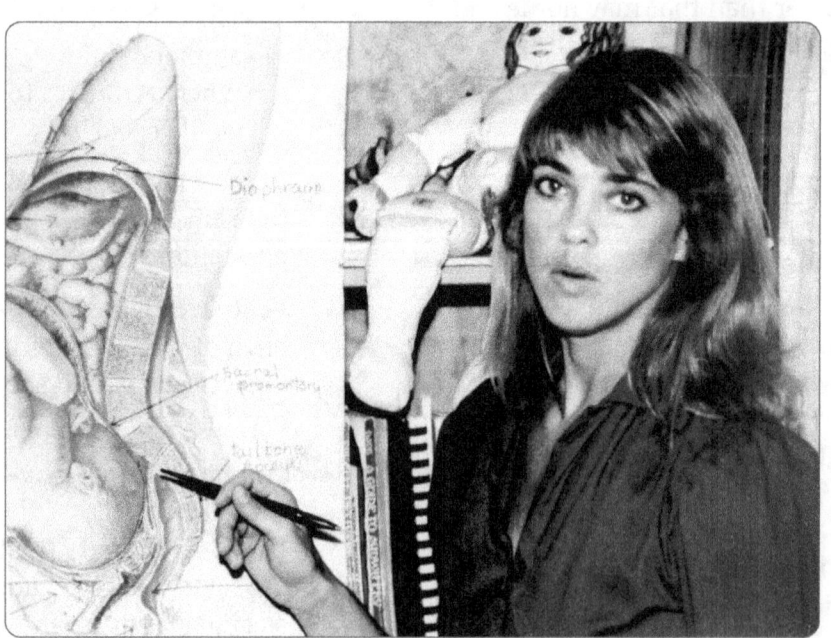

MariMikel Teaching Childbirth Classes in the Early Years of Her Midwifery Practice

Penelope: I signed up for and attended the childbirth classes at my local hospital where I was planning to give birth. They were extremely helpful and informative, not only about the birth process, but also about the hospital itself, which was useful, given that I would be laboring there. For one session they brought in a breastfeeding expert, and I'm so grateful they did. I learned so much in that one hour and it made all the difference in my breastfeeding success.

There are two other things I remember about that class in particular. One is that I was a single mother-to-be, and I was the only single person in the room. I did not have a support person with me. I invited my sister, who had followed me to Austin, to join me for one of the classes thinking that she might be good to have with me in the birthing room. The class she attended happened to be the one on complications and interventions, with very graphic pictures and descriptions. When the teacher described an episiotomy, my sister got up from her chair in horror and fled the room. So, I learned I would need someone else beside me in the birthing room.

The second thing I remember is that the teacher noticed I was alone. She pulled me aside after class one day, after she'd seen my sister flee, and asked me if she could introduce me to a doula friend of hers. She said the woman was like the sweetest grandmother that everyone needed to have, and that she thought this woman could really help me with my pregnancy and birth.

I didn't really know what a doula was, but I accepted her help, and met her friend, who turned out to be an angel among humans. I hired her and she was an immense blessing to me throughout the end of my pregnancy, labor, and birth. Knowing I was single and without insurance, she also charged a fee that, in retrospect, was way too low for everything she provided. Single mommas, especially if your besties aren't cut out to be your birth partner, HIRE A DOULA.

During my second pregnancy, my husband and I took a labor preparation class and that served as a good reminder and preparation for our second child's labor and delivery. One of the things that's lovely about smaller classes like that one, which was limited to six couples, is that you build relationships with your fellow pregnant classmates and their spouses. It has been 14 years since I took that class, but I still maintain friendships with some of those mommas.

I don't believe we took classes for our third child. I had three babies in five years and by the time we got to the third one we kind of felt like pros.

Aleah: When I got pregnant with my first baby, I had already been an apprentice midwife with MariMikel for more than five years, had taught childbirth classes for three years, and had read a huge portion of the birth and labor books in her lending library. I also had received a lot of training during my college education to become a social worker that centered around the development of children and models of healthy parenting. I felt very prepared to say the least.

Honestly, there was a big part of me that wanted to rebel and did not want to spend the many hours taking childbirth classes. I was working full-time at a very emotionally and physically taxing and stressful job. I didn't have a lot of time to give to myself or to the pregnancy.

But I knew that even though I had all this knowledge stored within me, my husband did not, and watching the classes on his own was not something I could ask of him. I knew it would be beneficial for us to take them together. They would give us some time to focus on preparing for the labor, birth, and welcoming of our new baby. My husband was not a novice when it came to birth. We had been together for almost 13 years, and he knew more than most men who have never had a baby before about labor and birth, as well as what a home birth entails, thanks to his close proximity to my mom and to me while I was her assistant midwife.

Even though we were in some ways "more prepared" than other first-time parents, we were both so glad we took the time to attend the classes and felt empowered, both with knowledge and in our partnership. It helped us to feel confident in our ability to face this experience together without fear, to surrender, and to trust the process.

No matter what route you take, I highly suggest you taking the time to empower yourself with knowledge through childbirth classes, with reading, and doing the breathing and relaxation techniques. It really can make a difference.

Babyproofing

By the time your newborn arrives, you want to ensure that your house is already safely set up to receive them. The best time to do all babyproofing in your home is before the baby is born. Ideally, start your babyproofing a few months before you are due to get it out of the way. Some babyproofing may take time and you don't want to have to be doing it with a small infant. It can also be easy to forget things during those first postpartum months when you are in the throes of this huge life transition and may not be getting a lot of sleep. So, I highly suggest getting it done beforehand so you can check it off your list.

Some of these items might feel a little premature, but your newborn will be capable of interacting with their environment before you know it and it will be a stress reliever to have this already crossed off your list of "Things to Do" as new parents.

Once your baby starts to crawl (around six to ten months), you'll need to do a second baby proofing sweep to make sure the house is safe for a baby on the move.

Below you will find a list of the most common baby proofing tips:

All Over the House!

- Be familiar with the settings on the hot water heater and make sure it is set to 120°F or lower, so your baby does not get scalded by someone accidentally filling the tub with water that is too hot.

- Make sure all fire alarms are in working order and that you have a UL listed carbon monoxide detector—at least one of each on every floor of the home.

- Cover electrical outlets.

- Keep all cleaning products behind locked *upper* cabinet doors. This way, even if your baby figures out how to get past the safety latches, they still won't be able to get to these typically toxic products.

- Remove heavy objects from tables so your baby can't pull them down on themselves or knock them off and cause injury.

- Block off staircases and rooms you don't want baby exploring with baby gates.

- Examine your windows. Tie up blind cords so they are out of reach or invest in cord safety wraps that attach to the wall and keep the cord safely up and out of baby's reach.

- Make sure all area rugs have non-skid material on the bottom.

- Cushion the corners of tables and other sharp edges in your home. (**Tip**: pool noodles are often excellent for this.)

- Fireplace safety—there are many ways you can ensure fireplace safety but one of the best is to install a baby gate in front of any fireplace you have. There are many different styles of baby gates; you may be able to find some that match your décor.

- Be careful with any water bowls for pets—any container with even a few inches of standing water poses a drowning hazard for small children.

- Check the house and yard for poisonous plants and move them out of baby's reach.

Penelope: My husband and I were chilling downstairs while our 9-month-old was asleep in his crib upstairs in our room, or so we thought. Suddenly we heard a loud sound, like a boulder falling and hitting the floor, and then a moment later we heard crying. We raced upstairs. My son had thrown himself over the railing of the crib. He was fine but do take this advice seriously.

Baby's Nursery

- Crib Safety—One of the most important things to ensure with the crib is that it's kept at the right height for their age and development. The older they are, the lower down the crib rail should be. When they are older, they can pull themselves up and potentially fall from a higher height. Do not have any bumpers, blankets, or toys in the crib, so there is no chance of them getting tangled up or suffocating.

- Check that none of the crib slats are more than 2-⅜ inches apart, and that all the bolts and screws are tight. Make sure there are no gaps between the mattress and crib.

- Place baby wipes and supplies where you can reach them from the changing table, but your baby can't.

- Place a thick rug below the changing table. Falls happen.

- Position the crib away from windows, heaters, lamps, wall decoration, and cords.

Test Small Objects

- Use a toilet paper tube—if an item can fit through it, then it's a choking hazard and should not be around your baby. Look around your house for small objects—if you have older kids especially, then you have to be careful about small toys and things like LEGO. Those should stay in an older child's bedroom or be safely put away where the baby cannot reach them.

Kitchen

- While cooking, turn the handles of pots and pans toward the back of the stove so they don't get knocked off and your baby can't reach them.

- Secure cleaning supplies and items such as knives, scissors, dish soap, etc. in drawers with locks or latches or on high counters or shelves.

- Use placemats instead of tablecloths. Tablecloths are easy to pull and can send glasses and sharp silverware falling to the floor.

- Secure the refrigerator and/or freezer door with a safety latch.

- Childproof the oven—The oven is one of the most dangerous things in the house due to it radiating heat when in use, as well as the gas or electricity that powers it. Even modern ovens with heat resistant glass can still pose a threat to young children, so you can do a few things to make them safer, including getting an oven guard, protecting the knobs, and keeping a lock on the door so it can't be opened by children.

- If your stove allows, consider removing the knobs and placing them out of baby's reach, especially if baby can turn the knobs and accidentally turn on the gas or burners. Many newer stoves have knobs that are made to be baby safe, but yours may not. Check in advance.

- Many kids enjoy playing with child-safe cups, bowls, pots, and pans. Consider designating a lower cabinet with items your baby *can* safely play with as you are cooking.

Bathroom

- Use a safety latch on the toilet—this will also help toys from getting thrown into a cool, new "pool."

- Make sure all cabinets that have any items the baby should not be getting into have baby locks on them.

- Make sure to keep hair dryers, curling irons, and other corded bathroom accessories away from the edge of the counter. Cords hanging down are tempting!

- Keep bathroom doors closed.

Living Room

- Mount larger furniture to the wall, if possible. As your little one pulls to stand up, they will reach for whatever's nearest to them. Make sure what they're pulling on is as sturdy as possible.

- When guests come over, place purses and bags high up where your baby can't get into them.

Laundry Room

- Keep laundry detergent and other toxic or dangerous materials on high shelves and out of children's reach.

Create a Safe Play Spot

- To make sure your baby is safe while you are making dinner or tending to chores, create a safe place for them with either an activity center that they are seated in or within a play pen area where they have safe toys that can keep them entertained while you tend to those things you need to do.

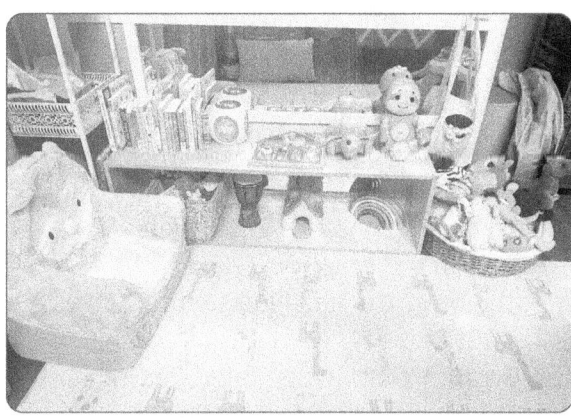

A Safe Place for Baby to Play

Eight to Twelve Weeks Before Your Due Date

To recap, here is a summary of what I'm asking you to pay attention to at this stage in your pregnancy. Refer to the corresponding section for complete details.

- Keep up your vitamins, healthy eating, and fluid intake.

- Buy and start to wear a belly support system.

- Start taking a childbirth class with your partner.

- Babyproof all over the house.

- Clean or change air conditioning filters. (Do this again right before the birth).

- Keep up your exercise, hydration, and spiritual practices.

Weeks 32 to 34
Do What You Can and Rest

By this time in your pregnancy, you probably are not feeling as well as you did during your second trimester. The halcyon days are over. Maybe your back hurts from the new demands on it. Maybe your feet or ankles are swollen. Maybe you're just achy or having trouble sleeping. You might be starting to feel the contractions your uterus has been performing since you became pregnant.

Give yourself permission to do what you can and to rest when you need to. Keep exercising, especially swimming, which will help you feel weightless and provide relief in addition to muscle tone and stamina. Exercise in the earlier part of the day while you still have strength. You do want to keep building up muscle now, while your body is primed to do so, because once your baby is here, I'm going to ask that you take a break from exercise for a little while.

Education and Reading List

This is a good time to really educate yourself. Parenting is such a tough job; it helps to learn how to do it more easily. Most people parent the way that they were parented, but you can improve on the model. I believe that reading a lot about children and their development is important. Our biggest goal as parents should be that our children are better people, parents, and partners than we are.

There are also a lot of good books on pregnancy info, preparation for birth, breathing and relaxation, pushing techniques, labor techniques, and coaching techniques. Please do a lot of reading as you deserve to have as many ideas, theories, and techniques as possible, so you have lots of choices for your own birth and the parenting journey beyond. My favorite book recommendations are listed in Appendix F.

Hypnobirthing

While there are several breathing classes out there, I want to call attention to Hypnobirthing because it does such an excellent job in helping women address their fears. Hypnobirthing is a childbirth preparation method that uses relaxation, visualization, and self-hypnosis to help women have a more positive and comfortable birth experience. It takes a holistic approach and proports that by changing the way we think about childbirth, we can change the way we experience it.

Hypnobirthing classes typically cover a variety of topics, including relaxation and visualization techniques, self-hypnosis, and other methods of coping with the sensations of labor.

Hypnobirthing is not a magic bullet, and it will not guarantee a pain-free birth. However, it *can* help women to feel more relaxed and confident during childbirth, which can lead to a more positive experience overall.

You can find hypnobirthing books and classes online to learn more about the techniques and how to implement them during your own birth experience. I highly suggest exploring hypnobirthing to be able to add this as another tool within your birth toolkit to help deal with fear and labor pains.

32-Week Exam

Since I implemented vaginal exams at Week 32 in my practice, I have been able to greatly lower the incidence of premature babies. It takes two seconds to check, but the information is vital. If you're at 3 centimeters, 100 percent effaced, and engaged and soft at 32 weeks, you're in trouble. If that is the case, you need to go

---

Penelope: I bought a used Hypnobirthing set on Craigslist for my first pregnancy because I couldn't afford to take the classes. I listened to the recordings religiously and found they really helped with the pain of labor for my first child.

For our second child, I told my husband that I was working with the word "peace" as a trigger for true relaxation. In labor, when I was in the thick of it and struggling, he would place a hand on my shoulder or back and say, "peace." Instantly my whole body would let go of that last bit of tension as it instinctively relaxed even more deeply, and I was able to ride the contraction out without as much pain. I imagine had I actually taken the classes it would have worked even better for me.

on complete bed rest and hopefully you will get that baby to 36 weeks and up to 5-½ or 6-½ pounds. Otherwise, the baby could be premature and end up in the hospital's Neonatal Intensive Care Unit (NICU) for a long time.

On the other hand, I have found women who do not at all seem ready. Their cervix may be very hard, and they are not experiencing the cervical ripening we would like them to have started at this point. If this is the case, there are some tricks to help improve ripening that I suggest to my clients, like applying evening primrose oil directly onto the cervix. The information from the 32-week exam can be very helpful as a guide for you and your midwife. Some women do not want to have exams done, and I totally understand this desire and am always one for following a woman's lead. You need to do what is right for you, but in my practice, I encourage this as a tool for guiding my clients to their ideal, perfect birth.

Prepare for a Hospital Birth

If you are planning a hospital birth, you may be able to have a prenatal appointment with each of the doctors in your OB/GYN's rotation, so you won't have a complete stranger attending your birth. Schedule a brief meeting with each of them to introduce yourself prior to potentially having them deliver your baby. Give each of them a copy of your birth plan and ask them to support your wishes so that you can have your ideal, perfect birth.

Prepare to Cease Working

Some women are really struggling by this point in their pregnancy. They have felt great up until now, but they're working, they are caring for their family, they have got all of their household chores—food, laundry, and bills—and they really need to start cutting back on their hours at work. If you're working a 40-hour week you might need to move to a 36-hour week and then a 32-hour week, so you are not pushing yourself too hard. I want you to remember that when you are pushed, your baby is pushed, and when you are stressed, your baby is stressed. We like to think we are superwomen and can do it all—and sometimes we can—but when we are aware we can't, it is critical to give in and make the necessary adjustments.

I ask that you completely stop work by 38 weeks. Now is the time to finish preparations for that exit from work. You will want to rest in preparation for the birth, and you will want to prepare for life after birth. You will find this time and space beneficial in shifting from your life as a Maiden to the perspective of a Mother.

In addition to making final arrangements with your workplace, you'll want to begin to marshal your resources for the postpartum period.

Keep Up with Childbirth Classes

You should be about halfway through your selected childbirth classes at this time. If you're behind on a video class, now is the time to catch up!

 Remember that the classes are critically important for your partner. Most men do not have a clue as to how to be with a woman in labor. Men's and women's roles in history have been very, very separate.

Throughout history most men were not involved in any way, shape, or form with anything having to do with childbirth—or children for that matter. It's only been very recently that we have formed more egalitarian relationships based on mutual respect, love, and fairness with an equitable division of labor. I have found that childbirth classes really help the partner to learn his role. There are some classes that may be appropriate for older siblings to attend as well. Check with your teacher to see if they recommend a specific class to help prepare your older children for the arrival of your newborn.

It is also incredibly important for your partner to learn the breathing techniques; he needs to learn what's going to happen—especially in a home birth where he's integral to your safety and comfort. Your partner needs to be informed so he can help if something were to happen that required you to be transported to the hospital or if you have a complication to deal with at home. There are lots of other things that he needs to learn as well.

He needs to know how to take care of you and the baby after the birth, because if you are taking care of yourself properly, you are going to be in bed. Everything that has to happen in the initial postpartum period outside of breastfeeding is his job, so getting prepared for this is super important, will help everything to go more smoothly, and will help the postpartum period to be joyful as opposed to stressful. Once you have finished this book, I suggest you move on and read *The Book of Birth Volume II: Your Postpartum Journey through the Fourth Trimester*, because that is right around the corner and there is so much to learn and understand about those first few minutes, hours, days, and months.

Belly Support System

If you haven't yet, I want you to start wearing a belly support system at this time. This will help to prevent pubic bone pain as the symphysis softens. Once your midwife is convinced the baby is in a good position, a belly support system will help to keep the baby in that position and help to prevent the baby from being able to move into a breech or other unhelpful position. The belly support system not only prevents stretch marks and backaches, but also helps to keep your abdominal muscles together while you are growing. It will help your round ligaments to not get pulled, and all of this is beneficial for your general well-being. It is also great to wear after your baby is born for support. You can find my suggestions for purchasing on page 308.

Kick Counts

At 34 Weeks I want you to start doing kick counts. These are designed to keep your awareness centered on the baby's activity. They help you notice if your baby is declining and needs attention. Women who experienced stillbirths have often said in retrospect the baby was moving less and less, but they just weren't conscious of it until they realized that their baby wasn't moving at all.

Kick counts help to make you more mindful, to make you more conscious. If you're not happy with your baby's movement, let your midwife know and ask to have an ultrasound done to see what's going on. I have had literally hundreds of women who were concerned, and I advised them to go in for an ultrasound. In all but a few instances the baby was absolutely fine. In those instances when the baby was not doing well, they had that baby c-sectioned out of there within 45 minutes of the ultrasound, and those babies were absolutely fine as a result. Intervention is brilliant when it's necessary.

It is normal for babies to have periods of stillness where they don't move as much. Also, as your baby grows, they get crowded in there and they just *can't* move as much. They sleep a lot. Your movement can mask their movement—there are lots of things that could make you think your baby's not moving appropriately when they're really doing fine. But if you get worried, call your midwife, and go in and check.

How to Do Kick Counts

Starting at Week 34, you should begin counting the movements of the baby each day. Before then, the baby is small enough that first-time moms especially may not feel their movements and may grow unnecessarily concerned.

You can't just pick a convenient hour and say, "Okay, baby. Start moving." You must pick a time when the baby is active. The baby's most active time is usually after dinner when you are not moving around. After lunch may be another opportune time to feel the baby move, but it's much more difficult to do this if you are also active. Regardless, whenever you feel the baby getting active, stop moving, note the time, and start counting.

In every 24-hour period, there should be a one-hour period during which you can feel the baby move 10 times. You can feel multiple movements in the same instant, for example, a kick and then a jab of an arm, elbow, or foot felt in two different spots would indeed count as two of your ten kick counts for that day. Count a roll as a single movement.

In every 24-hour period, there should be a one-hour period during which you can feel the baby move 10 times.

Your baby's hiccups do not count. Hiccups are characterized by rhythmic movements occurring steadily every few seconds, just like your own hiccups. They come for a few minutes regularly every five to ten seconds and generally you'll feel them repeated in the same spot.

If your baby moves ten times in a few minutes, you're done! You do not have to keep counting.

If the counts do not seem appropriate or if you feel that something is off, then you'll want to call your midwife right away. I did have one instance in the last few years where a woman was significantly past her due date, called me. and said the baby had been moving less. The woman had had an ultrasound a few days prior, but we went in again right away to do a biophysical profile at the perinatologist's office. We found that her water had decreased phenomenally in just a few days, and the baby was indeed struggling. They induced her labor right then, the baby did wonderfully, and everyone was fine. This can be a life-saving practice. At the very least, it will bring you peace of mind. Pay attention, and do your kick counts every single day.

Contractions

You're likely starting to feel the contractions that you've been having throughout your entire pregnancy. They haven't been painful and won't be until you get to the very end of your pregnancy, and for some women they aren't painful until they go into labor. It's different for everybody, but usually about this time you are feeling them come on a little stronger, and sometimes if you're having a contraction when you're walking, you'll actually have to stop and give yourself a moment.

This is part of how your body lets you know the day you'll welcome baby into your life is getting closer and closer. Those contractions are absolutely getting you ready, doing all kinds of important work to prepare your cervix. Use them as reminders to practice your breathing and to relax.

Six Weeks Before Your Due Date

To recap, here is a summary of what I'm asking you to pay attention to at this stage in your pregnancy. Refer to the corresponding section for complete details.

- ☐ Do what you can and rest.
- ☐ Keep up your vitamins, healthy eating, and fluid intake.
- ☐ Start doing kick counts.
- ☐ Begin to prepare to stop working at 38 weeks.
- ☐ Continue your childbirth classes with your partner.
- ☐ Clean or change air conditioning filters. (Do this again right before the birth).
- ☐ Read lots of books.
- ☐ Exercise faithfully.
- ☐ Say your affirmations and spend time in positive visualization and/or prayer every day.
- ☐ Drink your smoothie daily and get 100 grams of protein a day.
- ☐ Swim and practice hands-and-knees poses to keep your baby in the right position.
- ☐ Wear your belly band.

Weeks 35–36

Vaginal Culture & Bacteria Screen

At 35–36 weeks I do a vaginal culture to determine what kind of bacteria are present there. I've found e-coli, strep B, gonorrhea, chlamydia, and of course tons of yeast. If you determine what's present at this stage, you still have time to do something about it.

When I find strep B, the most common culprits are wiping incorrectly, sex from behind, and thong style underwear. The latter is like floss, except it wicks bacteria and other things from the rectum meant to exit the body and introduces it to the vaginal cavity instead. Isn't that lovely? I'm kidding, of course. Anal sex, vaginal sex where the penis rubs against the rectal area, and not paying enough attention to hygiene can also be factors that cause strep B to be present in the vaginal cavity.

If strep B is present, it's impossible to cure it with antibiotics. The only thing that can be done is to give the momma an IV bag with antibiotics during labor in the hopes that the antibiotics will protect the baby. A very small percentage of babies who are exposed to strep B during birth will die from that exposure. I tell you this not to scare you, but to help you understand why providers take this so seriously.

Over the last 20 years, it has been common for as much as 80 percent of women to have an IV with antibiotics administered during labor in the hospital. Of course, everyone who gets a c-section gets antibiotics to ensure there's no infection in the wound. Then anyone who was strep B positive got them, so that was another 25–30 percent of the population. They also administered it to anyone they thought might need it— if someone was in labor too long, if their waters had been broken for more than 12—24 hours, etc. Researchers have found immunologic issues in these babies, from asthma to allergies to failure to be able to properly digest breastmilk.[145]

I definitely don't do this IV treatment for most mothers who test positive for strep B, although I did for 15 years. If my client tests positive for strep B, they have had ruptured membranes for more than 24 hours, and are not in active labor, or if they exhibit any symptoms of infection, *then* I administer antibiotics via an IV in labor. Otherwise, there are other methods of protecting the baby that don't subject the mother and baby to the drop in good bacteria that antibiotics produce. If my client tests positive for chlamydia or gonorrhea, then antibiotics are definitely needed during pregnancy.

There is so much information available now about just how critically important gut bacteria are for the establishment of the baby's immune system, disease resistance, longevity, and overall health. At this point I see no reason to administer antibiotics to healthy women.

Blood Draw

I do a blood draw at 36 weeks to make sure that all of your values for hemoglobin, hematocrit, mean corpuscular volume, etc. are nice and high. I also look at your platelets to make sure that you have plenty of clotting factors. At Week 36 we still have enough time to fix many issues.

Partners, Clean Your Environment

 I do have to say in my 50 years of midwifery, 95 percent of the births I've attended have been in people's homes. There are people who are more clean and people who are less clean. There is something to be said for being conscientious regarding cleanliness, especially when you're going to have kids. Having a routine for cleanliness will help to prevent illness in you, your partner, and in your children as they grow. Even if you do not choose a home birth, you will be bringing your new baby with its newly functioning immune system into your home, and your space should be super clean. Develop better cleaning habits now if you need to.

I have long thought that American society does not have enough ritual or ceremony. It is kind of like everyone who came here— except for the Indigenous Americans who were here in the first place with their own wonderful practices around birth—came here from cultures rich with history, tradition, rituals, and ceremonies, but they wanted to leave those behind and become Americans in this new place. They abandoned all of the things that made them different and who they were in the Old World for what they could experience here in the New World.

Now we are developing birth rituals and birth ceremonies of our own. One of them that is so important is cleanliness, and I don't mean only physical cleanliness, though that is certainly critically important. You are warding off germs, negativity, and bad energy by building your practice of joy, building a clean space in your home, life, and heart. It is important to consider all of this and build more ceremony and ritual into this process. Doing this also helps build your spiritual connection to the process of birth.

You want the bedroom and bathroom to be very, very clean. This is a partner job. If you are financially able, you might wish to hire a professional cleaning service. No matter who is doing the cleaning, it should not be the pregnant woman. It is really hard for a pregnant woman to get down on her hands and knees this far along in the pregnancy and clean things like the floors, the walls around the toilet, the toilet bowl, and around and behind the toilets as thoroughly as they need to be cleaned.

I cannot stress enough how important this is. Partners, *this is absolutely essential and can be the difference between life and death.* In pre-modern times the most common cause of death in women of a childbearing age was childbirth or infection post-childbirth. Two of my great grandmothers

died from post-childbirth infections. Infections, hemorrhaging, high blood pressure, and malpresentation of the baby were the leading causes of death in childbirth. Now we have medical recourse for all of these things, including drugs and surgery, but bad infections can and do happen.

You want everything in your home to be as clean as possible. Women giving birth at home are going to get up just after the baby is born to go to the bathroom and they will sit down on the toilet. The uterus has a giant wound where the placenta was attached, and sitting on the toilet provides direct entry for germs into the woman's bloodstream and has the potential for causing septicemia.

Remember what we discussed about the germ problem in hospitals and the prevalence of nosocomial infections (see page 161). If you follow my recommendations, your home will be a cleaner, safer environment to give birth in than a hospital. Even if you are having a birth center or hospital birth, I suggest doing this deep cleaning to prepare for a healing postpartum period for momma and baby. You won't have time to clean when labor kicks in or after the birth, so do it now.

I suggest you use bleach products on the entire toilet, both inside and outside, as well as on the walls and floor surrounding it. Some people are hesitant to use bleach, but I want you to know it is critical to ensure that you're killing germs. Bleach evaporates completely within 12 hours. Make a mild solution of bleach and water—you can use ¼ cup of bleach to a gallon of water—

and wipe the solution all over everything, including the bath or shower, and let it dry. Everything will be so clean and as close to sterile as possible. Keep the door closed to keep any pets out. Use gloves and open the windows to facilitate ventilation of the area after cleaning.

Don't forget to deep clean the tub; lots of moms like to labor in the tub.

Also, do not forget to deep clean the bedroom. Pay attention to:

- Floors
- Walls
- Paintings
- Miniblinds/curtains
- Windows
- Ceiling fans
- Bookshelves and any decorations
- Bedspread
- Sheets
- Under the bed
- Dust ruffle
- Rugs
- Doorknobs
- Change air filters in your HVAC unit
- Vacuum air returns and AC registers as well as the intake vents for air purification systems
- Clear clutter, remove unnecessary items, and generally tidy the area

If you have carpet or rugs, have them professionally cleaned if you can. At the very least, rent a steam cleaner from the local grocery store and give your rugs a nice, deep clean. This will be such amazing prep for your sweet baby and will help to prevent allergies and keep them from getting unnecessarily sick or stuffy in those first few days and weeks of life.

Your family will be spending so much time in the bedroom those first two weeks after the baby is born, and you will all feel so much better if everything is as clean as possible.

Maintenance

It's great to do this deep cleaning at a convenient point toward the end of the pregnancy. Once you have done this deep cleaning, it will be easy to maintain. Perform daily maintenance and a weekly thorough cleaning until your pregnant partner goes into labor. Once she starts the labor and birth process, clean the toilet and bathtub again.

Practice Your Breathing

If you haven't started already, now is the time to begin practicing the breathing techniques described in the Movement chapter of this section (page 281).

Purchase Your Nursing Bras

Buy nursing bras four weeks before the birth. It is important to put a bra on within 24 hours after the birth to help prevent engorgement (the swelling of the breasts). You want to have it ready by purchasing it now in case you have an early birth. The reason why I ask you to do this now, and not after your baby is born, is that you should not go out in the world to get fitted for one right after the birth. You will preferably be down in bed, resting, bonding with your baby, and letting your uterus heal.

Find a place that specializes in nursing bras and that will measure you appropriately. It is best to have a professional fitting at a specialty store. Bras and belly support systems for pregnancy and postpartum are very unique to the body shape of each individual, you have got to try them on first. A bra, if not fitted properly, can cause blocked milk ducts and infections. Avoid underwires.

Buy a few of the bras (two for daytime, one for sleeping), so you can swap the one you're wearing for a clean one as needed (at least daily). Remember, your breasts will become larger, so make sure the bras are slightly loose in the cups now.

It's also beneficial to get washable cotton nursing pads, so if you do leak you don't have to take the bra off, the pad will absorb it (many women leak in the first few weeks after giving birth until their milk supply completely regulates). These pads will help to prevent milk stains on the front of your shirt. Wash these in the mild laundry soap you use for the bras.

Diapers

I'm just about to get into a long list of items for you to prepare for your birth and immediate postpartum period, and realized I really have a lot to say about diapers. They can't just be a line item on a list. I am a tremendous fan of cloth diapers for so many reasons. Disposable diapers are filling our landfills with nonbiodegradable plastic.[146] Many of the conventional disposable diapers have chemicals in them to help with absorbency, and this leads to a heightened incidence of diaper rash and an unknown amount of chemicals absorbed by the baby's body. More natural disposables are available, but they still require significant environmental resources to produce and are considerably more expensive than their conventional counterparts.

Meanwhile, cloth diapering has come a long way. Advances in cloth technology, closures, and the availability of form-fitting shapes and sizes make this option more attractive than ever. I think it's better to wrap babies in cloth the majority of the time. It is not only a matter of money, but it is a matter of safety and health, as well as environmental action.

I am loath to put disposable diapers on a newborn and actually just will not do it. I would rather use a washcloth or kitchen towel on them than a disposable diaper. They will have so much artificial and plastic

MariMikel: I took four kids for six weeks in a Suburban with a pop-up camper all around the country and spent two weeks at Disney World. The youngest was eight months old, and I also had a 3-year-old, a 10-year-old, and a 13-year-old. It was wonderful and a bit hard here and there. At the time I was fully committed to cloth diapers and natural baby food, and I took my cloth diapers with me.

After three days I mailed all the diapers home and switched to disposables. Anything else was insanity.

So, feel free to be flexible. If you're going to the zoo, maybe that's the time to use disposable diapers. If you're going to grandma's house for the weekend, maybe it's significantly more convenient to use disposable diapers for a few days. Make it easy on yourself and others.

exposure in their life as it is, and I believe it is a weird, unnatural sensation on their skin first thing after coming out of the womb. I strongly promote cloth diapers, especially for newborn infants.

Consider purchasing a month or two of a diaper service (or ask for it at your baby shower if you have one) to make your life easier as you adjust to motherhood. If you use a diaper service, ask for them to provide the infant size rather than newborn, or the second to smallest size, so they are big enough. The smallest diaper size generally does not fit or hold in much of the poops or pees that the baby will start to have after the first few days. You could also get just a week's worth of the newborn size and the rest should be the larger infant size. That way you have a range of sizes to fit your baby.

If you are going to wash your own diapers, you will need about four to six dozen on hand. Your baby will go through 12–15 diapers a day in the first few weeks and months. You want to have enough on hand so you do not have to do laundry every day. Go ahead and start purchasing cloth diapers in anticipation of your baby's arrival, as well as a cloth diaper sprayer, which is an attachment that hooks onto your toilet and provides a powerful jet stream of water to make cleaning the diapers easy.

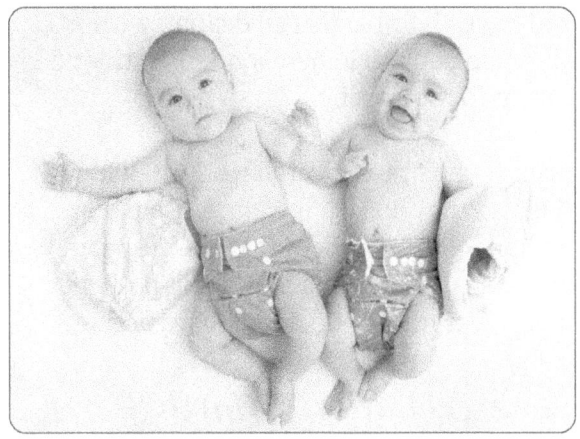

Modern Cloth Diapers

There are many modern brands of cloth diapers available. You can buy them new or look to resale marketplaces to build your stock of diaper covers. I know of many women who pass cloth diapers among their friend circle as a new baby enters the world. I think this is a lovely way to support one another as cloth diapers can represent a significant upfront investment.

Lately I have been telling families who are struggling to deal with the constant work of the postpartum period to buy really good quality natural disposable diapers for after the birth. Use cloth diapers for the first 24 hours, switch to natural disposable diapers for the first two weeks while you're down, and then go to a regime of mostly cloth and some disposable diapers after that. It's important to make it easier on yourselves in the postpartum period. Your partner

Robbie: I cannot even begin to count the many hundreds of times that I washed and folded cloth diapers. I was completely committed to using them, until I "lost it" and finally started using disposables when each of my babies was around six months old. The workload became too overwhelming after I returned to my teaching job at UT Austin. I did feel very guilty, but as MariMikel keeps reminding us, we moms have to care for ourselves as well as for our babies and children.

will have their hands full dealing with it all while you are in bed bonding with and caring for your baby.

Even if you are dedicated to cloth diapers, it is useful to have a few disposable diapers on hand. Reserve them for use on special occasions where a disposable diaper will make everything considerably easier.

Pack/Prepare Your Birth & Postpartum Supplies

 Now is the time to review what your midwife or care provider would like you to have on hand, and to order anything that's missing from your inventory. You'll want to collect all of those items and keep them together.

I have a series of lists in this section to help you out. Regardless of whether you'll be having a hospital, birth center, or home birth, gather the supplies from this first list, Supplies for All Births, then collect the supplies on the list that corresponds to your chosen birth environment: Home Birth, Birth Center Birth, or Hospital birth.

Buy everything for your birth and the immediate postpartum period at least six weeks before your due date, so if your baby does come early, you are prepared.

Supplies for All Births

These are supplies that you should have on hand regardless of where you give birth. Keep these with the supplies you want to have on hand for your labor and birth. You'll want to take these with you if you are having a birth center or hospital birth.

To Bring to or Have at the Birth

- ☐ **Birth plan.**
- ☐ **Camera** and film (or digital camera/phone) and **chargers/batteries**

I really recommend that you designate someone to take a lot of videos and pictures of the labor, birth, and the first hour or so. It's all saved on your devices, no one needs to see it if you don't want to share it. I have some women tell me they don't want pictures of their birth. I tell them, "It's not your birth, it's your baby's, and they may someday want to see what it was like on their very special first day. They may want to see the look on their father's face when he first sees them and catches them. They may want to see the first look their mother gave them, what their first cry sounded like."

TIP: I have had wonderful experiences with the parents giving any older siblings (if they're old enough) a disposable camera so they can take pictures during the birth. Their perspective is unique, and it can be something special for them to do during the birth of their sibling.

We have this absolutely amazing technology at our fingertips; it's a gift. No previous generation could record like we can. No one has ever told me they regretted taking pictures or videos, but I have had many, many mothers admit that they wish they had taken pictures, realizing after the fact that the opportunity will never come again.

THIRD TRIMESTER

If you don't like a particular picture or video, you can edit it or delete it. It's yours! Just because you video or take pictures doesn't mean you have to put it on YouTube or ever show anyone! It's for you and your child. And in the years to come, it can bring you a lot of joy and connection with your child. Don't let body image issues get in the way of documenting an amazing experience.

- ☐ **Heating pad for back pain** (if you planning a hospital birth they may or may not have this).

- ☐ **Extra pillows**

- ☐ Your **birth playlists** loaded on the device of your choice and a device/speaker to play them on. Make sure it is portable if you are planning a hospital birth.

- ☐ **Massage oil.**

- ☐ **Candles** (electric for a hospital birth)

- ☐ **Lip balm.**

- ☐ **Large exercise ball** (optional; hospitals and birth centers sometimes have these).

- ☐ **Acetaminophen and ibuprofen** Acetaminophen is a great fever reducer and mothers sometimes run a fever after a hard birth or when their milk comes in.

  Ibuprofen is a component of the Trick to help slow down warm-up labor in the middle of the night when you need to be sleeping. After the birth, it is also great for swelling, engorgement, a swollen bottom around stitches, or severe afterbirth contractions because of its anti-inflammatory properties.

- ☐ **Arnica** is a wonderful homeopathic preparation and will help the baby if there is any bruising or swelling on the scalp or face, which can be common. I also use it on the mom if she has any sore muscles after the birth. Anytime you have a fall or bump I suggest you put arnica on right away. It really works miraculously to help lessen bruises and pain. Get gel, cream, and pellets.

- ☐ **Electrolyte replacement drinks** (several quarts at least)—I suggest Recharge and you can buy it online, I know Amazon carries it. I do not like brands that contain chemicals and food coloring/additives that are not good for you. Read your labels. Coconut water is also good.

Supplies for a Home Birth

If you are having a home birth, work with your midwife to understand what she'd like you to have on hand and follow her instructions for preparation. Most midwives will have a birth kit you will be able to purchase with their guidance. These are supplies that a hospital would provide as part of their services, and that you will need to procure in advance for your home birth. I will share with you the things that I ask my clients to gather and prepare/sterilize in advance to give you an idea of what might be required. The birth kit I ask my clients to get costs approximately $100 and includes many of the items on this list.

Labor and Birth Supplies

- [ ] **Nitrazine paper** to test if your waters have broken. You can buy this online or at a pharmacy.

- [ ] **Povidone iodine**—this will be used to make an antiseptic solution that you clean yourself with if your waters break before you go into labor, as well as after the birth. We'll talk about this sterile technique in the next chapter. If you are allergic to iodine you need to have **Phisoderm or Hibiclens**

- [ ] **Combination hot water bottle/ douche apparatus**. This could be used for a douche or enema and will be used for sterile technique if your water breaks or leaks when you are not in active labor, as well as after the baby is born.

- [ ] **Thirty 23" x 24" disposable underpads**—used for double making the bed and protecting any space where you may be sitting while laboring. They are also used during pushing and the birth, and afterwards when you are bleeding heavily to protect your sheets, mattress, and furniture.

- [ ] **Two packs of sterile OB pads**—these are necessary because pads you can buy from a store are usually not sterile.

- [ ] **Twenty 4" x 4" sterile gauze pads**—to be used for hot packs on the perineum as well as to clean you up right before and after the baby is born.

- [ ] **Peri bottle**—used for sterile technique and after the birth to keep you clean once you are not bleeding as much. (Women sometimes continue to bleed for several weeks after giving birth as their uterus heals; this is not blood from the birth process itself.)

- [ ] **Twelve pairs of sterile gloves**—to be used for the birth and for exams. It is crucial your midwife uses sterile gloves, so no germs are introduced to your vagina and uterus.

- [ ] **Twelve alcohol prep pads**—to be used if you need to get an IV or to clean and sterilize skin during labor as needed.

- [ ] **Twelve packets sterile jelly**—it is important to use sterilized lubricating jelly while doing exams during labor.

- [ ] **Two plastic-backed paper sheets**—to help us double make the bed and protect the bed from any birthing fluids. These are each large enough to cover half of a king-size bed.

- [ ] **Sterile Povidone scrub brush**—used to sterilize our hands for the birth as well as some of the equipment. The scrub brush can also be used as a baby brush in those first few weeks to prevent cradle cap (a common skin condition that affects newborns).

- [ ] **One gallon pot with a lid** to boil water.

- [ ] A **small bottle of olive oil**—get the smallest bottle you can find. Make sure it is in a glass container. They are very cheap and an easy way to use for the birth to help lubricate the perineum and labia so the baby slides right out and doesn't cause you to tear. I have my clients boil the bottle of olive oil in a small saucepan to sterilize it. The contents of an unopened bottle are already considered sterile.

- ☐ **Four regular-sized bath towels.**

- ☐ **Four washcloths.**
  - ○ These will be used for perineal support—to hold hot packs onto the area, to bring blood to the area, as well as to distribute pressure evenly to prevent tearing.

- ☐ **Two sets of sheets** with a fitted bottom and flat sheet in each set that fit the bed you'll be giving birth in—unless you choose another location, such as a pool or your living room. Women sometimes give birth in surprising places! Wherever you give birth, you will still need these sheets for your postpartum family bonding. (Note that you'll need a third set to use in the meantime.)

- ☐ You need access to **ice**. If you do not have an ice maker, please send someone to buy a big bag of ice when your pregnant partner goes into labor. This will be used for ice chips if you are feeling nauseated during labor and/or for ice packs after the birth among other things.

- ☐ Make sure you have **food** on hand **for** both **the mother and father**, as well as for **the midwives**. For moms I have a rule—only eat what you are willing to see again, because women often throw up in labor. Things that are really easy are applesauce,

mashed potatoes, juice or Recharge, steamed rice, simple and well-cooked soups, chicken broth or stock, miso soup, yogurt, oatmeal, and tapioca or rice pudding. Please also have food on hand for your midwife; ask her what she would like.

- ☐ Trash can and **trash bags** for the birthing room—the birth creates a lot of trash.

- ☐ **Birthing Pool** (optional)

  Birthing pools can provide a wonderful environment for women to labor in. Getting into the water can bring sincere relief during an unrelenting labor. Research does not show an increased incidence of infections of the birth canal or uterus with their use.[147]

What to Buy

I discourage people from buying birth pools marketed as such because they are quite overpriced. There's an amazing **backyard wading pool** that's just as serviceable. It's huge and affordable and once you're done you can clean it out and put it in your backyard and have summer fun with it. The

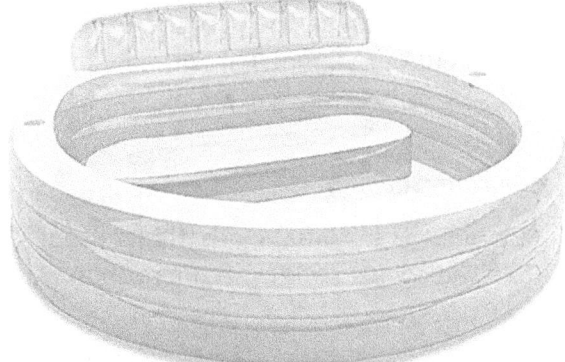

An Inflatable Pool Made for Recreation Can Make an Excellent Birthing Pool

whole family can fit in it. It's big enough for birth and shallow enough that the midwife can get to you and help with the baby. It even has a bench that you can sit on, lie on, or lean on. There's a backrest for when you're on the seat. **You must reserve this pool's first-time use for the birth**; don't put it in the backyard for a few months and then tote it into the house for your birth experience.

Buy a **brand-new hose** to fill the pool that will be used for labor and birth. A used hose could have bacteria that is dangerous. It is actually a law in Texas that only new hoses be used to fill birthing pools. The hose needs to be long enough to reach from the faucet to the pool (for filling) and from the pool to a safe area for disposal outside, usually through a door or window (for emptying).

You also need to buy a **fresh roll of clear plastic that is 4 ml thick and 10 or 12 feet wide by 12 feet long**. You can find this online or at a hardware store. You will need to put plastic under the pool so if it were to become punctured, your attendants could hold the edges up while the pool was being emptied and save your home from water damage. You will want to put a few towels on the floor on top of the plastic, so when you step out of the pool you will not slip on the plastic or get water all over.

Postpartum Supplies

- ☐ **Four traditional cloth diapers** (not the pocket style with microfiber pads).

- ☐ **An infant shirt**, preferably with snaps or ties, so you do not have to pull it over their heads, which are generally very tender from the birth experience.

- ☐ **A sleeper gown** that opens at the bottom.

- ☐ **A long sleeve footed sleeper outfit.**

- ☐ **Booties.**

- ☐ **Two newborn hats**—used immediately after the birth. Fluids from the baby might get on them, so we use these hats initially instead of your nice ones, so you can just get rid of them later if you like.

- ☐ **Two pairs of socks.** Babies can often have trouble regulating their temperature in the first twenty-four hours, so we want to have options as to what to put on them. Sometimes they come out and get cold quickly, so your midwife would put the diaper, shirt, footed sleeper, socks, and hat on them. Other times they may be very warm so she would just put the shirt and diaper on. You want to have options so you can tailor baby's first outfit to baby's first needs.

- ☐ **Four receiving blankets,** preferably cotton or flannel and not waffle weave, as that can imprint on baby's skin. Right after birth, I dry the amniotic fluid off the baby using one of the blankets. I put a clean blanket on them to cover them as they are skin-to-skin with mom, and we wait for the placenta to come out. Once the placenta is out, I use another blanket and help mom to turn on her side so she can begin breastfeeding. We use the fourth blanket when we do the newborn exam a few hours after birth.

- ☐ **Large cotton balls** and **alcohol**. These are used for your baby's cord care.

- ☐ **Hydrogen peroxide** is used to get blood out of anything.

- ☐ **Medicine spoon**—to be used to give the baby water, herbs, etc. if they get dehydrated.

- ☐ **DeLee infant suction set**—to be used to suction the baby if they have fluid in their airways right after the baby is born.

- ☐ **Sterile bulb syringe**—to clear the baby's nose and/or mouth out if needed after birth or in the first few months if they spit up.

- ☐ **Two pairs of stretch briefs**—these will hold the large sterile pads in place and save your underwear from getting blood on them. They can be washed in the sink and hung to dry and then disposed of once you are not bleeding as much—usually by about day three to five. You can also machine dry them in about five minutes.

- ☐ **Digital thermometer**—to take the mother's and baby's temperature after the birth.

- ☐ **Ten pairs of non-sterile latex gloves**—to be used for the birth cleanup and checking the placenta.

- ☐ **Two flexible drinking straws**—to help you drink when you are lying down.

- ☐ **Sitz bath herbs**—to help your bottom heal after the birth if you have a tear or stitches.

- ☐ **Sitz bath container**—a 4- or 5-inch tall, under-the-bed, plastic storage bin (medium size) works great for this.

- ☐ If you only have a bathtub, you need to have a **shower head attachment** so you can shower. You cannot bathe in the first two weeks as this can increase your chance of getting a uterine infection. You can do sitz baths if you have a tear or stitches, but not bathtub baths. With a sitz bath your bottom is the only submerged part of you, so the uterus is not exposed to germs from your feet.

- ☐ Two **one-gallon, resealable plastic bags**. We use these to contain the placenta after it has been birthed.

- ☐ **After Ease** tincture by WishGarden to use if needed—this helps to ease afterbirth contractions and can also be used for bad cramps during your periods once they resume.

- ☐ **Weleda baby cream.** This is a phenomenal cream that helps the baby's skin stay hydrated after they are born that I highly recommend.

- ☐ **Gentle shampoo** for your baby's hair (pH balanced as well as sulfate and chemical free shampoos are the best option for your infant's tender scalp and skin).

- ☐ **Nursing Bra.**

- ☐ **Nursing pillow.**

- ☐ **Soothies (gel pads) and nipple cream**—to help with soreness.

- ☐ **Diaper covers** are necessary with cloth diapers once your milk comes in. I do not generally suggest using covers in the first few days, though, because newborn babies dirty so few diapers and the covers can make their little legs spread out too far and be uncomfortable in the beginning.

- [ ] **Diaper pins or Snappis**.

- [ ] **A 4-ounce baby bottle** It's good to have a baby bottle handy in the rare case that your baby needs supplementation with breastmilk, formula, water, or herbs. If your baby is seriously dehydrated or if they become very jaundiced it may be necessary to supplement. If the baby is jaundiced the best remedy is to use cow's milk formula; soy will not work. The cow milk formula will bind with the bilirubin in the baby's blood and can help prevent hospitalization.

More typically what the bottle is used for is to put your own breast milk that you have expressed or pumped in it and then give it to the baby through a bottle. It can help them to get quick calories if they are struggling. The chances are very slim that the bottle will be needed, but it is important to have one on hand in case it is your baby who needs it.

- [ ] **One gallon of filtered water**—every now and then the baby needs water in the first few days if they are dehydrated, and filtered is the best option for their sterile gut. There is a medicine spoon in the birth kit, and we often use that to give the baby water if they are not peeing enough.

- [ ] A small container of **powdered, organic baby formula** in case the baby needs some. You don't want to be sourcing this in the moment. You need it right then, and it can be hard to find the good stuff at a moment's notice. Store this in the freezer to maintain freshness.

- [ ] **Co-sleeper** or **play pen.**

- [ ] If you are going to have the baby in bed with you, I recommend something like a **bed sleeper**, some sort of baby oasis. There are products that form a space with cotton or terrycloth covered foam cylinders. These work to define where the baby is, so no one rolls onto the baby and so the baby doesn't roll into anyone. Baby needs to be in the same room as you. It's hard on your baby to be in a room by themselves.

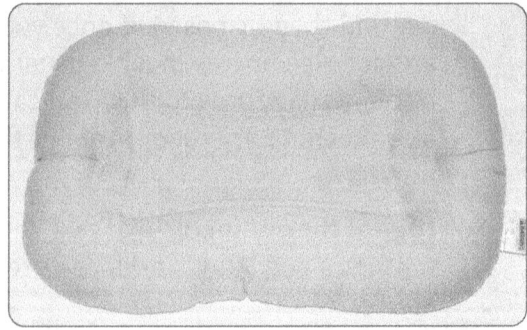

Baby Sleeper

- [ ] **Car seat.** You must never travel in a vehicle without your baby being safely buckled into a modern car seat. If you have a hospital birth, the hospital will not let you leave without one.

- [ ] You may find an **infant seat** exceptionally helpful. Put them in

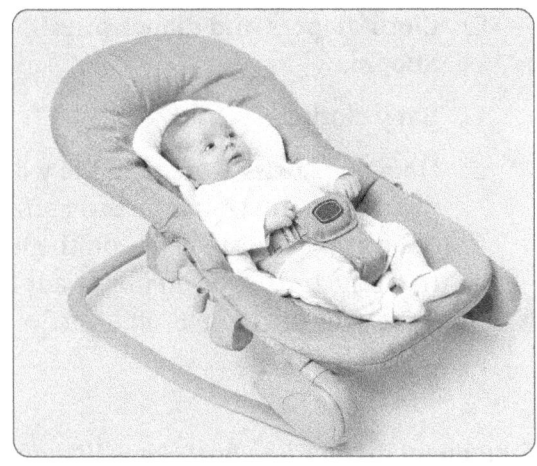

Infant Seat

there right after they nurse and they'll be able to keep the milk down rather than eating, lying down and then spitting up.

- ☐ **Swings or gliders** are also awesome after a few weeks.

Supplies for a Birth Center Birth

This is the time when you will want to find out how your care provider within the birth center handles everything when you go into labor: who will be there, what is expected of you, what you can expect from them, and what equipment you will need to bring with you, if any, for the birth. You can use the home birth postpartum list to help you prepare for your aftercare. Just work with your midwife to tailor it for your situation.

Supplies for a Hospital Birth

Following is a list of things that you will need to bring with you if you plan to have a hospital birth, or if you start at home or a freestanding birth center and find yourself in a situation where transport to the hospital is the best choice for you and your baby. It's good to review this list now and make sure you have these items on hand in either case.

You will want to leave most of these supplies in the car when you arrive at the hospital to be admitted. Some women arrive and then are told to go back home and labor for a while longer before checking in, so you don't want to lug everything up there only to have to drag it all back to the car. Most of these items will be used after the birth and will only be in the way for the staff and for you during labor. Your partner can go to get things from the car as needed.

Labor and Birth Supplies

- ☐ **Arnica gel, cream, and pellets.**
- ☐ **Vitamins.**
- ☐ **Pillows** for you and your partner. Pillows at the hospital are often terrible.
- ☐ **Toothbrush/toothpaste** for you and your partner.
- ☐ **Shampoo/hairbrush** for you and your partner.
- ☐ **Any other desired toiletries** for you and your partner.
- ☐ **House shoes** for you and your partner.
- ☐ **Loose, comfortable clothing** for you and your partner (e.g., sweatpants, yoga wear, pajama bottoms, T-shirts).
- ☐ **List of people** to call after the birth.
- ☐ **Books or magazines** to help pass the time.

- [ ] **Water**—**2-½ gallons of spring water** (if you prefer not to drink fluoridated water).

- [ ] **Food**—The hospital food is sometimes not very good, so bring an ice chest with drinks and good snacks such as yogurt, trail mix, fruit, etc. I also recommend Pacific brand soups such as butternut squash, tomato, chicken, or vegetable broth; light sandwiches; really any easy-to-prepare or already prepared healthy foods.

Postpartum Supplies

- [ ] **Car seat**—Important! You can't bring your baby home without it. Purchase a new, not used, car seat. The components of the car seat can degrade over time, and you never know if a used car seat was in an accident that damaged its integrity, so it's worth the peace of mind to buy new.

- [ ] **After Ease** tincture by WishGarden to use if needed—this helps to ease afterbirth contractions and can also be used for bad cramps during your periods once they resume.

- [ ] **Nursing bra.**

- [ ] **Nipple cream.**

- [ ] **Nursing pillow.**

- [ ] **Nightgowns/PJs** for you and your partner.

- [ ] **Weleda baby cream.** This is a phenomenal cream that helps the baby's skin stay hydrated after they are born that I highly recommend.

- [ ] **Cloth diapers and diaper pins/ Snappis.**

- [ ] **Baby clothes.**

- [ ] **Hats and socks**—the hospital will provide an infant hat directly after the birth. Fluids may get on them from the birth, so you may want to have your own to put on after.

- [ ] **Baby blankets.**

Equipment to Have Ready at Home When You Return from the Hospital

- [ ] **Soothies (gel pads)**—to help with nipple soreness.

- [ ] **Gentle shampoo** for your baby's hair (pH balanced, sulfate-free, and chemical-free shampoos are the best option for your infant's tender scalp and skin).

- [ ] **1 gallon of filtered water**—every now and then the baby needs water in the first few days if they are dehydrated, and filtered is the best option for their sterile gut. There is a medicine spoon in the birth kit, and we often use that to give the baby water if they are not peeing enough.

- [ ] **4-ounce baby bottle** It's good to have a baby bottle handy in the rare case that your baby needs supplementation with breastmilk, formula, water, or herbs. If your baby is seriously dehydrated or if they become very jaundiced it may be necessary to supplement. If the baby is jaundiced the best remedy is to use cow's milk formula; soy will not work. The cow milk formula

THIRD TRIMESTER

will bind with the bilirubin in the baby's blood and can help prevent hospitalization.

☐ A small container of **powdered, organic baby formula** in case the baby needs some. You don't want to be sourcing this in the moment. You need it right then, and it can be hard to find the good stuff at a moment's notice. Store this in the freezer to maintain freshness.

☐ **Co-sleeper** or **play pen**.

☐ If you are going to have the baby in bed with you, I recommend something like a **bed sleeper**, some sort of baby oasis. There are products that form a space with cotton or terrycloth covered foam cylinders. These work to define where the baby is, so no one rolls onto the baby and so the baby doesn't roll into anyone. Baby needs to be in the same room as you. It's hard on your baby to be in a room by themselves.

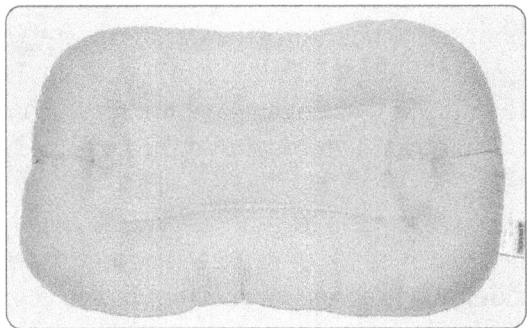

Baby Sleeper

☐ **Swings or gliders** are also awesome after a few weeks.

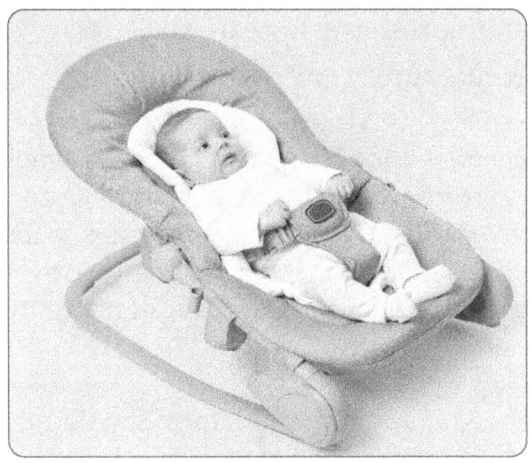

Infant Seat

☐ You may find an **infant seat** exceptionally helpful. Put them in there right after they nurse and they'll be able to keep the milk down rather than eating, lying down and then spitting up.

I have had clients ask me if they should prepare a bag to take to the hospital, in case they end up needing to transport from their home birth. I can understand this thought and wanting to be prepared for every situation, but my philosophy is that it is not necessary. Packing your hospital bag can put energy toward an end result that you may not want. If we do end up transporting, it is easy enough at that time to pack up the few things you may need before we leave or have another family member or friend bring you items a few hours later. Let go of any fears, surrender, and don't put any energy toward a hospital transport. There is no need to worry in advance.

Mitigating the Cost of All This New Stuff

Getting everything prepared for your baby can take a lot of time, attention, and money. A great way to mitigate the cost both to your wallet and the environment is to look at secondhand markets for gently used items. Fabulous places to look for free items are:

- Facebook: check for a Buy Nothing group in your area
- Freecycle.org

You can also check secondhand children's shops in your area, Craigslist, garage/yard sales, and Facebook Marketplace.

Don't forget to ask your friends and family for hand-me-downs. So many of the baby supplies we buy are used for a very short period of time, so hand-me-downs are usually quite gently used at this stage.

I do recommend you buy a brand-new car seat, but other than that, if you find all of this to be a bit financially burdensome, these are great avenues for you to try.

Perineal Massage

Perineal massage is a great thing to do starting four weeks before the birth. If you have never experienced anything unpleasant in your perineal area and suddenly you are faced with the baby's head dilating and stretching the perineum, it can be very difficult and scary and hard to surrender to. Perineal massage helps you to develop a conditioned response that allows your bottom to completely relax when the baby's head is stretching it out. It is most easily done with your partner's help. It can be done alone, but that is much trickier. The woman would need to use her thumb to massage the perineum if she's on her own, and it is so hard to relax when you do this by yourself.

It is important to separate perineal massage from sex. A few years back I asked one of my class groups how perineal massage was going and everyone snickered, which is when I realized they were all having way too much fun. Perineal massage should not be painful but should be just slightly uncomfortable. At least at first, it can be an unpleasant sensation on your perineum.

Have your partner wear non-sterile exam gloves; you can buy them at a pharmacy or online. A lot of men's hands are rough and provide too much friction, so this helps to avoid roughing up a sensitive area. It also introduces a sterility to the situation, and that makes you less likely to think of sex.

Use Vitamin E oil—not edible Vitamin E as it is too thick, but oil you can find at a pharmacy, health food store, or online (and get the highest IU's you can)—and apply the oil, then use one finger and press gently down onto the perineum until it relaxes.

Use two fingers to gently massage the perineum in a 180-degree arc going from side to side across the bottom of the vagina. The fingers should be inserted about an inch-and-a-half because you are trying to relax the pad of muscle in there called the perineal sling.

Start slowly and gently, then build the pressure up. Do not be rough and do not go fast; it should not hurt, but it should stretch and may be slightly uncomfortable.

While your partner is doing the perineal massage, you should practice your breathing and relaxation techniques. This is a time to go limp. Close your eyes and relax every muscle in your body and let your bottom go, let your rectum and butt go. Do not fight or tense up. Get comfortable feeling these uncomfortable sensations. Perineal massage and your ability to relax will significantly help in not tearing during birth.

If you want to prevent tearing, then do this faithfully with your partner. I suggest two to four times a week for 30–60 seconds a session.

Castor Oil Packs

Using castor oil packs to prepare the perineal area is also a great trick. You can apply one for about 20 minutes two to four times per week. You want to use a piece of flannel or cotton cloth; do not use terry cloth as it will absorb too much oil and not help to apply the oil to the skin. The castor oil helps to significantly relax and soften the area. It can also be amazing for scar tissue. If you had an episiotomy or tear with your last birth it can help to make that scar tissue soft.

Apply a small amount (1–2 tablespoons) of the oil directly onto the cloth and then put it in the microwave for about 15 seconds to heat it up. Alternatively, heat a small amount of the oil in a small, microwave-safe container or on the stove and then dip the cloth in it. Test the oil on the cloth with your fingers before applying it to make sure

it is not too hot and there is not one area that is hotter than the rest. I have made the mistake of failing to test for this and blistered my bottom—very unfun.

Sit on the cloth applied directly to your naked bottom and perineum with a disposable under pad underneath you to protect your couch or chair from the castor oil. You can reuse this pad; you do not need to use a new one each time you do it. If you can, keep the pack warm with a heating pad or hot water bottle under the disposable pad.

You can watch TV, read a book, or do anything else that keeps you stationary and distracted. Sit for twenty minutes. You do not need to wipe or clean the oil off. Once you are finished, it is mainly on the cloth, and what is on you will quickly be absorbed.

Air Filters

I suggest you clean or change your AC filters before the baby is born and change them faithfully every month to keep the air filtered and clean in your home. This will help to prevent allergy symptoms in the child and helps to eliminate pollen, dust, dust mites, dog, and other pet dander, and helps not only the baby but the parents and other children in the home. I also suggest getting an air purifier for your bedroom. This helps the air quality dramatically.

You may also be able to get your pediatrician or family practice doctor to write a prescription for an air filter so you can write it off as a medical expense with your taxes at the end of the year.

You should also use hypoallergenic mattress pads and pillows or cover pillows with hypoallergenic covers to help eliminate allergens on your bed.

Pets

Pets should be prepared as well, so everyone is ready for this great event for your family. When I arrive, pets always seem thrilled; they seem to know that I am a person of some authority who has come to help. I try to bond with them and prepare them as well.

Work in advance to prepare your pets for the new family member. You can show them the baby's things and talk about the baby. They understand our language far better than we speak theirs. Let them smell your belly and body. Let them into the baby's room to show them how you are preparing for the new life you will be welcoming into the world.

Sleeping with Pets

I think it's great to raise kids around animals. I think they turn out stronger morally, and become compassionate, empathetic, caring, and helpful because they've been around pets. However, our pets are covered with allergens and bacteria.

Now is the time to stop having pets sleep with you in your bed. In fact, it's best if they stay out of your bed entirely. There are a few reasons for this. One is that you cannot have your room clean enough. You want it to be as clean as possible for your baby, and so you want to stop some of those contaminants from entering the room at all. Once the baby is a month old their immune system is developed enough to be around your pets, but in the first little bit they are immunologically mostly helpless, and the bacterial load animals carry is a lot. Plus, you'll have a wide-open wound in your uterus that you'll want to avoid infecting.

Your pets may be a little sour with you about this new arrangement, but it's much better if you help them adjust now, so they are upset with you rather than blaming your new baby for the change. If your baby arrives and then your pet is booted from the bed, they may grow resentful of this new little usurper in the family.

Dogs

Humans genetically engineered dogs over thousands of years to focus on their specific human. Dogs consider themselves to be members of our families. Science has shown they have a wide range of emotions, similar to humans.[148] While this varies by breed, lots of dogs love, protect, and adore babies.

Dogs can smell the birth and then they're usually very happy with your new baby, though this can also vary by breed. I will usually let a family dog smell the first blanket that we dry the baby with after the birth. I'll put it down and let them fill their little heart with that smell. They understand their job now is to protect the baby.

When life goes topsy-turvy with a newborn, pets often lose that attention they crave from their human. It's important to remember that they are creatures with feelings, and they will need attention once your baby arrives, too. The vast majority of dogs pose no issues for your baby, especially if you take care not to abandon them in the process. Dogs want very much to be a part of your healthy family unit, and you must work to take care of their needs too once your baby arrives.

A few ideas for you:

- Change your dog's routine now. Go for walks at unusual times or switch their feeding schedule slightly to start them getting used to the idea that routines are going to be up ended.

- If they don't have one already, provide them with a safe space to retreat to when they are feeling stressed or anxious, like a crate.

- Keep your dog's vaccinations up to date. This will help to protect them from diseases that they could transmit to your baby.

- Provide your dog with plenty of attention and enrichment to help them feel loved and secure. Make plans now for how your dog will continue to get exercise and attention in those first few very busy weeks when you are occupied with your new baby. If you're hiring a dog walker, for example, have them start the new exercise routine before your baby is born.

Things will be different for your dog, and if you can work to change things now, they will likely be less resentful of your new baby because they won't associate the changes in their life solely with the newborn.

I don't want to give you false assurances. I have seen a very few instances where the family dog was not as welcoming of the new baby, and I have known a few families who had to part with their dog once their baby arrived due to the dog's aggression. Work now to prepare your dog, always supervise your dog with your infant, and hopefully this will not happen to you.

Cats

When it comes to cats, people's main concerns are cleanliness and safety. Keep your cat out of the baby's sleeping areas. This means anywhere the baby sleeps—the crib, your bed, the stroller … You can use a baby gate or door closer to block access to rooms. Cats will occasionally, especially in the winter, try to get up next to the baby because they're always looking for warmth. Get your cats a heated bed designed for pets before your baby arrives and they will likely seek warmth there instead of from your baby. Here are a few additional tips for you.

- Wear disposable gloves when cleaning the litter box and wash your hands thoroughly after you're done to help to prevent the spread of infection.

- Keep your cat's vaccinations up to date. This will help to protect them from diseases that they could transmit to your baby.

- Provide your cat with plenty of attention and enrichment to help them feel loved and secure.

Choose a Pediatrician

You'll want to start looking for pediatricians in your area who will work with a relaxed vaccination schedule. I highly recommend immunizing your child, but if you are breastfeeding (which I also highly recommend) you can start later and space out the immunizations. I'll talk a lot more about this in *Volume II*, but for now all I want you to do is locate a good pediatrician or three who are accepting new patients, who accept your insurance or are reasonably priced, and who aren't going to be dictatorial on the immunization schedule. It's important that you ask, because some doctors will not see you unless you will vaccinate according to their schedule.

Assessing the Baby's Position

By the seventh month things start to get very crowded, and the baby starts to curl up and flexion increases as the baby's chin tucks toward their chest. Engagement is also happening; the baby is moving down into the mother's pelvis. Most babies start to descend into the pelvis a little bit before labor. With first time moms it can be four to eight weeks before the birth. With women

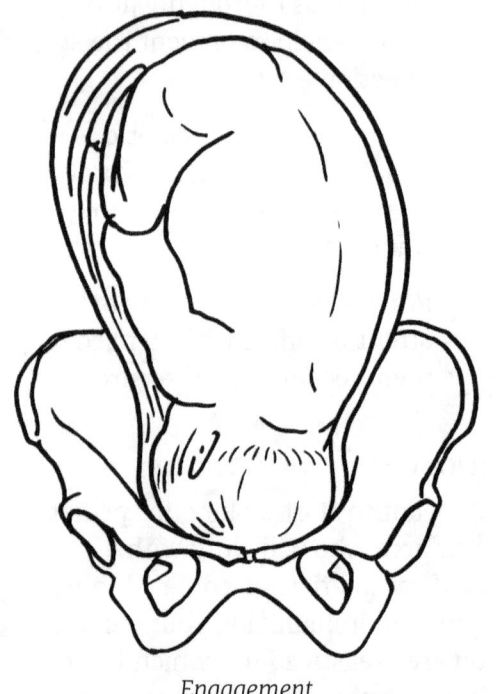

Engagement

who have had babies before it may be as soon as a few weeks before birth or even as they go into labor. I'm going to get a little technical here, so if you prefer not to go on this deep dive with me, you can refer to the captions for each of the images to get a quick summary before moving on to the next section.

The newborn skull is so cool to learn about. It has 33 bones, which is more than the 22 bones that make up an adult human skull. There are *fontanels* (also known as "soft spots") between the bones, and *suture lines* between the fontanels. The baby's head has an anterior fontanel closer to the face and a posterior fontanel toward the back of the head within the occiput.

The fontanels gradually close as the baby grows. The anterior fontanel, which is the largest, closes by about 18 months of age. The posterior fontanel closes by about 2 months of age. The combination of fontanels, less fused bones, and thinner bones makes the infant skull very flexible. This flexibility is important for childbirth and for the growth and development of the brain.

These suture lines and fontanels allow your midwife to tell the position of the baby when she does a pelvic exam. When the cervix is dilated to a certain point, I can examine the woman, feel these soft fontanels and suture lines, and be able to tell the position of the baby's head by where they are positioned in the pelvis.

Determining the baby's position is more than just feeling suture lines. The baby's body can be in one position and the head can be turned and in a different position, so your midwife will work to understand both of those aspects before helping the baby to be in the most optimal position for birth, if necessary.

The back and top part of the baby's head, called the occiput, is usually the portion of the baby's head that engages the pelvis. The occiput engages in one of four ways—right and left occiput anterior and right and left occiput posterior. These refer to the *mother's* left or right side, never the onlooker's right or left side. In the left

occiput anterior (LOA) position, the occiput faces the left front side of the mother's body and pelvis.

With the left occiput posterior (LOP) position, the baby faces the front of the pelvis, and the occiput is up against the back of the pelvis on the left side. In a right occiput anterior (ROA) position, the baby's occiput is facing the front right side of the pelvis. In the right occiput posterior (ROP) position, the baby's occiput is facing the back of the pelvis on the right side.

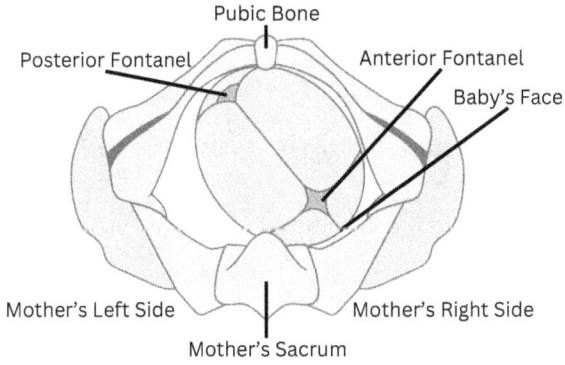

Left Occiput Anterior (LOA) Presentation:
If you are feeling your baby's kicks up against your ribs on the right, then the baby is LOA.

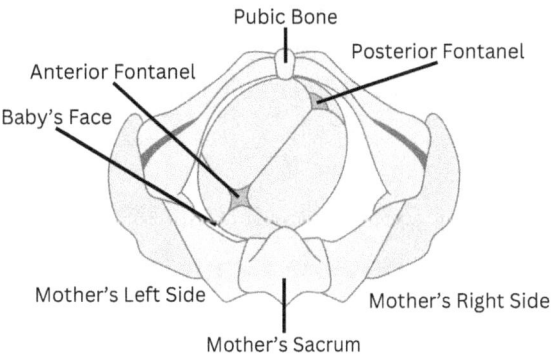

Right Occiput Anterior (ROA) Presentation:
If the baby is ROA, then you will feel the baby's kicks up against your ribs on the left side.

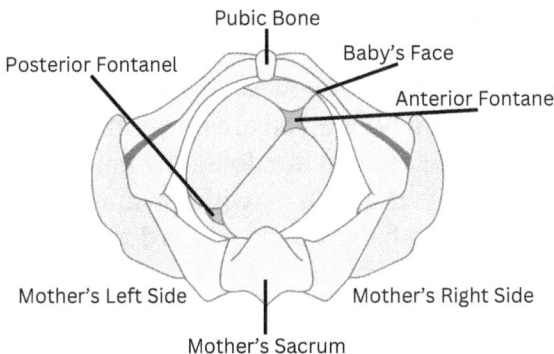

Left Occiput Posterior (LOP) Presentation:
If the baby is LOP you will feel your baby's kicks all on the front, right side of your body.

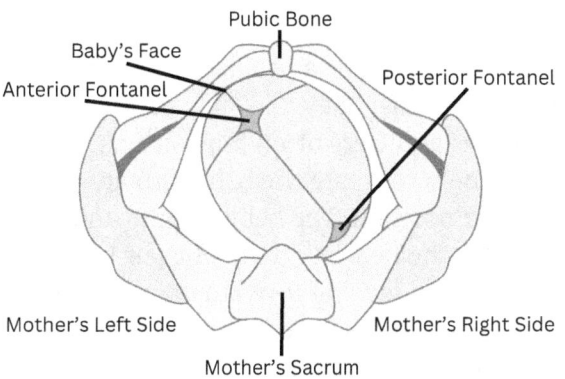

Right Occiput Posterior (ROP) Presentation:
If your baby is ROP, you'll feel their kicks out front on the left side.

THIRD TRIMESTER

MARIMIKEL POTTER, CPM, LM, RN-BSN ✦ 341

When the baby is LOP or ROP and the baby's occiput, or back of the head, is pushing up against the nerves at the back of the spine, it can be very uncomfortable for the mother-to-be. This is sometimes referred to as *back labor*.

It is very important to go into labor with your baby in an anterior position. Posterior positioning is one of the main reasons for prolonged labor and non-progression of labor because the diameter of the baby's head when it is being born in a posterior position is much, much larger, and therefore more difficult to be born and can sometimes not fit through at all. The more you sit, the more the baby will rotate to the back and to a less desirable position.

It is very important to go into labor with your baby in an anterior position. The more you sit, the more the baby will rotate to the back and to a less desirable position.

This used to not be a problem for primitive women because they had such active lifestyles and were often in positions that would help to rotate the baby into an anterior position. The baby's spine and head are the heaviest parts of their body, so if you are leaning forward on all fours (hands and knees) gravity will rotate those heavy parts forward, keeping them in that desired anterior position. Lying back, on the other hand, encourages the baby to rotate into a posterior position. One of the reasons why it can be less than optimal to be at the hospital is that you are generally kept in a bed on your back, so you can be hooked to monitors. This is not the prime laboring position as it can keep your baby in a less desirable posterior position.

The last weeks of pregnancy are a sacred pause, a moment of stillness before the storm of birth, where time seems to both crawl and fly, as you await the miracle of new life.

—Diana Korte, *The VBAC Companion*

What to Do

If your baby is in a posterior position, do whatever you can to encourage them to turn. If you feel your baby's feet all out in front, it is important to try to take steps to move the baby into a better position. Good activities for you to do are to walk and to swim. When you are down in a position where you are doing the kinds of movements that you do while swimming, it can help the baby's body rotate down.

The best position for you to try is the table position, where you get on your hands and knees and gently rock your hips back and forth while keeping your back flat and shoulders and hips level.

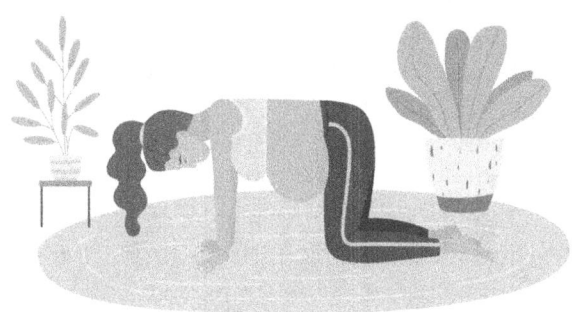

Table Position

This will also help to bring the baby into the anterior position. You can watch TV like this, or read a book or magazine, but you have to do it for about ten to fifteen minutes twice a day to get the baby out of the posterior position.

External Version

Most babies turn on their own between 30–36 weeks. If by Week 36 the baby is still in a breech position, I strongly encourage you to speak to your care provider about the option of turning the baby manually. This is called *external cephalic version* or external version for short.

I have done many external versions over the course of my career, with about a 70 percent success rate. The external version must be timed so it is attempted before the baby is too big to turn back to breech but big enough to stay in the head down position once turned. This is usually around 36 or 37 weeks. Prior to performing the external version, I have to know the exact position of the baby and placenta. Both are verified through an ultrasound. The position of the placenta is key to a successful version. If the placenta is positioned on either side of the abdomen, the version cannot be attempted.

I have the mom drink a glass of wine 30 minutes before the procedure in order to relax her uterine muscle as much as possible. When I start manipulating the baby through the uterine wall it causes strong contractions and can impede my ability to get the baby turned. I find that I have to get the baby turned as quickly as possible before the uterus begins to seize up under the pressure of the contractions.

I have the mother lie on her back with her legs extended and encourage her to

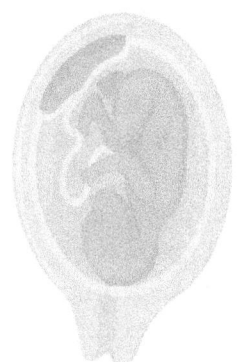

CEPHALIC

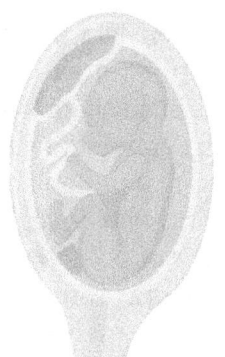

BREECH

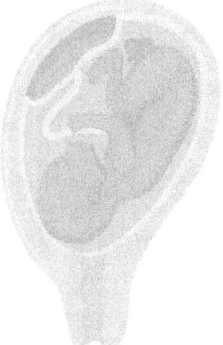

OBLIQUE

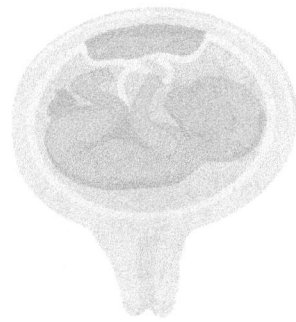

TRANSVERSE

Terms for the Baby's Position in the Uterus

deep breath and relax as much as she can. I have performed this by myself, but it is more successful when you have two skilled practitioners, one to lift the baby's buttocks, legs, and feet and the other to tuck and dive the baby's head down toward the pelvis. When performing version, it is imperative that the practitioner moves the baby forward, pushing the head down and pulling the butt/legs and feet up in a fluid motion. I put an oxygen mask on the mom and administer oxygen throughout and listen to the baby's heart tones as frequently as possible, so that I can monitor the baby and their response to the procedure.

External version is an uncomfortable procedure. How uncomfortable depends on the woman and how many nerve endings she has. It can be mildly uncomfortable to pretty seriously painful.

In a hospital, external versions are performed by an experienced doctor. They will start an IV and give the mother a drug called terbutaline, which relaxes the uterine muscle to stop the contractions that could interfere with the version. They are also prepared for the very unlikely possibility that the version could cause problems for the baby that would require an immediate c-section.

Breech Birth

According to the CDC, about 3–4 percent of babies in the United States are born in breech position. Of these, 93.8 percent are born by c-section. There are not very many doctors or care providers in the United States who know how to deliver breech babies. It is tricky. The head is the largest part of the baby's body, and with a breech birth the butt and body can fit through the pelvis, but the head can get caught up and not be able to be born. If this happens, the baby very likely won't survive. The chances of this happening are quite small, but you don't get to know if the baby's head will fit through the pelvis until the birth. These risks are why most breech babies are born via c-section.

In many states it is not legal to have a breech birth at home. You may be able to have a breech birth in a birthing center with a midwife certified to attend breech births. Some states do not have laws specifically prohibiting breech home births, but in other states you must be in a birth center or a hospital, or your care provider must have specific training and certifications to deliver a breech baby. Your provider will know what is legal in your state.

It is imperative to have conversations with your care provider about your options, and if you want to consider having a natural breech birth, confirm that your provider has plenty of education, experience with breech births, and adequate support personnel. When considering a breech birth at home, I am very careful to make sure the mother's pelvis has enough room and the baby is small enough to facilitate a successful natural labor. It also helps if she has had previous babies vaginally; we know her pelvis works. As long as her baby is not too big, it is something I and many other homebirth midwives will consider (if it is legal to attempt in their state).

As with some of the other risks and complications I discuss in this book, I say this not to scare you but to inform you. Knowledge is power and if you are going to do an external version or consider a natural breech birth, I believe it is so important that you understand all of these factors beforehand.

Four Weeks Before Your Due Date

To recap, here is a summary of what I'm asking you to pay attention to at this stage in your pregnancy. Refer to the corresponding section for complete details.

- ☐ Do what you can and rest.
- ☐ Keep up your vitamins, healthy eating, and fluid intake.
- ☐ Continue to do your kick counts.
- ☐ Continue to prepare to stop working at 38 weeks.
- ☐ Continue/finish your childbirth classes with your partner.
- ☐ Schedule a vaginal culture/bacterial screen with your provider if you haven't already.
- ☐ Say your affirmations and spend time in positive visualization and/or prayer every day.
- ☐ Drink your smoothie daily and get 100 grams of protein a day.
- ☐ Pack and/or prepare your birth supplies and gather your postpartum equipment and supplies.
- ☐ Begin perineal massage with Vitamin E oil two to four times a week.
- ☐ Start castor oil hot packs twice a week for 20 minutes each session.

- ☐ Partners, clean the birth room and bathroom (or arrange for it to be professionally cleaned).
- ☐ Purchase nursing bras if you haven't yet.
- ☐ Practice each breathing technique together two to four times a week for one minute.
- ☐ Keep wearing your belly band.
- ☐ Watch birth videos.
- ☐ Prepare your pets.
- ☐ Make an appointment with a pediatrician(s) for a prenatal consultation (if appropriate in your area).
- ☐ Work with your midwife to assess your baby's current position.
- ☐ Cut your fingernails. There's no corresponding section for this one, because it's as simple as that. I strongly suggest not having long fingernails with a new baby, you can hurt them or scratch your new little one easily in the course of providing newborn care. Now is a good time to cut or drastically shorten the fingernails on your dominant hand.

Week 37

Preparation Postpartum Nourishment

Now is the time to prepare your menus and begin to prepare and freeze home-cooked meals in advance of your postpartum period. See my guidance for this in the Nutrition section of this chapter.

Preparation for Postpartum: Room Setup

Set up the room so the partner can easily help mom and mom can help herself. The best way I have found to do this is to get the multi-function use Pack-N-Play that has the changing table at one end. You may want to wait until the day after the birth to set this up, but it is important that you have all these things ready to go beforehand, so you can set them up easily and quickly when the time comes. The baby is generally in bed with mom for the first day or so, but after that having this safe space for your baby to be in, as well as having all of your necessary and essential items on hand, gives you more options.

I suggest that you move the bedside table temporarily out of the room and push the Pack-N-Play with the changing table up against the wall where the bedside table was. You will need a cutting board that fits within the changing table section of the Pack-N-Play. If you place it there you will then have a stable surface to use as your temporary bedside table.

The area underneath the changing table is a great place for you to store some of the items that are so helpful to have nearby in the postpartum period like diapers, diaper cream, wipes, baby clothes, and baby blankets. It is also a great place to have a small basket with alcohol, thermometers, cotton-tipped swabs and cotton balls, arnica, Weleda baby cream, nipple cream and all the items that you will use frequently for baby or mom.

On top of the changing table with cutting board, I suggest you get a touch lamp with multiple levels of light (this can be a touch lamp or lamp with a dimmer on it). This is so helpful in the middle of the night when you may need to look at your baby quickly. It allows you to turn the light on dimly to not wake everyone up or turn it on brightly if needed.

You can set other items that are usually on your nightstand on the cutting board as well, like your water, chargers, etc. This area only takes up about a third of the top of the Pack-N-Play, leaving two-thirds available for the baby to sleep or be in between feedings.

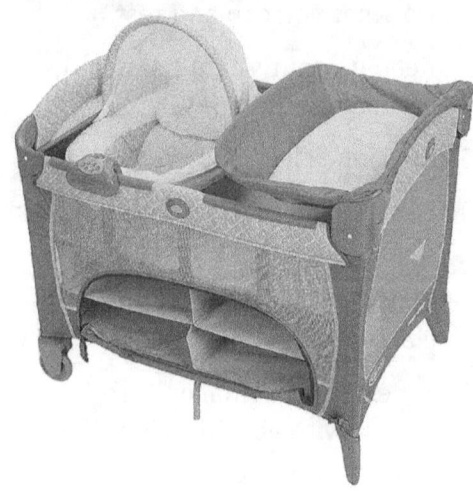

Deluxe Playpen

It is also handy to keep three sacks or bins on the floor close to the bed: one for dirty diapers, one for dirty clothes, and one for trash.

Preparation for Breastfeeding

It is really essential to prepare for breastfeeding. Just as you must prepare for birth, you must prepare to be a breastfeeding momma. It is challenging. It is a full-time job to make sure you are staying healthy enough to produce the milk that will help your baby to not only survive but thrive.

Furthermore, it is a learned behavior. For most of our presence on earth, humans have lived in tribes where breastfeeding would have been commonly seen. Women would have learned through repeatedly seeing it around them, as if by osmosis, and from each other, because it was such a commonplace experience. Women would have seen problems in other babies and seen how they were addressed. It was a very communal, hive mind knowledge.

This is not true anymore. Not at all. You must learn, and because breastfeeding publicly is often seen as taboo, we do not have the same space to learn from the mothers around us. While some women have a very easy time breastfeeding, for others it is not just a dreamy, la-la-la fairytale-like experience where everything just works blissfully. Some women struggle. Foreknowledge can wipe out many of the difficulties women face. It is very important to prepare, read books, watch videos, and go to La Leche League or other breastfeeding support groups or classes.[149]

It also is good to start to prepare yourself for the physical demands of breastfeeding. If you have very light-colored areolas or have significantly sensitive nipples, I have a few tips to prepare them for breastfeeding.

You can use a terry cloth washcloth to gently rub your nipples for one to two minutes occasionally after you take a shower to begin to toughen them up in the last few weeks of the pregnancy. While I am aware that some lactation consultants do not suggest this practice, In my experience I have seen it to be helpful. It is important to note that it should be done gently and should never hurt in any way.

If the climate and privacy are conducive, I also recommend sunning your breasts. This can help to darken the nipples and darker nipples will be tougher. You can sun your baby through your abdominal wall at the same time.

Another practice that is recommended to help prepare the nipples is to do a little bit of hand pumping a few times a week with an oil-based lubricant, like coconut oil, that you rub on the areola beforehand. This can also be used to help evert the nipple for moms with flat or inverted nipples.

When young girls begin wearing bras as their breasts are developing, the bras can flatten nipples as the tissue develops. If this happened to you and your nipple is a little bit on the flat side, you can pull it out or the baby will do it for you, which I don't recommend. So, pull it out as much as you can, possibly using an at-home breast pump to aid you, or look for a device called a breast shell or nipple shield.

Nipple Shield

La Leche League Meetings

Breastfeeding is sometimes so easy, and sometimes it is so incredibly hard, and you never know. You may have one baby who is easy to breastfeed, and the next baby is a struggle, but you just do not get to know in advance.

You will need a support system, and I am very fond of lactation consultants. La Leche League classes are usually structured to provide peer support—women acting in a surrogate tribal village to help each other with breastfeeding support and troubleshooting. Now, all this reading that you're doing is great, but it is not the same as getting together with other moms who are also breastfeeding. Meeting other women in the same stage of life gives you a wonderful network of support and camaraderie to be able to have people you can call and friendships with people like you. I strongly suggest you seek out a chapter near you now, and find out if they have classes you can take in advance of your baby's birth.

Men are not allowed at these meetings, so women can feel more comfortable breastfeeding and exposing their breasts as it's only women around them. If you are not close to a La Leche League, you may be able to find another breastfeeding support group in your area.

If you aren't able to specifically find a breastfeeding support group, look for a prenatal yoga group, childbirth classes, a mommy and me group, or any number of other supportive meetups for pregnant and/or breastfeeding mommas. There is a community that will suit you. And if there isn't, start one.

If it is not part of your midwife's practice, I recommend you find a lactation consultant in your area before you give birth so you have someone you can call on at a moment's notice. Again, sometimes breastfeeding is really easy and sometimes it is really *not*. Having your support system lined up ahead of time is a great idea.

Three Weeks Before Your Due Date

To recap, here is a summary of what I'm asking you to pay attention to at this stage in your pregnancy. Refer to the corresponding section for complete details.

- ☐ Do what you can and rest. Rest more. Rest more than that.
- ☐ Keep up your vitamins, healthy eating, and fluid intake.
- ☐ Make your menus and start to prepare your food for the first two weeks postpartum.
- ☐ Prepare your room for your baby.
- ☐ Prepare to breastfeed. Establish a support network.
- ☐ Continue to do your kick counts.
- ☐ Continue to prepare to stop working next week.
- ☐ Say your affirmations and spend time in positive visualization and/or prayer every day.
- ☐ Drink your smoothie daily and get 100 grams of protein a day.
- ☐ Continue perineal massage with Vitamin E oil.
- ☐ Continue castor oil hot packs.

- ☐ Practice each breathing technique together two to four times a week for one minute.
- ☐ Partners, maintain your home's cleanliness.
- ☐ Purchase nursing bras if you haven't yet.
- ☐ Keep wearing your belly band.
- ☐ Continue to prepare your pets.

Week 38

Stop Working If at All Possible

This is the time to seriously switch your focus. I dive deeply into why this is the time to stop working later in the Rest section of this chapter, but I wanted you to have a reminder of it here in case you are looking at this section independently of the rest of the book.

Assessing Baby's Position

Breech and Other Less-Than-Optimal Positions

By Week 38, most babies have turned, so they are head down. Your midwife will help you understand your baby's positioning and work with you to optimize it, but if you come to a place where baby just isn't cooperating, surrender to your care provider's advice and work with them to attempt to correct a less-than-optimal position. Refer to Weeks 35–36.

Set Up Your Birth Pool (Optional)

Select a Location for the Pool

Choose a place that meets the following criteria:

1. Privacy. Avoid high traffic areas like the living room or dining room.

2. You can walk around at least 65 percent of the perimeter—this way someone can always reach you as needed.

3. The placement is close enough that the hose will reach from the faucet to the pool and from the pool to the location of draining (usually outside through a window or door).

4. Where floorboards can support additional weight.

5. Where there will be room to get mom out and down onto the floor if needed.

A lot of parents have a designated nursery, which is often a great room for the birthing pool. It's cozy and private, you can close the door, and the pool often fits snugly in the center of the room. This can be a great choice.

If the pool won't quite fit in the nursery you can move some of the smaller furniture out, like a changing table or chairs and then the tub will likely fit. Moms are often so happy to be in such a womb-like, private space that it makes this effort worthwhile.

Inflating and Cleaning the Pool

It's a great idea to inflate and partially fill the birth pool prior to going into labor. You need to allow at least an hour to set the pool up in the room, position it, inflate it, clean it, and have it ready before then filling it with water. I suggest you have your pool set up but not filled with water by the time you reach 39 weeks.

If you have an older child, leave the pool empty until labor begins or have the pool in a locked room so your older child(ren) can't fall in. Use a hook and eye closure that is out of their reach on the outside of the door.

When setting up the pool, place the plastic sheet on the floor and center the pool on top of it to protect your floor. You will inflate the pool with an air compressor. **When filling the pool, please make sure to stand there the entire time to avoid over inflating.** My clients have lost several pools by not doing this. The pool may need to be re-inflated if it sits for a while.

After the tank is inflated, add room temperature water until you have a depth of 3 inches. Put this water into the pool ahead of time, so when you go into labor and your partner adds the hot water straight from the hot water heater to the pool, it won't melt the plastic. Add ¼ cup of bleach to keep algae from developing while it sits. The bleach evaporates completely daily so you need to add it every day.

If you don't do this before you go into labor, it can impact whether or not you are able to use the pool in labor. If you have a very fast labor, you may not be able to get the pool set up in time and your bathtub may be your only option. This is another reason to make sure your home is as clean as you can make it in advance of the birth.

Filling the Pool

It is important that your hot water tank is turned up *before* you go into labor. You want to be certain that you will have LOTS of hot water for your pool, showers, and clean up. Adjust the temperature of your hot water

tank to 140°F or more. It can be turned down to 120°F the day after the baby is born.

You should start filling the pool as soon as you think you are going into labor. You can always drain and refill the pool if you don't actually go into labor. It takes two to four hours to fill the pool if you have a 50-gallon hot water heater, longer if it's smaller. As you are filling it, feel the end of the hose occasionally and turn the water off as soon as it is warm instead of hot. If you let it get completely cool it will take much longer for the tank to reheat.

The size of a hot water heater is 30–50 gallons, and the pool holds approximately 150 gallons. When you go into labor, start filling with hot water only. You will have to empty the hot water from the heater into the pool, let the heater refill and reheat, and then empty again two or three times to completely fill the pool with the right temperature. It is very important not to get the pool too hot as it will raise your blood pressure. Aim for a very comfortable 98–100°F.

Two Weeks Before and Until You Go into Labor

To recap, here is a summary of what I'm asking you to pay attention to at this stage in your pregnancy. Refer to the corresponding section for complete details.

- ☐ Stop working if at all possible.
- ☐ Rest a lot. Now, rest more than that.
- ☐ Keep up your vitamins, healthy eating, and fluid intake.
- ☐ Continue to work with your midwife to assess baby's position and your overall health.

- ☐ Partners, set up the birthing pool.
- ☐ Finish your postpartum food preparations.
- ☐ Finish preparing your room for your baby.
- ☐ Prepare to breastfeed. Establish a support network if you haven't already.
- ☐ Continue to do your kick counts.
- ☐ Say your affirmations and spend time in positive visualization and/or prayer every day.
- ☐ Drink your smoothie daily and get 100 grams of protein a day.
- ☐ Continue perineal massage with Vitamin E oil.
- ☐ Continue castor oil hot packs.
- ☐ Practice each breathing technique together two to four times a week for one minute.
- ☐ Partners, maintain your home's cleanliness.
- ☐ Purchase nursing bras if you haven't yet.
- ☐ Keep wearing your belly band.
- ☐ Continue to prepare your pets.

Signs of Impending Labor

While you never know exactly when your true labor will start, there are several signs that the day is coming soon.

Hormonal Surge

The first thing that happens—the thing that gets the whole birth process going—is hormones start coursing through your body in increasing amounts. Estrogen, progesterone, relaxin, and oxytocin are all steadily going up in your bloodstream.

> **SIGNS OF IMPENDING LABOR**
>
> + Increased hormones
> + Ripening
> + Increasing contractions
> + Engagement
> + Effacement
> + Dilation
> + Emotional volatility
> + Increased amounts of vaginal discharge
> + Increasing or decreasing fetal activity
> + Increasing or decreasing maternal activity: nesting, lethargy,
> + Cramping
> + Mucus plug
> + Diarrhea and/or nausea
> + Warm-up labor

Ripening

The increased estrogen, progesterone, and relaxin will cause another sign of impending labor, *ripening*, which is the softening of the lower uterine segment, the cervix, the vagina, and the perineum. In reality, your whole body softens.

In the final weeks, you are a vessel of love, carrying dreams and hopes, feeling every flutter as you approach the crescendo of birth.

—Angela Gallo

Ripening is essential to the baby's emergence, but many of the complaints of late-stage pregnancy seem to come from this softening and ripening.

You can have more indigestion, varicose veins, hemorrhoids, and other ailments that come from your body being so soft. Even your eyeballs get soft, and you can have visual disturbances. Unfortunately, your body has not figured out that the baby will not be born out of your eyeballs. All of these things are normal but can indeed be bothersome. As far as impending signs of birth are concerned, we birth workers are especially interested in the softening of the cervix and the lower uterine segment at this time, so the contractions can pull the cervix open for the baby to be born.

Increasing Contractions

Another sign of impending labor is increasing contractions. Oxytocin is released all throughout the pregnancy and it makes you have contractions from the moment the placenta implants into the lining of the uterus until weeks after the birth.

When the pregnancy contractions happen, they gently but increasingly stress the baby to help prepare them for the real contractions of labor, they squeeze fresh blood into the placenta, and they build the muscle mass of the uterus. The pregnancy contractions are isometric exercises, so the muscle is strengthened and will grow to build the muscle mass. By the end of the pregnancy these contractions become very apparent.

You may notice that your abdomen is soft and then hard, and many think it's their

baby sticking an arm or foot out, but often it is actually contractions taking place!

Many times, the baby will move in response to being squeezed by a contraction. So, sometimes your baby's movements and contractions go hand-in-hand.

Engagement

The next sign of impending labor is *engagement*. This is when the baby's head moves lower into your pelvis.

The only way the baby's head can come down into the pelvis is because of the softening or ripening which has made the lower uterine segment soft enough that the contractions can push the baby down to engage with the cervix.

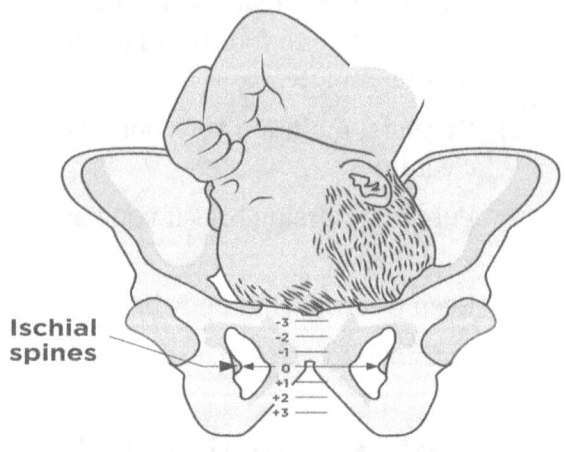

Pelvic Stations

When the baby enters the pelvis, it means that the occiput presentation is at -3 station, and as it descends into the pelvis it goes to -2, then -1.

When the top of the head is even with the ischial spines or mid-pelvis that is called 0 station, and as the head descends further it reaches +1, +2, and then at +3 the head is on the perineum.

The baby can also go in and out of the pelvis in those last weeks of pregnancy; it's very common. You may have a day where you are on your feet a lot more and the pressure and contractions and softening bring the baby into the pelvis significantly but then you have a day where you are off your feet and resting more and the baby floats back up out of the pelvis a bit and is not as low. For example, on a day where you are on your feet more and the baby is much lower, you could be 70 percent effaced and the baby is at +1 station, but the next day when you're resting you may only be 30 percent effaced and at a −2 station. This is a dynamic process.

A first time, or primipara (primip), mom often will engage about 4–6 weeks before birth, and for a mother who has given birth before (multipara/multip) this can occur anywhere from two weeks before to just before the birth.

Cervical Effacement

Another sign of impending labor is cervical effacement, which is the shortening of the cervix from the pressure of the baby's head coming down against the cervix. Effacement is spoken of in terms of percentages. When your cervix is 0 percent effaced, it is longer and not shortening at all. At 50 percent effaced it is halfway there, then 75 percent effaced, and so on, until it is 100 percent effaced, which means the cervix is completely thinned and there are no longer two oses. There is only one os and one opening for the baby to come through during labor.

Cervical Dilation

The next impending sign of labor is dilation. In reality, all of these impending signs are happening at the same time. The increasing hormones happen and because of that you have more and more contractions and softening. Because of softening and the contractions, the baby is pushed down, which helps the baby engage

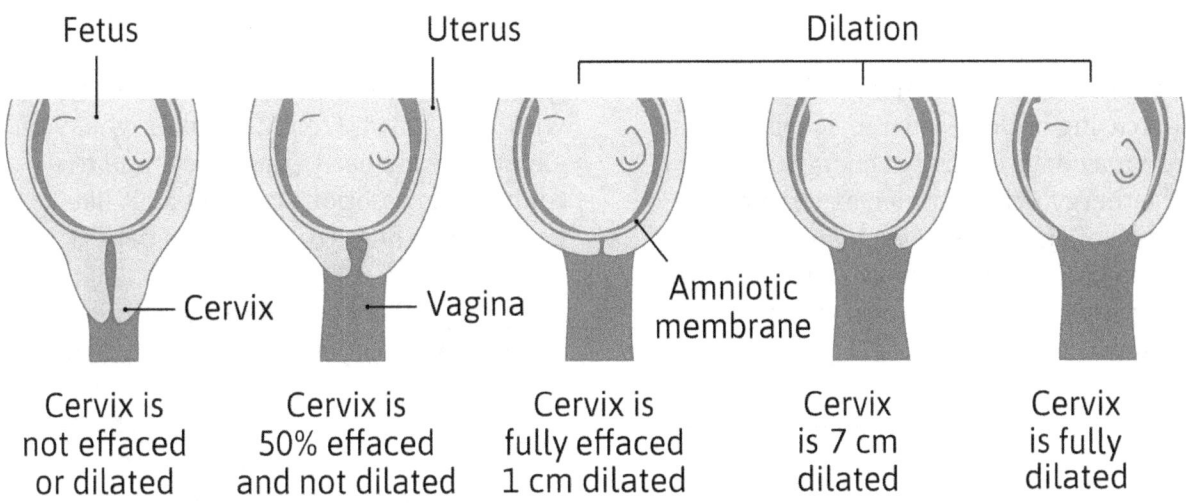

| Fetus | Uterus | Dilation | | |

| Cervix is not effaced or dilated | Cervix is 50% effaced and not dilated | Cervix is fully effaced 1 cm dilated | Cervix is 7 cm dilated | Cervix is fully dilated |

Stages of Cervical Effacement and Dilation

and the cervix to become effaced and dilated. Effacement and dilation generally occur together.

I love to see women reach 50–100 percent effaced and be 1–3 cm dilated when they go into labor. The dilation of the cervix is spoken of in terms of centimeters. With dilation you have 1 cm, 2 cm, 3 cm ... all the way up to 10 cm, which is fully dilated and means you are ready for pushing.

Dilation is somewhat dependent on the size of the baby's head. You are not going to have to dilate as much if your baby is 6 pounds versus 10 pounds, because the cervix will enlarge to the size of the baby's head.

At 5 cm your midwife can see the cervix shortening/effacing as well as dilating. At 7 cm it is about 75–80 percent effaced, and at 9 cm it is almost completely effaced, and dilation is nearly complete. The more warm-up labor you have, the more dilation you will have ahead of time.

Change in Maternal Activity Levels

The next sign of impending labor is increasing or decreasing maternal activity. You may have a burst of energy or a burst of lethargy. Many women experience these bursts of energy as nesting and are driven to repaint the nursery all of a sudden, or to rearrange all the furniture, or reorganize a closet.

Conversely, you may feel an urge to sleep more. Please give in to this urge! You don't need to clean anything or reorganize anything or finish anything else right now.

Change in Fetal Activity Levels

Another sign of impending labor is increasing or decreasing fetal activity. Many babies slow down a lot and are very still and just not that active, and other babies move lots and act like they are trying to kick their way out. Continue to do your kick counts every day (see page 318).

Vaginal Discharge

Increased vaginal discharge is another sign of impending labor. The vagina cleanses itself out, keeping any bacteria or pathogens away, so increased vaginal discharge is a very common sign that many women experience. It may be copious; you may have lots and lots of vaginal discharge or you may not see a big change at all (or anything in between). The mucus also serves to lubricate the vagina, so the baby slides by the tissues more easily without abrasions or tears.

Meteoric Emotions

As labor is coming nearer you may also experience increasing and decreasing emotional changes. You may be very happy or very sad; you may be easy to get along with or very hard to get along with. This may be reminiscent of what you experienced in early pregnancy, and the tumultuous emotions can feel a bit like you're on a roller coaster in the dark.

 Partners, please remember that you can make space for your pregnant woman to be emotional without becoming emotional yourself. Be the riverbed for her coursing emotions. Your assignment is to be calm and reassuring, and to give her

space to feel what she is feeling. Speak her love language to her. Be grateful that it's not your body undergoing all these radical changes. Remember, you have the ability through your support and love to help lift her up during this time. If you are feeling stressed or anxious, you can rest assured she is feeling that and more. Take a deep breath and be the supportive, guiding light through any dark or tumultuous times, so she has what she needs for the coming marathon of birth and the bringing of your sweet baby into this world.

Cramping

Another sign of impending labor is cramping. Cramping is always caused by contractions. In the last few weeks of pregnancy, you may feel like you are about to start your period. Some sharp stabbing sensations are quite common as the cervix effaces and ripens and the baby engages. In my own pregnancies, it felt like my baby had fingernails or some kind of sharp teeth that they would stab me with in my cervix. A way to tell the difference between the cramping that you feel at the end of pregnancy and the cramping of labor is that the cramping gets longer, stronger, and closer together, and the pain escalates. These types of pains can be very normal, but remember, if you feel anything that concerns you, call your midwife or doctor right away.

Nausea

You may also experience nausea as a sign of impending labor. Some women who are sensitive to rising oxytocin levels will experience a lot of this in early pregnancy, as labor approaches, and during labor. In these last few weeks, you may feel rushes of nausea due to increased hormones and oxytocin levels. Keep eating. It's easy to get low blood sugar by not eating frequently enough. Lay down in a cool dark room with no stimulus (TV, phone, etc.) and place a cold wet cloth on your neck. This is a great way to combat feelings of nausea.

Diarrhea

Diarrhea can also be a sign of impending labor. The nerves that innervate your uterus are the same nerves that innervate your colon, except that they branch off right at the end. Rectal nerves are stimulated by increasing contractions which can contribute to looser bowels as you get closer to the main event.

This is why you should not take laxatives, enemas, and colonics while you are pregnant. This is also why all women used to receive enemas when they went into the hospital in labor. It would stimulate the uterus and make labor proceed more quickly. Diarrhea happens as part of the process of your body cleansing itself in preparation for labor, so there is nothing in the way of the baby coming through the pelvis.

Mucus Plug

You may experience a mucus plug. I never did see a mucus plug with any of my labors, and most of my clients do not see one, but a mucus plug is present for most of the pregnancy. I think sometimes it is absorbed or it may fall out into the toilet. The plug looks like old mucus, not like vaginal discharge. It is like an old, solid chunk of mucus that may have some brown or pink in it. Seeing this drop out is a sign of impending labor. Your body is getting ready.

Warm-up Labor

The number one sign of impending labor is warm-up labor. You will never hear me call it false labor; I think that is an unkind characterization because there is nothing false about it. Women's bodies know exactly what to do and they practice a lot at the end. This practice is very important to get more effacement, more engagement, more dilation, and better molding of the baby's head, so it can better fit through the pelvis. All of this is absolutely essential, and you have to have stronger and stronger contractions in order to give birth. Practice your breathing when they come on strong.

You may find that you are going into warm-up labor at night, your body is acting like you're going to go into labor, but it's not quite true labor. Warm-up labor starts and stops. You'll find your body is practicing and trying to figure out what to do. This is a definitive sign that your time is getting close.

I'll do an exam on the pregnant momma (if they're not opposed) nearing the end of the pregnancy. If they're not effaced and not engaging, especially for first time moms, I'll put evening primrose oil on the cervix, and that is an incredibly great trick for ripening and softening the cervix, so contractions are more effective.

If you are having warm-up labor, take heart! Every contraction that you do ahead of time is something you don't have to do in labor. Your time is near now!

> If you are having warm-up labor, take heart! Every contraction that you do ahead of time is something you don't have to do in labor.

MariMikel: In three of my six births I had warm-up labor. On one of my last two, I knew the baby was coming soon. I had bloody show, contractions that were getting longer, stronger, and closer together, it was very painful, and I was doing the breathing to manage the sensations. I had had very fast births previously, so all the midwives rushed over, and they stood around waiting for my labor to kick in.

At about 11 p.m. I started yawning, so one of my friends and midwives suggested I rest for a bit. I thought, *Sure, okay*. I took what I thought would be a little nap and when I woke up, it was morning. There was no baby and everyone was gone. I was so embarrassed that I actually cried.

They said I had started snoring so loudly that they all stood and thought, *That does not look like a woman in labor*. It was obvious I was dead asleep and not moving, so they packed up their equipment and went home. I ended up having the baby three days later, and the intense contractions were exactly like what I had experienced when I'd called the midwives over.

The difference between warm-up labor and actual labor is that warm-up labor stops and actual labor does not.

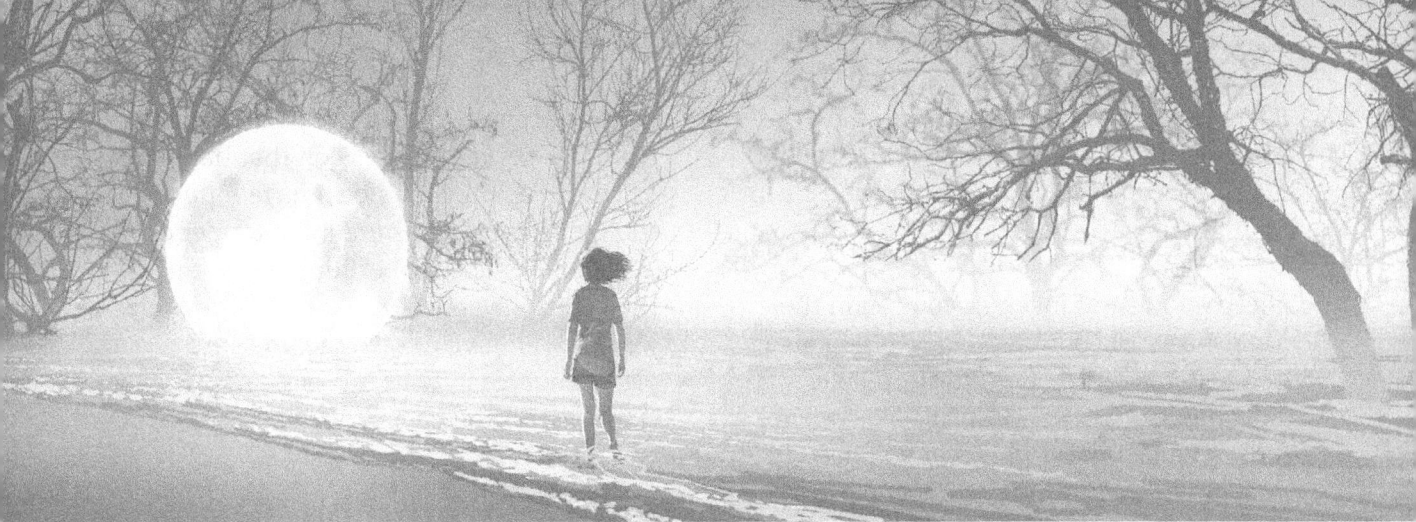

Rest

You will likely feel either an increase or decrease in your energy levels as you approach labor. Continuing to gain adequate rest as you approach the birth process is crucial.

The Four-Hour Rule

I had a client once who worked full time, and one Friday evening she came home and spilled some salad dressing. While she was cleaning that up, she noticed it took the wax off a small spot on the floor. She then got out the wax remover and scrubbed every inch of wax off her floor. She finished at 2 or 3 in the morning and, as she was finishing the floor stripping, her water broke.

She called me just weeping and inconsolable, asking, "How can I make this stop? I am so exhausted. What can I do to hold it off?" Unfortunately, nothing worked to slow it down, and she ended up having a miserable labor because she was so super tired.

Now I have a rule: if you grow a wild hair and want to go crazy with a project or

something during the last month of your pregnancy, you can only do it in four-hour increments, with at least one good break after two hours (at a minimum!). Do not go into the late afternoon or evening. That is the time for rest, not overworking or exhausting yourself. After four hours, you must stop and go back to it another day.

Rest and Decreasing Stress

You want to be resting deeply, as much as you can, in these final months. The marathon isn't over ... in fact, you've only just about made it to the starting line. Pregnancy and birth aren't the end of the demands on your body. It is so much more intense to deal with a newborn than it is to deal with birth. Birth is a day in your life, but parenting is forever. You will have months of interrupted sleep when your baby arrives, and you must build your strength and reserves for that now. Take luxurious naps. Relax in the tub. Lounge in the pool. Relax and take breaks. Rest whenever possible.

Listen to your body. Rest during the day if needed. If you nap, don't do it after about 1 p.m., because it can affect how you sleep at night.

Sleep and rest as much as you can in the final weeks of your pregnancy. If you are too agitated and restless to sleep, take advantage of pharmaceuticals like Tylenol PM or Benadryl. Do whatever you need to do. Melatonin or CBD works for some people.

Resting includes setting up boundaries to exclude people who are inadvertently checking in on you every few hours to see if you've gone into labor yet. Put your phone on Do Not Disturb when you are resting. It's important that you prioritize deep, uninterrupted rest.

One of the ways that you can deeply relax in this final stage is by trusting and knowing that you've done everything right. You've eaten fabulously, you've exercised regularly and deeply, you've made sure to get your rest, you are well informed, and living a healthy lifestyle. You're managing your stress and fear. You're working with the emotional, physical, medical, and mental components of what you're doing. You have done all you can do. Now, you can relax. You can let go.

Breathe.

Alleviating Hip Pain so You Can Sleep

By this point in the pregnancy many women experience hip pain when sleeping. In these final weeks as you are getting bigger and bigger, you're likely moving from one side to the other because lying on your back is no longer comfortable. Hip pain can result from the nerve compression that happens as you sleep on your side. I have found that getting an egg crate foam topper or Tempur-Pedic's topper for your side of the bed is a wonderful solution. It provides just enough give to take the pressure off the nerves in your hip that are being compressed and causing you pain.

Stop Working by 36–38 Weeks

Throughout your third trimester I want you to work to take things off of your plate. Then take more off of your plate. Take as much as you possibly can off your plate. Say, "No." Now is not the time to be taking on any further responsibility whatsoever other than the responsibility you have to the new life inside you.

> The last weeks of pregnancy are like the last chapters of an epic novel—every sensation, every movement, every emotion a poignant reminder of the incredible journey you've undertaken.
>
> —Laura Stavoe Harm

I very strongly encourage the women in my care stop working at 38 weeks. You may

Aleah: MariMikel is quite adamant about stopping work two weeks before your due date, and I know this can be such a difficult topic for so many women for a lot of different reasons. First of all, we only have so long in the United States for maternity leave. Typically, it's 12 weeks and most women want to spend that time with their newborn. It's usually unpaid leave. You may have vacation time stored up and can use some of that, so you either get a little money or can extend your leave, but some women have even less than that or don't even know that the family medical leave act (FMLA) is their right by law. Other women are single moms or in households that are paycheck to paycheck and literally cannot afford to take off that much time, so there are many factors that go into this.

We're a middle-class family. We're not necessarily living paycheck to paycheck, but we don't have much in the way of savings. It was hard for me to consider taking off work before I was due and having potentially less time with my baby after birth, so I struggled with it.

At about 35 weeks I was working 45 hours a week in a very high stress social work job, and my body came to a point where it sent a clear message of *no more*. I was at work and started having pretty intense, painful contractions. They didn't stop and were getting closer together. I had to breathe through them. I of course called MariMikel, and she told me to go home immediately.

She helped me to understand that my body was very ready, more ready than it should be at that point, or more ready than we wanted it to be. There was this impending sense that I was going to have the baby a month early, which we didn't want. The baby was very small by all guesses, and we wanted them to stay in longer. We wanted them to get bigger. They're just so much hardier when they are full term. They can breastfeed better; they have less likelihood of jaundice—there are just so many factors that come into play when a baby comes early.

I was put on bed rest. I really think my body was doing me a favor by saying *this is too much. You're pushing yourself too hard.* I had planned on working up until the end, maybe taking a week off before the due date, but I ended up having to take a month off beforehand instead. I was able to work it out with my manager, so I could work part-time from home on tasks I could do from my computer in my bed. I was lucky and glad they worked with me, but I wish I had slowed down during my third trimester, so I maybe could have worked until 38 weeks and then taken off, and so I didn't use all of my sick days beforehand.

We have such a sad state of affairs with our maternal healthcare system in the US. It is just backwards. We do not take care of our mothers, we don't take care of our fathers, and we generally don't do enough to support families with their real-world issues like family leave, support for childcare, broader support for breastfeeding, etc. If you look at European countries, you'll find many of them have policies that allow mothers to take a year or two off to take care of infants and young children. Fathers get significant paternal leave. And most of this is paid; it may not be a full salary, but it's enough to live on. This is the way we should look at families supporting families across the world. It is so challenging to leave a three-month-old and go back to work. I think there is a better way, and I wish we would talk about this more and change the policies in the United States to support families.

think you can keep going, and maybe you can, but know that it is incredibly hard on you and your baby for you to exert yourself. One of the reasons your baby comes out of your safe and comfortable womb is because your body has exceeded its capacity to provide what that baby needs in terms of space and nutrients from the placenta, etc. The end of pregnancy is as difficult for your baby as it is for you, and they need you to relax, rest, and give them the power and peace they need to go through the coming transition.

I do occasionally have clients whose jobs are truly not taxing, who are making good decisions about what they need to do for themselves, and they are able to work a little longer. There are also people who simply must keep working in order to make ends meet. I don't want you to feel bad if you have to keep working. Do what you can to mitigate the work stress in your life and surrender to the reality of the situation.

I encourage women to use this time to talk with their baby, reassure their baby, prepare their baby. Tell them about what's coming, and how they won't be alone in the dark for much longer. Tell them that soon you'll be able to look into each other's eyes and hold each other. Soon, they'll be nourished by the flowing breast milk that your body is preparing to make for them. Tell them to come for the milk, to come for the bonding. Labor is coming, and birth is coming, and it's going to be so wonderful.

Your baby needs as much from you in the two weeks prior to birth as they will in the two weeks after birth. All of these demands are going on inside of you, though, so it's very easy for people to not understand just how much energy your baby needs and is taking from you during the last weeks of pregnancy. You will certainly feel it, though.

You will have no problem dropping everything to nurse and care for your baby once they are out of the womb. Give your baby this same attention before birth. Relax, destress, let go of all of your "should-dos." Release any guilt that might arise from letting go of those things, too. You are putting your energy where it belongs.

Relax, destress, let go of all of your "should-dos." Release any guilt that might arise from letting go of those things, too. You are putting your energy where it belongs.

You will be shocked at where your mind will go if you give it the space to ride out the natural flow of these last few weeks. Instead of thinking about work-related projects, your mind will start going to the pregnancy, birth, and the new baby coming into your life. When you stop work and stop thinking about work and other external concerns, you are able to devote that mental energy to your baby, to what your impending life might be like, to motherhood and the experience in front of you. Make space for these important things.

Now, some women are so conditioned to feeling the corporate grind that it's a very difficult transition for them, and I would argue that for these women it is even more necessary to absolutely try to stop working by 38 weeks. There are of course single mommas who literally must work until they give birth and must return to work as soon as humanly possible after that just so they can survive. But if it is within your means, if your village can make it happen, I strongly recommend that you do stop working at 38 weeks. If your baby arrives early, they could join you in a few short days!

How to Sleep During Warm-Up Labor

With a planned home birth, the number one cause for hospital transport among my clients is exhaustion from warm-up labor, where the mother experiences long bouts of contractions that wear her out. Warm-up labor contractions are often 5–20 minutes apart. At that point there is not much to do aside from rest, eat well, drink water, and take your vitamins. Take care of yourself. Go to bed early.

If you are having warm-up labor during the day, go about your day as you normally would. I do not want you to march around, as that will wear you out. Once you are in actual labor, then you can definitely start moving around.

Warm-up labor can interfere with your sleep and exhaust you before actual labor begins. Sleep is worth its weight in gold at this time! Too many women are so excited to get on with the big event that when they experience warm-up labor, they expend a ton of energy walking and moving to stimulate actual labor. If your contractions are not escalating rapidly, are six or more minutes apart, or are not close together or painfully strong, chances are this is warm-up labor, and you should do the Trick to get yourself to sleep. It is fantastic and so amazingly effective.

The truth of the matter is, if you are truly going into labor, this trick will not stop it. Your labor will keep going no matter what you do. If it is warm-up labor there is nothing to do to stimulate actual labor, it will only serve to tire you out. I have seen women go through days and days of warm-up labor and end up in the hospital because they just got so tired.

The Trick

If you are experiencing warm-up labor and having difficulty sleeping, then I want you to try the Trick so you can rest and get some sleep. The Trick includes drinking a glass of wine, taking ibuprofen, and taking a hot shower or bath and lying down. Instructions

Penelope: I remember feeling a great deal of rage at my warm-up contractions. *Wasn't I already sore enough? Wasn't I already exhausted? Wasn't I supposed to be able to rest before real labor started?* Waking up several times a night wracked with contractions felt like practicing for something I did not need to practice for. It felt like I was unable to get any real rest, and it sucked. But I did know that it meant my time was getting closer and closer. I wish I had known then what steps to take to ensure that I got some sleep during those final weeks.

are below, but first let me talk about a few different aspects of the Trick.

The ibuprofen is there to help to take the edge off of cramping. It works for warm-up contractions (and PMS) that is just painful enough that you cannot sleep, so doing the two or three ibuprofen is absolutely essential. You may have heard that taking ibuprofen in the third trimester is not a good idea—and that is true *if* you take it for more than 24 hours.[150]

Next is the little bit of alcohol. First, I want to say that if you struggle with alcoholism and cannot have any alcohol under any circumstances then this is (I hope obviously) not an aspect of the technique that you should employ. I have a lot of people who have expressed concern about drinking alcohol because of their concern for the baby's health. There is significant stigma against drinking alcohol while pregnant in the US. Take comfort from the Danish study, reported on by the CDC[151] that documents no adverse findings in children whose mothers participated in low to moderate alcohol consumption during pregnancy (defined as fewer than nine servings per week!). The majority of the studies done on fetal alcohol syndrome looked at heavy, binge-drinking mothers and the effects on their babies. This I clearly and firmly do not recommend. But a small amount, taken medicinally, can really help you.

I have known women who were very opposed to alcohol consumption morally, and what I say to you if you are one of them is that this is not a recreational indulgence. This is *medicinal*, to help to prevent you from getting too tired during actual labor.

Alcohol is a smooth muscle relaxant. Your entire gastrointestinal tract is smooth muscle, which is why people drink a glass of wine with a meal to aid in digestion. Your heart is a smooth muscle, which is why you feel more relaxed when you have a glass of wine. The uterus is also a smooth muscle, so a little bit of alcohol can slow contractions down when they are annoying but clearly not strong enough yet to warrant staying up through the night. The alcohol really helps your chances of getting sleep in this early part of the labor process. Remember, we are talking about warmup labor, which is not actual labor. You can slow contractions down by 5–20 minutes—enough to sleep. If you can't sleep, doze. If you can't doze, rest deeply and don't move. Conserve whatever energy that you can because you're going to need it when true, active labor is upon you.

I've worked with women who have tried all kinds of alcohol, from hard liquor to beer to wine, and the alcohol works no matter what form it's in. That said, when women tried hard liquor, it tore up their stomach, when they tried beer, it foamed up and felt like a big ball of gas in their tummy, and when they were trying to go back to sleep, red wine gave them indigestion, but white wine seemed to work the best. It was the gentlest on their systems. That said, you can go to your drink of preference. It's the *alcohol* that works to slow the uterine activity down. It is dramatically effective when used this way, *medicinally*, so you can sleep—unless you're really in labor and then it's not going to do much at all ... you might be mildly relaxed for an hour. If labor has started, there is no stopping it.

Here is the protocol for the Trick:

1. Employ the Trick between 9 p.m. and 4 a.m. For women under 150 pounds, take 400 mg ibuprofen. For women over 150 pounds take 600 mg ibuprofen.

2. Take a hot bath and drink 4–6 ounces (depending on your tolerance) of white wine.

3. Immediately go back to bed.

Going back to bed is key. You cannot stay up and march around; that defeats the purpose. You have to lie down, even if it just slows your contractions down so they are 15 minutes apart, and you are able doze between them for several hours. This is the rest you need to be able to make it through transition, pushing, and postpartum (breastfeeding and bonding).

You can do the Trick again in the night, for example once at about 9:30 – 10:30 p.m., and again at about 2:00 – 3:00 a.m.

Let me say this again: If you are in warm-up labor, you will need the rest. If you think you are in warm-up labor and employ the Trick but you're actually in labor, your body will proceed with labor regardless. It can also be a great way to tell whether you are really in labor or not. If the Trick does not stop or at least slow down your labor, you are very likely in actual labor!

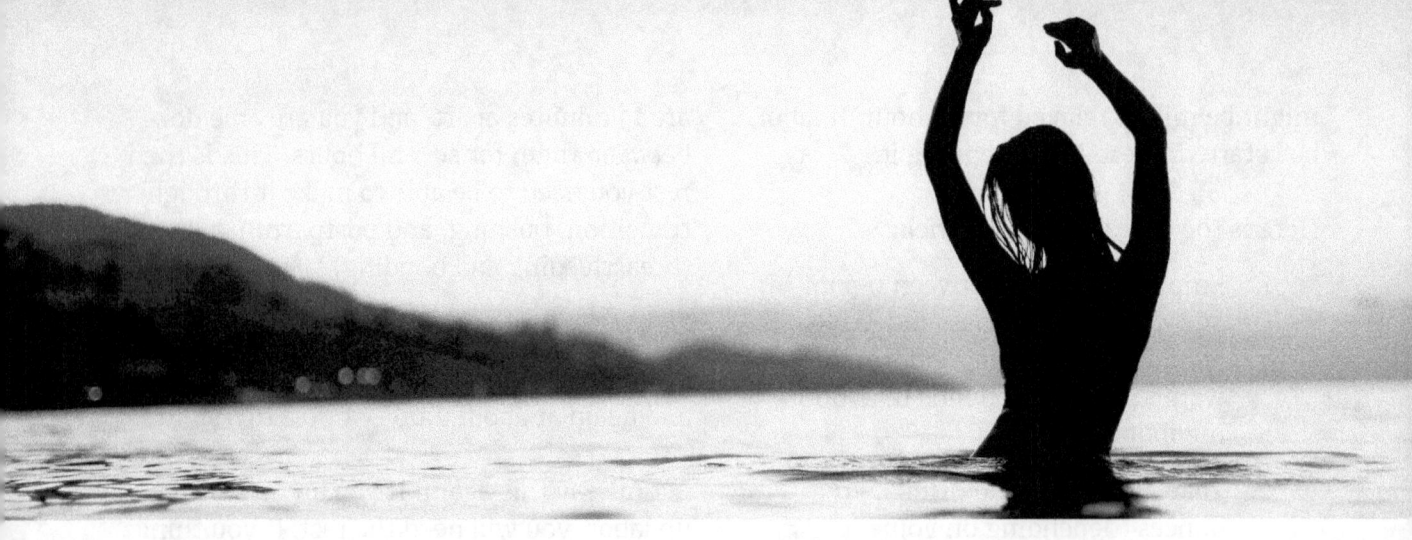

Joy

Make sure you do all you can to stay pumped up at the end of the pregnancy. If you knew that you were going to have the baby on Tuesday, wouldn't you take an extra nap, get a massage, eat perfectly, and take all your vitamins on Monday, so you are as prepared as possible? Since you don't know which day it will be, it is important to treat every day as if it is the day before your labor will start. Be prepared and do not let labor sneak up on you when you aren't in the best state physically, emotionally, or mentally.

Have fun and create joy in your life. At the end of pregnancy there is a lot to think about and so much to prepare for. It is easy to get wrapped up in the minutiae and forget to devote time to the joy coming and already in our lives. Many times, because of all that is going on, we forget to take time for ourselves and just have fun. Go on a date with your partner, go swimming, get a massage, or see a fun movie (avoid violence and horror)! Anything that makes you relax and have a good time will help you to have an easier and happier labor and birth.

> Anything that makes you relax and have a good time will help you to have an easier and happier labor and birth.

Boosting Joy in the Third Trimester

Continue to consciously and deliberately engage in the activities that nourish and rejuvenate you. Maintain your focus on self-care and things that make you feel good, lift you up, and fill your cup. Singing, dancing, and listening to music are great ways to continue to support joy and self-care practices.

Singing is a wonderful thing to do to connect with your baby. Your baby can definitely feel the vibrations of your singing voice from inside the womb. As their hearing develops later on in the pregnancy, they can hear the melodies and harmonies you sing. I used to put headphones on my abdomen and played music to my baby when I was pregnant. They really enjoyed it and would wiggle all around. I intuitively felt happiness and enthusiasm from them when I did this. Babies don't have a lot going on in their cozy apartment. It's pretty quiet aside from the constant white noise of the placenta and your heartbeat. Amuse and engage your baby with sound, and don't forget to shine bright sunlight on your belly!

Have Lots of Sex

Make time for sex. Sex is very important energy for you during the end of pregnancy. *The intimate energy that gets the baby in there is the same intimate energy that gets the baby out.* The endorphins that are needed to have an easier birth are the very same endorphins that are created during intercourse. Also, semen has prostaglandins that help to ripen your cervix and prepare for dilation. It's been suggested that having sex may be an effective method of helping labor get started. As I have said before, if your partner isn't into it for whatever reason, masturbation counts!

> The intimate energy that gets the baby in there is the same intimate energy that gets the baby out.

As always, if you are cramping, spotting, or have leaking waters consult your provider and refrain from having sex.

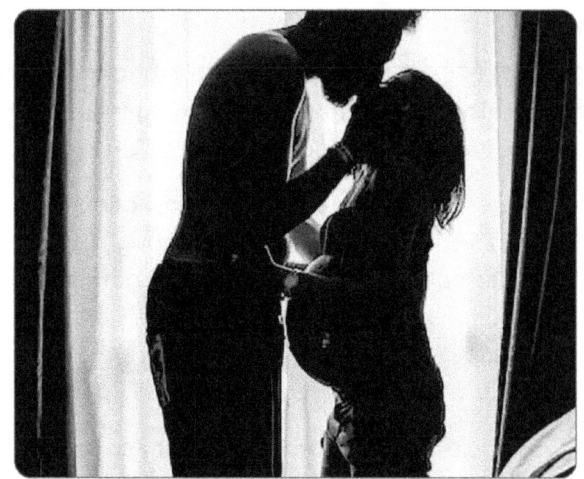

Continue to Deepen Your Connection with Your Partner as You Approach Labor

Spend Time with Your People

Re-focus your efforts on spending time with people you love who can help you to relax and have fun. Schedule time to chat, meet for a meal, or plan activities together that make you feel good. Share your thoughts and concerns. Allow yourself to be supported during this transformative time.

Continue to focus on building community around you that will help sustain you in your life as a mom or parent. Locate and try out breastfeeding groups, mom groups or create a new community of women from those you already know.

Your time as an individual without this new baby in your life is rapidly coming to an end. Use the third trimester to really enjoy yourself and be present in your current life stages. If you have other children and this is not your first baby, spending quality time with your older children can also be a great way to focus on joyful moments at the end of the pregnancy.

Pamper Yourself

As you near the end of your pregnancy, self-care becomes even more important to help you stay relaxed, comfortable, and emotionally balanced. Here is a friendly reminder of some self-care activities you can joyfully take part in during the end of your pregnancy:

Warm Baths or Showers

Enjoy warm baths or showers to soothe your muscles and help alleviate any aches or pains. Add relaxing bath oils or Epsom salts. Consider incorporating gentle breathing exercises or visualization techniques to enhance your relaxation.

Massages, Facials, or Manicures/Pedicures

Treat yourself to gentle body or foot massages to ease muscle tension and relax. Schedule a facial, manicure, or pedicure for yourself. You deserve it.

Mindfulness, Meditation, Breathing Exercises, and Prayer

Continue to practice your mindfulness and/or meditation practices that can support you during the birthing process.

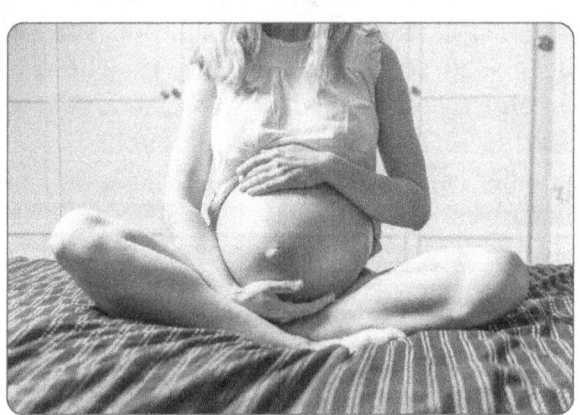

Meditate, Pray, Connect

Practice your breathing exercises to promote relaxation and emotional balance. Focus on deep, slow breaths, and use guided meditation apps or resources tailored to pregnancy to enhance the experience.

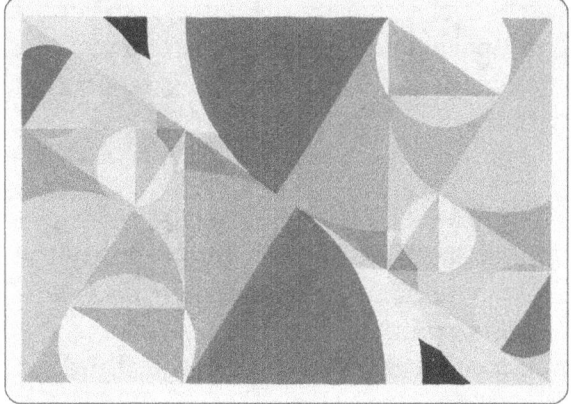

Joseph Schillenger's Area Broken by Perpendiculars

Prayer can be a wonderful refuge at this time, too.

Creative Expression

Engage in creative activities that bring you joy and allow for self-expression. Paint, draw, write, or engage in any other artistic outlets that resonate with you. Use this time to document your thoughts, emotions, and dreams for your baby and for yourself as a mother.

Prepare for Baby

Dedicate time to prepare for your baby's arrival. This can include organizing the nursery, washing and folding baby clothes, or packing your home birth supplies or hospital bag. Engaging in these activities can bring a sense of readiness and joy as you anticipate your baby's arrival.

Remember, self-care is about nourishing yourself physically, mentally, emotionally, and spiritually. Listen to your body's needs, honor your emotions, and be kind to yourself as you approach the end of your pregnancy. Take time for activities that bring you joy, relaxation, and a sense of fulfillment.

When you are decorating the nursery, pick out bold, colorful prints for your baby. Decorate for stimulation. Our primitive ancestors didn't develop inside of four white walls with a white ceiling. Our ancestors' homes were made from natural materials with all kinds of knots and whorls to look at. Think about what your baby can observe when they're lying down. You want them to be able to see so much more than plain white walls. Colorful posters are great additions to plain walls.

Go for Picasso's cubist era with all those primary colors. Matisse and Degas are also great.

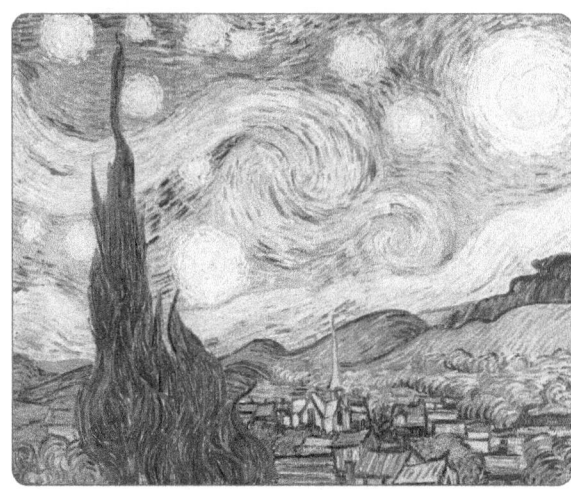

Vincent Van Gogh's The Starry Night

Use blue clay to hang the posters, so you don't poke holes in your walls, and you can change them out as your baby grows bored with them.

Connect With Nature

Connecting with nature is for me one of the most joyful, most rejuvenating things we can do as human beings. Here are ways you might connect with nature in your third trimester.

Outdoor Meditation or Mindfulness

Find a peaceful outdoor spot where you can sit or lie down comfortably, focus on your breath, and allow yourself to be fully present in the natural environment. You can practice mindful breathing, meditation, or simply observe the sights and sounds of nature around you as a way to let go of your mind and take in the beauty that surrounds you.

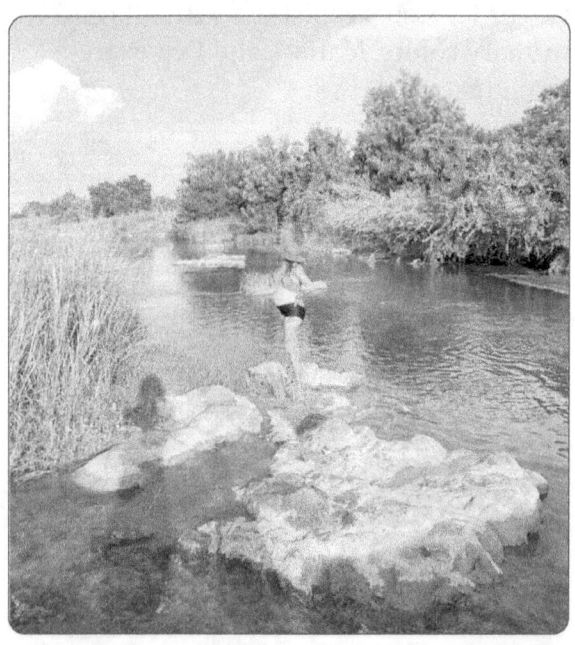

Enjoying a River Day in the Third Trimester

Forest Bathing

Take a leisurely walk or lie on a blanket in a forested area, immersing yourself in the sights, sounds, and scents of the surrounding trees and vegetation. Allow yourself to fully experience the calming and rejuvenating effects of nature.

Get to the Water

Spend a day at the beach, river, creek, lake, or ocean. Relax on the sand, listen to the rhythmic sounds of waves or water, and feel the soothing breezes. Take a refreshing swim if it's safe and suitable for you. Remember to use SwimEar afterward.

Wildlife Observation

Visit nature reserves, bird sanctuaries, or wildlife habitats to observe and learn about different species of animals and birds in their natural habitats. Bring binoculars or a guidebook to enhance the experience. Volunteer with these organizations with your older children to foster their social responsibility and values.

Birdwatching

Set up a bird feeder in your backyard or visit a local bird sanctuary. Observing and identifying different bird species can provide a sense of tranquility and connection to nature. I encourage everyone to have bird baths and fountains in their yard if they have one, and to fill shallow dishes like clay pot bottoms or old pie plates with water for wildlife and other creatures. If you do this, you will be treated to the joy of seeing these visitors in your yard.

Sunrise Or Sunset Appreciation

Wake up early to witness a beautiful sunrise or find a serene location to enjoy a breathtaking sunset. Take a moment to appreciate the natural beauty and the changing colors of the sky.

Remember to prioritize your safety and comfort during pregnancy. Stay hydrated, dress appropriately for the weather, always wear sunscreen when outside, wear a hat when you're in the sun, and listen to your body's signals. It is also always a good idea to consult with your midwife or healthcare provider about any specific concerns or limitations related to your pregnancy.

Focus on What You Can Control

As you approach the end of your pregnancy, it is so important to continue your practice of differentiating between things you have control over and things you do not. Focusing on what you can control can empower you and promote a sense of calm. Letting go of what you cannot control can help you to reduce stress and anxiety.

There are so many elements of the birth process that you do not have control over; the exact timing of labor, your natural progression of labor, unforeseen circumstances that are outside of your control, other people's reactions to your birth experience or decisions, and how your sweet baby will react to the new world once they arrive. With all of these unknowns, it is so beneficial to your mental, emotional, and spiritual well-being to focus on the things you *can* impact.

One thing you have control over is how prepared you are for birth. Focus your efforts on preparing for the birth. Educate yourself about the birthing process and revisit your birth plan to affirm that it fully reflects your preferences and values. Discuss your preferences with your midwife, attend childbirth classes, and engage in practices that help you feel prepared and confident. Clearly communicate your desires, concerns, and boundaries to your midwife and support team.

In the final weeks of pregnancy, time seems to bend, stretching the moments between each heartbeat as you await the arrival of your greatest love.
—Jennifer Jeane

You also have control over your immediate home environment. If you are planning to have a home birth, you can create a supportive and comfortable environment

THIRD TRIMESTER

for your labor and postpartum period by preparing your home, gathering necessary supplies, and discussing your needs and expectations with your partner and support network. If you are planning to give birth in a hospital, you will still need to prepare your home for your postpartum bonding period with your partner and your newborn babe.

By focusing on what you have control over and accepting what you cannot control, you can cultivate a sense of empowerment, resilience, and peace during the end of your pregnancy. Trust in your own strength and the support of your midwife, birthing team, and loved ones as you navigate this transformative time.

Baby Shower Ideas

Third trimester is typically when someone who loves you will throw you a baby shower. They may ask for your input as to what kind of shower you'd like. In recent years people have come up with lots of creative alternatives to the sometimes cringy traditional showers. Nowadays it's quite common for partners to be included. I've compiled a list of different ideas for you to consider ... this is a part of *your* ideal, perfect birth. Make your desires known.

- Provide cards at the baby shower for all the people gathered to **write encouraging notes** of belief and strength. Then post those prominently in your home, in your bathroom, on the fridge, etc. or bind them together into a little book of lovely wishes.

- Ask that people **buy books instead of cards** to help build your baby's library. Have them write sweet notes to your new baby in the book.

- **Onesie decorating.** Get a bunch of plain white onesies in varying sizes and have guests decorate them using fabric paint or tie-dye.

- Instead of physical gifts, have a **gifts of service shower** where people donate their time or services (gift cards for diaper service, maid, massage, etc.) instead of things. These can be great for moms with an older child(ren) who have all the gear but really need support.

- Virtual showers **online** can be great to include friends and family from far away.

- Consider having a **meal signup** during a baby shower to make sure your food is supplied in the weeks after birth. Mealtrain.com offers your network of friends and family the ability to see your dietary restrictions and sign up to provide your family with meals. You can arrange for a week, two weeks, or longer if needed.

- Moms with older children may opt for a "**sprinkle**," which is a lighter version of a baby shower that provides space for your closest friends and family to welcome your newest addition.

- Consider having your shower at a **restaurant or other venue**, so there's no cleanup, and you and your guests can enjoy time together in a neutral space that may provide more ease in the party planning (brunch, catered food, etc.) than at your home.

- Consider changing the party to a "**Meet the Baby**" party once your baby has arrived and their immune system has developed a bit, at two to three months old.

- Different cultures celebrate motherhood and transition in different ways. **Look to your own heritage** to see if anything inspires you. For example, *Godh Bharai* is an Indian tradition that celebrates pregnant mothers. It is typically attended by married women who come together to pray for the health and safety for both mother and baby. A Blessingway is a traditional Navaho ceremony that honors the woman's transformation from Maiden to Mother.

- **Candle blessing:** At the baby shower you might provide all of your guests with a candle. Ask them to light the candle, say words or prayer or affirmation or support for mother, baby, and family, and then blow it out. Ask the guests to keep the candle and when the mother-to-be goes into labor, have your shower host contact the guests and ask them to light their candles and send good thoughts and prayers as labor progresses.

Not all women want to open gifts at the shower, it can be uncomfortable at 7 months pregnant to have everyone staring at you while you open gifts. Others may revel in opening the gifts thoughtfully given by your family and friends; do what is right for you! If you do decide to open gifts at your shower, here are some tips for you.

- Make sure to have someone (most often the host) keep track of each gift and who gifted it. Writing this down will help the expecting parents to complete their post-shower thank-you notes and express their gratitude for their guests' gifts and contributions.

- It might sound silly but gathering and putting away wrapping paper and any extra materials as you go is helpful to do. Have a designated person help to gather trash after each gift is opened. This helps you to avoid a mountain of wrapping paper at your feet, and also ensures that any photos taken aren't tainted by a pile of garbage in the foreground!

- Ask your host to take pictures of you and your partner with each gift as you open it. Baby shower photos are a sweet part of many baby albums and are fun for couples to look back on long after their baby has arrived. Photos of the expecting parent(s) with their gifts can also be a nice addition to a thank you note.

Penelope: I moved to Austin from several states away and a week later found out I was pregnant. I was a single mother-to-be and knew absolutely no one. I didn't have a support network. I mentioned before that I hired a doula to help me. She was so cognizant of my emotional state, and she really wanted me to have a joyful pregnancy and birth. She knew I didn't have strong friendships built yet, and no one was planning to throw me a shower.

Unbeknownst to me, toward the end of my pregnancy she contacted another mother in her circle of friends whose twins had recently moved past their infant stage. The mother of twins gave her so many really nice things to share with me. She was so generous.

My doula went through the extra effort of gift wrapping every single item, and one day she showed up under the pretense of checking in on me. When I opened the door to greet her, her arms were laden with so many gifts. She threw me a shower all by herself. I must have opened 50 presents that day. She bestowed clothes and cloth diapers, a Boppy and covers, baby seats, slings, jumpers, even a wipe warmer ... She even brought cake. I'll never forget how she helped me to celebrate my journey. What a blessing doulas are.

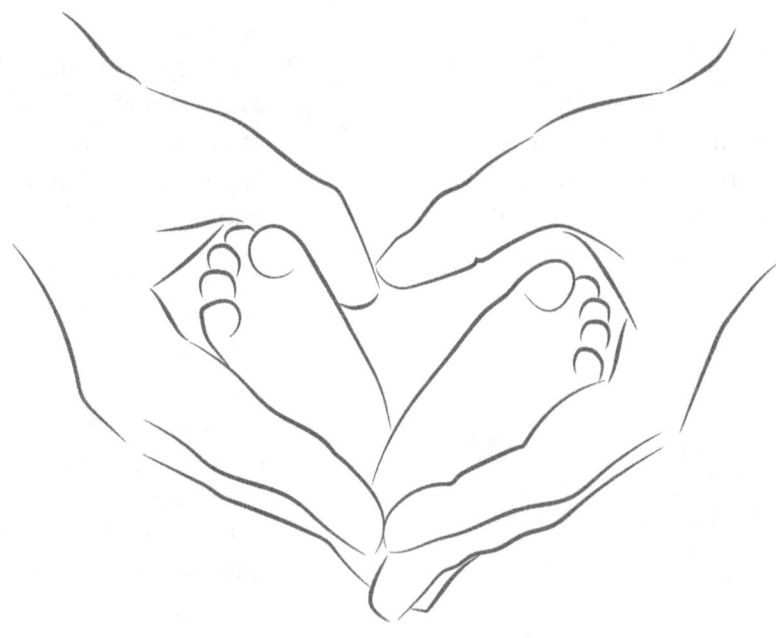

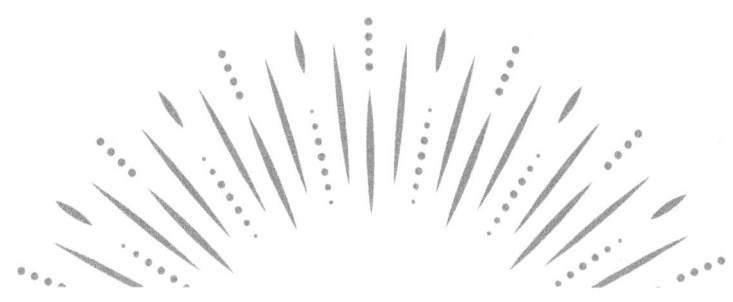

THE BIRTH PROCESS

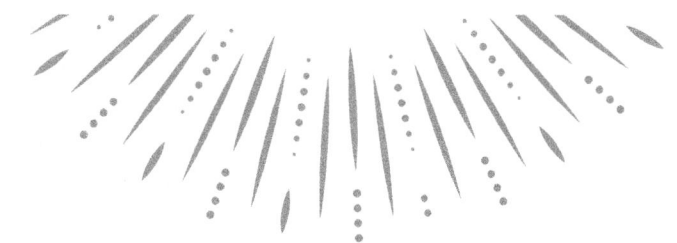

Introduction

This is it! You have reached your due range and the big event is very near. Maybe you are already experiencing warm-up or pre-labor. All you've been working toward is about to come to fruition in a healthy, incredible, transformative labor and birth experience. I imagine you are excited and likely a little anxious, and you are probably very ready to get on with it already and meet the new little person who is about to enter your world and life. Everything you have been doing over the long months of your pregnancy culminates in this glorious experience of birth, and at the end of it you finally get to meet your precious baby!

I'm going to diverge from how I've presented information to you in the previous chapters, because labor and birth is where the seven facets of the Sevenfold Approach merge and blend. So, instead of breaking this into seven sections as I have in the previous parts of this book, I'm going to talk you through what is happening at each stage of labor and birth, bringing in elements from each of the seven facets as appropriate. It's important to remember the bell curve of experience applies to the birth process as well. You may have an easier time than is typical or a more difficult time than is typical. For example, not every woman experiences pain in labor, but the vast majority of them do. I strive to share a typical experience in these pages. Your experience may be more or less intense.

In this section we'll cover:

- What to do between 39–42 weeks while you're waiting for labor to begin
- What to do if your water breaks
- Signs of actual labor
- Stages and phases of labor
- Birth
- Complications and interventions
- Sudden childbirth
- Partner's role (throughout each section)

On paper this important information about labor and birth begins to look a lot like a sterile textbook procedure, and I am less able to convey its incredible mystery and magic. There is a deep mysticism to this remarkable journey. Birth is an unfolding of spiritual time and space in a way that can transform women by the very sacredness of the process. I have sometimes felt at the hospital like I was surrounded by mechanics changing the oil. As I have mentioned before, I feel that due to the sheer number of births hospitals are faced with, they do not have the capacity for spirituality in every birth.

> Birth is an unfolding of spiritual time and space in a way that can transform women by the very sacredness of the process.

I also have seen birth workers creating sacred space even when they were exhausted, stretched way too thin, and dealing with people who had no inkling of the magic that was going on around and within them. I want each of you to bring your deeper awareness to the fact that *this is a transformational experience.* There is a quadrumvirate of beings within each woman. First is the Maiden, then the Mother, then the Queen, and then the Crone, and each of these life changes is accompanied by physical, intellectual, hormonal, and spiritual transformations. The Maiden is manifested at the point of menarche when a girl's periods begin. The Mother emerges in the moment of her first child's birth. The Queen emerges when the woman, having completed most of her child rearing responsibilities, comes into her full power in her workplace and/or in her life in general. The Crone appears when an older woman feels that she is ready to take on the Crone archetype. She is the wisdom giver and the knower.

I feel that some of the pain of labor is not just the cervix opening and the nerves crying out, but rather more like the cracking of a spiritual shell similar to an insect's chrysalis. The butterfly must completely dissolve its old self to become its bigger, newer self and so too must a woman shed her Maiden self for the Mother.

I believe this is a painful process on a spiritual level. When you observe insects splitting their old skin and wriggling free from their confinement into their newest manifestation, you can get a sense of how difficult it is. But if you cut open the chrysalis, the butterfly's wings won't develop fully, and it will never be able to fly ... if it survives. This is why the epidural rate in Japan is only 6.2 percent—Japanese women and their midwives tend to believe that labor pains are "metamorphic," meaning that they serve to transform the woman from Maiden to Mother.[152]

It is hard to shed the old self for the new self, one that has to be so much bigger, so you can open your heart and your life and your path to this new being who will take everything you've got and more, and who will give more in return than you can ever imagine. There is more going on here than meets the eye with this transformation. It's magical. It's mystical. It's sacred, and most women in an unmedicated birth cry out to the divine for aid and help to make it through. The moment of giving birth for me has always been the closest I've felt to divinity in my life. I gave birth six times and each time it was truly magic.

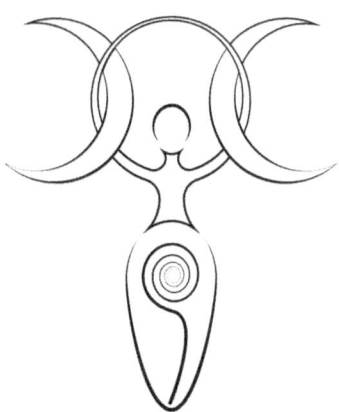

39–42 Weeks

What to Do While You're Waiting for Labor to Begin

Sometimes these last few weeks can feel never-ending. You feel so heavy all over, and everything is soft, and it hurts to move, and it hurts to not move. Your contractions are getting stronger, and it's difficult to get a good night's rest. Thankfully, there are a few things you can do to focus your energy in a positive direction.

Distract Yourself with Projects

It is very helpful at the end of pregnancy to stay distracted. There is an old saying that a watched pot never boils, and while it's not true, it sure does seem that way when you are obsessing about it. For many women in the final weeks of pregnancy waiting for labor to start is like waiting for that water to boil. Be creative in these final weeks. Do projects that are easy to do, that are not too stressful, and that do not take too much of your energy. But if you have things you want to get done before the baby comes, this is the time.

When you are distracted, time seems to pass more rapidly and you won't be dealing with as much longing for the pregnancy to be over, wishing for the baby to be here, stressing out over this concern or that concern, and it will make the ending of your pregnancy go more smoothly. Some of the things that you can do to distract yourself include:

- **Cook** more food to freeze and have on hand for after the birth, like soups, sauces, casseroles, etc.

- **Garden**—pruning, planting, cutting flowers, and harvesting vegetables feels so nurturing and in alignment with what your focus is going to be for a while. Plus, you can get in a hands-and-knees position to facilitate your baby's optimal birth position.

- **Organize** your closets or drawers: these are things you can do in smaller increments of time that are so satisfying and believe me, they will be much harder to find time for once you have the baby.

- Try arts and **crafts** like paint by numbers or a fun project kit from the hobby store.

- **Photo albums:** put together photo albums. If you are all digital, it can be really rewarding to put together a few photo books and have them printed.

- Write **thank you cards** to people for gifts that you've received for yourself or the baby.

- Get a **baby book** and begin to fill it in with the information you already know.

- **Bathe your pet** or have them groomed: it's a great thing to have your pets very clean and taken care of before the baby comes. Many pets are somewhat neglected after the birth; you actually have to work at making sure that they are not too neglected.

No matter how you spend this time, it's best to fill it with something other than anxious thoughts like, *When will my labor start* and *When will my baby get here?*

Have Patience

Now, there's an important point to be made here about patience. As a society, we have become more and more used to instant gratification, to getting exactly what we want exactly when we want it. The ability to wait is a dying art. The waiting that pregnancy, labor, and birth initiates and requires is a preparation for dealing with kids and raising them. A new baby takes so much patience, so much endurance, and pregnancy and birth are nature's way of preparing us to continually exhibit this patience. Motherhood is a journey of love through patience and surrender.

A new baby takes so much patience, so much endurance, and pregnancy and birth are nature's way of preparing us to continually exhibit this patience. Motherhood is a journey of love through patience and surrender.

The doctors and hospitals are very intense about the baby coming out before or at Week 40. Part of it is that their schedules are so tight because they are dealing with so many people, but the other important component is that most Americans are not really very healthy. They are not eating well, they are not drinking enough fluid, they are not

Midwives honor the sacredness of birth, nurturing the divine dance between a mother's strength and a baby's emergence.
—Gloria Lemay

exercising, they are not emotionally and spiritually empowered in their lives, and this impacts everything. Doctors are concerned because after 40 weeks, it does become more possible for complications to arise, even leading to stillbirth.[153] Most of this is due to placental insufficiencies.

I find that my clients give birth mostly between Weeks 41 and 42, and their placentas look gorgeous. This is because they are listening to my advice, taking their vitamins, eating well, exercising appropriately, drinking enough water, reducing their stress, and educating themselves on this process.

If you have the ability to eat well, take care of yourself, exercise, and drink plenty of water, I don't think you have to buy into the cultural demand of the medical profession that your baby must come out no later than 40 weeks. Your baby and your body should be working together in tandem to figure out the perfect time for the baby to come. This is not to say that I don't have to intercede in the process sometimes. Sometimes there are unknown causes why the baby is not coming, but mostly patience and understanding are all that's required.

There's a huge benefit to trusting in the baby's wisdom, in trusting that the baby knows the right time to come out. If you're buying into the message that the baby must come out at exactly 40 weeks, you may be putting yourself at odds with the natural process. It's imperative to understand from the beginning that you have a three-week due range from 39 to 42 weeks with 50 percent of my clients delivering around 41 weeks. I need to reinforce that 70 percent of my clients deliver one to two weeks after the "due date." This is SO normal.

Shift your mindset. Even a week can make an enormous difference in the baby's development. Consider that they've gone from two cells to a multicellular creature that weighs several pounds in the space of 40 weeks. They have to come out underdeveloped so they will fit through the pelvis, but they have to have enough development in their digestive system to avoid gastrointestinal issues, enough liver development to shed toxins, and enough strength to stay awake, so they can eat and bond (which is so incredibly important) ... up to a point, the longer the baby stays in the better.

A Message for Women Planning a Hospital Birth

I'd like to address those of you planning a hospital birth. The beautiful, transformative experience of natural childbirth is available to you in a hospital, just as it is to the mother birthing at home or in a birth center. However, this is the time when you may begin to feel some pressure from your OB to schedule an induction.

Women are told repeatedly in this culture that the sensations and pain of labor are not valuable in any way and should be avoided at all costs. This is simply not true. The sensations of labor and birth are a culmination of eons of evolution. This is no mistake. These feelings are empowering, strengthening, educational, transformational, and above all sacred. The women who experience natural birth more often than not end up transformed and have so much more confidence in themselves, in their bodies, and in life in general.

We are living in a throwaway society where it is easy to walk away or avoid hard or painful things. Remember that you are not being damaged by this beautiful albeit painful process, but you are going to have the opportunity to see yourself as stronger, more capable, and able to stick it out in tough situations whatever they may be.

Before you choose an induction or epidural, I implore you to consider making use of the suggestions in this book for how to handle natural birth. Use them as a guide.

Shift Your Energy Toward Your Ideal, Perfect Birth

I understand feeling like you are ready, and you want things to move along. Activity is helpful at this time. Here are a few ideas:

- Pray or meditate.

- Sleep.

- Eat incredibly well and eat plenty of foods that are easy on your system.

- Turn off your phone (or notifications) and tell your friends and family you need to be left alone for now. They only increase your anxiety if they are continually asking if you are in labor or have had the baby yet.

- Clean your house.

- Walk.

- Have sex to stimulate the cervix and amplify your oxytocin levels, which can help to stimulate contractions and endorphins (the body's natural painkillers).

- Visualize and Bless: Open your heart to how important blessing is. It can really help. Bless yourself. Bless your coming child and any older children you may have. Bless your family and your spouse. Call down blessings for your labor, your baby, your safety, and the whole process becomes a form of affirmation.

  Visualize being blessed by life, by love, the divine, whatever you want to call it. You can say, "I am being blessed every day to have a safe and healthy pregnancy and birth," and then visualize white light starting at your toes and circling around you all the way up your body until you and your baby are a glowing cocoon of divine beautiful energy and wrapped in divine love, power, and safety.

Do your best to distract yourself. Be well prepared intellectually. Review the books you've read so your mind can rest and not be anxious about the changes going on in your body. Know what's coming so the lack of knowing doesn't create an additional layer of stress during birth. You have to have enough

information so your mind will shut off. You don't need to have it saying *What's that? What are you doing? Am I safe? What's happening? Is that good? Is this normal? What does that mean?*

When your mind is spinning, you can't get to the zone. You want to go to the zone. It's a primal place. It's the same place you get to when sex is really good. You want to enter the place where you are in another world, a place where you lose self and time, and you are fully present in your heart and body. There is oneness with the universe in that place. Getting that connection is getting to the zone and that is better achieved in a more private, familiar, and relaxed environment.

Most of all I urge you to relax and trust the process. Don't give space for fearful thoughts to circle around and around in your head. Distract yourself. You are going to be the mother who chooses health for her body and her baby. You're going to be the momma who understands that if her baby goes to 41 or 42 weeks, it's because that's what is normal and needed for your baby. Enjoy these days as much as you can.

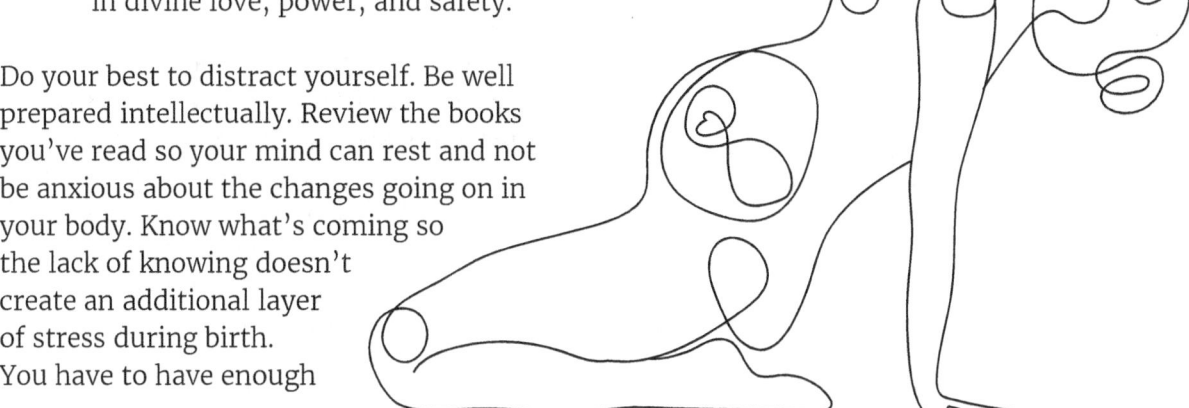

This is a great time to connect more with your doula. If you are going to have your baby in the hospital or your midwife doesn't provide labor support, then a doula is a wonderful helper along with your partner. The closer you get to labor, the more you want to connect with her and with your partner, so your relationships are deepened, and the trust and camaraderie is there to make all your communications easier during the birth process.

Movement

Movement is one of the most effective ways to keep your body primed for labor to happen at the perfect time. It is easy to want to do less at this point in pregnancy when the baby is taking so much out of you every day. Your body is also preparing for labor and trying to conserve energy. You likely feel like resting quite a lot, but there is a balance, and as much as you can keep moving is good. Notice I don't call this "exercise." I think you have to conserve your energy enough that walking miles, swimming laps, or doing cardio or weight work is not a great idea anymore. It's too easy to use up too much of your energy at this point and go into labor depleted. The baby is taking an enormous amount out of you at this point in the pregnancy.

I believe that one of the reasons you give birth is because your body can no longer meet the needs of the baby on the inside. So, the baby has to come out and start getting milk, which ultimately will feed them better.

That being said, you do have to try to keep moving. A short walk is lovely. Some gentle, stretching or yoga is a good idea. Anything that feels good in short segments of 15–20 minutes. I encourage you to get in water; it is so incredibly lovely at this point (you're weightless, no one can bother you, and you are cool!). If you're in the water, just lounge. Float. Be weightless. Enjoy it. Don't feel like you need to work out at this point.

Sex

I encourage you to have as much sex as you're comfortable with. If you have a partner who doesn't feel comfortable having sex because you're hugely pregnant and you have a baby inside you, then there are a lot of things you can do yourself to stimulate oxytocin and get the hormones flowing. Anything you can do at this stage to keep the sexual energy flowing is very helpful. Try masturbation, or gentle walking, swimming, yoga, and/or squatting—just remember not to push yourself too hard or hurt yourself.

Rest

To reiterate, it is as much a blessing to receive as it is to give, and it is as important to relax as it is to move. Find the times to let yourself be refreshed and renewed by good food, good friends, funny media and movies, great music, singing, gentle dancing ... all of these are ways to distract yourself, which is critical. Don't jump up and down till the cows come home ... There's no way to make labor start before the baby's ready—unless you choose to have an artificial induction of labor in the hospital, which I believe to be less than ideal because the Pitocin used for labor inductions stops your normal flow of natural oxytocin—and there is no way of holding back the tide once it starts.

Engage Your Spirituality

This is a time to reach out to spirit, to whatever you think of as the divine in our universe. Connect to it. The veil between you and the divine is very thin at this point. I think that's so the baby can come from its spiritual home to its physical home, and there is some thinning of the wall between this world and the spiritual world in these late stages of pregnancy. You have an opportunity to connect with divinity in ways that are difficult to find at other points in our lives. Open your heart. Pray. Meditate. Affirm the positive and continue to surrender and breathe.

Signs of Actual Labor

Bloody Show

Sometimes the cervix will bleed a little bit at the end of the pregnancy. It is called a *friable* cervix—another medical term that simply means it bleeds easily and the tissues are a little bit delicate. Bloody show is a little bit of pink or red-tinged fluid in vaginal discharge or a small amount of blood. This can happen easily in the final stages of pregnancy as additional pressure is put on capillaries in the cervix, but if you have bloody show in conjunction with contractions that are longer, stronger, and more frequent, this is an indicator that you may be headed into labor. It means that the cervix is changing more rapidly than those blood vessels can stretch.

There is a reason that it is called bloody show; they don't call it heavy bleeding because that would be worrisome and could be indicative of serious problems. Bloody show however is normal and even kind of a good sign, because it lets you know that the cervix is getting more ready. It can happen during warm-up labor, at the very beginning of labor before things get going or in the very early stages of labor. Sometimes bloody show does not happen until late labor when the cervix is dilating very rapidly. All of this is normal. If you do see heavy bleeding, like a heavy period, that is more than you want to see and needs to be checked out immediately with your midwife.

Quality of Contractions

The number one sign that labor has started is contractions that are painful, and are getting longer, stronger, and growing closer together. With warm-up labor, your contractions will get longer, stronger, and closer together for a while, but then plateau or recede. Your contractions must continue to escalate for you to be considered in active labor.

The number one sign that labor has started is contractions that are painful, and are getting longer, stronger, and growing closer together.

It also (usually) has to be painful. I have women call me who say, "This is it! I have contractions. Things are moving right along; they are five minutes apart and a minute long." I ask if the contractions are painful. If they respond, "They are powerful and intense but not painful," chances are excellent that it is not yet *it*. Generally speaking, no pain, no baby. Labor is painful most of the time. And it gets more painful—remember, longer, stronger, and closer together.

Most women feel contractions as if they were menstrual cramps. But there are other ways you can feel contractions—some people can also feel back pain or gas pain or stomach-flu-like symptoms. Some even feel them way up high in the abdomen, though that is fairly unusual.

Most women experience all the sensations of labor down low, in the vagina, behind the pubic bone in the middle. That is another thing you want to be paying attention to. If weeks before you are due you start feeling things in that area, you need to let your midwife know.

I had another woman in my practice who only experienced the feeling of contractions in her big toe. It was not even in both big toes, just one of her big toes. At first my team and I were thinking, *Wow, how interesting.* But after a while she was in such agony with that one toe that we were trying everything we could to alleviate the pain—massage and ice packs and heat—but nothing worked. It just got worse and worse. The pain in that toe was very serious for her until she had the baby, and then the pain went away. I am convinced that the baby's head was pinched up against a nerve in her pelvis that was connected to her big toe.

So, you can experience contractions in many weird ways because of your nerves and how they are connected. I never saw another big toe labor but know that labor can present in strange ways. The bottom line is, if you feel contractions or *any other*

sensations that are painful, longer, stronger, and closer together let your midwife know! You are most likely in actual labor, though it may still be early.

Tracking Contractions

 As your warm-up labor intensifies, you'll want your partner to start tracking your contractions so you can monitor if you are approaching actual labor! Have your partner take note of the time and duration of your contractions. They can do this on paper if they like or with one of the many available apps for your smartphone. I've included the chart that I provide to my clients in Appendix G.

When you chart, write the hour, minute, and second that the contraction begins. Next to it, on the same line, record the minute and second that it ends. Record the next contraction on the next line in this same fashion. *You do not have to track every single contraction.*

Tracking contractions too early can make you feel like this process is going on forever when actually it's just your observation of minutiae that's going on forever. When tracking contractions, you do not want to start too early. If it's very mellow, maybe briefly notice approximately how far apart they are, but don't time contractions until they really are starting to take over and you cannot distract yourself from the sensations. You also don't want to do it too often. It's sufficient to track fifteen minutes every few hours until the contractions get strong enough that you need to breathe through them. Don't do this too much or too early. You'll stress yourself out.

Partners, you can tell the beginning and the ending of each contraction by the deep cleansing breath your woman takes as bookends to her contraction. Remember this is a signal to you that the contraction is beginning. Some women want certain things during the contraction, like quiet. This way you don't have to say, "Is it starting?" You can listen to her breathing and know, and you can get into your contraction support role. With that deep cleansing breath everybody knows to stop talking, to start pressing on the mother's back, to get the cold cloth ready for her throat, to not move in her field of vision, etc.

You'll know you're getting close and it's time to call the midwife if you haven't already when contractions are lasting about a minute, occurring every 4–5 minutes, and this pattern is sustained or intensifies over a few hours.

Other Signs

There are other things that can go along with labor and make you aware that this is truly it. One is diarrhea and another is lots and lots of mucus discharge. There can also be nausea and vomiting, as well as hot and cold flashes. There is a lot going on in your body!

This is such an exciting time. The baby really is coming. Before you know it, your baby will be here. Labor and birth can be scary, but you have prepared, and labor is just a matter of hours or a few days in your life and then your sweet baby will be here forever. The magical process of birth has begun, and you are a bringer of love and light into the world.

> The magical process of birth has begun, and you are a bringer of love and light into the world.

I want you to remember that so much of labor is surrender. This can be a huge challenge for driven, results-oriented people who are used to getting what they want in life through sheer force of will. I had a mother who was screaming out in labor, "I want this to be over. I want this to be over!" I told her I heard her, I wanted that for her too, but it wasn't over yet. She needed to surrender.

The process of pregnancy and birth also serves to teach us skills we will need in the next phase of our lives. There can be a lot of discomfort and unpleasantness. You must exhibit patience. Surrender is one of the biggest lessons that every woman has to learn. You have to surrender to your kids all the time. There will be days when they won't go to sleep when you want them to, no matter how much you need them to. You have to surrender. Ride the waves and breathe.

When to Call the Midwife

It may be hard for you to know if you're just having warm-up labor or if the contractions you're feeling are the real deal. If you are experiencing one or some of the following symptoms, please call your midwife.

- Bloody show
- Contractions that are getting longer, stronger, and closer together

Don't ever worry that it may be too soon to call. She'll be happy to listen and gauge your progression at any time. If she doesn't know these things are happening and you call after the fact, she could miss the birth and you do NOT want that to happen.

These are the questions I ask when my clients call me.

1. When did you start to have contractions that felt like labor and how far apart were they?

2. When did your contractions get stronger and how far apart and how long were they then?

3. How far apart are the contractions now and how long do they last? How strong are the contractions?

4. Are they painful? Do you need to use breathing techniques to get through them?

5. Have you been able to sleep or eat?

6. Are you drinking enough water or electrolyte replacement drinks?

7. How are you feeling emotionally?

8. Have you had any bloody show or leaking waters?

9. Is the baby moving minimally, moderately, or lots? (It is normal for the baby not to move in labor, they are generally very still.)

10. Are you ready for me to come to you?

Your midwife needs as much data as you can give her. If my client is a first-time mom and it seems early, I will often come

out first by myself and check her, and then my apprentices come in waves. It is very important not to overwhelm your space with a lot of people early in labor. I work to preserve the intimacy of this event in your life.

If my client has had other babies or quick labors, I will often have everyone come right away when they call because it will likely move faster, and I want to make sure my team is prepared for them and for the baby's arrival.

If you are working with an OB/GYN or midwife at a birth center, they will advise you on when to come to the hospital or birth center.

What Your Partner Should Do When Labor Starts

 These are the instructions for a planned home birth. The majority of them are also applicable for most planned hospital births. If you want to avoid the cascade of interventions and prefer an unmedicated labor and delivery, it's best to go to the hospital later in your labor. Use the techniques you've practiced to help your woman manage the sensations of labor. Here are the steps to take when you believe labor has started.

• Call your midwife immediately.

• Continue to time your laboring partner's contractions and record them on the "Tracking Contractions" sheet (Appendix G) or on an app. Your midwife or other care provider needs information to gauge where your partner is in the labor process, but not a continual data stream. I've seen partners get fixated on tracking every contraction and recording pages and pages of contractions. This made both the laboring woman and her partner feel like labor had been going on forever, when in fact they were still in the very early part. It's really only necessary to track three to four contractions at a time every hour or two.

- Regarding informing family and friends whom you have invited to attend the birth: If your partner is in early labor and it's late at night, let your friends and family sleep. You can call them in the morning so they will be fresh and able to help her when she really needs it, when labor is moving along strongly. I usually suggest contacting them when your woman is between 4 and 6 centimeters.

  If you have older children, this IS the time to inform the people who will be with them while your partner labors. It's super important that kids be taken care of by somebody other than you. You need to focus on the mother, the baby, and the labor. You need to set up support for your older children ahead of time. Have a Plan B for this in case your first choice ends up not working out for whatever reason (illness, other conflict, etc.)

- Make sure the parking spot closest to your home's entrance is available to your midwife.

- Get out any equipment your midwife has instructed you to prepare for the birth.

- Get out cameras or recording equipment and batteries/charging cords if you're documenting the birth.

- Put on a big (at least 1-gallon) covered pot of water to boil. Once it comes to a boil, let it boil for 20 minutes with the lid on, and then turn off the burner and move the pot to the back of stove to sit. Leave it covered. It is now sterile water.

- Unless labor is progressing very rapidly, take the time to clean the birth room and bathroom again very thoroughly. Vacuum or mop the floors, wipe things down, and focus on the bathroom so it is really clean for your partner after the birth.

- Both of you should take a shower and get clean.

Penelope: We are very lucky to have my husband's very large family near us in Texas. His aunt and uncle watched our 1-1/2- and 3-year-old while I was in labor with our third child and kept them for several days postpartum. They all had a grand time together. They did visit to meet the new baby a few hours postpartum. My husband's mother was available to be with us and to help us out postpartum as well, and it was a blessing to have that tribe of support.

- Be aware that anything your partner eats now may come back up, so keep the calories gentle. Have her try a bowl of soup or broth. Mashed potatoes with no skins. Bananas, applesauce, yogurt … These are all easy to digest. As I like to say, your partner should not eat anything in labor that she isn't willing to see again, as vomiting is very common. Some women are sensitive to the advanced levels of oxytocin produced as labor intensifies, and the increase in hormones can also be nauseating.

If your partner finds that she becomes nauseated during labor, suggest she switch to ingesting ice chips over calories. It's important that she does not deplete the electrolytes she does have, and depletion is triggered by vomiting.

Remind her not to drink juice; it will make her throw up if she is queasy.

- Your partner should not take vitamins during her labor. Vitamin C can be okay if she takes it really early on, but it can be acidic to the stomach. And if she takes some vitamins in early labor because she feels really good, make sure she takes them with food.

- You both need to rest. If it's late at night, and her labor is in its early stages, try to sleep. You will need to be rested for the work ahead. Even if you can't sleep or doze, resting is better than nothing.

Enjoy yourself and think positive thoughts. Soon you will meet the newest member of your family!

Aleah: Growing up with a midwife for a mom is definitely a unique experience. Pregnancy and giving birth were all very normalized for me very early on, and I knew from a very young age I wanted to have kids. I also always knew that I wanted my mom to be my midwife.

I had the incredible pleasure of working with MariMikel for five years as an apprentice midwife in my twenties, and it was such an amazing experience, and it also gave me such a strong foundation of knowledge for my own pregnancies and births.

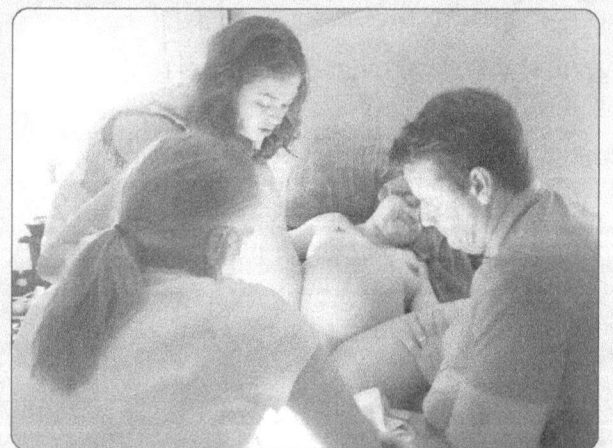

Aleah and MariMikel in Attendance at a Birth.

When I found out I was pregnant with my first baby I called my mom. She was the first person I told, even before I told my husband.

She asked me, "Where do you think you want to give birth?" and "Will you use a midwife?"

I said, "What are you talking about? Of course I'm going to have a home birth and you're going to be my midwife, silly!"

She said, "Well, I just didn't want to assume. It is totally a personal choice, and some people may not feel comfortable with their mother in the birthing room."

I laughed and said I wouldn't feel comfortable any other way. I told her I would be honored to have her as my midwife and would feel the safest and most secure knowing that she was that person for me.

As I neared the third trimester, we started talking about the birth more and what my birth plan looked like, what I wanted, what I didn't want, and one thing she brought up to me was the fact that some of her midwife friends did not feel comfortable being the midwife for their daughters. They'd said there is an energy to watching your own daughter in labor and giving birth, and there may be a disconnect from her being her best midwife self, so we discussed having another midwife present in case that happened to her.

I was incredibly lucky to have Varshna willing to assist at my birth. Varshna is a skilled and amazing midwife in Austin. She was one of MariMikel's former apprentices and very good friends. She came to a few of my prenatal visits, and I felt instantly connected to her and deeply grateful to have somebody else present for the birth. While my mom was the main midwife during my birth, Varshna was the main support person.

There were moments where Varshna stepped in, and it was really wonderful. My birth happened very quickly and when I started pushing there was some part of me instinctually that was like *Oh, hell no! This is too intense. I don't want to do it.*

I kept backing off because it was incredibly painful. My mom kept assuring me. She was very sweet and not pushing me at all, just saying, "You're okay. You've got this. Just listen to your body. You're doing great, love."

I remember at a certain point, probably after 15 minutes, Varsha chimed in and said, "Okay, honey. It's time. Open your eyes. You're going to do this. You're going to push this baby out. Your baby is *so* ready to come out. You have this. You just have to bear down a little harder and push through the pain."

I heard the authority and intensity in her voice and knew that it was time for me to let go of that fear of the pain and just get the baby out.

I am so incredibly grateful to have had my mom as my midwife, but Varshna was amazing, and both were in attendance for the birth of my second baby as well. I am grateful that my mom did listen to her midwife friends, and we came to a place that felt really comfortable for both of us. Getting to fulfill that deep bond and lifelong dream of mine to have my mom as my midwife was one of the best experiences of my life and I would never ever change it for anything. I was so lucky to have the wisdom and knowledge of her decades of catching babies, and her love and support as both my mother and my midwife. All of this, coupled with the care I received from Varshna, the lovely apprentices, and my sisters, my best friends, and my husband was exactly what I needed to help me through my own ideal, perfect birth.

When Your Water Breaks

Your waters can break with a moderate to large gush of fluids or it can be an occasional trickle. If you have a big gush of fluid, it is because the bag is truly broken and there is nothing between the baby and the vagina anymore. However, if it's a trickle frequently the bag is not truly broken, but rather there is a small hole up high in the uterus where the fluid leaks out and runs down outside the bag and the inside of the uterus until it comes out of the cervix. One of the ways that trickles can happen is by a very strong contraction where the baby shoves its foot out and pokes a hole in the bag up high.

Both urine and amniotic fluid come out of the vagina. Often when your waters have broken, it feels like you're peeing. Sometimes you think your waters broke, but it's only urine. So, it is important to test with a pH kit or nitrazine paper (available online). If you suspect your waters are leaking or have broken, call your midwife, and then employ the Sterile Technique in the following section (which will help you determine if your waters are truly broken and keep you as clean as possible).

Also know that it is *normal* for waters to break. My waters broke with four of my six births before anything else happened, so I thought that was how you knew you were going into labor. The majority of my clients' waters do not break due to all the vitamins I recommend. These help the amniotic sac to be stronger and if the amniotic sac stays intact and does not rupture that will actually help the baby's head to be protected by the cushion of amniotic fluid.

I've had about 20 babies in my practice that were born with the bag still intact. It's called being born *in the caul*. It looks like you've given birth to a giant pearl except there is definitely something moving in there underneath the surface because the baby wiggles all around. You have to break that bag really quickly because they're going to start breathing because of the release of pressure on their chest and you want them to fill their lungs with air, not amniotic fluid.

If your waters break, you are considered to be in labor, though you may not exhibit signs of labor yet. I want you to allow your body time to figure it out and relax into the process. I think it's best to go about your day as your normally would, with a few exceptions. You cannot have sex or put anything up in your vagina. You can't go swimming. You can take a shower, but not a bath—until you go into labor (see Signs of Actual Labor, page 381). Once you're in labor you can be in water, but not before.

Even if you're not contracting, if your water leaks or breaks you are considered to be in the birth process. It's important to avoid an examination (much loved by hospitals) at this stage because that can introduce bacteria present in the vagina to the cervix, and that then puts you on a timetable. If you don't introduce those bacteria, there's less of a race against bacterial propagation and less possible introduction of dangerous bacteria to the newborn baby. Once your water breaks it is absolutely a sign that this is it, you are going to have that baby!

Once your water breaks it is absolutely a sign that this is it, you are going to have that baby!

Once you are fully dilated, the cervix is completely out of the way, and the head is moving through the pelvis, there is nothing that will protect the baby's head from the bones of the mother's pelvis. So, at that point the bag becomes less important. It is really helpful if the bag stays intact as long as possible in labor. If your waters break before you go into labor, the hospital practitioners tend to want to induce you after 12–24 hours. Midwives tend to give you more time than that, but it does become problematic if your waters have been broken for an extended amount of time and you do not go into labor.

Make sure to contact your midwife if your waters break or leak. See the Sterile Technique section below for the kind of

Robbie: I want to reinforce MariMikel's point here by sharing part of my own birth story. During most of the first two days of my at-home labor, I was absolutely convinced that I was in real, active labor because my contractions hurt so very much and were coming every four minutes or so. As I mentioned in a previous chapter, my two midwives would come to check on me, shake their heads, tell me that I was still in latent labor (which Marimikel calls "pre-labor"), still at 4 cm of cervical dilation, and go home. I was furious! But in the late afternoon of the second day, my contractions suddenly stopped completely, and I was able to rest and even to get a good night's sleep. I woke up early in the morning of the third day to startling pain. I called my midwives, and by the time they got back to my house, I had dilated to 5 cm and was in truly active labor.

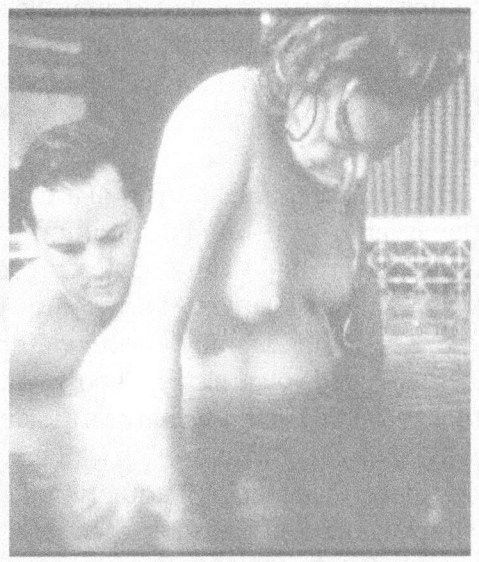

Robbie Laboring in the Birth Pool

I was absolutely stunned by the difference between latent and active labor! The contractions were so much stronger, lasted so much longer, and came much closer together, just as MariMikel explains above. While my latent labor had lasted for around 32 hours, my active labor took only 7 hours, and pushing out my 10-pound baby boy took only around one hour. When you are in latent labor, it is very easy to think that you are in real labor, but you're not. Your midwife will help you to know the difference.

But for my first birth, which was in a hospital, I never dilated more than 4 cm, and ended up with a cesarean for "failure to progress" after 26 hours of what I now know was only latent labor, which means that I should not have been admitted to the hospital at all, as I never achieved active labor. But most hospital practitioners don't recognize the extreme differences between latent and active labor. So, if you plan to give birth in a hospital, please don't go there until you are truly in active labor! If you choose to have a doula, she can be with you at home. She's not allowed to do vaginal exams, so she can't tell you how dilated your cervix is, but she will have other ways of knowing when you enter real, active labor, and that's when you should head to the hospital, not before.

information that's helpful to provide when you call.

If your waters have been broken for 24 hours, I also draw another tube of blood to look at your white blood cell count, because if you're developing an infection your white blood cell count is going to dramatically rise. Now, almost everybody whose waters break sees a rise in their white blood cell count. It shows a responsive immune system. But if it's a drastic rise, that can indicate an infection, and I would likely start my client on antibiotics if she did. I recheck every day until active labor begins.

When your water breaks and you are not in labor, after 24 hours, I do another vaginal culture and strep B screen to look for anything that could be worrisome and require antibiotic therapy. If your waters are broken and you are strep B positive, the situation is different. I would start trying to get labor going with every trick I can think of. I would start IV antibiotics after 12 hours. I would also transport them to the hospital after 24 hours to be induced. After 24 hours with no contractions, I ask that you listen to the baby's heart tones, and take your temperature and pulse every four hours, day and night. You have to remember that this is a process, and it can take a while of contracting, even painfully so, before it really gets to the active stage.

If there's any question whether you could be leaking or if your waters have broken, it is imperative that nothing be introduced to your vagina. Do not have sex and avoid the urge to put fingers in the vagina to see what's going on. Nothing goes in the vagina. I don't do any exams until the mother-to-be is in active labor. As soon as you establish that your waters have broken or are leaking, I strongly suggest you start doing what I call sterile technique to stay clean and help prevent infection.

Sterile Technique

Once your waters break, I want you to initiate the sterile technique. If your waters leak or break before you go into labor, it is very important for you to maintain a serious level of cleanliness. Most of the bacteria in the vagina is normal and poses no threat, but there can be bacteria—in particular strep B—that can create significant issues. I have you use a hot water bottle because it provides a large volume of water to try to really get your labia, perineum, and pubic hair as clean as possible to prevent anything traveling up the vagina and getting through the cervix and into the womb where it can infect the baby. You take the hot water bottle and use the tubing with no tip attached.

Here are the steps for sterile technique. If your waters break with an unmistakable gush, go directly to Step Three. If they are leaking, begin with Step One.

1. Test a trickle on your leg or outer labia (not on your panties or internally) with about a centimeter of nitrazine paper. If the paper turns dark blue or black, continue to Step Two. If it tests any other color, the fluid coming out of you is not amniotic fluid and your waters haven't broken.

2. Cut off the used piece of the nitrazine paper. Pee in a cup and test your urine with another small piece of unused nitrazine paper. If the urine also shows a blue/black test result, it is very likely that it is only urine. Your urine can have a very high pH and look the same as amniotic fluid sometimes. If the urine tests a different color, that is an indication that the trickle is amniotic fluid; go to Step Three. If the trickle continues, it is likely to be amniotic fluid.

3. Remove your clothes and underwear. Shower very thoroughly. Pay particular attention to the folds of the labia and around the clitoris. Do not put your fingers into your vagina.

4. Clean your hot water bottle with one teaspoon of bleach, a squirt of dish soap, and very hot water. Shake well and run it out through the tubing without a tip on it. Rinse with hot water until you can't smell the bleach in it anymore.

5. Put one tablespoon of povidone or betadine solution and warm water into the hot water bottle. This is an antiseptic solution that helps rid the area of bacteria. Shake the bottle to mix the contents. Sit on the toilet with your legs spread far apart and rinse off your labia and perineum, using the *entire* bottle. Be very careful not to touch the end of the hose to any part of your body. This is an external wash only. Drip dry. Do not wipe. Do not use soap, just rinse with this solution. Do this every four hours during the day and every six hours during the night.

6. Leave the bag hanging upside down in the tub or shower so it can drain between uses.

7. Put a sterile sanitary pad on. Change it every four to six hours or when wet. I recommend pairing this with the mesh underwear I suggest buying in preparation for birth.

Repeat Step 4 every 24 hours.

TO DO

Call your midwife immediately and let her know:

- The color of amniotic fluid
- The approximate amount of fluid
- If it had any particles
- The time of discharge
- Also note how often you are changing sanitary pads and how soaked they are

She'll likely want to see you to assess the condition of the baby, listen to the fetal heart tones, and check the fluid. If the fluid is clear and there's still plenty of it in the sac, you don't usually have anything to worry about. The baby's head comes down and acts like a cork, which prevents the majority of the water from coming out. Two to four cups of fluid is completely normal; there's usually plenty left if you expel that amount when your waters break.

The main source of amniotic fluid is the baby's urine. Of course, this is absolutely tied to the mother's hydration. If the mother is significantly hydrated, the baby will be also, and they pee into their environment, which builds the fluid level.

The placenta adds all kinds of nutrients, hormones, and electrolytes as well. Amniotic fluid and the baby are sterile in utero. There is no bacteria in the uterus at all. The baby comes out and must be inoculated by the mother. This occurs by contact with the vagina, the mother's breast, and all of the wonderful kisses that the baby gets.

Keep in Mind

- DO NOT wipe, except after a bowel movement—and then only wipe front to back and be sure to rinse. Drip dry and give a little shake, and then put the sanitary pad up against your vagina.

- DO NOT take a bath or swim, no hot tubs—don't submerge your body — showers only (until you are in active labor).

- DO NOT put anything in your body— no tampons, fingers, etc.

- DO NOT use soap in your vagina. Only use it around your labia and the folds.

- DO NOT engage in sexual activity below *your* navel or above *your* knees.

- DO NOT touch your labia and do not submit to any exams until you are in active labor where contractions are under five minutes apart and getting longer, stronger, and closer together.

I ask that you continue to use the sterile technique after birth, especially if you have stitches or tears; this will help to keep the perineum and vaginal area clean. I'll mention this again in *The Book of Birth, Volume II: Your Postpartum Journey through the Fourth Trimester.*

As you go about your day, be sure that you are super hydrated and super well fed. Labor is an ordeal and it takes a huge toll on your body. A lot of women, as they get closer and closer, get more and more nauseated, and as this happens, they can no longer eat. You want to make hay while the sun shines and get some food in your body while you can. Try for a meal like salmon, squash, and baked potato. Load that potato up with some cheddar, grass-fed butter, and sour cream to give your body great fats. If your water breaks early in the day, you could be in labor by dinner, so aim to have a big meal in the early afternoon. Be sure to take your vitamins, too (if you are not feeling nauseated)!

Get the Support You Need

 You may want your partner by your side as you are waiting for labor to start, or you may want them to stay at work or away. Make your wishes known and get the support that will make you the most relaxed. If it's better for you when your partner is there, they need to be there for you. If you are going to be more relaxed not being watched, then blanket yourself in solitude and enjoy your day.

This is a wonderful moment to ponder the miracle that is unfolding in your body and life. To recognize that this is the last moment of your life without another person's dominance of your time and energy. Enjoy these last moments. Think deeply. We each need to not just reach for the heights in our life but also reach for the depths of emotion and spirit that are available in these profound experiences.

Take a Nap

It would be wonderful if you could eat a good meal and maybe have a glass of wine and try to take a really good nap. It's an exciting time, so if alcohol is something that works for you, it may help to wind you down enough so you can get that nap in before labor begins in earnest. The key is to do it early. If you take a nap in the late afternoon and ruin your ability to sleep at night, labor will be more difficult. Same thing goes for your partner.

After your nap, go back to enjoying your day. Catch up on a show you've been wanting to watch, read a book, do whatever you like that doesn't overexert you.

Use the Trick

In the evening, close to when you're ready to go to bed. I'd like you to get another glass of wine, take three ibuprofen, take a nice hot shower, and go to bed by 10:00 or 10:30 p.m. If you've had a glass of wine more than four hours ago, you're fine to have another one now. I find that many, many labors, even if they're moving right along at 11:00 p.m., start flagging by 1:00 a.m., and they go very slowly till dawn. When the light comes up, all of a sudden the energy rises and labor kicks in. I tell most people to not try to make things go in the middle of the night if they're not dilated. Do everything in your power to sleep, doze or rest deeply.

Do your level best to get a good night's sleep. You may wake up in the night and find that you're in labor.

Mechanisms of Labor

For some time now you've likely been experiencing signs that labor is impending and now it is here. Your baby is coming. Your body is moving along a pathway that's been mapped into the very fiber of your being. You are going to be feeling a lot of big emotions as you move through labor; let them come and go like ocean waves. They are temporary; just as with contractions, I advise that you ride them out and let them pass.

> You are going to be feeling a lot of big emotions as you move through labor; let them come and go like ocean waves.

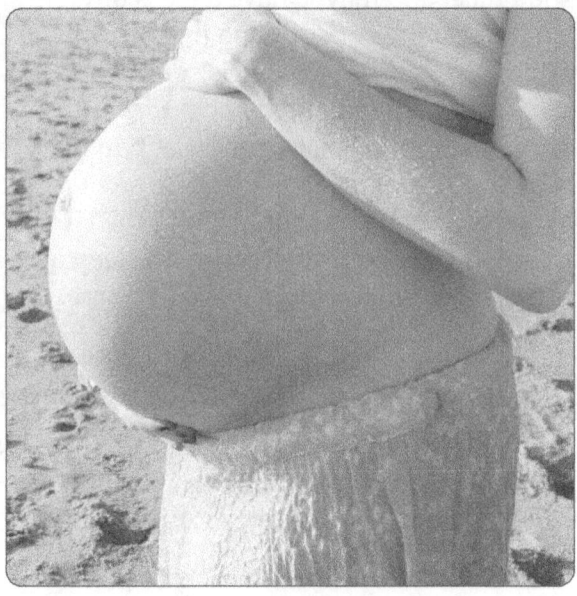

Full Term Pregnancy

Take a moment to reflect on all your body has done for you and your baby over the last nine to ten months. You are a vessel of divine creation. And you're probably way past ready for that baby to get on out so you can meet them already.

I'll be talking a lot about the technical aspects of birth in this section, but I want to remind you that what's physically happening in your body is only one aspect of the transformation that is taking place. This transformation is happening simultaneously on a neurological, hormonal, emotional, intellectual, spiritual, cultural, and tribal level.

But, very broadly, regarding the physical aspects, your body must first thin and then

dilate the cervix, so it is big enough for your baby's head to fit through. This is the 10 centimeters that I'm sure you're familiar with. Once you reach 10 centimeters (over the course of several to many hours), you must then use your stomach and abdominal muscles to push the baby's head out. Once your baby's head has emerged, the body usually comes through more easily. Shortly after your baby is born, your body will birth the placenta.

Let's break this down into a little bit more detail by examining the mechanisms of labor, or how the head and body of the baby gets through the mother's pelvic bones. The first and second mechanisms of labor, flexion and engagement, may sound familiar, because I discussed them briefly in the Third Trimester chapter. By the seventh month the baby starts to get very crowded, and as they curl up, flexion begins. The baby will not be able to descend into the pelvis unless their head flexes toward their chest. When it does, the skull goes through the pelvis easily.

The next mechanism of labor that happens is engagement. The pelvis is heart-shaped, which means the baby cannot come in there in just any way; there are specific ways in which the baby's head can engage and come into the pelvis. Most babies start to descend into the pelvis a little bit before labor. With first time moms it can be four to eight weeks before the birth. With women who have had babies before, it may be as soon as a few weeks before birth or even as they go into labor.

The next mechanism of labor is the baby descending. It descends facing slightly to the right or left side. It will descend until it comes into contact with the sacral curve and cannot go down any farther.

The baby will then rotate until their face is facing straight down. Internal rotation always takes place during pushing, but descent may take place some in labor and some in pushing.

Next, the baby's shoulders are right up against the pubic bone and will stay there until the head extends and is born, also called extension.

After that external rotation happens immediately after the head is born, which allows the shoulders to fit through the pelvis, and that allows the body to be born.

The mechanisms of labor are flexion, engagement, descent, internal rotation, extension, external rotation, then the top shoulder is born, and finally the whole baby is born! Let's take a look at a few images to help you to see the mechanisms of labor a little more easily.

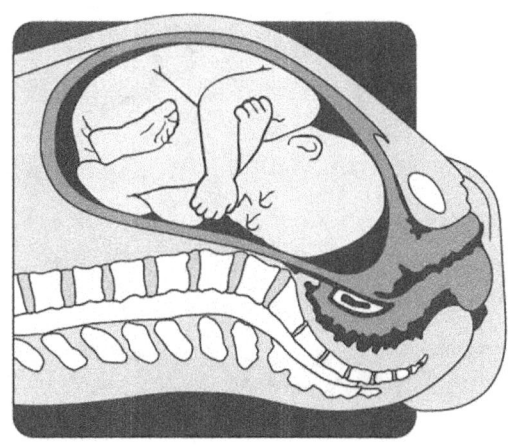

Head Floating Before Engagement

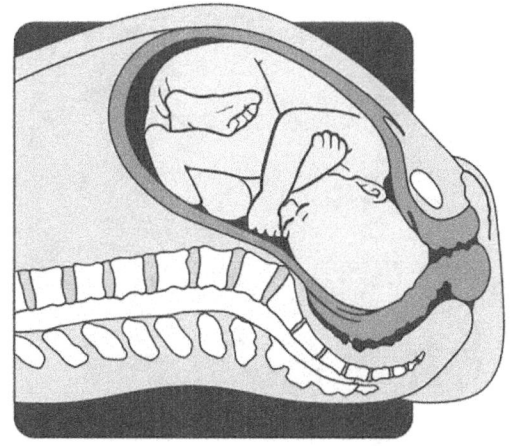

Engagement, Flexion, Descent

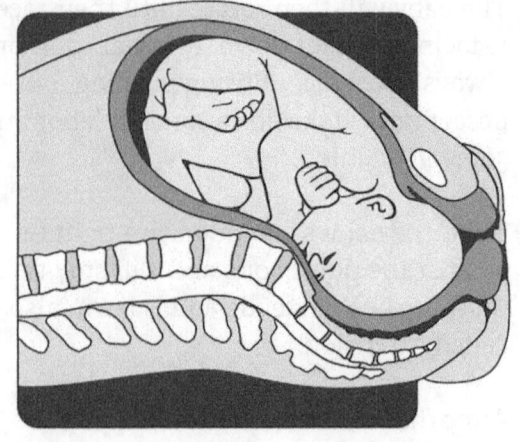

Further Descent, Internal Rotation

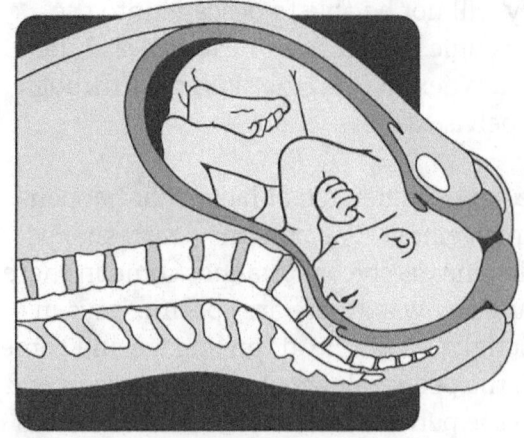

Complete Rotation, Beginning Extension

You can see in the first few diagrams the baby's face is looking to the side but in the next few diagrams you can see the baby's head slowly rotate to directly face the back of the mother's body and the bones of the sacral curve.

Then you can see the baby's head is beginning to extend now and the chin which was against the chest starts to come off the chest to prepare for the birth of the head. The head is being born by the mechanisms of extension.

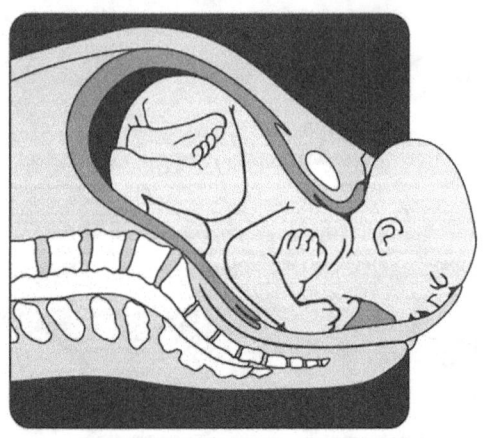

Complete Extension

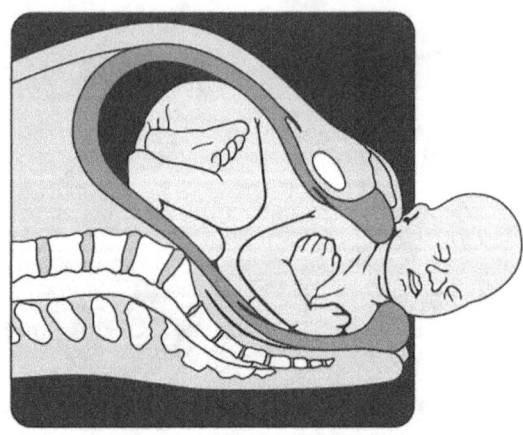

Restitution (External Rotation)

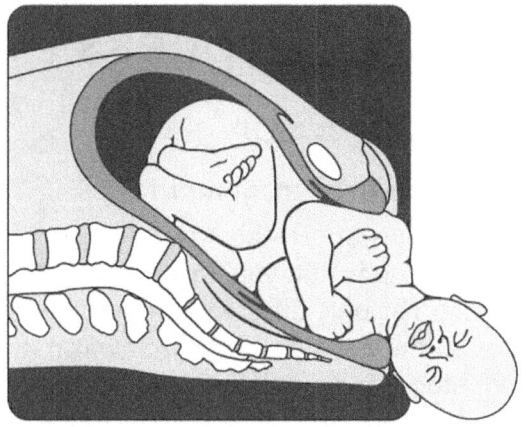

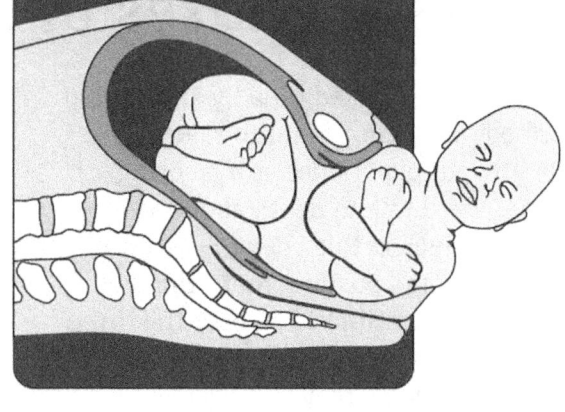

Delivery of Anterior Shoulder

Delivery of Posterior Shoulder

The baby comes out looking straight down but then immediately rotates back in external rotation to face the side of the mother's body, so the shoulders of the baby can fit through the bones of the pelvis. They most often turn back (restitute) to the side they were facing in pregnancy and labor. So

most of the time, you can accurately predict which way they will rotate.

After that, the anterior, then posterior shoulders are born, and then the rest of the baby's body is born.

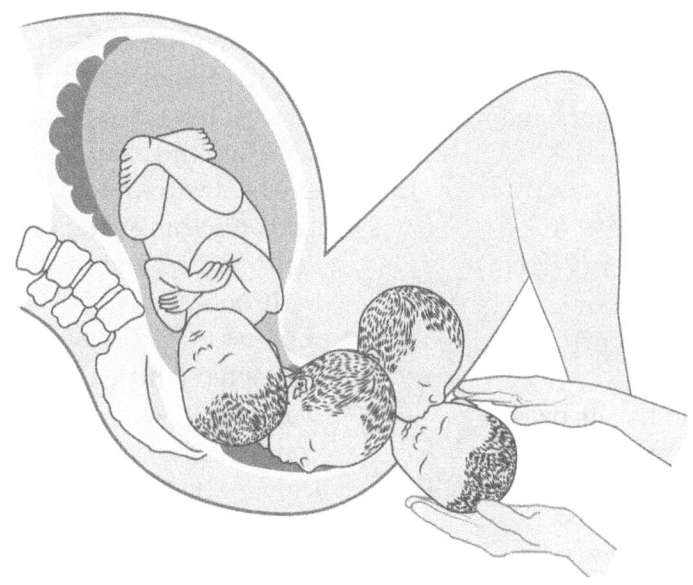

Summary of the Mechanisms of Labor

Stages & Phases of the Birth Process

Now that we've talked broadly about what your body is doing, I want to talk you through your experience as a laboring woman: We'll talk in depth about the first two stages in this chapter, because it is dilation and pushing that bring your baby into the world! We'll cover the three final stages in *The Book of Birth Volume II: Your Postpartum Journey through the Fourth Trimester*, because they happen after your baby is born.

There are five stages in the birth process.

1. Dilation
2. Pushing
3. Birthing the Placenta
4. Involution
5. Breastfeeding

Stage 1: Dilation 1–10 cm

The first stage of labor and birth is dilation. It is where the body opens the cervix, so it goes from 1 centimeter to 10 centimeters of dilation. Dilation usually takes from six to twelve hours and has several phases.

- Pre-labor
- Phase I: Early Labor (1–4 cm)
- Phase II: Active Labor (4–7 cm)
- Transition: (7–10 cm)

Each phase of dilation has its own characteristics and there are different strategies for handling each, which I will share with you.

Stage 1 Pre-Labor

Keyword: Discouragement

The thing about pre-labor that is discouraging is that you are not really dilating. The only difference between pre-labor and warm-up labor is that warm-up labor stops, and pre-labor does not. Pre-labor leads to early labor. Not everyone experiences pre-labor.

I once had a woman in pre-labor who was planning to have her baby at my birth center. When I went to her home to check on her, she was 1 centimeter dilated and 50 percent effaced, and the baby's head was a little high. She was ripening, but not fully ripe. I said, "Well, you are definitely in labor. Everything is moving along, but it is early, and it will probably be a little while."

Six hours later she called and said her labor had gotten really serious and she was going to come to the birth center. We got ready, and when she arrived, I checked her out. I had to tell her that she was still 1 centimeter dilated, but now 100 percent effaced, totally ripe, and the baby was very, very deeply engaged with the waters bulging a bit. The only thing she heard me say was "one centimeter," and then she headed to the bathroom.

I gave her a little time, but I could hear she was crying, so I knocked and asked if I could come in. She was a math professor at the University of Texas and was a phenomenal genius. She had her notebook with her. I asked her what was going on for her and what she was feeling, and through her tears she said, "I am still one centimeter. I have had four hundred and thirty-eight contractions, and at this rate I'll have to go through another nine thousand, six hundred and forty-eight more contractions before I can hold my baby."

I took that notebook from her and told her she was not allowed to look at it any longer. I told her that the process of birth is not math, it is beyond math. This is a miracle, this is magic, this is an astounding situation that doesn't follow any laws. Just because she was only one centimeter didn't mean the birthing process couldn't proceed quickly from there. She needed to stop thinking about the birth because she was not going to *think* that baby out. All she was going to do was disrupt the process and slow things down with all her upset and anxiety.

The process of giving birth is not a head thing, but a heart thing. You have to let go and let God and trust the process. Amazingly, she let go of her fear and did exactly that, she surrendered to the process and got into it.

The process of giving birth is not a head thing, but a heart thing.

Her contractions were intense and very close. One hour and forty-five minutes later, her baby was out. All of the effacing, engaging, molding of the baby's head, and ripening of the cervix—all of that had been the major work of her labor and because she had done all of that for six hours, the remainder of her labor was quite short.

Her life was transformed after this experience, and she went on to do some experimental math because it inspired her so much. All of this is to say, you will not get the baby out with your mind but with your body. All you can do is to surrender to it, relax, and let go.

What To Do When Pre-Labor Starts

Labor is usually easy in the beginning. You can still take an easy breath in and out, and you don't yet need your breathing exercises. At the beginning, distract yourself! Watch a movie, take a casual walk, play a game or cards. What you are trying to do is keep your mind distracted, so you aren't fighting the sensations. Continue to relax into the sensations of the contractions when they come. That is essential and will help you to continue to relax once things are much more intense.

Stay Nourished

You really need fuel for birth, so eat now and fill your tank. Stay away from wheat, red meat, dairy, sugar-laden foods, and gut-irritating foods like tomatoes or citrus. Don't eat anything heavy.

If you do end up going to the hospital, they often won't let you eat until after the baby is born. Too often I have seen births go poorly simply because the mother was too depleted going into the experience. Stay fully nourished.

Stay Hydrated

It's super important to be hydrated and stay hydrated throughout labor. Partners, make it your job to keep your woman hydrated throughout the labor process. Keep handing her water. Keep encouraging her to drink it. It is your job to direct her focus to hydration. Measure how much she is taking in.

I have found that many women respond really well to coconut water at this stage. It is easily digestible, has high levels of potassium, and provides some of the minerals that help her to function well. Partners, it is also your responsibility every hour to remind her to go to the bathroom— it makes more room for baby to come out!

Take a Shower

Be sure to clean the labia and in between the labia. Pull the folds of the labia and clitoris back and be thorough.

Revisit Your Affirmations

Here are some affirmations you might like to use during labor and birth:

- I am willing to open up to my sensual birth experience.

- It is safe for me to have a perfect healthy baby at the perfect time, in the perfect way, surrounded by the perfect people.

- Labor is a time that has both pleasure and sensations of pain. There is nothing to be feared.

- Breathing and intense sensation can combine to create the most joyful and transcendent experience.

- Everything I do, say, or feel in the birth is approved of by everyone. I can be myself.

- Contractions are my friend, and each contraction brings me closer to the birth of my baby.

- I am calm and relaxed. The baby feels my calmness and shares it.

- My baby and I are rested and ready for the work we will do.

- My baby is naturally doing just what they should.

- My uterus is contracting by itself on its own timetable. My body knows what to do.

- With each contraction my cervix dilates more.

- The contractions of my uterus are massaging my baby and hugging them.

- My belly feels as if it is suspended in warm water, floating lightly.

- My abdomen feels almost as if it were separate from the rest of my body. I can watch the contractions come and go as if they were slow waves breaking on a shore.

- My breathing is slow and even.

- My legs, hands, and jaw are loose. My belly and bottom are loose. The baby and I rest deeply in between one contraction and the next.

- In a while my baby will be here. The baby and I are doing beautifully.

- The baby is descending naturally. With each contraction my baby descends a little more.

- My baby's head fits perfectly in my pelvis.

- It feels good to push. It is wonderful, exhilarating work.

- My vagina stretches tight as the baby's head crowns, then emerges. I think of coolness.

- Pain is my friend! This is not pain that hurts me but helps me to bring my sweet baby into the world. I welcome the pain of labor. Pain teaches me to be brave, strong, and to persevere.

I must not fear.

Fear is the mind-killer.

Fear is the little-death that brings

total obliteration.

I will face my fear.

I will permit it to pass over

me and through me.

And when it has gone past,

I will turn the inner eye

to see its path.

Where the fear has gone there will

be nothing. Only I will remain.

—Frank Herbert, Dune

Rest

Lie in bed. Find a comfortable position. If it's evening, encourage your partner to get some sleep before the real show begins. You can handle this on your own for now. Relax. Sleep if you can. Labor will get stronger and harder. Resist the urge to march around at this point. Later it will help. Right now, your job is to fuel up and rest.

Labor can be exhausting, and there could come a point when you simply need to surrender. When you're alert, awake, and rested earlier in labor your mind can wreak anxiety on you. It poses questions like *What if?* and *How much more?* and it tells you, *I don't know if I can do it ... I don't know if I want to do it ... Can I still have that epidural?* If you're planning for a natural, vaginal birth but you are exhausted when you go into labor, this stage can make you want to give up. Please don't put yourself in that position.

Get the rest you can when you can, even during labor.

I've seen it far too often that women get excited at this stage, and they want to get down to it. They march around, go for walks, practice squatting thinking they'll be able to speed things up. But then, when they really need that stamina, they don't have it. Their spirit is willing, they're saying, "I can do this!" but their contractions are petering out. They're getting shorter, farther apart, and they're getting less intense because their bodies are so tired. Please relax in early labor. There's not much you can do at this point to make it go faster, so save your strength because you may need it.

What to Do for Nausea/Vomiting

Nausea and vomiting are fairly common issues in labor. Movement, bright light, and strong scents make nausea worse. Most women are very sensitive to smells while in labor. There are a few smells that tend to be repulsive to some women in labor. Here's a list of smells to avoid:

- Tobacco
- Meat cooking, especially bacon
- Coffee
- Garlic, raw or cooked
- Any other pungent or strong smells (advise those you are inviting to the birth to not wear any strong scents including perfumes, hair product, or body lotions).

Partners, work to minimize these triggers and make sure to check in with your woman that any aromatics in the room like candles or diffusers remain pleasant for her.

Move quickly if she tells you she feels nauseated. Once she starts throwing up it can be difficult to stop. Take these steps if she says she's feeling nauseated.

- Immediately put a **cool, wet cloth** on her throat. Use tap water until you can do the next step.

- **Fill a bowl with ice water.** Put a washcloth in it, pull it out and wring it out, then place it on her throat. The vagal nerves, which run down your throat, make you feel nauseous. You can chill them and slow down the firing of the nerves, which can lessen the urge to vomit.

- **Get a trash can** or other large, clean receptacle and put it next to her for her to easily vomit into. Don't have her stand over the toilet.

- **Darken the room, be quiet, and be very still.**

- **Have her lie down** and prop her up slightly on a pillow. If people are in the room, have them step out.

- Encourage her to take **deep breaths** in through the nose and out through the mouth slowly to help calm things down. Breathe with her.

- For some, it is sometimes better to just get it over with, capitulate to the nausea, throw up and move on. As I mentioned earlier, make sure you're eating things that are easy on the way back up. Avoid acidic foods.

- **Peppermint essential oils** may also help. Put a few drops onto the temples or under the chin over the lymph nodes (directly under the outer edge of the chin bone).

- **Try ginger.** Using all natural ginger lozenges, candied ginger, real ginger ale, or ginger lollipops made to help with nausea might help to calm her stomach.

Stage 1—Dilation
Phase I: Early Labor 1 -4 cm

Keyword: Excitement

The keyword here is *excitement*. The time has arrived! It's happening! Your brain can still take in day-to-day events and focus pretty easily on the world around you, but it is very obvious that something big is happening inside of you and the contractions are noticeable. There are smiles and laughter in the room.

Early Labor takes you from one to four centimeters in dilation. This is often the longest part of labor, with contractions usually lasting 30–45 seconds and ranging from five to twenty minutes apart according to the charts (Though I believe if the contractions are 20 minutes apart you are likely still in pre-labor.). Some engaging and effacing is happening in this phase as well. First time mothers generally dilate 1 centimeter every two hours and multips dilate about 1 centimeter per hour. Things happen slower in early labor, and it can take time to get to 4 centimeters.

Prior to going into active labor, your body will work to initiate cervical dilation. Early labor is considered complete when the cervix reaches 4 centimeters in dilation.

Joy During Early Labor

Remember, labor is not one long contraction. You have periods of rest in between. Early labor is a great time to revisit some of the things you have been working on through your Joy practices. In early labor you have not yet been completely taken over by the all-encompassing intensity that generally happens in active labor and transition.

Think positive uplifting thoughts to yourself and revisit your affirmations and visualizations. This is your perfect, ideal birth unfolding around you.

If you made a birth plan, have your partner or a birth attendant go over it, so you can focus on the sensations of early labor, trusting that they can help your plan

come to life. I don't recommend doing this yourself as it will pull you into your head, where you don't want to be.

Smile, it will release hormones that will aid you as you embark on this journey. Remember this is the culminating event you have worked and prepared for during pregnancy. Be kind to yourself. If you begin to have feelings of doubt or fear, feel your feelings, and try to then let go of them, like water flowing over the rocks of a riverbed.

Rapid Birth

It is important to talk here about rapid birth. About a third of the births that I see are very fast, so this is significant. We tend to talk more about the labors that take longer, but sometimes it does go quickly. I had one of my babies in 45 minutes, one in two hours, one in three hours, and one in three-and-a-half hours. The rest of them were longer, but the active part was still very short in all of my labors.

If labor is proceeding very quickly, I don't encourage you to march around. I don't encourage you to try to put more pressure onto your cervix. I don't encourage you to try to make it stronger when it's already obviously very strong. In those cases, I try to get you to slow it down a little bit, mellow it out a little bit.

The pressure on the baby is much greater when there's not a lot of time between contractions and they are very intense. They recuperate in between each contraction. If the contractions are very long and very close together, you can take some of the pressure off of the baby's head by lying down on your left side. This will increase oxygen to the baby and really help to slow things down so the baby doesn't shoot out, which I assure you actually can happen! If labor is going quite quickly for you, you need to lie down the whole time and just try to keep there from being too much pressure on the baby. This will also help to make it less intense for you, which is really helpful if things are rushing along that quickly.

Early Labor at the Hospital

When you are having your baby in the hospital the first step when you think, *This is it*, is to call the number the doctor has given you. Let them know what's going on and they will advise you as to when to head to the hospital. They will also usually advise the hospital that you are on the way.

 Partners, make sure you put your packed bags in the car. Drive safely and carefully, and as slowly as possible. Avoid any bumps in the road if at all possible.

When you arrive, park in their parking garage, and walk to labor and delivery. If you are farther along in labor, you can drop momma off at the entrance, park, then go to meet her inside so she does not have to walk as far. If she is feeling fine, a gentle walk from the car to the inside of the hospital is not going to hurt. Ask her what she wants. I suggest you leave almost everything that you have brought with you in the car until you figure out exactly what's going on. Every now and then they will decide it really is still too early and send you both back home. You don't want to have to bring everything in and then bring it all back out immediately. So, leave it in the car and you can get it as you need it.

When you arrive at labor and delivery, they will take you to the room that you will be laboring in and ask you to change into a gown, which they will provide. They often will ask you to provide a urine sample and then situate you in the bed.

They usually attach two monitors to your abdomen—both are discs that are attached with wide elastic bands. One is situated higher on the abdomen to monitor your contractions and one is placed lower on your belly to monitor the baby's heartbeat. In some places they will allow you to monitor intermittently instead of constantly, but it depends on the hospital, their policies, and your care provider's choices. You may need to ask about this ahead of time. Intermittent monitoring allows you to be up and out of the bed and moving around to facilitate your labor when the monitor isn't hooked up.

Most practitioners start an IV catheter at this point. They will not necessarily hook you up to IV fluids, but they need a line in your blood vessel in order to handle any emergencies that could come up. Some places will allow you to just have the line in and other than that you're really free to move. The IV catheter will only be utilized if necessary. In other places they are not going to allow you to eat or drink, and they want you hydrated, so they send fluids in to help with that.

If you are having an induction or a scheduled c-section, you will definitely be getting the IV fluids as soon as you arrive to make certain that you are very well hydrated for either of these procedures.

Either the nurse following your care, the nurse midwife in charge, or the doctor will palpate your abdomen to make a last-minute determination of the size of the baby, the position of the baby, the amount of amniotic fluid that's felt around the baby, and then do an exam to see where things are at in terms of dilation, effacement, and pelvic station. From there they will make a determination as to how to proceed.

In the hospital they often want you to lie down. Those who get an epidural aren't standing because they cannot feel their feet. Not moving makes birth a passive experience that slows it down and increases complication levels. Staying up and active is the key to moving things along with your labor.

In the hospital most of the time they try to give you a lot of privacy. You can call for the nurse anytime you need her or have questions. They do a wonderful job of being intuitive and knowing when to be with you and when not to, unless they have a significantly high number of patients at that time, in which case they are watching you through the monitors on your abdomen in the nurses' station. They may also put on a blood pressure cuff that will automatically take your blood pressure. They are looking to see if the contractions have faded or picked up, whether the baby's heart tones are normal, if your blood pressure is elevated, and these indicators will tell them if they need to come and help.

In these instances, having a doula at your side could be incredibly valuable to you and to the process. They will be supportive of you, able to help your partner to be supportive of you, and on hand to give information to the hospital staff.

This is the time when you want to move around your room or get in the shower or water at the hospital. Listen to your doula's, your partner's, and the nurses' suggestions for how to manage the situation and what you're feeling. Most doctors do not stay with you much during labor. They often will meet with you in the beginning, but not always, and then they come again part way through after a few hours, and again at the end. Remember, this will be the on-call doctor for your OB/GYN's hospital. It may or may not be your OB/GYN in attendance on the day you go into labor.

Shift Changes

One thing to prepare yourself for mentally when having a hospital birth is the possibility of shift changes. This can occasionally be disconcerting, but it doesn't have to be. Most everybody has your best interest at heart and wants to help you to have a great experience. If ever you get assigned a nurse you don't like or the energy just does not feel right between you, you have the right to advocate for yourself (or better yet, have your doula or partner advocate on your behalf) and ask for someone else to assist you.

Early Labor at a Freestanding Birth Center

The midwives at your birth center will also tell you what signs to watch for and when to come into the center. You will have a number to call when you feel that labor has become active, and the on-call midwife will consult with you and meet you at the birth center to assess how far along your labor is. Again, leave your belongings in the car until you determine if this is really *it*. They will show you to your room and in most situations, especially with first-time moms, they'll assess vital signs—take your blood pressure, listen to the baby, have you provide a urine specimen, and palpate your abdomen.

During this process they will time your contractions and feel the intensity of the contractions through your abdomen. Contractions are spoken of in terms of indentible—where the uterus is softer when palpated during a contraction—and unindentible, where it feels very hard and cannot be indented when you gently squeeze it. Perhaps needless to say, the contractions are stronger when they're unindentible. Knowing the intensity gives your care provider significant information about the strength of the contractions. In most instances they're going to ask to do an exam within the first hour to determine if this really is it and how fast things are moving.

If you arrive breathing furiously and looking very serious, especially if you've had a baby before, they are going to do everything much more rapidly because you could arrive in late labor and be almost about to push the baby out and give birth. It is very important for all care providers to know how fast they need to move around to set up for the birth and get you situated appropriately for where you are at, get you in the water if you're having a water experience, etc.

Shift Changes

At the birth center, it is more likely you will be attended to by the midwife you have been seeing over the course of your pregnancy. She will be checking on you and or part of the team that's going to attend your birth. Her attendants may experience a shift change while she is working with you, and that is something to be prepared for. Recognizing that you are getting fresh help from people who are there to lend their strength may help alleviate any distress you feel.

Early Labor at Home—Midwife's Role

Just a quick note here to say that the "we" in this section either refers to "we midwives" or "I and my apprentices." It is by no means a royal we. No midwife is an island, and while I have attended births on my own, it is always better to have a team. While I have said before that not all midwives offer the same standard of care that I provide, many do.

I ask all of my clients to call me when their contractions are slightly under five minutes apart, a minute long, painful, and have been going on for a while. This is usually the time that they need some support, and they need to have information about what's going on with their body, so they make an informed choice about what the best course of action is from there.

Usually at this point they are 1–4 centimeters dilated, which is an excellent time to start listening to the baby's heartbeat, taking the mother's blood pressure, and getting ready for the birth. Sometimes it takes a long time and sometimes it is incredibly, unbelievably fast. I load almost 175 pounds of equipment into my car, just in case it's needed, and head on over. I walk into my client's house with my vibrant, loving energy, a small oxygen tank, and my home visit bag.

Just in case it's not clear, any care provider that you have is going to tell you when to get in touch with them and when to go to the hospital or birth center. They will let you know if it really is too early to be there and may send you home with instructions on what to watch for, so you know when to come back if you are not planning a home birth. If it's too early for your midwife to be there, she may opt to return when things intensify.

Initial Assessment

The first thing I do when I walk in the door is get out my doppler and listen to the baby's heart tones. If there is something off with the heart tones, I will put oxygen on momma immediately and jiggle her tummy around to try to move the baby. I will have her lie on her back, roll her onto her left then right side, and then have her get back up. All of this will be done very quickly. This is to hopefully dislodge the baby from pinching the cord with a shoulder or other body part. If that is the case, usually these quick movements will dislodge the cord and they will return to normal.

If this is unsuccessful and the baby's heart tones continue to be of great concern, I would opt to transport the woman to the hospital at that point. I will talk more about that later. For now, I want to reassure you that every educated and/or certified midwife is trained to assess the birthing mother and baby at every stage of the process to ensure their health and safety.

Blood Pressure Check

The second thing I do is take the woman's blood pressure. If her blood pressure is high, I will have her lie on her left side and possibly administer homeopathic or herbal remedies. I bring a full homeopathic kit and an herbal kit with me to the birth with all kinds of homeopathic and herbal medicines we use in different circumstances. These homeopathic remedies can be very effective for blood pressure problems during the birth. If these techniques do not work, I might also in that circumstance choose to transport the woman to the hospital. Sometimes blood pressure can be a bit high at the beginning because the mom is so worked up and anxious about her labor starting, but once the midwife and her birth team are there, often the anxiety fades and blood pressure will go back to normal. If the blood pressure issues do not subside, the hospital can quickly and effectively bring this under control with an epidural or other medicines.

I know this might sound scary. I want to remind you that 90 percent of the births I attend have resulted in a beautiful natural birth at home without major complications.

Assess Labor Patterns

I will assess the mother and her labor patterns as soon as I arrive. How quickly things are moving will indicate how quickly we need to move to set up and get everything prepared for the baby's arrival. This will also help me to decide what needs to happen first, second, third, and so on. I will ask the partner to unload my birthing equipment from the car in preparation for the birth.

Vaginal Exam

I will always do an exam when I arrive so I can both make sure nothing is wrong, evaluate where things are at, and give you an educated guess as to how long things will take. I will let you know how dilated you are, how effaced you are, how engaged the baby is and what is the position of the baby's head, as well as how flexed it is. I will also assess if your waters are intact or bulging. Things can change significantly between a contraction and no contraction so I will usually do the exam through a contraction as well.

I had one woman in my care who was 4 centimeters dilated when I checked her in between contractions, but she felt very soft and stretchy. I waited for a contraction to come, and when I checked during the contraction, she was at 8 centimeters! As soon as the contraction stopped, she went back to 4 centimeters. She had the baby 30 minutes later. If I had not checked during the contraction, I might not have realized how close she was and not been set up and ready for the baby to come. I have also seen a woman whose cervix clamped down during a contraction and went from 4 centimeters to 2 centimeters.

This is all just to say you never know how quick it is going to go, so we need to do everything we can to assess labor and be prepared. I might suggest that you rest at that point. If I get there in the middle of the night and you are 1–2 centimeters dilated, I will almost always suggest that you lie down and not march around. Even if you just rest or hopefully doze in between contractions it will help you in the end.

Equipment Setup

I will set up my entire birth kit as well as the birth kit you purchased. I get my pressure cooker started on the stove with water and the instruments I will be using during the birth. This sterilizes them. We have instruments to clamp and cut the cord, instruments to suture a tear, as well as instruments to do the occasional episiotomy. I never expect to do an episiotomy, but occasionally it can be a good choice. Once the equipment is fully sterilized, we leave it to cool.

I make sure to have my ambu bag with me, just in case the baby is not breathing well at birth. I also set up our oxygen tanks. I have a large oxygen tank as well as a smaller one that I arrive with. I always carry multiple spare tanks of oxygen in case we should run out of one of the tanks.

Birth Notes

I begin writing the birth notes shortly after I arrive. My team keeps excellent notes and I write down everything that happens in great detail, so my clients have comprehensive documentation of not only every medical fact, but also the complete accompanying story of what happened before, during, and after the birth. I document what was happening in the days before the birth, how they went into labor, when they called and what I suggested, when I arrive, what the mother does and says, what their partner does and says, what their family does and says, and

> **Robbie:** Because I was so exhausted when the time came to push out my 10-pound baby, my midwives gave my husband an oxygen mask to hold over my nose and mouth in-between the pushing urges. The extra energy that I received from the oxygen really helped me to make it through!

much, much more so they have a wonderful journal of the birth to reflect on later. This is a common practice among midwives and doulas, though it may come in less detailed forms than mine.

Continuing Assessments

I listen to heart tones every 1-2 hours in early labor, approximately every 30–60 minutes in active labor, every 15–30 minutes in transition, and every contraction or two during pushing. I am very careful, and if I ever hear anything that is concerning, I listen much more frequently and transport to the hospital if necessary. Every so often I will listen through a contraction and for a while after the contraction as well. An exam usually takes 10–30 seconds. The baby could be having heart tone decelerations that only occur during the contraction, but your provider will want to understand this fully.

I take my client's blood pressure every four hours, as mandated by state law. If a woman's blood pressure seems worrisome in any way, I also check her blood pressure more frequently and transport if necessary.

I try to be very intuitive in a woman's labor to know when to encourage her, when to guide her, and when to be quiet. I also ask women what they want. Most women say, "Please guide me," or "Please encourage me," (or both) but occasionally I'll have someone who says they'd prefer not to have guidance and I respect this ... up to the point where it starts to get complicated. Your health and safety and that of your baby always comes first.

I continue to do exams every two hours and I do time them with a contraction, as it can

make such a difference. This information is so helpful and gives us the medical data we need to adequately assess progress during labor. Almost all women do not want labor to go on longer and longer. It can be a hard and painful process. I spent the early decades of my career not doing very many exams during labor and not encouraging women to do what they could to advance their labor because I felt that they needed to follow their own internal guidance.

In the early years of my career, after six hours a woman might finally say, "Okay I would like to go ahead and do an exam to see where I am at," and I'd find that she had not progressed at all. It was very depressing news for her at that stage. She hadn't been doing what was required by her body to keep things moving along. I realized that these women hired me so I could help and support them through a safe experience. I was there to support this process and to make it go as quickly and easily as possible, but I needed to have data to make that happen. So, now I encourage earlier exams in labor. I am very quick; my exams usually take about 10–30 seconds. Information is power, and performing exams when a woman is in labor allows me to give my clients more information faster, which gives them the power to make choices in alignment with their vision of their ideal, perfect birth.

Exams may also provide reassurance that you're doing just fine! If you have been lying down and you progress two centimeters an hour, then you can stay down and do whatever feels good. If you have been lying down and you only dilate half a centimeter in two hours, I will likely suggest that you get up and move around to move things along. Many women want to lie down during labor as it makes things milder and less intense than when you are upright.

Cervical Massage

Every now and then I will do a little cervical massage if there is a little band around the os. This band can be stiff and tense, but with that cervical massage it goes right away and can help to progress and move things significantly faster. I have additional information about this in the interventions section, later in this chapter.

Special Services

In my practice, we perform a lot of additional services as well as providing great midwifery care. We cook and clean, do the birth laundry, take great pictures and videos, choreograph the family and friends, aid the children, and much more. This is one of the reasons we work in teams of three or four, as it is essential that we have enough people present to support this process and the health and safety of the mother and baby. If your midwife doesn't provide these kinds of services, they can often be handled by a doula.

Open the Windows

Sometimes when I arrive at people's homes, they have all the curtains drawn or blinds closed, because they're afraid of being seen without clothes on. You need the light on your body and eyes during labor in order for your pituitary to be stimulated appropriately, so you need to not stay in the dark. During the day you need to be in the light. I can't tell you how many times we have gone out into the yard to prove that you can't see into the windows at all from the yard. If this concerns you, check out the view of the room you plan to labor in from

the outside during the day ahead of time to reassure yourself. Now, at night you do need to close the blinds or draw the curtains shut or the room will be on full display.

> *Midwifery is the art of holding space for a woman and her family during one of the most magical and transformational times of their lives.*
>
> —Sister MorningStar

Early Labor Anywhere
Be Active and Change Positions

Keep moving. Your goal is to make all the sensations stronger. Whatever you don't want to feel, you will have to feel at some point, so *go for it*. More pain is better. It will make it go faster, and this is good. The longer your labor takes, the more exhausted you'll become. Work to keep it shorter.

I hear some women and some midwives say that labor should never be helped along but I disagree. The constant squeezing of the baby for many hours and the pushing of the baby's head down into the pelvis is hard on the baby. I fervently believe anything that you can do to aid the process to not be as long and hard for either of you is a good thing.

Often what we naturally go for in labor is whatever we can do that makes it less painful, less intense, less close together, and this is always going to make it take longer. As it does, the woman and the baby are getting more and more tired. As you get more and more tired, you are able to access fewer and fewer coping strategies and you have less ability to withstand the increasing pain and strength and intensity of labor.

I do find that shorter is better up to a point, but don't ever wish for a two- or four-hour labor—you might get one, but it is very hard. It can be like a runaway train, hard to get a handle on, and hard to stay on top of. Having an 18- to 30-hour birth is also a very difficult experience, and so we strive to find a balance.

You can try a variety of positions and shift to something new whenever you like. You might try some of the following:

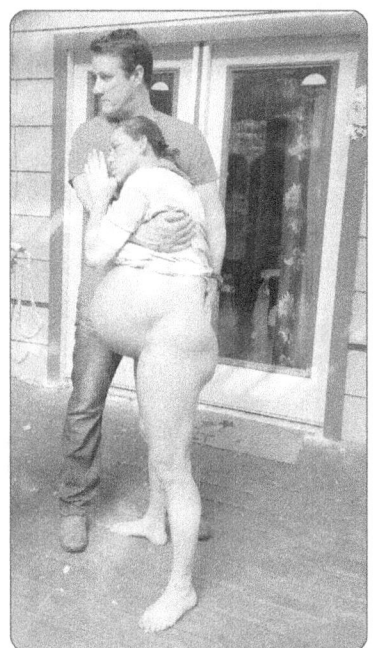

Laboring at Home

- Get on your hands and knees.

- Be up and walking.

- Stand and rock in place.

- Hang around your partner's neck or on a door frame in a hanging squat.

- Rock in a chair.

- Spend time in the bathtub, shower, or birthing pool.

- Sit on a birth stool.

- Sit on the toilet—this can be a great place to have contractions. Every single time you've sat on a toilet, you've relaxed, so it is a place where you sit down and let go by reflex. The more you let go, the more the baby moves down, which makes the baby come down faster. This can

often make labor more painful, but anything that makes it more painful is *good*! It usually means that the cervix is dilating.

- Place your chest on a couch, chair, or bed with your knees on the floor on top of a pillow. You can rock your hips a bit in this position.

The next two pages show a variety of Positions for Laboring.

Deep peace of the running waves to you,
Deep peace of the flowing air to you,
Deep peace of the quiet earth to you,
Deep peace of the shining stars to you,
Moon and stars always giving light to you.

—Ancient Celtic Prayer

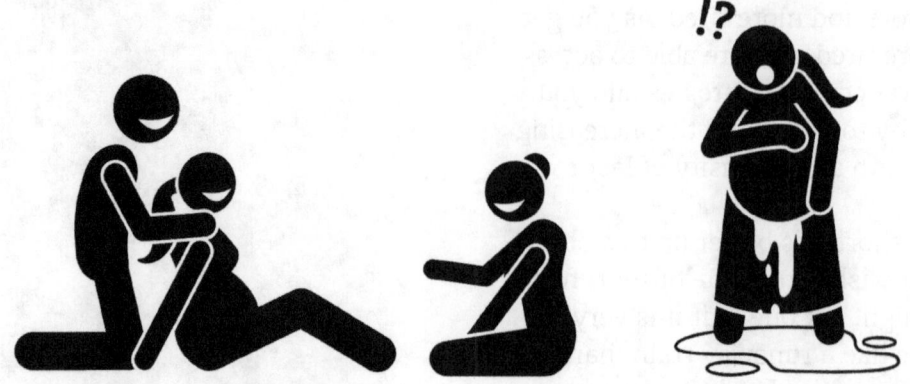

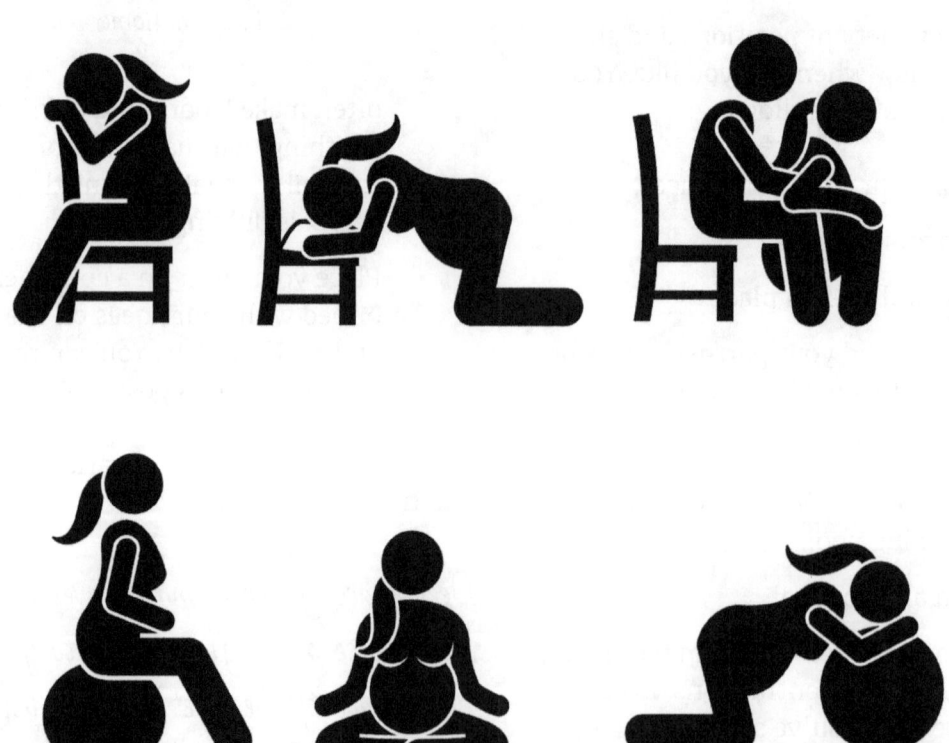

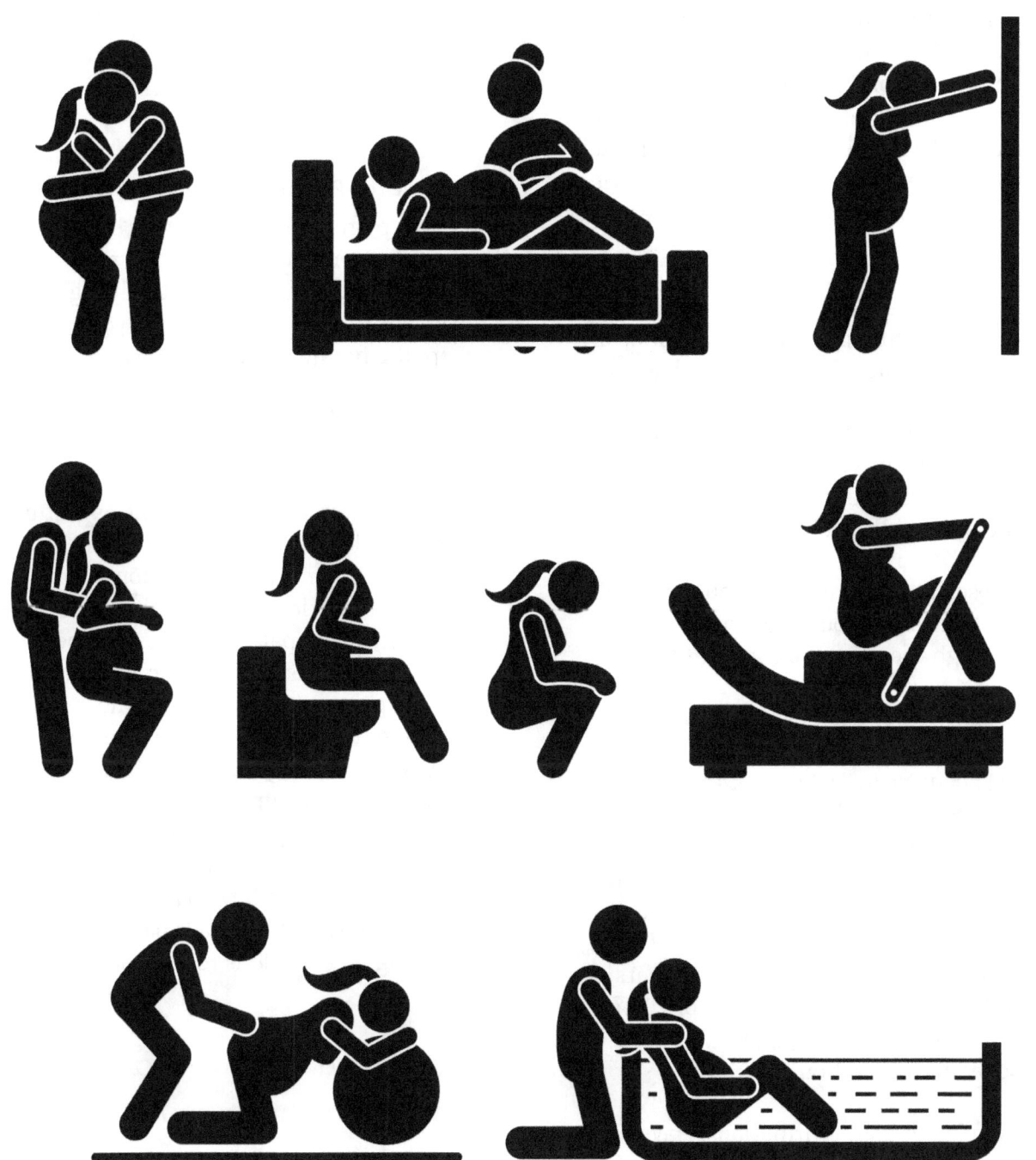

Don't Back Away from the Sensations

Years ago, I was playing at the beach, and I noticed that contractions are very much like waves. They start out, build to a crescendo, and then ebb. What I realized is that there are three typical ways people play with waves. They might give a little jump, sail up over the front of the wave, and slide right down the other side, carried by the power of the wave.

Then there are bigger waves, and they might dive right through them aerodynamically and shoot through to the other side.

Then there are the times they stand up against the wave and its power smacks them down, they tumble and are spat out the other side, choking on sand and water.

These are the three ways you can handle contractions—you can go over them, through them, or you can fight them.

I highly recommend going over or through. I did try fighting them at first. I thought, *I am not going to do this breathing stuff. I am just not going to do it,* but that lasted all of about half of one contraction before I realized that it didn't feel good and doing nothing was not working. I wanted to run around, scream, and get away from what I was feeling ... which, my dears, unfortunately also does not work. You cannot escape labor (unless you choose to schedule a c-section).

Remember your affirmations. Have others encourage you and believe their words. Everyone is proud of your courage and strength. I am proud of you. You are a beautiful, divine woman, flexing your creative birthright.

> You are a beautiful, divine woman, flexing your creative birthright.

Welcome the Pain and Surrender to It

Usually, pain is a sign from your body that something terrible is happening, and you need to be very afraid and get help right away, but this is the one time in your life where it's not quite that way.

I need you to know that pain is your friend during labor.

You know, pain is such a trip in this culture. We do not deal with pain very well nor do we experience much pain. We don't have rickets or do serious manual labor that gives us the aches and pains that most of the world experiences. We just don't experience as much pain as is the norm for most of the women in the world who have given birth. So, typically the biggest physical challenge that we ever come up against as women in this culture is the pain of labor, and you have got to remember that pain is your friend. If you do not have pain, you do not have the baby. You will have pain and the best thing you can do is to surrender to it.

> Pain is your friend. If you do not have pain, you do not have the baby. You will have pain and the best thing you can do is to surrender to it.

I swear I could summarize my entire approach to birth, parenting, and life in that one word, *surrender*. You prepare, you make plans, you get ready, and then you let go and let God. You surrender to this process, and you surrender to the pain.

Yes, it hurts. For some women it hurts more, and for some it hurts less. But without pain there is no baby ... That is how it works, and you have got to decide that it is going to be okay. You have the tools you need for this, and you are going to work through it.

Your strength as a woman is in your ability to *allow*, not to control. Trust the process. Trust your baby. Trust the wisdom of the millions of women in a long line who have come before you. Trust that you can take your position among them with grace, dignity, and faith.

Your strength as a woman is in your ability to *allow*, not to control. Trust the process. Trust your baby. Trust the wisdom of the millions of women in a long line who have come before you. Trust that you can take your position among them with grace, dignity, and faith.

Use Your Breathing Techniques

Most women at some point will not be able to handle the sensations without some focus. You may not be there yet, but if you are, what I think is the most helpful in early labor is deep breathing.

Remember to take your deep cleansing breath, breathe in and out connecting the inhale to the exhale, equalizing the inhale to the exhale. Completely inhale and completely exhale. Focus on relaxing on the exhale. Let every muscle go with every exhale. Visualize yourself getting on top of the contraction and just letting go into it.

Let the sensations be big, let them get stronger, this is exactly what you want. The point is *not* to make it less, but to relax enough to ride through what is happening.

Deep breathing is like going right through the contraction. The pant and the pant-blow feel to me like you kind of go up over the waves of the contractions. You build up and go down with the force of the contraction. Reserve those for when it gets a little more intense.

The deep cleansing breath is not only oxygenating at the beginning and the end of every contraction, but it will be a signal to everyone present in the room that you are having another contraction. You may want them to stop or start whatever they were doing. Communicate. If they are applying lower back pressure, you may want them to stop or do more as the rhythm of the contraction asserts itself. Make your wishes known. This is all about you right now.

Everyone should stop and focus on you again when you take that deep cleansing breath. It is also most importantly a signal to *you* that there is a beginning and end to every contraction. It can be a little hard to believe that at some points during labor because the sensations are so powerful that you start to feel like you have been in labor forever, and you will continue to be in labor forever. It's not true.

I promise you; your brain is lying to you. There is an end to this. Your baby is coming. This will not last forever. No pain, no baby. Stronger pain means you're getting closer. And remember, *you were built for this.*

Partner's Role

Be There for Her

 You have to take breaks to pee, drink water, and eat, but otherwise, no whining. She's doing the exceptionally difficult work here. Be present and available to help however is needed. You do have to take care of yourself. If you are not hydrated and pumped up it is impossible to take care of anyone else. I work hard to remind partners to take care of themselves, but it is important for you to remember to attend to this because the midwife's first priority is always going to be the mother and baby.

Breathe with your partner if she wants you to. She may or may not want you to,

but it's important to know how. Be sure to practice together ahead of time. Love her. It's your love that's really helping her. Visualize her being bathed in white light and unconditional love.

Ask her what she wants, what she needs, and how you can help. Make suggestions for her.

Say positive things to your woman. She's working very hard and needs to know that you love and support her. Let her know how strong and beautiful she is. It is so helpful to hear your beloved tell you how strong and brave you are, how beautiful you are, give encouraging words, ask what you can do to help.

Make sure to do this in between contractions, it is not very helpful to talk when they are in the midst of a contraction; let her concentrate. But in between, build her up, give her that support and pour your energy into her to lift her. Ask her what she wants, what works best for her, and then do that.

Keep her hydrated. Remind her to pee.

Stage 1—Dilation
Phase II: Active Labor 4-7 cm

Keyword: Serious

Active Labor is the stage when your cervix goes from four to seven centimeters in dilation. The keyword here is *serious*. Your demeanor will shift. This is hard, hard work and it demands your full attention. Smiles evaporate as concentration takes over and the realization that you may not have a painless childbirth hits you. After a

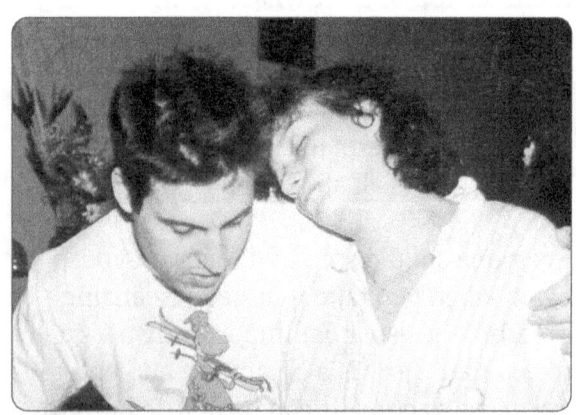

Partner Supporting Laboring Woman

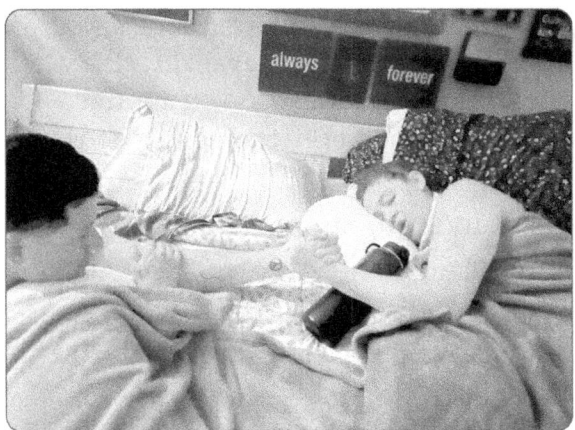
Aleah in the Throes of a Tough Contraction

certain point it is very difficult to relax and distract yourself as you did in pre-labor and even early labor. When you are feeling intense sensations in your lower abdomen and pelvis, it can be very hard to let go and relax in spite of that. At this point in labor, you won't be chatting much during contractions. When labor becomes intense and it's too uncomfortable to do anything else, use the breathing methods you've been practicing. I especially want you to not hold your breath, as doing so decreases the oxygen to the baby.

If you get stuck in your head it can be a quick path to major intervention, because birth is a body-spirit phenomenon, and it is not in your head.

This phase is a bit quicker on the timetable. I typically see women dilating 1–2 centimeters per hour with contractions lasting 60 seconds and being two to four minutes apart at this phase. Try to let go of your need to control. SURRENDER! You are never given more than you can handle, and you are not alone, you have your partner and your support staff with you. You are the end product of an unbroken line of

successful birthing women going back into the misty dawn of time.

There's a feedback mechanism that's happening between your cervix and your brain, and additionally all this biochemical activity is happening in your uterus and your vagina and your cervix, and it's extremely dynamic. The joy and wonder of natural birth enables this dynamic connection, and the resultant rush of wonderful hormones facilitates the incredible bonding that occurs between you and your baby when your hearts are fully open after such a deep and profound experience.

Once you get to 4 centimeters, wow! Gravity works. Find some balance. Work to be up and laboring actively 40–50 minutes out of every hour and then rest for 10–20 minutes. When you rest, lie down, just chill, and let all your muscles relax. Rehydrate. Communicate what you need.

It may be nice to be on your hands and knees in a tabletop position for a few minutes. A lot of women like to do this because it makes labor easier. When you do this, what's happening is the baby falls forward and it comes off your cervix, so it isn't as painful for you. As your midwife, I would let you do that for 10–15 minutes and then we'd talk about it. The chances are when it's more comfortable, you're not progressing as quickly. Your baby's head needs to press down against the cervix to progress. If you're in a position that brings the baby off your cervix, chances are your labor may not be progressing as well. Now, if you're okay with that, then do what you want, but I at least want you to have the information that often when you're making it less, you're making it longer.

The number one reason I transport women to the hospital is either exhaustion from warmup labor, pre-labor, or exhaustion from a prolonged labor, so I'm now pretty proactive and let women know that staying on their hands and knees is not something they want to be doing for too long, unless they are progressing fine. Then they can do whatever works for them.

> When you're making it less, you're making it longer.

Things that will make it more intense will make you progress faster. It's not a race, but you don't want to stall out. Keep moving and keep changing positions. Things to make it more intense include sitting on the toilet, standing in the shower, rocking in a chair, kneeling by the bed resting your upper body on the mattress, walking, and then squatting with the contraction. Get on your hands and knees in between contractions if you like, but then during contractions try to get the baby down against the cervix. Whatever makes the contraction more intense is good.

Know that while it feels better for you, it can be harder for the baby to stay in longer, and if you continue to back away from the sensations of labor it will prolong the birth process. Your baby is as challenged during labor as you are. You are going through this together. I think it is better to not let fear be your guide here, but to focus on surrendering to the pain so you can meet your sweet baby. You're going to feel it all at some point, so call on your strength and your resources and get to it! The bottom line is that this is your birth process, your body, and your labor. You can do it the way you want, but I want you to be informed and understand the effects of your choices.

What to Do to Support Yourself in Active Labor

Some of the things that are exceptionally helpful at this stage are:

- **Walking**
- **Swaying.** Drape your arms around your partner for support, spread your legs slightly, and bend your knees to open the pelvis. Relax your pelvis. Lean into the opening so the head can really come down with the contraction. As the head goes down onto the cervix, the pressure helps to open the cervix and not only that, but with the contraction the uterus pulls the muscle back and pushes the baby farther down, helping to open the cervix even more.
- **Sit on the toilet.** When you sit on the toilet, you relax your bottom and your vagina. When you do this in labor, your muscle memory will kick in and help you to relax your glutes and vagina. A lot of women have a lot of difficulty relaxing completely, so this is a way to trick your mind into letting go and relaxing, so it lets go of the tension on the pelvis. It will feel unnatural and strange. It may be uncomfortable. But relaxing is important to the process. Relaxing will shorten your laboring.
- Get into clean **water.** A shower, a big tub, pools ... Water helps to relax us and helps everything go better

at this stage, unless it slows it way down. Avoid natural sources of water at this time (creeks, ponds, rivers, streams, lakes, oceans). You need to be in chlorinated water.

- **Affirmations.** One of the biggest causes of tension at this stage is fear. Fear creates tension, which creates pain, which creates more fear. It's a cycle that you need to break. If you are knowledgeable and have enough information about what's going on, you can relax your mind. This allows your body to relax more. Repeat your affirmations. Trust that you've done enough to prepare.

In the throes of active labor, there is a point of realization that labor is upon you, and it is something that you cannot escape. While in early labor you may be able to take moments to call on your joy more actively, active labor is more intense, and it can be a little daunting. Continue to think positively, use your affirmations, visualize your body doing exactly what it needs to do to help your labor progress. Imagine the baby continuing to come down into your pelvis, pushing on your cervix to open, and helping to dilate you. Welcome the contractions and the pain. Remember, pain is your friend, you are not being damaged. This is the path to bring your baby into the world and you have all the love, strength, and power within you to have your ideal, perfect birth.

In active labor, I get concerned if we aren't progressing. Slow progression is fine, but the cervix needs to be opening. If it gets stuck it's often due to the baby's positioning. I try to establish the position

of the baby early in labor and guide the woman to different positions to optimally position the baby in the birth canal. A baby being in a posterior position is one of the things that will slow labor down the most. Posterior means that the baby is facing up toward the front side of the mother's body instead of facing down. (Anterior is facing down, with the face looking at the mother's sacrum). Babies in a posterior position present a much larger diameter to the cervix and are more difficult to give birth to.

Water in Birth

Mothers-to-be should get into the birthing pool whenever they want to during labor.

Know that immersion in water can slow labor down, so if labor seems to have slowed or stopped your midwife will likely encourage you to exit the tub until regular or stronger labor is reestablished.

 It's important to note that immersion in a warm tub of water while laboring can lead to loss of body fluids through perspiration. Partners, encourage your laboring mother to drink 8 ounces of clear fluids every hour.

For most women, water is an amazing soother. Sometimes when you're on that trek up the Mount Everest that is labor, you need a little break. Getting into water helps to slow things down and gives you the space to take that break. You can catch your breath and get a second wind. At some point you'll be ready again to work on helping that baby come out, you'll exit the water, and the work will resume. For some women, entering the water allows further relaxation, which makes everything go better. Not always, but it's worth experimenting with.

If you're at a birth center or a hospital, find the water options there, the shower, the bath, and a birth tub or tank are all great options.

I am not enthusiastic about hot tubs because I think it's hard to keep them sanitized to the level that is appropriate for birth.

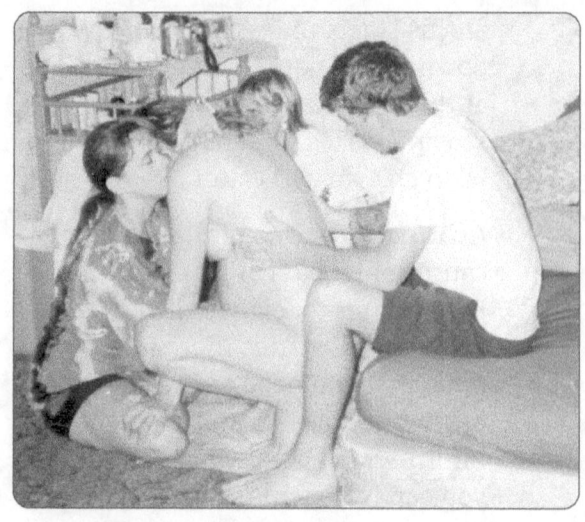

Supporting a Squatting Woman in Labor

Partner's Role

 Most women prefer that it be quiet in the birthing room because they are lost in the zone. To get pulled back into their head with questions, then have to find language, and then verbalize the answer to those questions pulls them away from the zone, where they had lost track of time, space, and language. Ask your woman what she wants in the moment and give her the option for a nonverbal response. You can say something like, "Nod if you want me to keep talking to you right now or shake your head if I should be quiet."

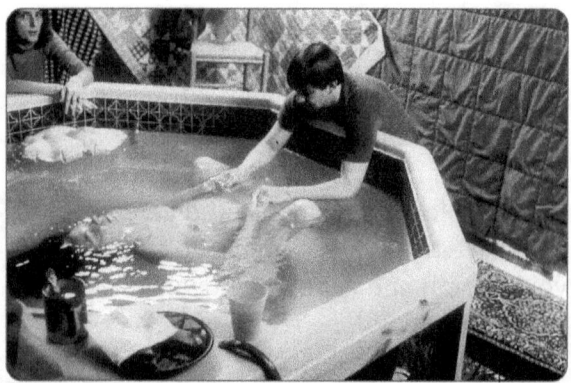

A Partner's Support is Invaluable Throughout Labor

Squatting

 Partners, remember your role here is to provide support at your laboring woman's direction. She'll let you know by saying something like, "Here comes another one," "Now," or by taking her deep, cleansing breath, and then you're going to support her as she squats. Take on her weight. She will then work through the contraction. Let her shoulders down a little bit. When you hear the final deep, cleansing breath, stand and lift after a count of three. This is where you have to work to coordinate because you must work as a team. Moms, you've got to use your legs, so your shoulders don't get out of whack. Partners, don't exert too much force underneath her armpits as you lift.

Aid in Relaxation

 Help your laboring partner to deeply relax in between contractions. Remember the squeeze and stroke technique you learned in the third trimester (see

page 285). Use your body language, not your words. If you tell her, "Just relax, honey," she's likely to want to yell at you, which is of course unproductive.

Respond immediately to her cues. She may want you to stop stroking, or to never stop stroking, or somewhere in between. Listen to her. I've had women who were fine all through labor as long as they were being stroked, and the entire team took turns to keep her comfortable. I've also had women who didn't want to be touched at all, by anyone. As with all things, there is a spectrum.

You never know what's going to work for you. Experiment. But know that most woman want their beloved to be very loving, close, and present. If she's not yet in the zone, whisper your terms of endearment in her ear, let her know how amazing she is, how much you treasure the work she is doing for your family. That energy raises the oxytocin level and can help her access the zone where sex and birth come more easily.

I use intuition born of decades of helping birthing women to respond to a laboring woman's cues. Maybe she's red-faced and I apply a cold, damp cloth to bring relief. It is likely that your midwife will be just as intuitive in her responses to your partner, and that she will help you to help your partner. Don't be afraid to ask her what you can do to help.

How to Help with Back Pain

 Back pain can be severe in labor as the baby exerts pressure. Here are a few tricks you can use to help your partner.

Apply counter pressure by placing the palms of both hands against the spot that's bothering her. Push in with contractions and let off in between. She will tell you exactly where to lean in and how much pressure to apply. See the bottom left-hand illustration on page 413.

Some women like heat, some ice, some massage with a tennis ball or massage device. Massage tends to be better between contractions. Pressure tends to be more preferred during a contraction.

Ask her what she wants! Good communication is key to comforting her.

Midwife's Role at a Home Birth

I talk a lot over the course of a woman's pregnancy as I get to know her and her partner. I talk and talk and talk to empower my clients, to educate them, to create a relationship between us, and to bring love to the process, but by the time I get to the birth I want to be quiet, and I talk very little.

It's very surprising for people, because I'm usually such a chatterbox, and I'm teaching and teaching and teaching so much that for me to be quiet is a different experience for them. I find that what most women want is for their beloved to be right by their side. They need the support of their loved one, and they want a sense of privacy, quiet, and intimacy. Everyone except for your partner needs to be very much in the background until the baby is coming out.

It is my role as a midwife to stay in the background, and to provide as much privacy as I can. I work to be unobtrusive, even if I have to listen to the baby. I pull my energy within and just completely focus on how the baby is, and once I see that everything is okay and you are working in tandem, I will retreat to the background again, until I am needed or wanted. Most midwives do the same, including hospital-based nurse-midwives.

Hospital Birth

The care you receive during active labor (as well as transition) in the hospital is very dependent on staffing. If they are really busy with lots of births, you are not going to get as much attention. This is one of the reasons that you will be monitored, so they can watch your and the baby's vitals from the nurse's station.

For the most part, they leave you alone a lot. This is not a bad thing. It is a great time for you to put on your playlists, take advantage of the birth ball or peanut ball that many hospitals will have or will allow you to bring. (A peanut ball is shaped like a peanut and fits snugly between your legs. This helps to increase the progress of labor and to facilitate the descent of the baby's head.)

Most hospitals only have showers available, but those are lovely and are a great way to use water to help you relax during your contractions. They often have a stool for you to sit on in the shower and you can allow the nice, hot water to run on your back.

Some hospitals allow intermittent monitoring, and some have Bluetooth monitors, so you are not tethered to cords. If they allow intermittent monitoring, you are typically connected to the monitor for 15 minutes out of every hour. When you're not hooked up, you can move freely around the room, and sometimes the halls. If the hospital has Bluetooth monitors, you are then able to freely move around while being continuously monitored.

Remember, active labor is about allowing your cervix and uterus to open. Use any of the suggestions I mentioned at the beginning of this chapter that feel good for you. Active labor is also a good time to eat, but only if you are not feeling nauseated. Remember to only eat lightly and to consume things you do not mind seeing come back up.

Hospitals differ on their policies on eating during labor, so it is another question to ask beforehand. The reason why they are concerned about letting you eat is due to the potential risk of having food in your stomach in the slim chance that an emergency surgery with general anesthesia needs to be performed. If you have food in your stomach and vomit during the procedure, there is a risk of dying of aspiration pneumonia. So, it is common practice for food not to be administered in hospitals prior to a situation that could result in surgery. My point is that they are not just being mean or unreasonable, they are being cautious.

I am confident there is a minimal chance of you needing to have an emergency c-section with general anesthesia (c-sections almost always use local analgesia) and I think it is incredibly important to eat so you can keep your energy up during labor. Just food for thought.

THE BIRTH PROCESS

Most hospitals do not conduct a lot of vaginal exams during active labor. Your provider's preferences and your situation may indicate a need for more frequent exams. Remember that you have rights, and it is important for you and/or your partner to know what your birth plan is and to advocate for your wants and needs.

If everything is moving normally, it is okay to only do exams every few hours. You may also have to remind your nurses that you do not want to be offered anything for pain and that you will ask if you want it. If you have a doula, it may depend on the hospital as to whether they will allow her in the room with you. Check beforehand with your doctor so you know and can be supported by anyone you want by your side during the birth.

It is important that I mention shift changes again. The doctors and nurses caring for you work either eight- or twelve-hour shifts. It is possible for you to have as many as three different sets of people caring for you over the course of your labor. This can be a little difficult to adjust to at times, but if you are prepared for this eventuality, you are less likely to be thrown off-kilter by it. Again, this is where a doula can really help to provide continuity of care.

Birth Center Birth

The care you receive during active labor (as well as transition) in a birth center falls somewhere between what you experience at home and what you experience in a hospital. As compared to a hospital, it is a more relaxed environment, there are fewer people, you usually have bigger rooms, and many birth centers have birthing tubs for you to use during the labor. Depending on the protocols in your chosen freestanding birth center, you may be able not only to labor but also to give birth in the tub. You will very likely not have as many shift changes, and you may or may not know the people attending you, depending on the birth center.

Most women will be monitored the way it is done at a home birth, with a midwife or apprentice using a handheld doppler to listen to the baby occasionally and increasingly in the later stages of labor. Depending on the birth center, their policies, procedures, and their midwives, you may experience a labor and birth that is much more like what you would experience at a home birth as I've described, or you may have an experience that leans more toward what you would experience with a hospital birth.

Stage 1—Dilation
Phase III: Transition 7-10 cm

Keyword: Psychedelic Discouragement

This is the stage where your cervix goes from 7 to 10 centimeters in dilation. Once you achieve this, your body is ready to push your baby out, and it's very exciting. But this last stage before you get to pushing is usually the hardest, and it is usually more painful. The biggest thing to do to prepare yourself is to decide that it's all going to be okay, and that this is the good pain of birth, not the bad pain of a broken leg or appendicitis.

Think of the pain of labor as a rite of passage. There is a quadrumvirate of female archetypes: the Maiden, Mother, Queen/Matriarch, and Crone. With your first birth, you move from Maiden and become the Mother and it is a huge life change. You are coming out of your old self into your new self and there is existential, spiritual pain to that movement and that enormous growth, because you are a different person as a mother. You are being remade. With one event, somebody is now totally dependent on you. It's amazing and challenging, and sometimes it's hard and even scary, but it's also incredibly wonderful.

Birth is a profoundly emotional experience in women's lives. Not every woman is emotional. There is a bell curve, as there is with pain. Some are very emotional, and some are not at all, and most people are somewhere in the middle. The zone that you go to in birth exists within that place of pain, surrender, and survival. In that place your defense mechanisms evaporate. This state of heightened and altered awareness sends you off to a completely different plane and gives you a unique and special experience, so you can more fully and completely devote yourself to your baby when you come out on the other side of it. It was important for the survival of humanity for nature to create a mechanism that would transform a woman from an independent someone to an interconnected nurturer, devoted to protecting and growing this new life, even to her own detriment.

No matter how many people are in the room with you, birth is a solitary experience. There is only you. You are the one contracting and experiencing the sensations in your body, the depths of your emotion, and your spiritual awakening as a Mother. It's not to say you can't be supported, but you are all alone on an intense ride that will not stop and that you cannot get off of until the baby is born. Let go.

Surrender.

Breathe.

Robbie: I once read a wonderful book called *Water Dancer* by Jenifer Levin. A young and very determined woman swimmer trained for many months, and then set out to swim a very long distance across the ocean. On her first attempt, she kept asking the people in the boat beside her how much longer she had to go, and she failed to reach her goal. On her second attempt, while her mind told her that it was impossible, her body knew that she could always take one more stroke. She entered a timeless dimension—which MariMikel calls "the zone"—and kept total focus on taking each stroke, until, to her amazement, she hit the sand on the other side. That book inspired and supported me during my three-day labor. I let go of my fear that I would end up in the hospital, entered laborland/the zone, and took it one contraction at a time. I never knew for sure whether or not I could actually give birth, but I *always* knew that I could flow through just one more contraction—until, to my own surprise and amazement, I was actually pushing my baby out of my body and into our new lives together!

Focus on handling the contraction you are experiencing right now. It's the only one that matters. You can get through this one.

> Focus on handling the contraction you are experiencing right now. It's the only one that matters. You can get through this one.

The reason I use the keyword *psychedelic* is because oxytocin is a very interesting and wild hormone. For a lot of women, labor is a psychedelic experience. I have seen women whose pupils were completely dilated, and I could not see their irises at all. Many women say that they feel very altered, they can't get their words out, they see colors around lights and around people (also called auras). It can feel very disorienting, and that alone can induce fear, especially if you've never had another experience like it. If you understand that it's a potential for

---

PSYCHEDELIC RECEPTORS

I experienced very altered states during birth, and I have had many clients who also felt the same way. When I was trying to explain the emotional state of transition, I called it *psychedelic* because of this altered state, and *discouraging* because for most women it is definitely the hardest part. I then did research and found that oxytocin, Pitocin, ergot, and LSD were all linked. The connection between them is that they all interact with the same receptor in the brain, the 5-HT2A receptor, which is a type of serotonin receptor, and it plays a role in a variety of functions, including mood, perception, and behavior.

Ergot is a fungus that grows on rye and other grains. It contains a number of alkaloids, including ergotamine and lysergic acid. These alkaloids can have a variety of effects on the body, including vasoconstriction, nausea, and inducing hallucinations. LSD is a synthetic drug that is derived from lysergic acid, which comes from ergot. It is a powerful hallucinogen that can produce a wide range of effects, including visual distortions, altered perception, and changes in mood.

Oxytocin is a hormone that is produced by the hypothalamus and released by the pituitary gland. It is involved in a variety of biological functions, including childbirth, breastfeeding, and social bonding. Oxytocin also has some effects on the brain, and it can increase feelings of trust, empathy, and bonding.

Pitocin is a synthetic version of oxytocin that is used to induce or augment labor. It is also used to control bleeding after childbirth. Pitocin is produced from ergotamine. While Pitocin will induce contractions and even make you have a baby and stop bleeding or hemorrhaging it will not produce any of the same emotional and behavioral effects as oxytocin. When Pitocin is given to the mother it attaches to all of the receptor sites that oxytocin would during a natural labor, and my belief is that this can limit the production and availability of your body's naturally occurring oxytocin. If the receptor sites are not available, then oxytocin cannot work its magic. This can have effects for both the mother as well as the baby.

The link between ergot, LSD, oxytocin, and Pitocin is still being studied, but it is clear that they all interact

(continue on page 426)

THE BIRTH PROCESS

you to go to a strange and different place, it will be easier for you to not be overly alarmed if it does occur for you.

If you do experience this, and it feels like a roller coaster ride you just can't wait to get off of, I want you to know that as soon as the baby is born this altered state dissolves completely and instantly. Adrenaline hits and wipes out those feelings and effects so that you can be present in the moment with your new baby.

Discouragement is also part of transition because most women are challenged by this stage. It pushes them to their absolute limit. I believe this is actually very important. When you are not medicated and you feel the sensations, you feel the pain, it becomes a transformational moment and makes you absolutely expand spiritually. You need to expand spiritually because you are moving from Maiden to Mother.

This is the most difficult, but often the shortest part of labor. It can be very quick, usually lasting between 30 minutes and a few hours. Sometimes it can take an hour per centimeter. The contractions can be 60–80 seconds long and are usually about one to four minutes apart in this phase.

There's a point where the fear can intensify because the pain is just so intense. I see the light in women's eyes dim as they realize how much this hurts, how inexorable it is … for some women giving birth is the first time they've really ever felt real pain.

At this point you're no longer thinking *How much longer? Is this one going to be a hard one?* You're not thinking about anything. It's definitely an altered state but I wouldn't exactly call it euphoric, because you're in a lot of pain, and pain precludes euphoria. But *your baby is coming.* You need to keep reminding yourself that you're having a baby, that there's a method to this, and that you're not being damaged. *Your body is made to do this.*

Labor helps you to realize how incredibly strong you are. While a small percentage of women do need support through intervention in labor, the vast majority of women can have their baby without medical intervention; it is just left up to them to decide whether they will or will not. I have had fewer than thirty women in my whole history of thousands of births, who have said, "Nope, I am not doing this, and I want help." And we then go to the hospital, and

THE BIRTH PROCESS

we get an epidural and that is the perfect path for them and the right thing to do.

In a typical sample of one hundred of my clients, six or seven women go to the hospital for necessary help, one woman finds herself on the wrong end of the pain bell curve and goes to the hospital to get an epidural, and the rest of them have a natural vaginal delivery at home with or without minimal intervention from me.

When you experience the sensations of labor, you get through transition, pushing, the birth of your baby, and come out the other side, you are truly transformed as a being. I believe this is so important and makes you stronger. It is so easy in our society to quit things. We are the throwaway society and anything that is hard, we say, "Well, let's just not do it." Labor helps us do the hard work later, too.

The pain of labor is nothing you cannot handle. I have had a lot of unpleasant physical stuff in my life—several major surgeries, and other extremely painful experiences—and I can tell you, for most women, there are a lot of things that are much worse to experience than the pain of labor. The key is to surrender, do not fight, do not tense up. Allow your body to go limp; ride the contractions with your breath. Transition is a road to courage. Keep reminding yourself to be a noodle. Relax into the intensity. Don't fight against the waves of the contractions, work with them, allow them, welcome them.

The pain of labor is nothing you cannot handle.

Partner's Role

It's the midwife, doula, nurse, and partner's role to continue to reassure the laboring woman. Make sure there is at least one person in the room who will take on this role for you. The experience of labor and birth when you have a partner who is involved, caring, and supportive of you during the labor and birth process is transformative; this is an opportunity for the two of you to deepen your bonds. It can make you better friends, better partners, better lovers, and better parents. Most men in the world have not had an opportunity to be very involved in birth, and this is changing in America. Now we have men who actually want to be a part of this process. They want to be a help to their beloved during this trying and miraculous moment, and this enriches each of you and helps you open up to your deeper selves and each other in a way that might not otherwise happen.

Partners, between contractions most women relish encouragement and tenderness. They may still want you to be quiet, so ask first. If they are welcoming of your verbal support, be very loving with your words. "I love you. You're doing so well." Here are some more words you can use that will help.

"I'm right here with you."

"You can do this. I'm so proud of you."

"You are incredible."

"You are amazing. I see how incredibly strong you are."

"This is a good sign."

"Remember you are safe; it is supposed to feel like this."

"This is exactly how we meet our baby."

"You're doing everything perfectly."

"I know it hurts. I love you so much. What do you need?"

"What can I do for you?"

"Let's try something different. How about we get in the shower/take a bath/try a new position."

Breathe with her. Remember to keep her hydrated. She will at times be in another world. She may be in the zone. Continue to offer her water, coconut water, or Recharge in between contractions.

Remember this can be a joyous process, albeit a difficult and challenging one. Face the rising and falling contractions with joy in your heart, let go of fear, release doubt, and continue to surrender to what is unfolding. If you start to feel fear and doubt rising within, talk yourself up. Let your partner and midwife know what you are feeling. They are there to help you.

Midwife/Home Birth Experience

 I believe that an ideal, perfect birth is one that elevates and empowers your partner as much as it elevates and empowers you as a woman. When you are deeply connected to your partner, you share energy. That's very powerful. It requires a lot of privacy; it can be harder when you have a bunch of people standing around gawking at you to make it to that intimate place. It requires getting really quiet and being alone together. My role as the midwife—unless you or the baby are having a hard time—is to occasionally listen to the baby's heartbeat and otherwise stay in the background. My apprentices and I give you privacy so you can experience the birth intimately, working together.

I always listen to the baby very carefully and increasingly as labor progresses. I continue to take your blood pressure. We do an exam every few hours to make sure that things are progressing—unless it's just obvious that things are progressing, in which case there's no need for an exam. I am there as a guide. If my clients need more support from me in this or any stage, I am there in an instant to provide it. I strive to allow the natural process to unfold, for you and your partner to experience it together, and for us all to find the rhythm that is right for you so that you have your ideal, perfect birth.

How to Get in the Zone During Labor at the Hospital

Give yourself the benefit of spaciousness. You want to have a bubble around you that just can't be messed with. Each intrusion from a staff member is a threat to your psyche, even if just for a moment, before your conscious mind recognizes why that being has invaded your space. This is where your birth plan and self-advocacy come into play. When you arrive at the hospital, ask for as much space as you can possibly be given. This is not a physical space as much as it is privacy to labor as you desire.

Consider having a sign ready to tape to the door that says, "Please knock before entering," which serves subtly to give you a sense of ownership (this is your room, they are at least announcing their presence before crossing the boundary of your domain) and perhaps also changes the demeanor of staff, preventing them from just barreling into your birth or postpartum environment.

 Partners, stay present. You don't want to be distracted. Turn off the television. Put down your phone. Stay on guard and be an advocate for your woman. Listen to her. Be attuned to her. It may be that labor's been going on for hours and you want to check in on the game or take a nap. Don't. She doesn't get to take a break. Know that this is your marathon, too.

Stage II: Pushing

Once you are completely dilated, the next stage is pushing the baby out. Pushing usually takes a first-time mom one to two hours, though it can be shorter or longer. A woman with a big pelvis and a small baby will not have to push as long. A woman who has had a baby before usually takes between 10 and 45 minutes.

Make sure the bedroom thermostat is set quite warm for the baby's arrival: 80−85°F. Sometimes you just need to close the AC vent in the birthing room. Bring in a heat lamp, space heater, or heat dish if necessary.

Pushing is a powerful activity, and it is a learned response. You will have an urge to push, but the *way* to push is something you

learn. You have an instinctual response to push when completely dilated or very close to it, but the way you do it is not instinctual. First time moms have to work harder to get the baby out. It does get easier and easier with each subsequent baby. I love to tell moms that the first time you push a baby out you are also pushing out every other baby you have after that.

You are going to push the baby out with your stomach muscles, and you truly do need them to be successful at pushing. You pull the stomach muscles in and bear down to force the contractions to work for you and move the baby down and out. You can see why it is important to be in good shape and have good muscle tone.

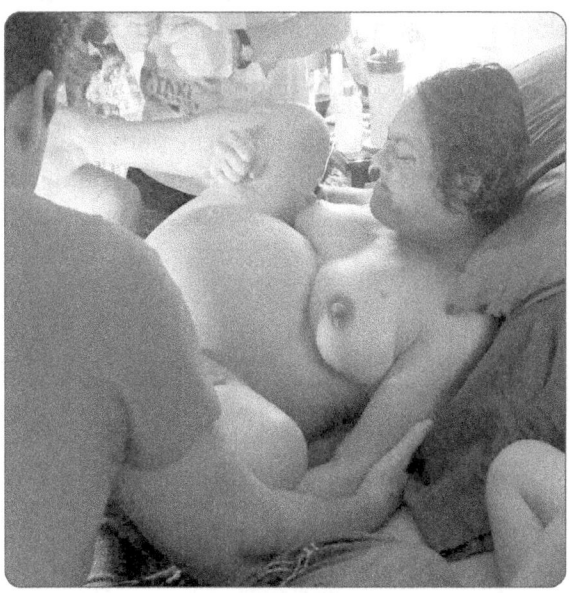
Pushing is Hard Work

For most women pushing is not painful, although it is very hard work. You have to contract your muscles, and bear down with all your might, but it usually doesn't hurt until the baby actually comes out. That pain may last for a few minutes at the very end. If you have a very rapid pushing stage of less than 20 minutes, sometimes that's pretty intense because the tissues don't have enough time to really stretch, but for most women, during the hour to two hours it takes to push the baby out, the tissues are very slowly stretching and it's not actually painful, though you do feel a lot of pressure. You can look forward to this stage! Sometimes the parts of your pelvis can hurt as the baby's head stretches them out as it comes through, but, again, this is pretty rare.

You are usually lying down at the very beginning of this stage because your midwife needs to make sure your cervix is completely dilated so you can push. You cannot push if there is even a little bit of the cervix left in the way because it will tear or swell.

When you are ready to push, I use betadine scrub, sterile water, and sterile gauze to clean all along the outside of the vaginal and labia as well as the upper thighs. If I arrive and your waters have already broken, I will likely scrub you up right then. This helps to prevent infection from bacteria if you have a tear or abrasion. So, after the cervix is completely dilated and scrubbed, I have the mom give one good push and then, if it feels like the baby is coming very quickly, the mother can stay lying down, but most of the time I suggest that first-time mothers get up and push in the squatting position. Gravity is your friend.

Squatting

If you push in the squatting position, it can help to decrease the pushing time significantly. This is not always the case, but usually it's going to make a difference. It will increase the oxygen to the baby during the pushing time and help you to stay focused and keep your energy up through the hard work.

Squatting while pushing helps to use gravity to aid in bringing the baby down into the pelvis so your body doesn't have to work so

Robbie: My own homebirth experience contradicts what Marimikel says above, so I must be on the outer edge of the bell curve she talks about when it comes to this. I started out thinking that pushing would not hurt as much as labor, so I was shocked and upset to discover that it actually hurt a whole lot more, possibly because I was pushing out a 10-pound baby!

My pushes were ineffective until I found the right muscle to use—it was located at the top of my uterus, and once I figured out how to bear down in the right way using the right muscle, my pushes suddenly became much more effective.

I do believe that this kind of body learning is permanent. For example, once you learn how to ride a bicycle, your body will always remember how to do that, even if you haven't ridden one for many years. I think that it's the same with pushing—once you learn how best to do that, your body will always remember. When I look inside myself today, I can still feel that particular muscle—it was one that I had never used before, which is why it took me around 20 minutes to find it during the pushing stage of my labor.

hard during pushing. It can be an arduous task to push your baby out, especially if it takes two hours, so we use gravity to help you. Imagine yourself as a 2-liter bottle with a marble the size of the diameter of the bottle's opening inside of it. Imagine the bottle on its side and attempting to get the marble out of that hole. You can imagine how difficult that would be, how much muscle power it would take. Now, tip the bottle up so the opening points down. This is the path that squatting provides for your baby instead. All of a sudden, gravity and physics are in your and your baby's favor. The marble can slide right out.

Sometimes it is super easy, and you don't need to bear down at all. I have read things about how no one needs to push, and all babies will eventually come out on their own. Michel Odent, an incredible French obstetrician (his books are absolutely amazing and well worth reading) talks about the fetal eject mechanism. This proposes that if you just leave everything alone and you don't do anything at all, eventually the baby will shoot out. After complete dilation, the contractions slowly, slowly work the baby down, and once it gets to a certain point of pressure on the rectum, the body involuntarily ejects the baby in one reflexive or several reflexive pushes.

Having served as a midwife for nearly 50 years and having attended well over 3,000 births, I do not believe this to be true, generally. I have seen way too many babies who required hours of pushing to get them out. I'm uncomfortable even talking about this, but I think with a first baby it's far less likely to happen the way that Odent suggests. You are more likely to experience this with subsequent babies. Assume that

> **Penelope:** My first baby took about 45 minutes to push out. I'd had an epidural and was pushing on my back. My second, a 9-pound baby, came out in three pushes. I was also on my back on a hospital bed. It would have been two pushes, but the nurse-midwife coached me to slow down so I didn't tear. I squatted for my third and she slid out with a single push.

you will need to do some work here. But pushing is nothing like the work of dilation. You have done the hard work. Now the end is so, so close.

What to Do

If you are having the baby in the hospital and have had an epidural, you will not be able to be upright for pushing. They will position the bed to help you to be as upright as possible. Your legs are often supported by stirrups, which are very helpful to properly position the legs. Sometimes pushing takes longer with an epidural because you're not getting the feedback mechanism of the baby's head against your rectum. You have to just visualize and push anyway. The doctor will help you to get the baby down and out.

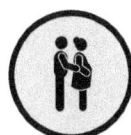 In the beginning, pushing while upright really helps to use gravity to bring your baby down and out. Squat with the contraction; stand in between. Your partner should be sitting on the edge of the bed with their knees facing out and you stand in between their legs facing out as well. Practice this ahead of time so you can work as a team. You can say "One, two, three,"

as a cue and then your partner will use their arms to help you down, into the squatting position. After each contraction the partner will use their muscle and power to support you in standing up again. Shake your feet out when you stand so they do not go numb. This is much easier if you have practiced squatting together before the birth to get the hang of it.

Try to relax your face while you push. Put your chin on your chest, curl up into a "C" shape with your whole body; your spine forms the core of the "C." Don't arch your back, it works against the bones of your body and the baby's body. Point or tilt your pelvis forward and upward.

Take a quick deep cleansing breath in and out and then fill your lungs completely as the contraction starts. Don't let any of the air out, you want to hold your breath during each push! It is very helpful to have your lungs filled first, then bear down with your stomach muscles working in tandem with the contraction. This builds the inner thoracic pressure, so the intra-abdominal pressure is increased. That means you have more power and leverage to push your baby down against the pelvis and vagina. You want that baby out!

> Take a quick deep cleansing breath in and fill your lungs completely as the contraction starts. Don't let any of the air out, you want to hold your breath during each push!

In between the contractions you want to try to keep the pressure on in your abdomen by tightening your stomach muscles. It will help the baby to stay where it has advanced to during that push. If you relax your abdominal muscles and let up on that pressure, the baby will move away from the cervix, and you end up working much harder. You must then continue to use your stomach muscles to push. You have to push through the pain and not back off of it. The sensations are so very intense, but the only way to get it over is down and out. It takes tremendous work, but you can do it!

Contractions are much shorter during pushing, so work to get three good eight- to-ten-count pushes in with each contraction. Don't back away from the sensation of labor and birth. Your body will deliver a hormonal storm to help you. I know it doesn't feel good to have the head come through, but you have to push past the pain. Push harder than it hurts. You need to tighten and pull in your stomach muscles, so the force of the contraction bears straight down on the abdomen rather than straight out in front.

Many women in traditional societies, including contemporary ones, gave or continue to give birth in standing or all-fours positions. In fact, legendary midwife Ina May Gaskin learned about what she later called the Gaskin Maneuver—hands and knees/all fours—from traditional Guatemalan midwives, who learned it from watching birthing women instinctively adopt this position during pushing.[154]

Getting Back in Bed for Birth

When the head is showing and crowning significantly, the midwife's birthing team will often lift you from the squatting position and lay you gently back on the bed. You can of course give birth in the squatting position, but there is a higher chance of tearing if you have the baby come out in that position. Also, many women tell me their feet are also in a lot of pain at this time and they are ready to get off of them.

I typically get you back in the bed right before I think the baby is going to be born, in enough time for you to relax and let go at the very end. I aim to also not add a lot of time to the pushing process; most women and babies are pretty fatigued at this point and getting it over with is a great idea.

Lying down slows your labor enough so the head does not pop out quickly, which can cause tearing. You can also relax in between each contraction when you are on the bed, which helps to make sure your bottom is more relaxed and also is a preventative measure for tearing.

There are many positions in which to push out the baby. I prefer semi- sitting/lying because I have experienced it being easier on the mom and resulting in fewer tears, but you can push the baby out on your hands and knees, you can push the baby out on your side, you can push the baby out standing with your knees bent supported by others, you can push the baby out while squatting as we've discussed...there are many other ways.

I have caught babies in all of these positions, but I want you to know that I have received tons of feedback about a certain disconnect when the mother could not see her baby come out and/or the father could not see the baby come out. In the end,

this is all just food for thought, and you should do whatever feels good to you in the moment.

Push with the contraction. *Try not to scream.* I have had women who tore their throat up screaming and couldn't talk for days, and then I've had women who chose to scream because that was part of their therapy process, and those babies came out pretty upset with elevated heart rates.

One time I got a call for a birth that was happening quickly. It was this mother's third baby, and I dashed over there as fast as I could. I ran up to the door with my most important equipment and found it locked. At that point I could hear the mother screaming at the top of her lungs and I could hear lots of other people screaming as well, including children and bystanders. It was absolute bedlam. I realized they really needed me, so I broke a window adjacent to the door, unlocked it, and ran into the room just in time to catch the baby. Everyone was so frantic that when the baby came out, the fetal heart tones were almost 200 beats per minute (bpm) (normal is 120–160 bpm).

While this story has some funny overtones to it, I don't think it was very funny for the baby. I think it scared them. This is why breathing through the process can be so helpful to avoid the urge to scream. It's not a joke—you may well feel this strong urge.

 Once you are back on the bed, it is usually another five to fifteen minutes before the baby is born. It is helpful if the partner and someone else you've invited or one of the apprentices will hold and support each of your legs for you for those final pushes.

I apply sterile hot packs to bring blood to the area, which helps prevent tearing, as well as sterile olive oil. Some of that may be done while you are squatting as well if it is needed. The hot packs are supported with a washrag to equalize the pressure across your perineum. There is a point of least resistance on your perineum which is the point that is most likely to tear but with the pressure and support of the hot packs it helps to evenly distribute the pressure across the perineum and makes it much less likely to tear.

Lying in the bed also allows you to watch the baby being born with a mirror if you would like to see their emergence. You and the father can also reach your hand down and touch the baby's head when it is crowning. This really helps to allow you to *know* you are almost finished and the baby is truly almost here.

I have had many moms pull the baby out by themselves, reaching down with both hands. This will only work in this position.

The Umbilical Cord

It is normal for the cord to be around the neck, and it is most often benign and easy to correct. The cord is around the neck in about 25 percent of births, and usually we slip it over the head as the baby is born and it's just fine. Every now and then the cord can be more tightly wound around the baby a and can decrease the oxygen to the baby. Sometimes this happens because there are multiple loops of cord around the neck.

Sometimes the cord is short and as the baby comes down farther and farther in the pelvis it tightens up more and more. Just know that most of the time *fetal distress due to a lack of oxygen* has something to do with the cord. It doesn't necessarily have to be around the neck, it could be wrapped around a part of the body or the shoulder as well. This is one of the things that we watch for regardless of where you give birth to make certain that your baby is doing well and handling the push safely.

The only reason I would advise you to squat for the actual birth of the baby is if the baby is in distress and there is a need to get them out quickly. It is very common for the heart tones to drop at the very end due to head compression, it is called a vagal response. The pressure on the cranium and vagus nerves causes a drop in heart tones. That associated drop does not last long and will not harm the baby, but it is hard to tell the difference between that and the drops in heart tones resulting from the baby's cord being around their neck, which in some instances can be a potential problem for the baby due to oxygen being cut off.

We will talk more about what we do when there is any sign of fetal distress later in the chapter.

The Moment Before Birth

I talk the mother through a guided visualization at the very end. I will ask her to open her eyes, then I will meet her gaze and say, "Sweetie, look at me, let's work together here ... Can you relax this muscle ... Oh, that's perfect ... Just like that now. Just keep letting go and on the next contraction the baby's head should be born ..." When I can work with a woman eye-to-eye I am able to make incredible inroads to helping her to not lose control in those last serious moments. It's okay to lose control, and I've had hundreds of women do it, but many of them afterwards conveyed some unhappiness or discomfort at that loss. I found I could help them to stay in control and be present in the moment and not recede into the panic of *Oh, my God, I'm splitting apart.* (You are not splitting apart.) Work with your midwife. Let her know your fears and how you'd like to be supported at the final stages. Feel free to communicate in the moment as well. Remember, this part lasts a very few minutes. It is nothing that you cannot handle.

Mothers who have had babies before can usually just push lying down and it generally takes about 10–45 minutes. The bottom line is you can push in any way you want; these are ideas, techniques, and theories but you are in charge of your labor and birth.

Birth

Once the baby is actually getting ready to come out, I help the mom to go more slowly, and I work to keep the baby's head flexed so the smallest diameter comes out, which helps prevent tearing.

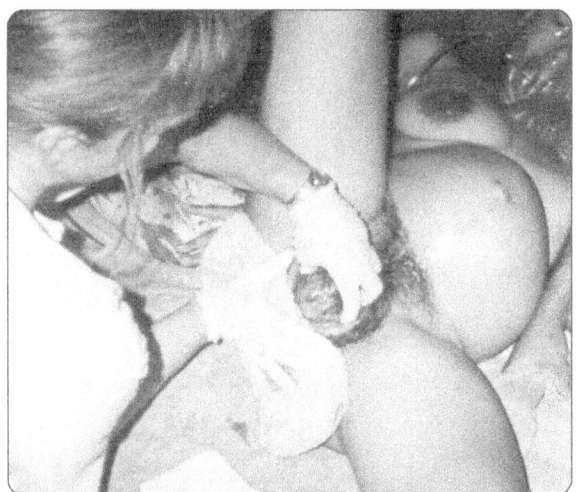

MariMikel Applies Pressure to the Perineum as the Baby Crowns

It is optimal for the whole baby to be born in one contraction, so the head is not stuck out of the perineum until the next contraction comes. If this happens, the baby often turns blue, and their lips turn purple, and it can be much harder on them. This is the point where the baby can get little broken blood vessels in their eyes. So, when they are fully crowning, I have the laboring woman stop and blow through it until the next contraction comes. Once it comes, she takes a deep breath and can start pushing again.

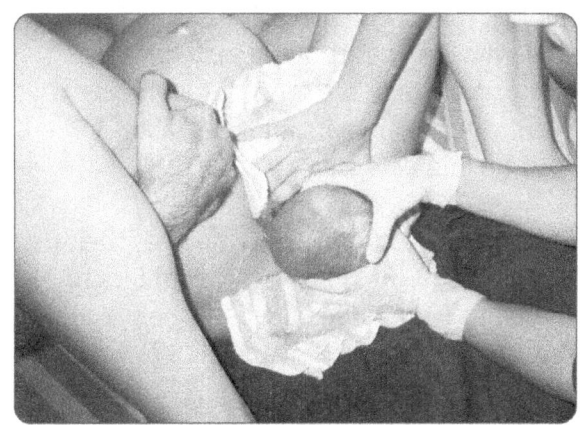

Head Is Being Born

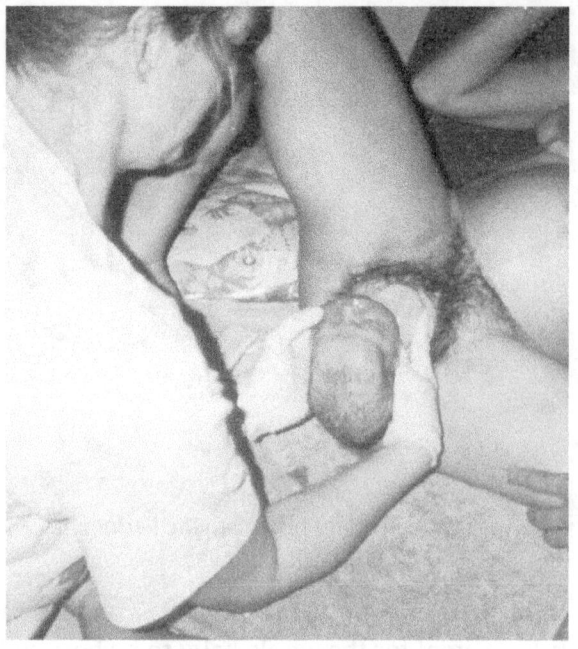

Helping to Turn Baby's Shoulders

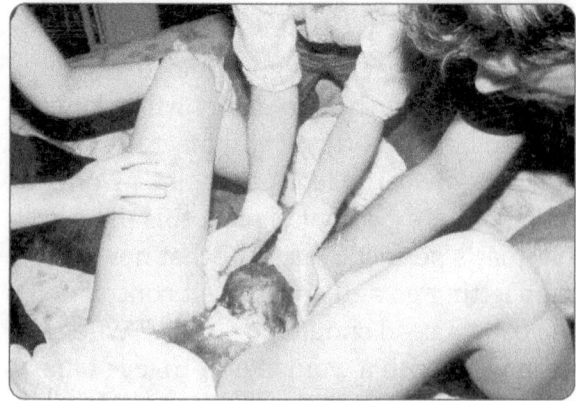

Dad Moves into Position to Catch the Baby

The Ring of Fire

 The head and the shoulders are the most intense part of the stretching of the opening to the vagina during the birth. When you push out your baby's head, you may or may not experience what is often called *the ring of fire,* which is a very rapid flash of a strong burning sensation in your perineum. Don't worry, it will go away quickly, but it might catch you by surprise and you might scream a little, as this is a very different sort of pain than the ones that you have been experiencing during your labor and your pushing stage.

First the head completely emerges, then the head rotates, and I help the shoulders to come out from under the pubic bone. I let the partner know they can reach down and catch the baby if they would like to. Ninety percent of the partners in my practice catch their babies. There is usually no blood or anything like that because they are coming out of the amniotic fluid, which is just salt water. The only way they have blood on them is when you have a significant laceration or an episiotomy.

Baby Arrives and Goes Skin to Skin

There is nothing more delicious in the world than feeling those little feet slide by as it is over, and the baby is laid up on your chest. I encourage women to be unclothed at this stage so the baby can go immediately from the vagina onto her belly or chest (depending on the length of the umbilical cord). She is very, very warm from the effort of the birth, which

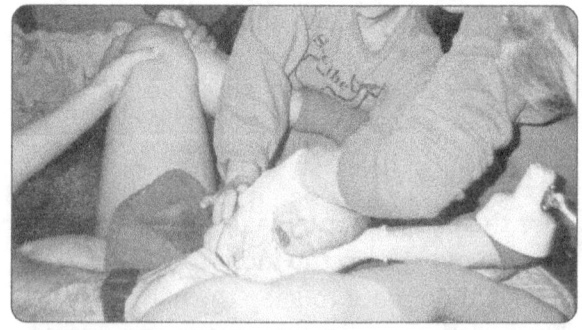

The Midwifing Team Supports Baby on Their Way into the World

> *The moment a child is born, the mother is also born. She never existed before. The woman existed, but the mother, never. A mother is something absolutely new.*
>
> —Rajneesh

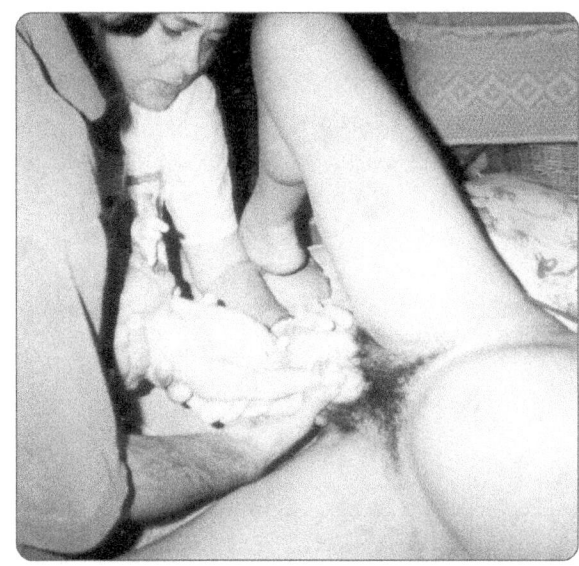

Baby Emerges into Father's Waiting Hands

is wonderful for baby, and this way she gets to see her baby's first breath and first opening of their eyes. The baby being against your skin and not cloth is important.

In other positions that I've mentioned it takes us a while to get the mother into a position where the baby can go into her arms, and she can be comfortable. You can experiment before the birth to figure out the ins and outs, so you're prepared to make the choice that works for you when your baby is entering the world. These are all just ideas, not a blueprint for how you have to do it. The true joy comes the moment the baby is out, laid against your skin, and has taken their first breath, and you are beginning to relax into this new mystical moment of mothering.

Sometimes it really molds the baby's head to come through the pelvis and the baby can come out looking like a tiny torpedo. Don't worry, its normal and the conehead appearance will go away.

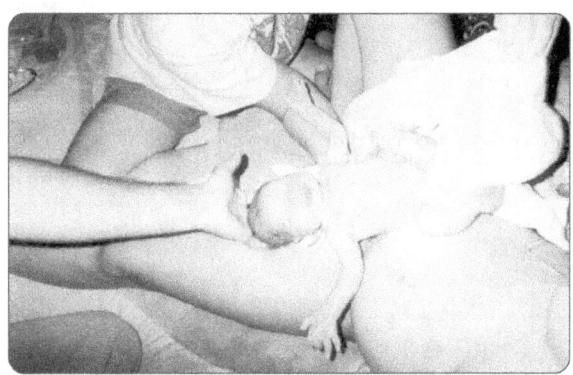

Seconds after Birth

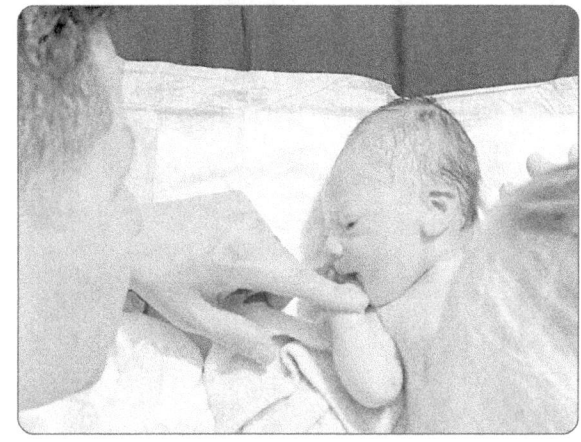

Conehead Baby. Don't Worry, It Goes Away.

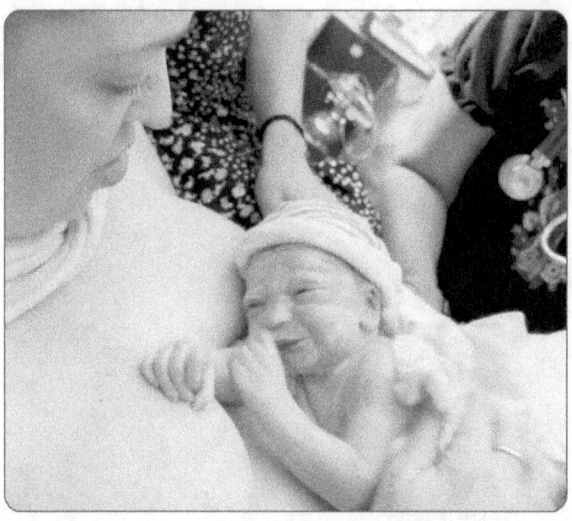

Aleah and Her Daughter Moments after Birth

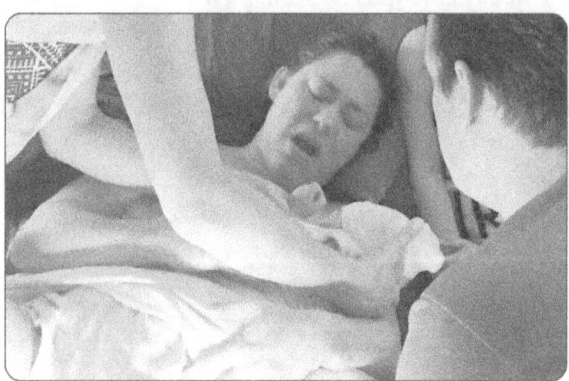

Baby Goes Skin-to-Skin and a Cap Is Donned to Keep Them Warm

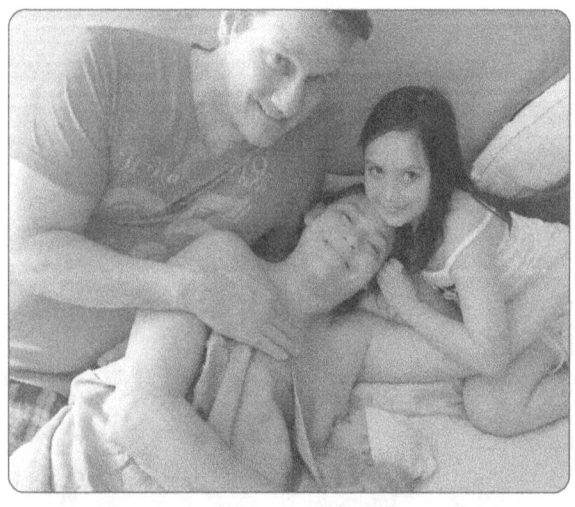

Now We're a Family of Four

Birth Stories

Hospital Birth: Sarah's Story

My name is Sarah, and this is my birth story. I had a very easy pregnancy. I took a prenatal supplement and ate very carefully. I knew a lot of women who had used their pregnancies as an excuse to eat whatever they wanted, and I didn't want to do that. I chose to do a food combining diet, which was something I had practiced before, so I was familiar with it, and I ate really healthy stuff. I didn't eat a lot of junk or have any real cravings like you always hear about. I gained about 25 pounds over the course of my pregnancy. I was hardly sick. I wasn't tired until the very end.

I had people asking me if I was okay all the time, and I kept wondering, why? They made me feel like I had cancer because they were asking how I was doing so often. I was like, "Look, I'm fine." I did kind of have a small belly for my term, and when I look back on pictures now, I'm like, *Wow, I looked like I was like six months when I was about to give birth.*

My little kid did not want to come out on his due date, so I went in for a checkup a few days after. I had chosen this little boutique clinic right across from the hospital that was closest to my house. Both were really close to me, which was a major factor in my decision.

I felt like I got really good care from that clinic. They've since been bought out by a larger company, but anyway ... I went in and they put some kind of belt around me. I think it was a heart rate monitor for the baby, and they found my baby's heart rate was all over the place. I didn't really know what was going on. I was a little bit clueless when it came to this whole process. I did not really care to have a home birth or look into anything that was a little bit more natural. I would have been really happy if a stork had dropped my baby off. I was pretty much like a deer in the headlights throughout my pregnancy in terms of knowing what to expect.

Anyway, my baby's heart rate was erratic, and the doctor said, "You need to go to the hospital for monitoring. You might need a c-section."

I'm laughing at myself now because I said, "Can I get a cheeseburger first?" No, I couldn't have a cheeseburger because I guess it's not good for you to eat when you're possibly going into surgery.

I went to the hospital, was put in a bed in a room, and they put this monitor back on me. I stayed there for a while. At one point I supposedly had a five-minute-long contraction. Well, I didn't feel any contractions, so if these contractions were happening, I had absolutely no clue. They said that the five-minute contraction was cutting off the oxygen to my baby, because I didn't have a whole lot of amniotic fluid. They said, "We can induce you, but this might end up in a c-section anyway. If you want, we can just do a c-section." I agreed to the c-section.

Once the c-section was decided on, it got a little scary. All of a sudden six nurses showed up and before I knew what was going on there was an IV in my hand. Everyone in the room was very stressed, and I was picking up on that stress. I didn't really know what was going on. They were trying to remain calm, but it felt like a swarm of bees around me. I remember really wanting my dog to be in the delivery room with me. I'm ridiculous, I know, but I really wanted to be comforted by my dog, because it was a little bit scary, but then most of the nurses left and everybody was so friendly after that. This was a hospital that's really well known for women's care. I didn't know that at the time. I mean, it was just the hospital across the street. I didn't put much thought into it.

Then, I got an epidural. That took a little more time, but it went fine. I was wheeled to surgery and my baby was born at 8:10 p.m. I went into the hospital at 2:00 p.m., so I never really experienced a true contraction. I didn't have any expectations of what my birth would be like, so I wasn't really disappointed or happy one way or the other. I really feel very neutral about the whole experience.

Afterward I stayed in the hospital for four days, because I was 40 years old when I gave birth, and they keep women who are over 35 for longer.

I loved the hospital food. I liked being served. We got a lot of care from a lactation consultant there who helped me and helped the baby to latch. I remember all of the nurses were so lovely and wonderful ... except one of the night nurses maybe should have had a day shift or maybe not have been a nurse. I don't know if she was just exhausted, or babies just weren't her jam, or whatever. I do specifically remember the last nurse we had was just exceptional. She had been a delivery nurse for a really long time—like over 20 years.

My husband and I had a little side hustle on eBay. He wanted to be near me during my recovery, but the orders were backing up and needed to get shipped out. So, he would go get the inventory we had sold, bring it to the hospital, and pack and fulfill orders from our recovery room. This last nurse saw what he was doing and told me, "You know, *you* should just do this business for a couple of years. That way you can stay at home with your baby." I looked at her like, *Lady, you're crazy. I'm a working woman and I'm not going to work some work-at-home job.* But, you know, as we fell in love with our baby, and we realized that our life was going to change, and already actually had changed, I realized I really didn't want to go back to that stupid job. I took her advice and turned that side hustle into a very profitable business. I don't know if I would have ever

really thought about it had she not said something, but it was almost like a message from the heavens that she was there to deliver.

I think hospital births are terrific. As I mentioned, I didn't really know what to expect. When people would ask me, "What's your birth plan?" I'd say, "The birth plan is to have the baby."

Anyway, that's my birth story. You know ... I think the only little weird thing is .... I know that c-section rates are really high in America, and I think I felt maybe a little bit rushed. Like, *Why is this so serious?* I'm not a doctor, so I just decided to leave it in the hands of the people who do this every day. I have a healthy little boy and that's what I care about.

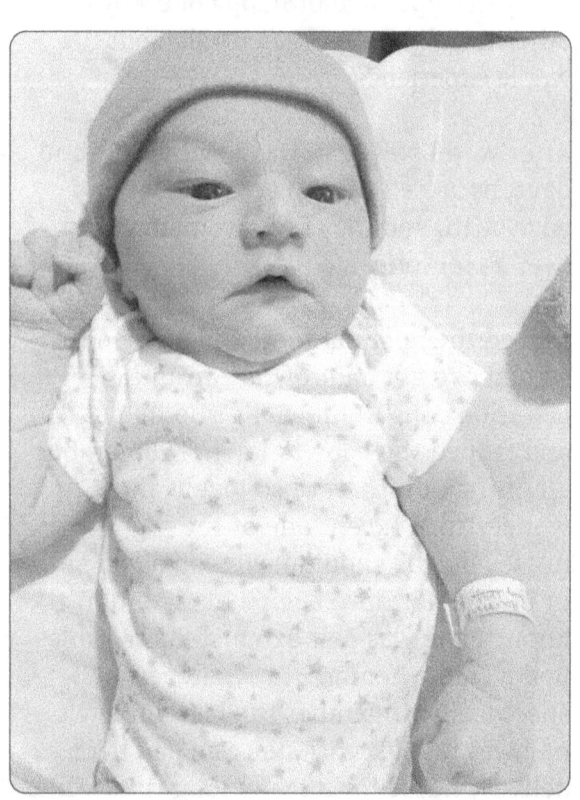

Sarah's Sweet Little Boy

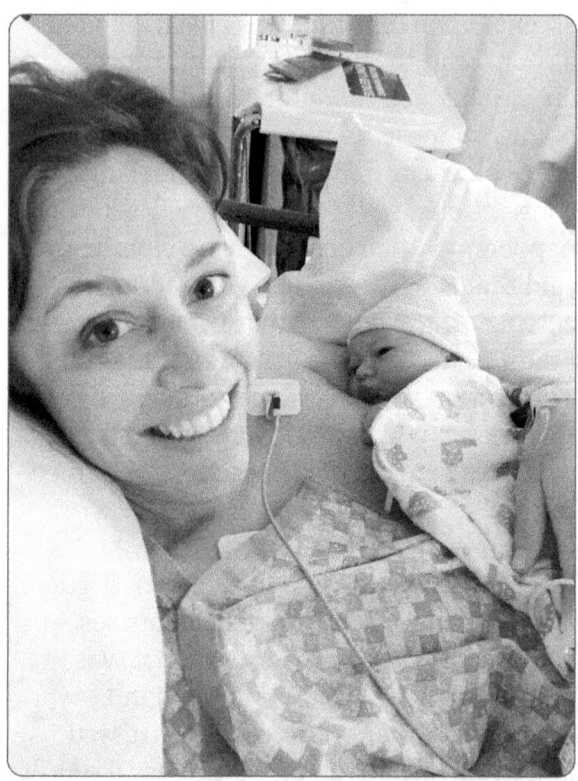

Sarah and Her Baby Boy

As for the c-section recovery ... I think I've kind of blocked it out because it was brutal. I felt like my body wanted to pull apart. There was a lot of tension, and initially a lot of pain. It's almost like a sore muscle, but it's more like a twinge or like a pulling sensation. They say the recovery is supposed to take six weeks, but it took at least two months for me. I have friends who healed faster than I did, but I was a little bit older, so maybe that was a factor.

They gave me some pain medication, and I remember needing more of it. The doctors wanted to make sure I wasn't addicted; they seemed really aware that I was asking for more. It was strong stuff, but I needed it. I was in a lot of pain. I think they eventually had me switch to ibuprofen or Tylenol for the pain, but it was hard.

I remember a girlfriend asked me out to go to the lake with her. Three weeks had passed since my delivery, and I could still barely move. It was awful trying to do anything active. I was really glad we didn't have stairs in the house at the time. It was hard, but I also didn't have a lot of family around. I didn't have a mother-in-law or mother around. I didn't really understand that I might want to have help.

I remember getting acupuncture eventually to help with the healing of the wound. The incision is very small; they do it right above the pubic hairline or pubic bone, so it's not like people are having these giant scars across their bellies anymore.

The scar did itch now and again, and that was kind of a weird sensation that went on for some time, but eventually it healed and that was it.

Hospital Birth: Penelope's Story

Over the course of my pregnancy, I was inspired by Ina May Gaskin's books and planned for an unmedicated, natural delivery. I had read about the possible side effects of epidurals, and I wanted to go through the beautiful, transformational process of natural birth that Gaskin described. I told my doctor this, and I remember he sort of laughed at me and said, "You'll last ten minutes. It's okay. I'll be ready with the epidural when you ask for it."

My baby was due on Halloween. When I reached my due date, my warm-up labor had been going on for weeks. A few days into November the pre-labor contractions I'd been having intensified, and I had bloody show. It was a Friday afternoon, and I called my doctor. He assured me it couldn't possibly be labor and told me to check in with him on Monday. I was a single mom-to-be, and I didn't want to be alone. I felt that this was it, and called my doula. She took me at my word and came to be with me.

A short while later I started peeing involuntarily. I made it to the toilet and just kept peeing continuously, the longest stream ever. It felt like it went on for 20 minutes but was probably more like three or four. Needless to say, my water had broken, and for quite some time I just waited for the contractions to intensify. My doula and I watched Netflix together for several hours. She suggested I eat and get some good rest. She slept next to me in bed that night, and rubbed my back when I was moaning.

The next day, when 24 hours had passed since my waters had broken, my doula encouraged me to go to the hospital to avoid the risk of infection. I had recently moved, and the hospital that was once nearby was now a 45-minute drive away. My contractions were strong at that point, and I remember the drive as sheer torture. Every bump hurt. Everything hurt.

I was admitted to the hospital, and entered armed with my birth plan, expecting it to be adhered to. I didn't understand the hospital landscape and how futile it was to try to have a natural birth in an intervention-rich environment.

My doctor was not available, and the doctor who attended me at first ended his shift about two hours after my arrival. The next doctor in the rotation was someone I had met previously at my OB's insistence. I had not gotten on with her. She'd seemed very judgmental to me, making disparaging grunts when I'd told her that my baby's father was not in the picture.

Shortly after she started her shift, the nurse came in and told me the doctor had decided to put me on Pitocin. I told her I didn't want it. She said she'd make it a light dose. I said I didn't want it. She said the doctor ordered it and started me on it anyway. Over the following hours each time a nurse came into the room they would up the dose, crank up the meter. It didn't matter that I didn't want it.

By the time Saturday evening rolled around it felt like there were demons inside of me trying to claw their way out. I was squatting through contractions and resting in between, up and down, up and down, for hours. Sometime in there, my mother arrived from Arizona. I remember her being present, but I also remember that it was very difficult for her to watch me in such pain for so long. At some point I think it was too much for her, though she bravely stayed by my side. Also, at some point— after the Longhorns' game had finished in overtime—the man I was dating (now my husband) showed up to support me.

I remember talking to my doula about whether or not I should invite him, and her telling me that it was a big deal, and that if he showed up that was something to pay attention to. She was right. He held my hand and supported me through every stand and squat. His assistance, his words, and his muscles leant me strength to keep going.

At about 11:00 at night the nurse came in and told me that I needed to get an epidural and relax because, "If you don't get this baby out," she told me, "the doctor is going to cut you open."

Determined to have a vaginal birth, I acquiesced to the epidural. The anesthesiologist came in and administered it, and I was able to sleep for about 45 minutes while the Pitocin continued to open my cervix. I do remember the anesthesiologist being incredibly kind. My mom said something like, "You're my hero," to him, and he looked at me and said, "She's the hero." I fell asleep for a little while.

The doctor I didn't like woke me up when it was time to push. Though her shift had ended, she had returned to catch this baby so she could get paid for it, although I didn't know that at the time. I remember her screaming at me to, "Push! Push!" and me telling my brain to bear down, but not being able to feel anything whatsoever from my abdomen to my knees.

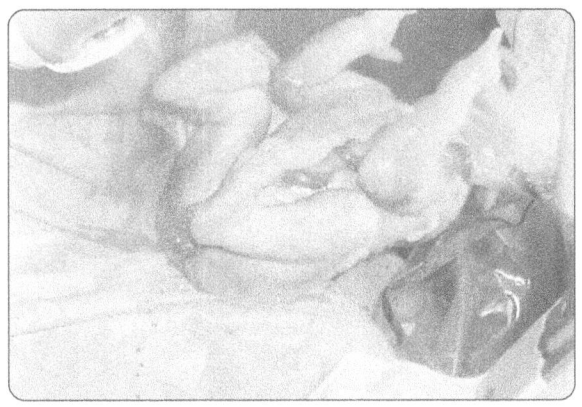

Penelope's Newborn Moments after Birth

My mother yelled back, "Look, she's blue in the face, she's pushing!"

And I remember the doctor shouting, "I have to cut you," before she gave me what my OB later said was the biggest episiotomy he'd ever seen.

My baby came out and the nurse said, "Oh Doc, isn't it wonderful, this is the moment we all wait for.

And the doctor said, "I'm kind of over it. I'm in menopause."

They quickly cut the cord and took my baby away from me. I remember reaching my arms out and crying out, "Where's my baby? I want my baby!" and my doula assuring me that they just needed him for five minutes to clean him up. Those were the longest five minutes of my life and I still cry when I think about them.

But then he was in my arms, and everything was finally okay.

We were then stuck in the hospital for two days. It was impossible to rest with the noise and the lights and the constant interruptions. I was exhausted. When I'd finally fall asleep, I'd sleep so hard I didn't even hear my baby crying, and the nurses would have to wake me up so I could breastfeed my baby.

The recovery rooms were a joke in terms of comfort. The hospitals did a great job creating a beautiful labor & delivery room and selling people on that. What they didn't tell us is that as soon as they could move us after I gave birth, they did. The recovery room was cramped and uncomfortable compared to the labor room. My husband's legs extended two feet past the end of the cot they provided for him, and to this day he describes the pillows as, "Five pieces of gauze held together by hate." I wanted so badly for our new family to be home. I felt trapped at the hospital.

Even given our first experience, my husband really wanted the comfort of the hospital's lifesaving equipment on hand for my second and third births, and I didn't have the right information to present to him with as to why my desire to have a home birth with a midwife would be just as safe, if not

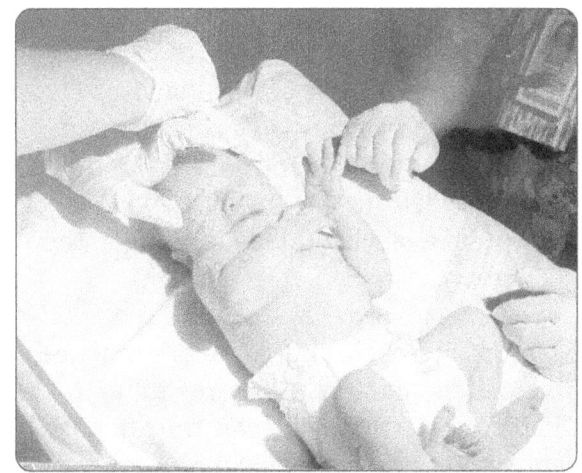

Waiting for Baby, Waiting for Momma

safer. We compromised and I began to work with an OB who had five nurse midwives on her staff and was supportive of the natural birth process. I could be attended to by a midwife in a hospital. I am grateful that Christina Sebestyen, MD, made this type of care available in Austin.

This was better. I was able to labor naturally and did not have Pitocin or an epidural or episiotomy performed on me in either of my two subsequent births. It really is true that you push out all of your babies with your firstborn. While I had been in labor for 46 hours before delivering my first baby, my second arrived in well under 10 hours and with my third I believe it was about six hours.

What I remember most about my second child was how my body knew the process and I really didn't need to do anything other than follow its directives. I spent a lot of my labor alone while my husband slept, and I remember taking refuge in the shower many times to let the water pound on my lower back. I remember waking him when my contractions had reached a certain frequency and telling him, "It's time to go to the hospital."

He drove me, and one of the midwives I was familiar with from my OB's clinic was on call. She checked on me from time to time, but mostly left me and my husband to labor alone with a playlist I'd made going in the background.

I labored at the hospital for another hour-and-a-half, and when I became fully dilated, my body knew it was time to push. I remember being taken over by a primal force and roaring as I bore down. I felt

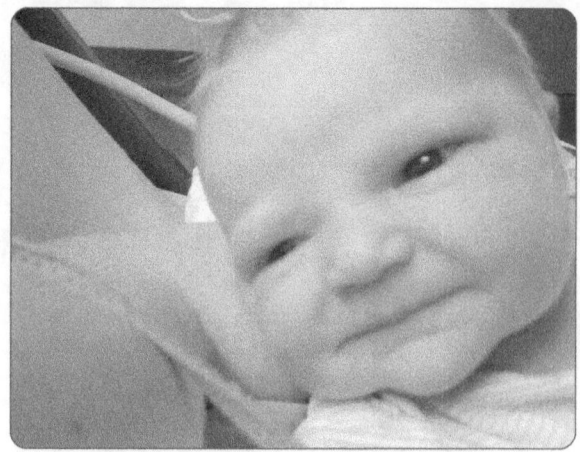

Penelope's Few-Hours-Old Daughter.

incredibly powerful. And I'll never forget that feeling of completion when my baby girl was first put up on my chest and later into my arms and I first got to look into her gorgeous eyes.

By the time my third child was ready to come out I remember feeling irritated with the hospital staff at that point. I felt like I knew what I was doing, and I didn't need to be monitored so much or poked and prodded so much. A nurse would come in and hook me up to a monitor for fifteen or thirty minutes at a time. They were so busy that it was easier for them to just leave me hooked up. Toward the end of my labor, when I really wanted to be up and about, my husband encouraged me to just take the monitor off myself. I couldn't bring myself to do that. I don't like going against authority figures, I guess.

I remember at one point needing to go to the bathroom and the nurse telling me, "I don't want you to go to the bathroom. You're going to pee your baby out into the toilet!" I guess I just got tired of how crass so many of the nurses were throughout my

THE BIRTH PROCESS

pregnancies. Maybe it was just a day on the job to them, but it was a sacred event in my life and my husband's life. I don't want to pollute your brain with the worst of what they said, but their words definitely brought out the momma bear in me.

I didn't pee my baby into the toilet, but my bladder did make room for her to just fall out. I remember walking back to the sort of half bed, getting up on it, facing the back of it, squatting, telling my husband, "Baby's coming," and then pushing her out in a single push. My husband was up near my face, holding my hand. It was three in the morning and my midwife in attendance was dozing on a chair in the room. She came to in a start when she realized what was happening but did not make it to the bed in time to catch our baby, who landed on the bed instead of in somebody's arms. Don't worry, she's fine. We snatched her up right away and I turned around and put her on my skin immediately. It was such a moment of peace as we looked at each other for the first time, like a knowing that we were both in the right place now that we were together.

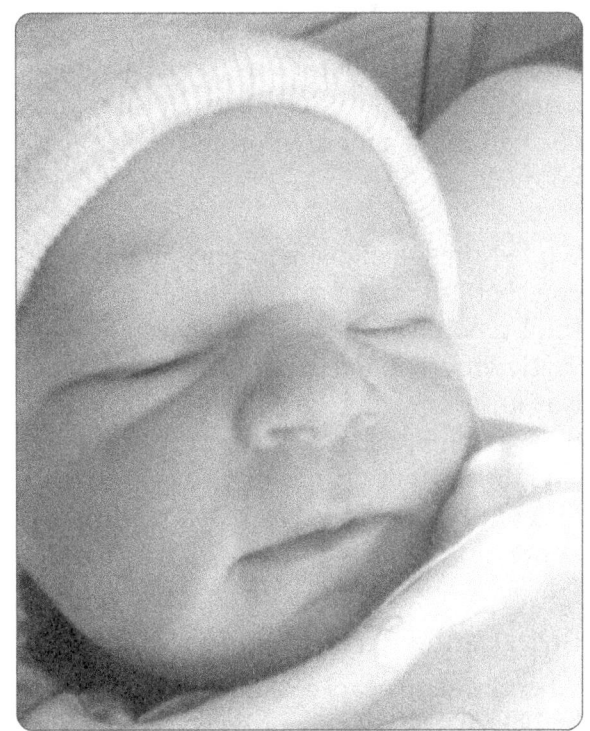

Penelope's Youngest

I think the biggest lesson for me was that I was not a strong enough advocate for myself and my own desires for my own pregnancy. I did not adequately stand up for my desires, and I let myself believe that a midwife in a hospital was just as good as

MariMikel: There are still plenty of hospitals who remove the baby from the mother after the birth for observation. The hospital that I work with does not do that any longer. They allow the baby to stay with the mother as long as everything looks good, and they provide minimal support like suctioning and warming while the baby is on the mother's body.

Remember, you do have the choice to refuse anything. Once your baby is born, if your hospital care providers think that you are refusing care that is vital to the baby's health and safety, they are going to ignore you because at that point it is about the health of the baby. Nevertheless, it is important to remember that you can refuse anything.

Most hospitals in larger metropolitan areas now have labor, delivery, and recovery rooms known as LDRs. This means that you don't get moved around like Penelope did. Find out ahead of time what your options are and what the hospital's policies are.

a midwife at home. It was better than an OB in a hospital, but it was not as good as being at home. I can't go back in time, but you can make a more informed choice for yourself.

While I think a midwife in a hospital is eons better than no midwife at all, I really think a home birth would have been a vastly different and better experience. I was lucky enough to get off of the factory birth assembly line for my second and third births, but I truly wish I had chosen differently and birthed all of my children at home.

Birth Center Birth: Juliana's Story

When I was 16 years old, my oldest sister had her first baby. When she got pregnant, she told us that she was planning to stay home to have her baby. None of my family really knew what that meant. We of course had a lot of questions because who has a baby at home anymore? Her experience as an L&D nurse over the years had shown her that she didn't want the interventions or the environment that comes with hospital births, and she felt safe and comfortable at home.

When she went into labor, she called our other sister and me, and we went to her house to wait for the baby. We didn't get to see much, but I found it so exciting anyway to wait for the baby, and to hear his first cries when he finally came out. Afterward, I remember we made her a special bath, and I made her a big breakfast that she ate on the couch with her baby. I guess it all really stuck with me, because when it was finally my turn to be pregnant, I knew I wanted a midwife and a homebirth, too.

When I got pregnant, I knew right away that my oldest sister, Elise, would be my doula. From there I just had to find a midwife. It took a couple tries but I finally found a great midwife, Varshna, who didn't seem too nervous about me being a first-time mom, and she answered all my fiancé Ethan's many questions. I was about to enter grad school but planned to travel back home over the winter break to my mom's place to have my baby.

As the pregnancy went on, we decided that it might be best to move our birth plans to Varshna's new birth center, so we might have more room and not have to worry about adding too much mess to my mom's environment. The birth center was close to my mom's, and it seemed like a good alternative.

As I prepared for the birth and my baby, I did a lot of research. I read tons of articles, watched all kinds of birth videos, breastfeeding videos, took a birthing class, and listened to hours and hours of pregnancy- and birth-related podcasts. I was constantly consuming birth and baby media. I also prayed a lot. I prayed for help, guidance, and support. I prayed and meditated so that I would be able to hear my body's needs and have a warning if something ever felt off.

Mostly, I asked for my people to be there for me and my growing family.

On January 11th, I woke up around 4 a.m. to a semi-painful contraction. During the last weeks of my pregnancy, I'd been having tons of Braxton Hicks contractions, and in the last few days every time I woke up at night, I was having one, but this one was a little stronger. I went to the bathroom and couldn't go back to sleep right away, which had become usual. I had allergies, and, while I was leaning over in bed and grabbing tissues, I felt a little *pop* and a small gush. I knew my water had broken. It wasn't much but there was definitely liquid on the bed. As I got up to go to the bathroom again, I was still leaking, so I woke Ethan. He called Varshna to let her know what was happening.

I tried to rest and go back to bed but we were too excited. I had some cramping and contractions, but not much. We tried to wait awhile, but we ended up calling my sister at 6:45 a.m. and told her what was happening. She arrived at about 8:45 a.m. Since my contractions weren't yet very hard or close together, we went to the grocery store, cleaned up the apartment, made breakfast, and ate. I felt mild/medium contractions on and off all day and continued to breathe through them.

Varsha called to check in every 4 hours and at the 4:30 p.m. call she told us that since contractions were still not close enough together, we should try the breast pump at home to see if that would stimulate them. I felt she was getting concerned that my water had been broken for 12 hours already, and active labor hadn't started yet. She also instructed us to take my temperature every two hours to spot any sign of infection. So, I pumped and then and again later, at about 6:30 p.m. for 15 minutes each time. This started some contractions, but they stalled and separated again.

I did NOT like the breast pump and I kept asking when we could stop. At 8:45 p.m., she finally told us to come into the birth center to use her stronger breast pump and to take some herbs to really try to get contractions going.

During the first round of pumping with the stronger pump I started feeling really emotional. The tears started flowing. I was going to miss having this little life inside of me, and I was nervous for this change, but I knew I had to let her come. It was inevitable. The time for our new chapter was coming, and I could be afraid, but I could also be excited.

We did a last round of pumping for 20 minutes, and I took the herbs. Finally, stronger contractions started. That's when I started throwing up. I laid in the bed at the birthing center for a while, breathing through contractions. At about 10 p.m., Varshna checked me and told me I was at 2 cm.

We decided to send me home to try to get comfortable and labor there for a while because it was still early. Contractions got very consistent and stronger all through the night. I could no longer just breathe through them and started with a low moan through each one (sorry apartment neighbors!).

Elise stayed with me the whole time and sent Ethan to rest because she could tell we had a lot longer to go. She laid in bed with me and talked me through each contraction as they got more intense.

I started throwing up again. I had three more rounds of throwing up and contractions got to be 5–6 minutes apart for a while, so Elise finally decided to call Varshna again and update her. At this point I want to add that I just felt so miserable. I had no idea how I was going to get through each contraction. I was really trying to just stay in the moment and not think about anything in the future, because I knew in the back of my head that we had a long road left.

Throughout my life, every time I've thrown up, I get major petechiae (burst blood vessels) and face swelling, and I cry from it all. This time was no different. Actually, it was probably worse. So, at 4 a.m. on January 12th we called Varshna to say contractions were very consistent and I was throwing up a lot. We went back to the birthing center at 4:45 a.m. so she could give me some Zofran and I could continue to labor there. I took the Zofran, and it was a lifesaver. I kept contracting strongly and moaning through them, but I wasn't puking and crying anymore.

Just before 6 a.m. I decided to get into the birth pool. Varshna checked me before I got in and found I was 7 cm dilated! I know the numbers don't mean everything, but I was ready to be so disappointed and instead I found it encouraging. I got in the birth pool and labored there for a while. I really think it helped with contractions so much.

As the water started cooling down, I got out and labored in the bed, then the birthing ball, and then the toilet. After I got out of the pool, Ethan was able to put counter pressure on my hips, and it helped so much. At every contraction I called for him, and he'd come right away and do the counter pressure. I could tell he was getting tired, but I didn't care, and he never complained. How could he?

At about 10 a.m. I got checked again. I was at 8 cm—maybeeee 9 cm—it was stretchy.

I was a little disappointed, but we moved around, and I got back in the pool with Ethan this time. I laid on him in the pool and kept low moaning/yelling through contractions. We got out and went for a little walk and back inside again to try different positions.

At one point, as we were moving back to the bedroom from the bathroom, I looked up and saw a crowd of people had formed around the bed. Lined up along the wall and by the bed I saw different people in all different styles of clothes as if they were waiting. I knew right then that my prayers were being answered. My people had come to help welcome my baby and guide us through. When I looked up again the room was normal.

> My people had come to help welcome my baby and guide us through.

At about 2 p.m. I was fully dilated and effaced. Varshna said she wanted me to labor down for a while and tell her if I started to feel rectal pressure. So, I laid down on the bed again, with the peanut ball to labor more. Contractions were more intense and longer than ever, but around this point I felt like my brain flipped a switch and, all of a sudden every pain was exciting.

I felt my baby coming down and closer to being in my arms. My moaning even felt like it changed tune, and I was looking forward to the peak of each contraction to try to feel the pressure to push. I could also hear my sister during every contraction telling me, "good, good, good."

I could hear Ethan telling me, "keep moaning low," that I was "doing so good," and it made me feel good. I felt like I had tunnel vision on the contractions and bringing my baby down, but their voices were little lights showing me how. I felt ready for the contractions to hurry up and get my baby out already.

My mom had also been there the whole time and was doing a good job staying out of the way. At around 2:30 p.m. she took my sister to get lunch for everyone and to let our dog out. A second midwife, Kate, was called in, and she got there at about 3:30 p.m. I was getting uneasy while my mom and sister were gone, and worried; I didn't want them to miss anything.

Luckily, they didn't take too long, and returned at about 4:00. At this point, I was extremely dehydrated from the vomiting I'd done, and I hadn't really had an appetite all day. Varshna wanted me to have energy for pushing, so she gave me an IV with fluids. I was hoping not to have an IV, but I understood the need.

Then they moved me to labor on the toilet backwards. They had Ethan sit behind me with a rebozo around my waist and lightly pull it back during contractions to try to pull my tummy in to maneuver the baby to drop better. Honestly, this was a really miserable moment in the process. I hated laboring on the toilet and the rebozo combination made me feel almost annoyed and added so much discomfort.

After a while I was moved to the birth ball. They told me to bounce on the ball through contractions, with Ethan again behind me pulling in my tummy with the rebozo. I

thought I hated the toilet version, but this was something else. The combination of contractions, bouncing, and pulling felt so rough. I kept asking, "When can I get off? Can I please get off?"

But also, it totally worked, and I am so grateful for it.

I started feeling a lot of pressure building and finally felt that rectal pressure they kept asking about. I was also feeling a lot of the contractions in my hips and lower back as well as my tummy area. At this point, Varshna felt I had labored down a long time, and was a little concerned that I still didn't have the urge to push, so she checked again, and my baby was at a +3 station!

She decided to go ahead and put me on the birth stool so I could start pushing. I felt a pause where my body stopped and relaxed. I felt everything winding up and then a contraction came, and I pushed a little.

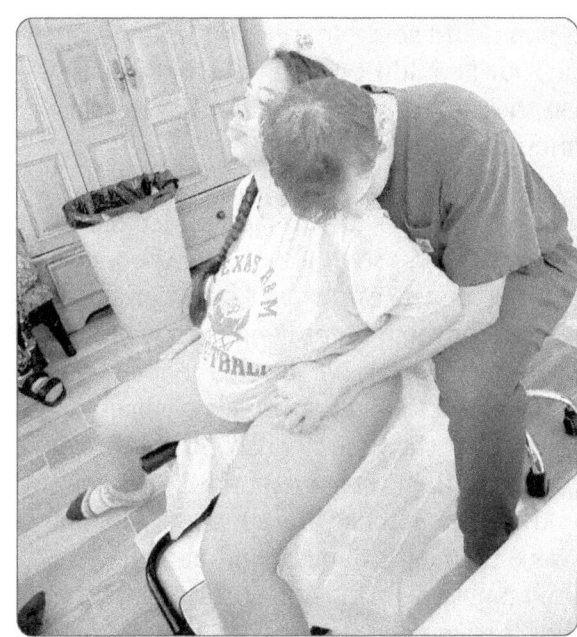

Juliana Pushing on the Birthing Stool

The baby was coming down, so we moved straight to the bed. I got on the bed, and she told me to push with my contractions. I rested a bit and then tried some coached pushing. Everyone got so excited and said it was working, so we kept going. I was on my back, Ethan and Elise held my feet and I held the backs of my knees and pushed with everything I had at least 3 pushes per contraction. Varshna counted to ten while I pushed, and I would take a breath and push twice more the same way.

Once the contraction faded, we'd wait for the next and try again. I heard everyone cheer when they started seeing her head, and then she was crowning, and I touched her slimy head and then pushed again, and she crowned a little more.

They had me stop right at the ring of fire to let me stretch out, let her head mold to prevent tearing. We waited for another contraction, and then went again. When I got her head out, I heard something about a hand, and some small commotion going on, but I couldn't really tell what it was. On the next contraction I got her big fat shoulders out.

The rest of her slid out and I pulled her right to my chest! 5:38 p.m.! She pooped right when she came out. I held her and we waited for the placenta and then we took so many pictures. We learned that she had a nuchal hand and that may have been why I never got the urge to push. Ethan cut the cord, and then we stayed in bed a while, and ate. She latched after a while, too. She was 8 pounds, 4 ounces, and 21 inches. I only had two small, skin surface tears that didn't even need stitches. We basked in amazement at her and her extreme cuteness

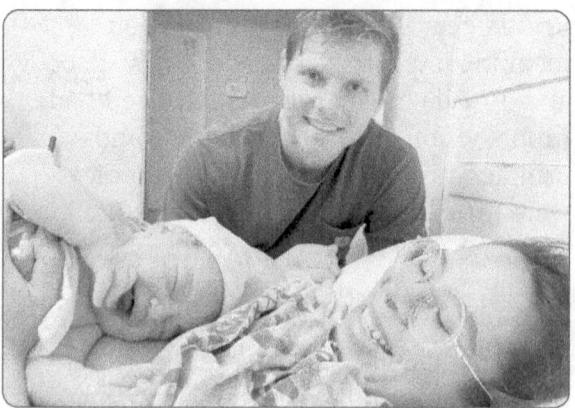

Juliana and Ethan Welcome Their New Baby Girl

and then got ready and went home at about 10 p.m., so exhausted.

A few days later I went over the labor experience in my head, and I started to just cry and cry. It finally hit me how overwhelming it had all been. At the time I kept trying to stay in each specific moment and not think about what was left, so I wouldn't get discouraged. I finally allowed myself to soak in how incredibly hard it was, but at the same time, I felt so proud of myself and so proud of my baby and so thankful that we were able to have the perfect labor and birth. I never had a moment where I thought I couldn't do it. It helped that the baby's heart rate was steady the whole time and never dropped, even while I was pushing.

That allowed me not to worry about her too much. So, while I definitely gained an understanding of why people choose to be medicated, I also understood why that wasn't for me. I'm nothing but grateful for every feeling and every bit of our experience. I'm also grateful we had a lovely and comfortable birth center to have our baby, but I do hope we can be in the position to stay home for our next baby.

Birth Center Birth: Monica's Story—a Journey of Love and Empowerment

In the quiet stillness of the birthing center, surrounded by soft lighting and soothing sounds, my husband and I embarked on a remarkable journey—the birth of our second child. It was a journey filled with mindfulness, gratitude, and an unwavering trust in the process of bringing life into this world.

Unlike our first birth experience in a hospital, this time we had chosen the serene embrace of a birth center. Working closely with a dedicated midwife, we discovered a path that minimized potential risks associated with medical interventions, fostered a homelike and comfortable environment, and supported natural pain management.

From the moment we walked through the doors of the birth center, we felt a warm sense of belonging. The midwives, like our own guiding stars, understood and respected our needs, creating a nurturing connection that went beyond medical care. This personal touch was the very essence of what we had envisioned for our second childbirth journey.

With my husband by my side, serving as my partner doula, we embraced the experience together navigating the ebb and flow of labor. It was an intimate dance of support, empowerment, and love that transcended words.

The birthing room itself was a haven of serenity and tranquility. I had prepared for this moment with meditation and affirmations, which infused the room with a soothing atmosphere as they played.

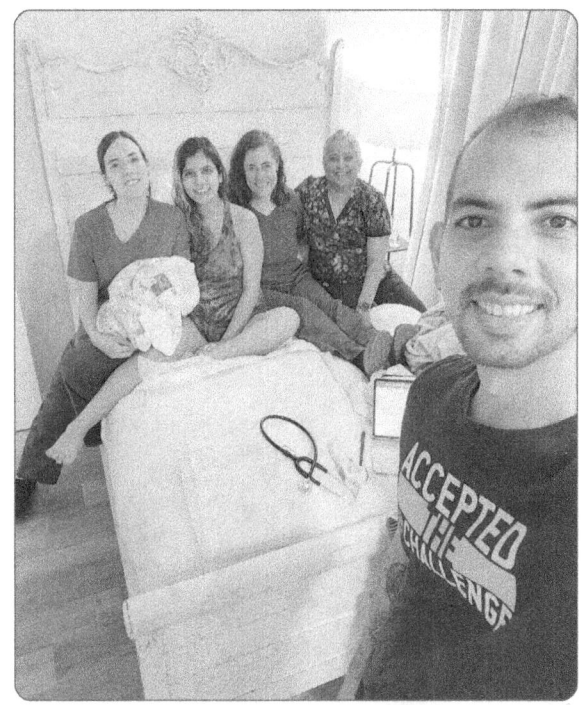

At the Tranquil Birth Center

In the stillness of that birthing space, I felt a profound connection to my inner self, the precious life growing within me, and to the unwavering support of my husband. As we navigated the waves of labor together, my meditation practice allowed me to stay centered, grounded, and fully present in the moment.

The affirmations that had been my companions throughout pregnancy echoed in my mind, reminding me of my strength and the incredible capabilities of my body. They became my mantras, guiding me through the intensity of labor with a sense of calm and empowerment. With each contraction, I visualized our baby's arrival, drawing strength from these positive declarations. With each surge of a contraction, I would gently close my eyes, focus on my breath, and silently recite these affirmations, feeling their profound impact.

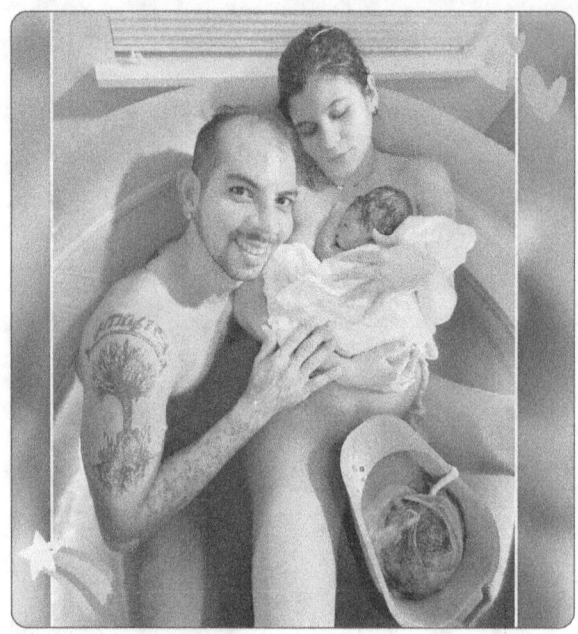

Welcoming Our Baby

As I settled into the birthing tub, the warm water enveloped me, offering the natural pain relief of hydrotherapy. The gentle pressure of the water against my body provided comfort and ease. It was as though the universe had conspired to create the perfect space for this sacred experience. In that warm and tranquil haven, with the loving presence of my husband, we shared smiles and whispered words of encouragement between contractions. Our connection, already strong, grew even stronger as we witnessed the miracle of our child's arrival together.

The midwives, a universe of wisdom and calm, guided us through the labor with grace. Their reassuring presence reminded us that childbirth is a natural process, one that our bodies were designed for. Their encouragement echoed in the room, reminding me to listen to my body and trust its innate ability to bring our baby into the world.

With each contraction, my husband stood by me, offering his love and dedication with unwavering strength. We felt like a team, partners on this incredible journey. It was an experience that deepened our bond and solidified our sense of teamwork, an invaluable gift that we believe can be best cultivated in the comforting embrace of a birth center or one's own home.

And then, in a moment that felt both eternal and ephemeral, our baby arrived, welcomed into the world with abundant love and tenderness. As I cradled our newborn in my arms, an overwhelming wave of gratitude washed over me. Gratitude for the little being who had chosen me as their mother, for my husband and his unwavering love, for the midwives and the support they provided, and for our loving family, sending their energy and love from afar. The midwives and the birth center had created the ideal space and support for us to craft an intimate and empowering birth experience. It was within this sanctuary that

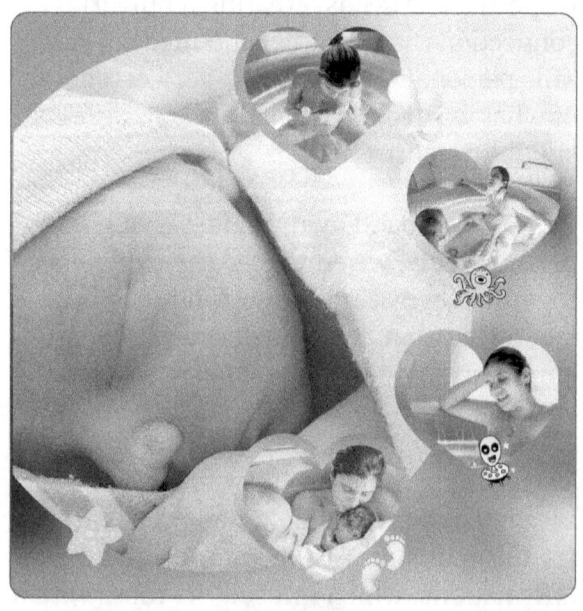

The Journey into Motherhood Is Transformative

we welcomed our precious baby into the world—a moment forever impressed in our hearts.

To all the courageous women setting forth on this incredible journey, I offer these words of encouragement: Listen to your body, believe in its extraordinary capacity to bring forth life. Embrace the nine-month journey of pregnancy and engage in activities that connect you with your body and the life blossoming within. Delve into practices like yoga, meditation, visualizations, mantras, and mindful breathing.

In our mindful and grateful journey at the birth center, we discovered the beauty of bringing a child into the world in a way that honored our desires, beliefs, and the sacredness of childbirth. May every woman find the path that empowers her and may love and mindfulness guide her on this extraordinary voyage of motherhood.

Birth Center Birth: Justus's Story

Walking up and down the path beside the birth center at night, I wait with anticipation for the next contraction to wash over me. The moon has outlined my belly's silhouette as I watch a gray fox dart out in front of us. It's 11:00 p.m.

"It's your third? Oh, that baby will slide right out," everyone said.

I tried to push their words from my mind hours after arriving at the birth center with little success. The beauty of it was, I felt no pressure from the midwives. No, "Well, why don't you just go home for a while." No, "Let's give you something to speed this up." No rushing. I didn't feel like an inconvenience to the birthing team.

Everyone waited, with joy in the process. It was right and beautiful. That's the gift of a birth center, which I had experienced twice before. Everything was flowing the way it was meant to. Everyone trusted my body to do what it was made to do.

Sleep met me hours into the process. Contractions slowed, and still no one felt bothered. It's 1:00 a.m. The birth center has a quiet, dark room, with no bright lights and no tubes, no interruptions. I slept peacefully next to my husband, feeling safe, and ready for what was next. As my body labored on, waking me up with each contraction, I felt immense gratitude for the environment of peace and support. As the hours passed, my midwife offered some natural tinctures and movements to encourage the little one out.

6:00 a.m. The contractions intensified. Each wave came and I was held up by encouragement and support. As my body grew weaker, the team grew stronger. They helped me into the bed, and we realized this baby was ready.

I was unable to think, but the team moved my legs, and coached me through the last few deep breaths and pushes. And he was here. 9:00 a.m.

Perfect, sweet angel. He never left my side in the comfort of the birth center room. The midwives cared for us both with communication and compassion. We slept in peace, ate, and bonded. Being at Lotus Community Birth Center felt like home. The prenatal process felt like family. The options before me felt like educated decisions. I was empowered every step of the way. After having three natural birth center babies, I can confidently say that it is a process filled with joy, growth, and empowerment. I felt known and supported. This route gives you a beautiful passage into the wild, brave adventure of motherhood.

Home Birth: Aleah's Story

I'd been pushing myself too hard at work and found myself having warm-up contractions and labor-like symptoms at only 35 or 36 weeks. I called MariMikel and told her what was going on. We wanted our baby to stay in the womb longer and to develop more, and so I was put on bed rest.

After a few days of being down the baby rose back up and out of my pelvis, so I was a little bit less effaced, a little bit less dilated, and my baby was less engaged. After a few weeks, I was taken off bed rest although not cleared to go back to work.

At 38-½ weeks I had three nights in a row of really intense warm-up labor. It started on a Thursday. I remember my husband, Frankie, and I were watching a Dallas Cowboys game and they scored an amazing touchdown. I jumped up and down, and then I thought that maybe my water had broken a little. I had a trickle down my leg. I called MariMikel and she had me use some nitrazine paper to test for amniotic fluid, but the result wasn't really clear. She said she thought it was probably just a little bit of pee, which can happen.

I had lots of warm-up labor that night and was not able to sleep well the next two nights either. Sunday morning MariMikel came and checked me, but nothing had changed. She said, "Honey, you're probably just having lots of warm-up labor, but it could happen anytime now."

I had even more intense warm-up labor that night and so she came Monday morning to check me again. We were in constant communication at this point. We really thought this was going to be it because my contractions had been more intense than any other night, but she said, "No, I'm so sorry. I know you were thinking that this is it, but you're still the same; there's been no major change." I think maybe I was a little bit more effaced, but other than that there was nothing, no more dilation, the baby was a tiny bit further down into the pelvis, but pretty much the same.

I was really disappointed and very tired. I was at this point so ready to move into the labor and birth process and looking forward with immense anticipation to finally greeting my sweet baby earthside. My mom had cleared her schedule for the day because she thought it was probably going to be it as well and she said "Well, I cancelled all my appointments. I'm here for you. Let's do something relaxing and fun. What sounds good to you?" We decided to go out to lunch and then to a movie.

We went out for Tex-Mex. I had chicken soup because I was still not feeling great and, mind you, I was having strong contractions every 30 to 45 minutes at that point. My brother and sister-in-law happened to be at the restaurant next door and saw my mom's car. They came inside and ended up sitting with us for a little while. My brother asked me "How are you doing sister?" and gently touched my shoulder and at that very moment I had a really hardcore contraction, strong enough to where I could not open my eyes, could not talk to anybody, and had to deep breathe. They looked at me and said, "Are you in labor?" My mom and I both responded, "No," and I said, "I've been doing this for a few days now, but it's not labor yet. We're going to go see *Ad Astra*.

Ad Astra is an incredibly intense Brad Pitt movie about a space station above Earth. The first two minutes of the movie are people falling off this space station in the stratosphere. It was so intense I had a huge contraction right away and was gripping my mom's arm.

Over the course of the 2-½-hour long movie I had contractions the whole time and definitely was having a really interesting time just watching this crazy, weird, wild movie. My mom at one point maybe an hour in said "Are you okay?" because I was squeezing her hand like I was going to break it. I assured her I was.

It was dark in the theater while the movie played, and when the lights came up at the end, I realized I was in another world. I had sunk into the dark cozy space of the theater and the story to the point that I didn't realize what was going on, but when the lights came up, I thought, *Oh, I think I'm in labor, like real labor.*

I said to my mom, "I need to go to the bathroom, and I think I'm in labor. I think this is it. I feel very different, and I've been having contractions this whole time." They were still maybe 20 to 30 minutes apart at the end of the movie, which is not usually indicative of active labor. When I went to the bathroom, I saw that I had bloody show, which is another sign that you could be going into labor. I remember I yelled out, "I'm bleeding!"

MariMikel said "Shh, it's okay, but there are people in here. We need to get you home so I can check you." I could barely walk down the hall to the car.

My contractions were on top of each other, suddenly happening every three to four minutes and I remember moaning "Oh God, Mom. Oh God, Mom," and she said, "Shh, I don't want people to call an ambulance for you." I laugh now as I think about how loud I was in the bathroom yelling about bleeding and how I must have looked, wide-eyed and waddling down the hallway of the movie theatre.

We made it to her car and were luckily only 10 minutes from her house. We went in and she checked me and said, "Oh, honey. Yeah, you're 4-½ centimeters. This is definitely it. You're in labor. Let me get my birth kit together; you call Frankie and get him home. We'll meet him there."

I called Frankie and I remember saying, "I'm sure it's going to be hours. You can finish your day." It was about 3:15 at this point.

He said, "No, I'm going to leave now. I'll meet you there."

It was my first baby, and we had every expectation that it would take a while, so it seemed to me like my mom took her sweet time getting all of her stuff together. My contractions were really intense. I was still in a completely different state of being, feeling as though time had both stopped completely and was flashing by at a lightening pace. I was hanging on door frames, going from deep breathing to the pant-blow and just full-on in the thick of it. We got in the car and got to my house at about 4:30. The 30-minute drive in traffic was even more intense for me. I could not stand being seated and strapped in by the seatbelt. Every bump was torture and I just wanted so badly to be up and free to move as my body guided me.

Frankie started to get my mom's equipment out of the car as soon as we pulled in the driveway and my mom said, "We need to check you again."

We went inside and she found that I was at 9 centimeters. I had gone from 4 to 9 centimeters in just over an hour. MariMikel said, "Frankie, you need to get everybody here right now."

In my birth plan I wanted my sister, sister-in-law, and three of my best friends present at the birth. She said, "Call everybody, get everybody here if they can, and you and I need to get everything together right now."

Frankie and MariMikel rushed to make the bed for the birth and to put water on the stove to get all the instruments sterilized and to get everything set up. My mom said, "We need to put you in the bath so we can try to slow this down, otherwise nobody's going to make it here in time for the birth. My apprentices aren't going to make it, none of the people that you planned for your birth are going to make it, and you're going to have this baby right now."

I got in the bath, and I was basically laboring alone the entire time, so it was not at all like the experience I had planned for. I was completely in the zone though and was able to let my heart and spirit open to this as my perfect birth, even if it was not what I had expected. I felt strong and one with my body and my baby. It continued to be incredibly intense. I was completely in another world. The bath was amazing and totally slowed my labor down and made it feel more manageable.

One of my best friends arrived—thank God—and was able to hold my hand and to be a support person while I was in the bath. My other best friend and my sister-in-law got there soon after. I was in the bath for about 20 minutes when I started having feelings of involuntary pushing. My mom heard the change and came in and said, "Do you want to have your baby in the bathtub?" I didn't, but it took me a few contractions to actually be able to get out of the bath and onto the bed. Once I was there my mom checked me again, and sure enough, I was complete. I wanted my sister to be there so much ... My mom was the midwife for both of her babies, and I was there for both of my nieces' births. and I remember kind of holding back as much as I could. I didn't want to have the baby without her there.

Also, pushing was so painful for me. It was totally the Ring of Fire. I'd start it and think, *Oh no, Oh no, no, no. I'm not doing this. Nope. I don't think so. Nope. Nope, not gonna do it. You can just stay in there.* I know now that she was basically on the perineum right when I started pushing, so that Ring of Fire happened right away and was all I felt at first.

After about 15 minutes my sister walked in. I just started crying when I saw her, I was so overjoyed that she was there and overwhelmed with the experience, and she came and got in the bed with me.

Varshna, the second midwife in attendance said to me then, "Okay Aleah. Open your eyes. It's time. You can do it. You've got to bear down a little harder, but you've got to get the baby out now. She's ready. She's right there. She's been crowning for a while. You've just got to push past this last bit of pain and then you're going to have your sweet baby in your arms."

I remember thinking, *Oh, okay, right. Alright, this is what you learn about. This is the end game. I have to do it. I can't say no. I can't keep her in. There's no going back ...* and two pushes later my sweet baby girl was born and with me, and it was just the one of the most joyous occasions of my life. I felt like I could do anything after giving birth. The strength I found within myself was like

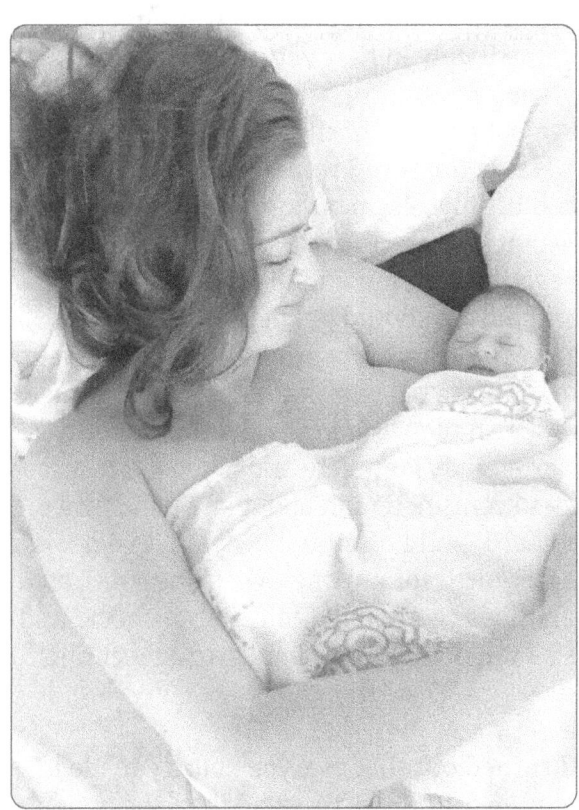

Aleah and Baby Téa

looking into a mirror and seeing the divine looking back at me and saying, *I am you, you are me, WE are one!*

With my second baby I was in complete denial that I was in labor and that afternoon I went to a party with a bunch of friends and all our kids, figuring the contractions I'd been having were just pre-labor. Two of my best friends had come back to Austin from Prague to be there for the birth. One had her little boy with her and they stayed with us while she visited. The party included our whole group of friends that had been together for 20 years and with our friends back from overseas it was like a reunion. It was a great time and helped to distract me. I was having contractions every 30-45 minutes during the party but would just pause whatever I was doing, take some deep breaths, and then continue on. I do remember one contraction that felt different from the others, I had to close my eyes and kind of gripped the wall I leaned on and when I opened my eyes everyone was looking at me. I smiled and they all asked if I was okay. I told them I was, and it had been like this for days. One of my friends said to me, "Girl, that one looked intense, you got all red in the face and everything!". We packed the kids up to start making our way back to my house. I was driving home at 7:30, all the while still having contractions, and my friend said, "Maybe you shouldn't be driving. Why don't you let me drive?"

I said, "I've got this. It's ok, I promise." In retrospect, I don't advise this.

She said, "I don't know, you seem different." We got home, we put the kids to bed, and my contractions started getting closer together. She said, "We need to call your mom."

I said, "No, no, no. We don't need to bother her."

She said, "Aleah, we need to call your mom." She and Frankie started getting everything together, boiling water, and getting my birth kit all prepared.

I called my mom at around 8:45 p.m. On the phone she said she needed to call Varsha and I said, "I don't think it's it yet, you don't need to call her."

She said, "Aleah, she lives an hour away. We need to get her here. This could be it, and you could go even faster than last time."

I remember telling her I would feel bad if this wasn't it, and she said "No, don't feel bad. I'm going to call her right now."

My mom got there quickly and when she checked my cervix I was about 4 centimeters dilated but she felt a band around the cervix that was very hard and tight and asked me if she could do some cervical massage. I didn't want that to hold labor back, so I agreed and in just a few seconds it was gone. The contractions were so intense at this point I was having trouble breathing and decided to get in the tub, which was so wonderful and really made it more manageable for me I kept reminding myself that *I was strong and I could do this*, *pain was my friend*, and *surrender, surrender, surrender*. These words were like a lighthouse in the night for me, lifting me up through a dark storm, guiding me back to myself when I started to lose my way.

It was so lovely to have my friend from Prague with me; she was just an amazing support to me, and I'm so glad she was able to be there. She wasn't able to be at my first birth because she lives so far away and her son was not even six months old at that time, but we had planned to have her here for this birth, and it was just the best. Frankie was such a good labor support person too, and unlike during the first birth he was able to really be there with me for the short labor I did have. He held my hand, breathed with me, and talked to me in a sweet, gentle, and empowering way.

It was so fast that I definitely felt I was on the runaway freight train MariMikel talks about with rapid births. It was so hard to stay on top of my contractions, every wave crashed down on me with no respite before the next, again and again. I was almost immediately in that very altered place you often get to during transition. I leaned against the side of the tub as I labored, and it was so intense I think I wanted to try and lift myself up out of the pain. I started feeling an urge to push soon thereafter and began having involuntary pushes. My mom asked if we should get back in the bed so she could check my progress. I did not want to have the baby in the water, and she knew my birth plan. When she did the exam, I was already complete and had gone from 4–10 centimeters in about an hour. It was so hard, and I often tell people I do not wish a fast birth for anyone. When she confirmed that I was complete I felt a bit of shock, and also relief. I knew I would get to meet our sweet girl so soon.

It turned out that everyone barely made it in time for this birth. I had the baby about an hour after my mom arrived, but no one

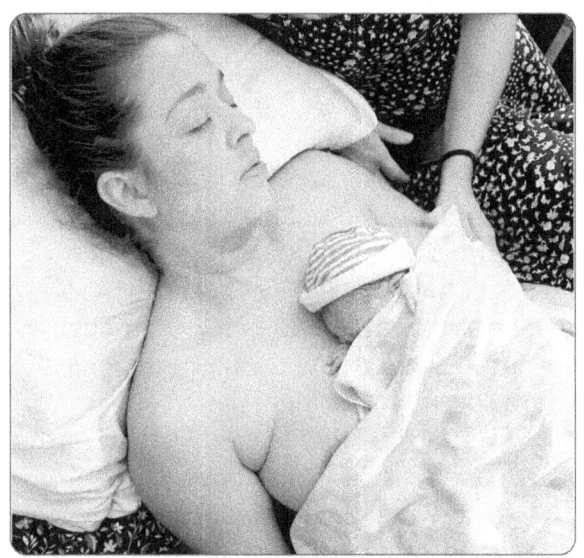

Aleah and Her Daughter Moments after Birth

else made it in time for the birth except for my sister-in-law, and she slipped in and made it by about two minutes. I pushed twice and she slid out and was up on my belly, she was tiny and perfect, and I was overwhelmed with joy and love and extreme gratitude for my team and for this new healthy girl that had joined us. My sister and my niece who was fourteen came in right after the baby was born thinking I would still be in labor. I remember saying "She's here!" and I remember the look on their faces, like *What do you mean?* It had only been 30 minutes since they were called, and the baby was already out. My other two best friends also didn't make it, one of whom had also come back from overseas to be with me for the birth. It happened so quickly. My second daughter is a year old now and knowing her spitfire personality, it makes sense that she made such a quick and grand entrance into the world.

My home birth experiences with both of my girls were incredibly transformative and magical. Not to say it wasn't the most difficult thing I have ever done, because I believe birth is not made to be easy, but it changed me for the better in ways I cannot fully convey in words. The level of education, care, love, and support I received from MariMikel was exactly what I needed to feel empowered and have the full, deep level of belief in myself that having a natural home birth was something I could not only do, but it was also a challenge I was up to, it was a challenge I wanted and accepted and took into myself as a powerful life changing event.

If you can, I strongly encourage you to find a midwife in your area, someone that you trust and connect with. Home birth is not only safer, but you are also in your most comfortable space, which allows you to

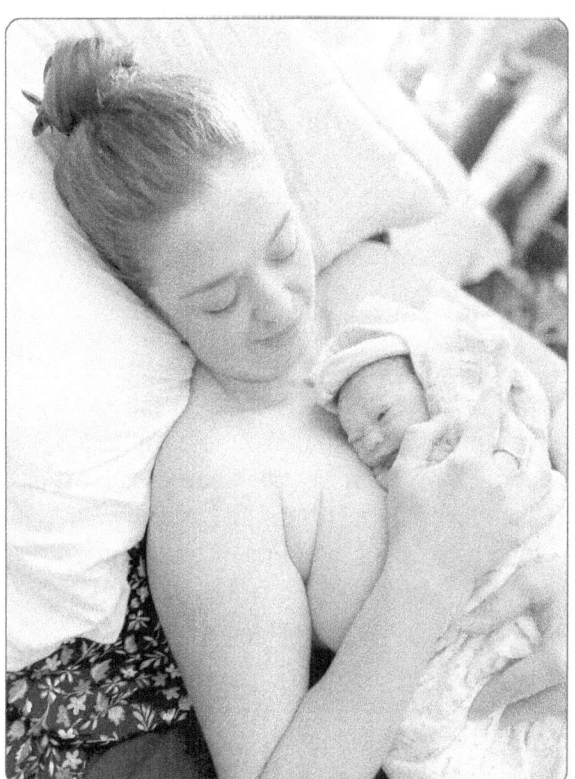

Aleah and Her Daughter Ava

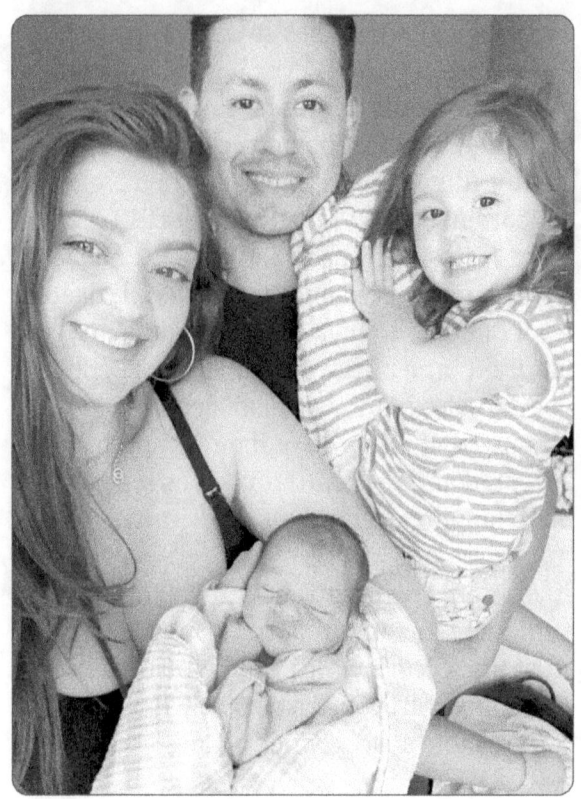
Our Beautiful Family of Four

"You know there's two in here, right?" the technician said. I almost fainted.

I immediately called MariMikel and told her. I made it clear that I still wanted to be under her care. Still, a twin pregnancy and birth is different in that it is higher risk. But, if MariMikel was committed to me, I was committed to her. Even though she is an expert midwife, she persuaded me to consider a hospital delivery to avoid complications related to twin births. For the safety of my darling baby boys, I agreed. She assured me that she would be right there in the hospital advocating for me the whole time! I was relieved.

During the months of check-ins, she would tell me "You've got to eat more!" After that visit, I went to the Olive Garden and ate a tour of Italy and stopped at P. Terry's for a burger on the way home. I ate everything in sight.

On the night my water broke, I went to St. David's hospital and Marimikel was there, advocating for me as promised. I went home three days later with two beautiful, healthy baby boys, Sagan Lux and Solen Veritas, who were of a hearty birth weight for twins at 6 pounds and almost 6 pounds!

release fear, let go of all the heady stuff, and lose yourself in the deeply profound, mind-body-spirit experience of birth more easily.

Home Birth: Sheryl's Story

In 2012, after helping throw the Austin-based Learning Man festival, I made a wish upon a pinecone around a bonfire to become a Mother. My wish came true after I discovered I was pregnant, and I was referred to MariMikel Potter by my good friend and recent mother, Daniela. I had a reassuring phone chat with MariMikel on the banks of the Colorado river, and I was elated to have someone with so much experience to guide me on my path. Later during a sonogram, I found out I was pregnant with twins. Game changer!!

Home Birth: Andrea's Story

I had a home birth with MariMikel on Feb 23, 2013.

When I found out I was pregnant, a friend recommended her, as she'd heard great things about her.

We set up an appointment to meet and get to know each other—to see if we were a great fit. I showed up with terrible morning sickness and right away MariMikel started taking care of me. She told me I looked pale and needed calories. She went into her kitchen and brought me an apple and I knew she would be my midwife.

My care was intense, specific, and thorough.

I was told to walk/swim, drink a gallon of water a day, eat well, take my vitamins, and rest.

These lessons were hard pressed into me at every single appointment. MariMikel could be a hard ass about how this all was going to go, but I knew I was in great hands and that there was a method to her madness. I truly felt like I was training for a marathon. I did everything MariMikel told me to do—except for buying the brand of vitamins she wanted me to (because I worked for a vitamin company and was very loyal to the brand)—and I didn't eat mild food the day before my birth (which I massively regretted during labor).

I started swimming a lot (like MariMikel), drank tons of water, walked a lot, took my vitamins, did prenatal yoga, ate well (when my morning sickness subsided), and enjoyed the quiet days with my husband.

MariMikel was kind, intuitive, warm, comforting, and told me she was there for me whenever I needed to hear the heartbeat or just check in about something.

I remember when we were getting close to the birth, I got scared that she would be bored by my labor pains, and impatient with me because this was just another one of her thousands of births. She reassured me this was not true, that every birth was a miracle, told me she prayed on the way to each birth, and that she was honored to be at every birth. I totally believed her.

Dan and I woke up on Friday morning, February 22nd, and immediately something felt different to me. My due date, Monday, February 18th, had already passed. Dan decided he would not go to work that day. We planned to run a bunch of errands together. What was I thinking? I could not go anywhere. I did insist that Dan go to this one Target in North Austin (we lived in South Austin) to get this one monkey laundry hamper that they only had at that location. What a trooper—he did it. Otherwise, we had a very lazy day at home playing backgammon, and eating, etc.

Dan also had to finalize setting up the birth tub. I was getting contractions throughout the day, but nothing regular. At around 4 p.m. we called MariMikel to let her know what I was feeling. She told me to stay home and rest and not to take a walk or do anything active, so as not to bring on labor during the night. Since the contractions were longer than a minute, she was pretty certain they were not dilation contractions, but rather my cervix dropping. At my last appointment on the previous day the baby was at a +2 station, but there was no dilation, and she said my cervix was still in Dallas (which was better than New Jersey, where it had been the week before). Dan and I didn't listen to MariMikel, because we wanted to get out and take the dog for a walk.

We didn't get very far. Once we were on the walk, the contractions came on stronger, and were getting closer together. We realized why MariMikel didn't want us walking. We would be bringing on labor in the evening.

We went home, had dinner, and did what MariMikel calls "the Trick." I took two ibuprofen, drank a glass of wine, took a bath, and went to bed. It was a very interesting evening. I know that Dan and I slept. And I know that I was having contractions all night. Some I could take lying down and some I could not. Sometimes I only needed to move my hips around to deal with the pain, and some contractions brought me to my hands and knees in a cat-cow and then child pose position to deal with the pain. Some I handled on my own; some I woke Dan for so he could support me.

Going to the bathroom was difficult, every time I transitioned out of the bed I would have a contraction and I was getting the chills when I got out of bed. It was a long night—BUT, I was falling back asleep in between each contraction, and that was really important to me. I didn't want to call the birth team until the morning. I also had it in my head that these were not dilation contractions, and it was just my cervix moving down to Central Austin.

At 6:30 in the morning, Dan and I decided to call the team, MariMikel, her assistant, and our doula. Everyone arrived by about 7. When my doula walked in the door, it was ON!! She got me on the birth ball and started helping me through the contractions.

I had a moment at that point when I got sad and cried. I realized how I had been laboring for so long, practically by myself, and how

much pain I was in. Then the midwife arrived. She had been calling us and we hadn't picked up the phone. Dan's car was in the driveway blocking her car, so when she arrived, she had an intensity about all of that, but once she settled, she went into nurturing mode.

Soon after she arrived, she asked me if I wanted to be checked to see where I was in my labor. YES!

Amazingly, I was at 6 cm. Holy shit—I was so encouraged, and in so much pain. I was throwing up, crying, breathing, moaning, humming along to music, everything. I was in full-on labor. It was an altered state. I felt vulnerable and afraid, and I remember wondering, *Why the hell was I not having an epidural or c-section?*

But my team was outstanding. My husband, the doula, my midwife—I felt so taken care of and supported in every way. They kept telling me how great I was doing, and how beautiful I looked, which was amazing to me because I really felt like I could be dying.

Then at some point my contractions slowed down to about four-and-a-half minutes apart, and I was so happy to have a slight break. My midwife was not—she very clearly and calmly told me that in order for this labor to keep progressing I had to move my body in such a way to bring the contractions closer together again. This was hard to hear.

More pain? Closer together? I have to make that happen voluntarily? But I did it. I wanted to get this baby out in the shortest amount of time possible, and I really trusted my midwife and everyone supporting me. So, I moved my hips around, sat on the toilet, sat in between my husband's legs, and puked some more. I started to feel real pressure in my perineum.

It was working.

The next exam showed I had made it to 9 cm. OMG—yes!! MariMikel asked if she could do something internal to help me get to 10 cm—OMG yes! More pressure down there, more pain, more moaning; it's getting intense, getting rough. More crying. One more puke.

Time to push. I was so scared to push, but I knew somewhere in me that I would be a good pusher. So, as depleted and scared as I was, I was ready!! Because I had been throwing up during labor, I was only allowed ice chips, but now that I was about to push, I was able to drink, and I was thrilled. The ice-cold coconut water tasted AMAZING!

MariMikel had Dan stand behind me near my bed, and when I felt a contraction Dan would drop me down into a squatting position and I would push. After the contraction was done, he would pull me back up to a standing position. I'd gyrate my hips to bring on a contraction, repeat and on and on. After about 20 minutes of this we could see the baby's head, and we knew I was almost there. Next, the team helped me to move onto my bed for the final pushing. After two more rounds of contractions/pushing, Dan and I pulled out our baby boy (it's a boy!!!) at 11:19 a.m., four-and-a-half hours after the team arrived, with 30 minutes of pushing and no tearing, no medication, nothing. Oh, happy day! It was everything I could have ever hoped for my birth. Safe, happy, healthy, extremely challenging, rewarding, home birth. That's my story. I am grateful and newly in love with Henry Wolf. 8bs, 21 inches. Full of red hair.

MariMikel was the perfect blend of tough as nails, intuitive healer, and nurturing storyteller. She was there for us when we were having relationship problems, were frustrated with our parents, and offered words of advice like "young parents have tons of energy, but older parents are wiser parents." We were in the "older parents" category and felt insecure about it at times.

I felt like I was 100 percent in great hands, even though it felt hard at times to be working so hard during my pregnancy—the water, the swimming, the supplements, the preparations.

MariMikel had us come to her for our 2nd after birth checkup. She was so smart; she told us to take our baby in the car and drive and go out for lunch. It would have been weeks upon weeks of staying in the house had she not pushed us to take him out. She was also adamant about me "staying down" after the birth—so my uterus didn't fall out—which was amazingly helpful because I'm a "do-er." I really let others take care of me while I took care of my baby and stayed in bed as much as possible.

When MariMikel was at my house for the birth she was hands off and let me, my husband, and my doula go through the labor process. She stepped in at the exact right moments with words of encouragement and special tricks only her experience attending thousands of births could bring to the moment.

She has a special place in my heart and in our family.

Unfortunately, I was not able to get pregnant again, and didn't get to have MariMikel deliver our next baby. Fortunately, we adopted a beautiful baby boy, and we get to run into MariMikel at the grocery store every once in a while, and hug hello.

Newborn Pictures
I love sharing pictures of the babies I have helped bring into this world.

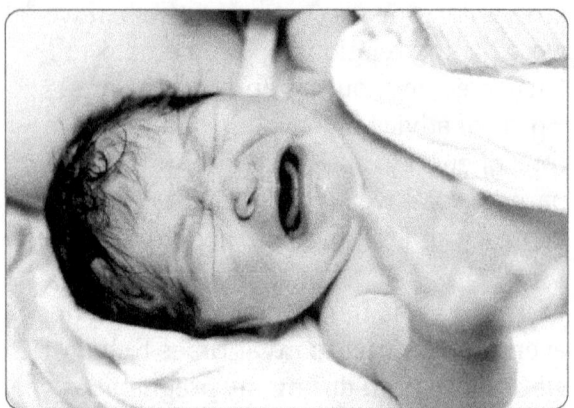
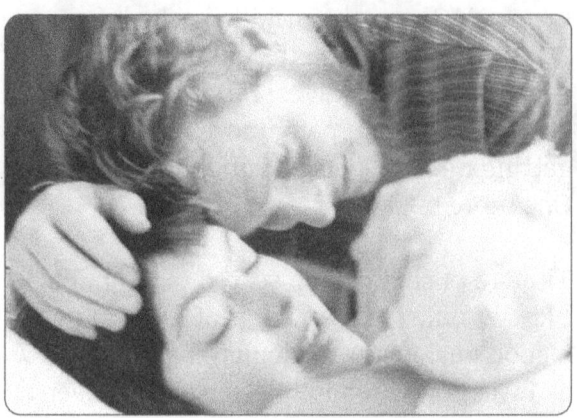
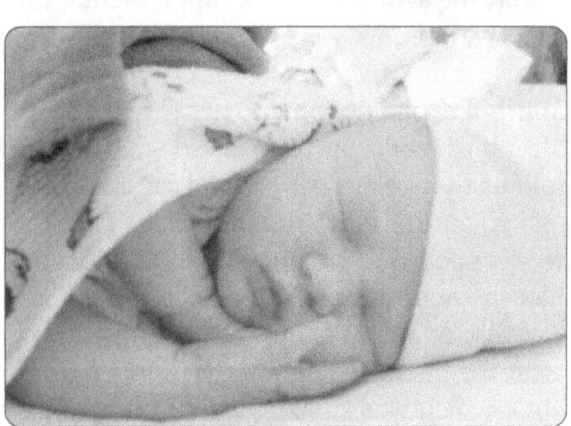
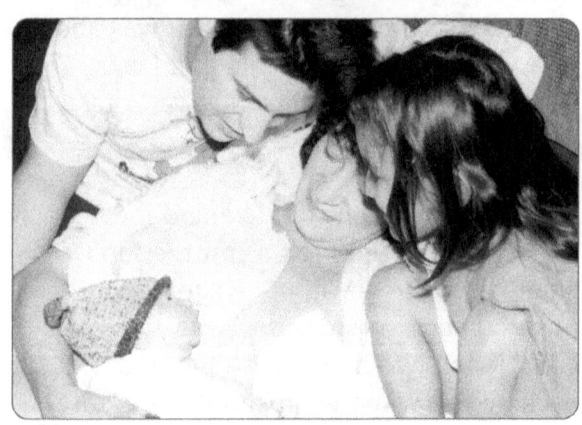
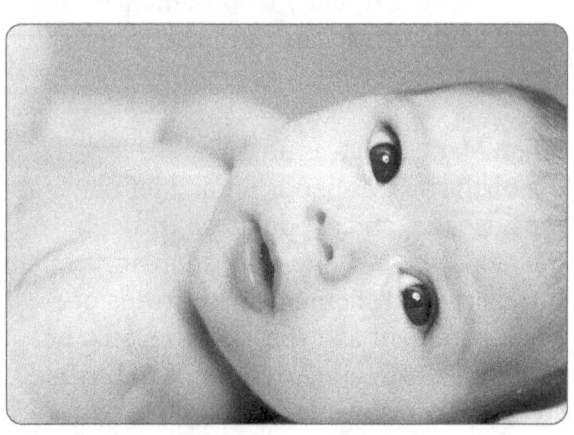
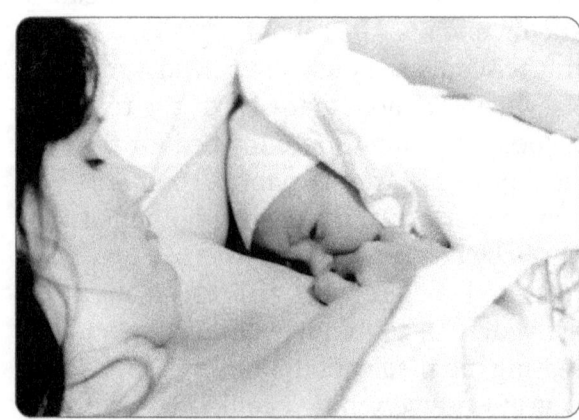

Moment

There's this moment just after someone is born, where time stands still and, if you pay attention, you'll feel the universe bend and shudder. It's the briefest moment, just before the baby takes a breath and the parents take a breath, just before the baby starts to cry and the parents start to cry, just before we are all returned to earth, and the now. The sensation is somehow one of both rushing forward and catching up, like standing at the shoreline and watching the waves roll in and the tide go out around your feet all at once, as if the universe is making space for what is new and every story that led to it to meet. I don't know what exactly happens in that churning, foamy brine where what has been and what is to be intermingle. But it is holy and humbling and deserves protection.

—Small Things Grow Home Birth

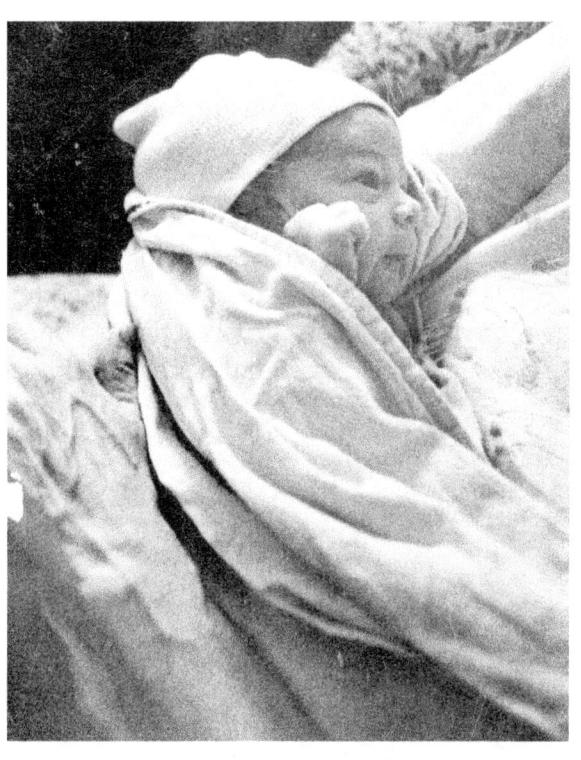

42 Weeks

If you make it to 42 weeks without going into active labor, there are steps we can take to make sure the baby's still doing alright and then to encourage them to come on out.

Ultrasound

If you reach Week 42, the state of Texas mandates that an ultrasound be performed to assess the condition of the baby and placenta, the heart rate, respiratory movement of the baby (babies breathe amniotic fluid about six to nine times per minute), overall movement, and how much amniotic fluid is present. Other states have similar mandates, and your midwife will be familiar with your state laws. This ultrasound allows providers to assess if it's time to get the baby out through more direct measures. I think it is a very good idea.

If you reach 42 weeks and are going to go in for an ultrasound, drink several ounces of juice right before you walk into the office to give the baby a good jolt of sugar, which they usually respond to by showing a lot of activity, indicating they likely don't need to be forced out just yet. If they don't respond to the sugar, that's a sign that they likely

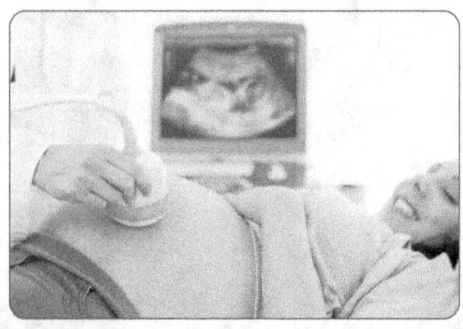

Getting an Ultrasound

need to get on out of there and it's a good thing you checked.

There have been a few times where things didn't look great for my client's baby or there wasn't enough amniotic fluid present, and we went to the hospital to be induced. If this happens to you, one thing they may opt to do at the hospital is to pump IV fluids into your uterus to help cushion the baby. When you have a contraction, the uterus seizes down around the baby so tightly that—if there is not enough amniotic fluid—it can constrict the baby's cord, causing oxygen deprivation. These fluids serve to avoid that issue.

If your placenta is fine but your cervix isn't ready, it may be that you actually need to be induced or may need medical intervention. As a midwife, I would work with you to try to get the baby out for a full week, or until it looks like there is a problem or complication, but if you get to 43 weeks, that's when it's time to go to the hospital.

Pumping and Herbs

If my client reaches 42 weeks and the ultrasound says everything is just dandy, but her labor hasn't started yet, I start her on a regimen of pumping her breasts with hospital grade equipment coupled with herbs to attempt to stimulate labor.

This is sort of like starting an old motor that hasn't been turned over for a while. You've got to rev it for a bit to get it going. The first time a woman pumps her breasts, she may have a minimal response. Sometimes it's miraculous. I've had women who put that pump on and after 15 minutes their labor shot into the stratosphere and they had their baby four hours later. I've also had women who put the pump on and when they took it off everything stopped. We put it back on and pump during pushing and then again after the birth to get the placenta out, because for some women, nothing happens without the pump. I also can't tell you how many times I've had a client just go and take a look at that intimidating machine and then go straight into labor. Their bodies decided they were definitely not doing *that*. I have also had women for whom the pumping didn't work at all. But for most women it helps to stimulate active labor.

Another amazing thing is that whenever you pump there is way more milk for the baby present after the birth, way more colostrum. It's really awesome. You'll see colostrum as you're pumping and soon there will be more and more and more. You may have the impulse to save this for the baby, but I don't recommend this. The colostrum is prone to getting bacteria in it. Don't worry, you're going to make more. You're going to have plenty for your baby.

If you find yourself in this situation, work with your midwife to understand what she recommends.

Breaking Waters

One of the things I will try if the pumping and herb regimen doesn't stimulate labor is to break the waters (with the mother's consent). If the herbs and pumping don't work on their own, as a last resort I break the bag with what looks like a long crochet hook with a tiny barb on the end. It is sterile and made of plastic. I catch the bag with it and poke a little hole. If this doesn't work

within 24 hours, we will go to the hospital to get their help. In labor, I will also break the waters if the head is really high and there's a bunch of water in front of the baby. In that scenario, if the bag breaks while you're upright, the cord can prolapse (meaning that it can get in front of the baby), which is a really grim thing.

There are some midwives who do not agree with this method. They believe in a more hands off approach, no cervical stimulation or breaking of the waters. I think if you are at the 42-week marker and wanting to have your ideal, perfect home birth and this feels like something you want to try to stimulate labor then these methods, if employed under the care of your midwife, are a great and effective way to get things going. In the end it is up to you to make an informed choice as to what you want to do, what feels right to you for you and your baby and family. Sometimes, when all signs and vitals are looking good at 42 weeks, I may decide that the baby is not actually 42 weeks gestationally, that it just needs more time, and we wait patiently. There are also times when the mother makes the decision not to intervene. It is important to note that these methods are used to best serve the health and safety needs of the mother and baby, who could be at risk after a certain point of gestation. Midwives generally prefer not to intervene, but we do want to prevent complications.

Other Methods

If nothing works and it seems like it isn't going to, then we go to the hospital and use their approach. It's really difficult to do Pitocin without an epidural, so if you're going through the relentless, brutal nature of Pitocin, I understand and support your choice to get help with the pain.

Complications and Interventions

Your beautiful baby has entered the world! The long-awaited moment of birth has arrived. You are likely feeling elated and exhausted and overwhelmed and such a strong, strong desire to hold your baby so close. Absolutely everything in your life has changed, and we're going to talk about all of that, starting from the very first second of birth, in *The Book of Birth Volume II: Your Postpartum Journey through the Fourth Trimester.*

However, there are a few more items I should cover before we proceed. The vast majority of my clients never experience any of the complications and interventions I describe in this section. Mostly, your body knows what to do and does it. You have deep instinctual knowledge and have done everything you can to prepare for this. Most women have a beautiful experience that matches their desires. But I think it's kind of important to know that these are the potentials when things don't quite go as expected. I talk to all my clients about these possibilities, so if something happens, they know there's a plan. Then, if they encounter one of these situations, the fear is lessened because they have this information.

That said, if you find yourself growing anxious while reading this section, put the book down! Walk away and recenter yourself. Remind yourself these complications are the exceptions, not the rule. Further, remember that if your experienced provider deems them necessary, then they are making the best choice for your health and that of your baby. When you return to reading, instead of imagining yourself in these situations, imagine a stranger in your place. Depersonalize it.

I do believe it is important to at least review these topics, so you can refer to them if you need to. If you are planning a hospital birth it may be even more important, as there is a higher likelihood that you may experience some of these interventions.

Oxygen

The most common intervention that I do at home is administering oxygen. If you have a drop in fetal heart tones at any point during labor or pushing, I administer oxygen. It is common for heart tones to drop in labor, sometimes it can be due to head or cord compression, but we do not know which it is until the baby comes out, so we always just have to act in the best interest of the baby as much as we possibly can. If it's the cord that's being compressed, the baby's oxygen level drops and this can be dangerous. Head compression is not as worrisome, but you cannot tell until the baby comes out which it is, so I use oxygen just in case.

Sutures for Tearing or Lacerations

The second most common complication I handle at home is a tear or laceration. If I believe the tear is not severe and you have the option to either repair it or let it heal naturally, I discuss this with my clients. The only thing to consider in those moments when it could be an option is that sometimes the tear or laceration may not heal exactly the way it was before, which is not a big deal, just something to consider.

If you do the repair you will not only have it heal exactly the way it was anatomically speaking, but you will also have less stinging or burning when you pee, there is less of a chance of getting any kind of infection in the wound, and it will heal quickly and effectively (especially if you stay down after the birth).

Breaking the Waters

The third most common thing I do is break the waters of the amniotic sac. I do not routinely break waters, as the amniotic sac can protect the baby's head from the cervix during labor, and you are less likely to see bruising or swelling on the scalp, abrasions, and/or excessive molding when the bag remains intact. I do have women who have their babies born in the bag, it is actually not that uncommon. Once the baby's head is coming through the pelvis though, there is nothing that really will prevent their skull from the pressure and contact, and the bag of water then becomes superfluous.

I will only break the water if it is preventing the baby from engaging or coming through and is stalling labor or if I believe the bag

is going to explode all over the birth team when the baby is born. If the former is the case, I will give you the option to break the bag so labor can continue to progress at a quicker pace. It is always going to be your choice, but I will say I have never had a woman in a stalled labor say no to this option. If the latter is the case, I will still discuss it with you first, but it is a hazard for my team to have those fluids splatter all over us, and we have to protect ourselves from that exposure. At a hospital, they wear a significant amount of protective gear that we do not wear at a home birth.

I also ask to break your waters if I think that the baby is in distress. If there is meconium (baby's first poop) present in the amniotic fluid, the baby can inhale it, and it can cause very serious damage. If I know there is meconium in the fluid, I work with the mother to have the baby's head born at the end of a contraction, so I have enough time to deep suction as much of the meconium-stained fluid out as I can before the baby takes their first breath.

Suctioning these babies provides an incredible benefit to the baby. Meconium-stained fluids are very acidic, and can cause a lot of distress. Issues can include seriously increased mucus production in the baby's respiratory passages, often preventing the baby from being able to nurse or even breathe adequately. When there is really severe, thick meconium staining in the waters we go to the hospital because they have a wonderful intervention of inserting a tiny tube into the uterus and pumping IV fluids in. This process washes the meconium out, decreasing the viscosity and particulate count. It is a fantastic intervention that can really prevent the baby from being very negatively impacted by meconium aspiration.

Suctioning

The next most common intervention is suctioning the baby. I probably use a DeLee suctioning apparatus about 10–15 percent of the time. Suctioning the baby takes 15–20 seconds. This entails putting a small tube down the baby's throat and sucking out the mucus and fluids in the passage. It is another intervention I do simply because it seems to make congested babies so much happier to have mucus and fluid out, and it helps them not to struggle as much after the birth. This does not harm them, and this intervention allows them to be able to focus on bonding and nursing more rapidly instead of working the fluids out on their own, which can take a long time.

Stripping the Membranes

The amniotic sac can be stuck to the inside of the cervix. This can hold labor back and keep it from really getting going. In these instances, I utilize an ancient technique called *stripping the membranes* or *sweeping the membranes* to help (with the mother's consent). This technique requires the woman to be slightly dilated, at least a few centimeters, because I have to get my finger between the inside of the cervix and the outside of the bag and gently rotate it in a 360-degree arc. I am able to feel if the bag is adhered, and if I can get it unstuck, it is a great trick for helping labor to initiate soon.

I often try sweeping the membranes at a little over 41 weeks to try to avoid getting to Week 42, because people in your orbit may start to exude anxiety around you. Having anxious family and friends around you does not help you to go into labor. If the ancient mother perceived a threat, most of the time her body did not go into labor. You need to be peaceful for this to unfold in a good way, so I usually do try these things before we have to resort to the ultrasound and everything that follows at Week 42. Check with your care provider or midwife to see if they are familiar with this technique.

I have had women who went immediately into labor by just separating the bag from where it was adhered to the inside of the cervix. I don't go in very far—it's about an inch all the way around the inside of the cervix—but this can be all it takes to get labor going, and it's certainly better than going to the hospital and being induced when you are wanting to have a home birth. It doesn't always work, but when it does it is much less invasive than Pitocin or breaking the waters.

Stimulating the Cervix/ Cervical Massage

There can be scar tissue around the os, which is the opening to the cervix. It can come from previous births, previous cervical surgeries, abortions, or miscarriage, and it can form a membrane that prevents the cervix from opening to completion in labor. I am able to gently massage this scar tissue and help it to stretch so you dilate more effectively.

You cannot push if there is a lip, and if I just massage it back a bit, often it will go away, and then you can start pushing. Early in my career I transported women with non-progressive labors to the hospital many

Aleah: When MariMikel arrived during my labor for my second birth, she checked me and found I was only four centimeters. She said, "You have a bit of a cervical lip here. It's a little hard. Are you okay with me doing some cervical massage, so we can get past this, and you won't sit here at four centimeters for a long time?"

I said "Sure, go ahead."

She did cervical massage for maybe 10 seconds before telling me, "Oh yeah, it broke right up. You're good! You're maybe four-and-a-half centimeters now, but you can get in the tub, do whatever you want." I got in the bath and within 15 minutes I was having involuntary pushes. My mom said, "Are you pushing?"

I said, "Oh, I think so. Yes, something's changed."

I got back on the bed, and she checked me again. Sure enough, I was 9-½ centimeters. I'd gone from 4 centimeters to 9-½ centimeters in a very intense 15 minutes.

After that, my baby came out in a matter of minutes with a gush of amniotic fluid. I was happy to have had MariMikel be able to do the cervical massage and make sure that there was nothing in the way of things progressing naturally.

---

times and each time the doctor said, "Oh we just need to get this band out of the way." They were able to massage it and it opened right up, and I learned how to do this from them. It is a wonderful aid for women who have this issue.

I fairly frequently have to hold back an anterior (to the top front of the baby's head) cervical lip while the mother pushes to get the baby down far enough that the lip is not in the way anymore. If you don't do this, the mother's cervix can tear, and it can hold the baby back, keep the baby from coming out at all, or become very, very swollen.

Not everybody practices these techniques, but I do know plenty of doctors and midwives who do, so you want to talk to your midwife about what her skill level and inclinations are. You want to pick people to

aid you that you feel confidence in and that you feel are going to do what you want in your birth.

Administering Fluids Intravenously

Another possible intervention is giving IV fluids. I carry IV fluids, both large bags for blood loss and/or dehydration and small bags that I can add antibiotics to if you are strep B positive. I check every mother for strep B at the end of the pregnancy. I only use an IV with antibiotics now if you are strep B positive, your waters have been broken for 24 hours, and you're not yet in labor. If I can avoid interrupting the establishment of the baby's gut flora and immune system, which can happen when they are exposed to antibiotics in labor, I will. You are more likely to receive antibiotics in a hospital during labor than in a home birth.

A 2023 study published in the journal BMC Pregnancy and Childbirth[155] found that 44.2 percent of women who gave birth in a hospital received antibiotics during labor, compared to only 18.2 percent of women who gave birth at home. The study also found that the most common reason for antibiotic use in the hospital was cesarean section, followed by premature rupture of membranes (PROM) and chorioamnionitis.

Another study, published in the journal BIRTH in 2012,[156] found that first-time mothers who planned to give birth at home were less likely to receive antibiotics than those who planned to give birth in a hospital, even when the same midwives were providing care.

I use an IV catheter that allows you to continue to be mobile during labor, so you are not resigned to staying in bed during the administration of IV fluids. You cannot get rid of strep B ahead of time, unfortunately. Douching can help to take it down but generally will not knock it out.

I also commonly administer IV fluids in the case of significant vomiting during labor. Vomiting can produce serious ketones, which make you feel horrible. If you can drink water or other fluids to stay hydrated that is ideal, but when you are sick you often cannot keep anything down and IV fluids can help to combat dehydration.

Occasionally, women lose a little too much blood during the birth and can feel quite faint, and that is another, albeit rarer, time that I would administer IV fluids.

Episiotomy

One of the most uncommon interventions that I perform at a home birth is an episiotomy. I do not perform very many episiotomies, I have about a 1–2 percent rate with my clients, and I have only ever performed one episiotomy on a woman who has had a baby before. She needed the episiotomy because she had been sewn up more tightly than she should have been during the repair of an episiotomy by the doctor who assisted her first birth.

I don't like doing episiotomies. It seems like a subtle assault. When they are necessary, they are extremely helpful, though. I opt for them when in my judgment the fetal distress is too high, and the episiotomy will help and not harm. I pray as I'm preparing to perform them, and I think loving thoughts to the woman as I am cutting her, because it is an act of love, support, and help. But there's always a little mixed feeling for me of doing something that serious to someone. I don't perform them lightly. Usually when it comes to that point, the woman is grateful for the choice.

I talk gently and lovingly to the woman in labor, explaining exactly what I will be doing and why, and get her agreement and support, which makes everything go better. I always use numbing medication, so the woman doesn't feel anything when I do the episiotomy.

The most common reason for administering an episiotomy, true for about 90 percent of the episiotomies I perform, is fetal distress and not because the mother is not or will not stretch to accommodate the baby's head. Every now and then I will perform one when it is evident that a woman is going to tear so incredibly badly that an episiotomy is a better choice.

More frequently, a tear is going to heal much better than an episiotomy would as the perineum generally only tears a tiny bit to allow the space needed for the baby's head to be born. Often if you do an episiotomy it will continue to tear as the baby's head comes out, making it a much larger wound than it would have been if the body tore naturally. So, I take episiotomies very seriously and only do them if I really feel it is necessary.

I also always go slightly off to the side with the incision. An episiotomy right at the middle of the perineum is situated at the point of least resistance, and it is much more possible for the episiotomy to extend into the rectum, which is less than desirable to say the least. I do very small episiotomies as well. I find they don't need to be very big to do exactly what we want, which is to let the baby out.

Herpes in Labor and Delivery

I have had a number of women who have had an outbreak of type 2 herpes at the time that they went into labor. There are many doctors across the United States that will automatically perform a caesarean section on any woman who has an outbreak of herpes at the time of the birth. There is evidence that women who have had repeated outbreaks also have antibodies to herpes and pass those on to their baby.[157]

I knew a supportive doctor who said what he did for 50 years was cover any lesion on the mother with a heavy coating of petroleum jelly and sterile gauze, then had someone hold it in place as the baby was born so the baby didn't come in contact with it.

If you have an *initial* outbreak of herpes at the time you go into labor, you simply must have a c-section. You have no immunity, there is no immunity being passed to the baby, and the baby can get it and become ill enough to die.

But if you have had herpes for years and have infrequent outbreaks, I think this is a safe approach. I also recommend women start Valtrex at the first sign of an outbreak.

Hospital Transfer

I prepare all of my clients for the slim possibility of going to the hospital, so they are informed, cooperative, and grateful for these amazing people who are helping in a situation that cannot be handled at home. The doctors, midwives, and nursing staff should be respected and admired for their expertise and their willingness to help in these difficult moments. If your midwife transports you, it is because the miracle of modern medicine is something you absolutely need to take advantage of, and it is such a blessing that you have access to it.

Always remember, when you planned a home birth but need to be at the hospital, it's because you have a complication. It is an absolute miracle, a blessing, and a phenomenal gift that we don't have to die in childbirth because of something our medical professionals now know how to fix.

> Always remember, when you need to be at the hospital because you have a complication it is an absolute miracle, a blessing, and a phenomenal gift that we don't have to die in childbirth because of something our medical professionals now know how to fix.

If I deem it necessary to go to the hospital for complications during the birth, I go with my clients and stay with them. I run interference, I interpret, I work with hospital staff to inform them of the mother's wishes, and I serve as an advocate the whole way.

It is important, however, to understand that once you are at the hospital, your midwife is no longer in charge. The relationship between doctor and midwife may be at times adversarial. Ultimately, we need to be grateful that we have somewhere to go in these times of need, and we need to be cooperative.

If you are planning a hospital birth and experience these complications, the response from the hospital will be the same.

Reason for Hospital Transport: Non-Progression of Labor

The number one cause for going to the hospital is **non-progression of labor**. This is where you are actively in labor and contracting continually, but dilation is just not moving fast enough for the baby's safety, or not moving along at all.

Exhaustion

There are many reasons for non-progression of labor, but the most common cause is **exhaustion**. I can't tell you how many people I have had to take to the hospital because they have had days and days of warm-up labor with no sleep that just wiped them out, and they did not have the energy it took once they were actually in full-on labor.

Baby Is Too Big

The second reason for non-progression is having **too big of a baby**. If you do have a baby that is too big to fit through your pelvis, we will do everything we can, the hospital will do everything they can, but most of the time if that is the case you are more likely to get a c-section.

Poor Positioning

The third reason for non-progression is **poor positioning of the baby**, which can also create a stall in labor. Every now and then the baby will come down through the pelvis in a weird way, with the head off to the side, which is called *asynclitic*. If that is the case, it makes for a very, very difficult labor. Sometimes I can reposition the head during a vaginal exam. A posterior baby can also make labor be much more difficult. I always work to reposition the baby before resorting to transport.

Fear

The fourth reason I see for non-progression is **fear or resistance to pain**. Occasionally I do see women who just have a very hard time with their fear or with dealing with the pain, and they just can't handle the feelings or intensity. You know, every woman's path is different and sometimes this does happen, and you just let go and get help, and remember that you can always try again and do it differently the next time around if you choose to have more babies. I do not want you to judge yourself if that ends up happening. I really believe exercise, sex, affirmations, visualizations, meditation, education, and communication are ways to build your confidence and find a way to surrender to this process. If you are unable to work through the fear, the hospital has interventions that can help you.

Gaining Too Much Weight or Not Being in Good Shape

The final reason I see for non-progression is due to **not exercising adequately during the pregnancy or gaining too much weight**. Remember, exercise and sex are the ways to create oxytocin and endorphin production. Endorphins are your body's natural pain killers and oxytocin is the hormone that controls and produces contractions. You want to build your endorphin and oxytocin production through exercise and sex, and when you do so it is much more likely you will have an easier, faster, and less painful birth.

Reason for Hospital Transport: A Blood Pressure Problem

The second most common cause of going to the hospital is **blood pressure problems**. To prevent this, do not gain too much weight (I recommend 20–40 pounds; 20 if you are over your ideal weight and closer to 40 if you are underweight), exercise regularly, eat well, drink lots of fluids, and take your vitamins. All of these things will help to prevent blood pressure issues. High blood pressure is very serious, though, and can cause seizures that can detach the placenta and kill both you and the baby, so we do not take it lightly.

If we cannot get your blood pressure under control at home and do have to go to the hospital, they will administer an IV with drugs or magnesium sulfate and/or give you an epidural. Both of these lower your blood pressure significantly and work very well to alleviate risk. If your blood pressure gets too high, a c-section is necessary.

Reason for Hospital Transport: Fetal Distress

The third most common cause of going to the hospital is **fetal distress**. This is pretty rare, though. Fetal distress and blood pressure problems make up fewer than 10 percent of my transports, less than 1 percent of my total clients.

Cord Compression

Cord compression is the number one cause of serious fetal distress. Cord compression decreases the oxygen content going to the baby and depresses their respiratory and neurological functions.

When the head is born, I feel for the cord, and if it is indeed around the neck, I slip it around the head the opposite way to release it from the baby's neck, then the partner can still catch the baby. Having the cord wrapped around the neck is actually quite common; about 25 percent of babies are born this way. Occasionally the cord can present a problem, though, and sometimes it can even be wrapped around the neck a few times, causing distress to the baby and I have to really work to unwrap it. On rare occasions I have had to cut the cord to get the baby out, but that is very rare indeed.

Placental Insufficiency

Placental insufficiency can also cause fetal distress and that is where the placenta is just old and used up and not adequately supplying the baby with oxygen like it should. This is one of the reasons doctors are all up in arms about babies being "late" after 40 weeks. They very well may have patients that are malnourished and not in shape. You are different from a typical hospital patient, though, because you are taking all the supplements, eating well, drinking your fluids, and taking really, really good care of yourself. You are armed with the Vitamin E, C, essential fatty acids, and omegas that are phenomenal for keeping the placenta healthy during this process.

Reason for Hospital Transport: Bleeding

The fourth most common cause of going to the hospital is **bleeding**. I cannot remember the last time I transported anyone to the hospital for postpartum bleeding, but I have had a few clients who were bleeding in labor in a way that concerned me, and I transported them. There is a situation where the placenta can partially pull away during labor, it's called a partial abruption.

There is also a condition called placenta previa and it is where the placenta is down low and as the cervix opens an edge of the placenta is exposed and more bleeding occurs than is normal. Postpartum bleeding is the least common cause for going to the hospital because I have many of the drugs available at the hospital on hand with me and use them as needed at home. Hidden **internal bleeding** somewhere that you cannot see can also cause fetal distress, but this is also rare.

Reason for Hospital Transport: Placental Problems

Placental problems are the next reason you might have to go to the hospital. I cannot remember the last time I had to go to the hospital for that, but very occasionally there is a defective part of the placenta that is permanently attached to the uterus, called *placental accreta*, and occasionally a part of the placenta that has fused itself through the muscle completely, *placental percreta*. There also can be a succinct lobe, which is an extra lobe formed off the main portion of the placenta and when the placenta comes out, the lobe stays, and you have to have a surgical procedure to have it removed.

Reason for Hospital Transport: Infection

The sixth reason you might have to go to the hospital is due to an **infection**. If your waters have been broken or leaking for an extended amount of time it is possible for you to get an infection. I have not had that happen. The only infections I have seen in my clients are with waters intact and it has always been a weird fluke of an infection. In this case you would go to the hospital and get IV antibiotics and generally this would take care of any infections.

There are a few other very rare things that can happen that would also need hospital intervention.

What to Expect at the Hospital

If I must transport a client to the hospital, I go with them and take my lovely spiritual energy along with us. In my experience they start an IV immediately and the doctor or nurse/nurse midwife comes in soon after to check the woman out. They do not stay in the room; they come and go as needed. The nurses are generally very nice but can change up to three times during your labor as they generally have eight-to-ten-hour shifts. If for any reason you get a nurse who is not nice or whom you do not like, ask for someone else to attend to you.

I always bring my client's chart with us and try to go through as much of the health histories and paperwork with the nurses as possible. If we go in for non-progression, they always give you an epidural and Pitocin in an IV and then hook you up to a fetal monitor. Almost everyone going in for a complication is going to have a monitor on and you need it, it is very important to watch the baby closely.

A fetal monitor is used extensively in a hospital birth. The monitor has two sections typically, each comprised of a belt and a disc, each connected to the receiver. One belt holds a disc onto your abdomen and monitors your contractions, and the second is placed toward the bottom of your abdomen to monitor the baby's heartbeat. Most of the time these monitors are synced with displays in the nurse's station so the baby's heartbeat and how the contractions are going can be watched at all times, even

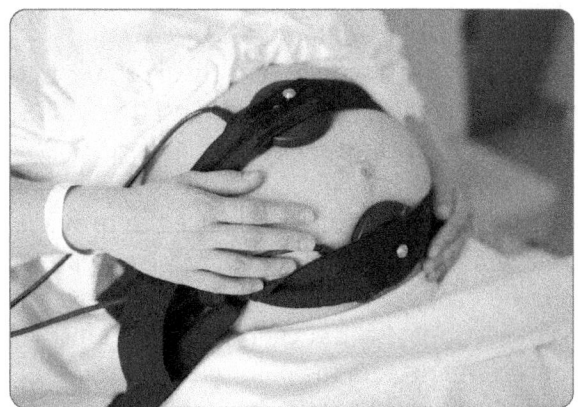

Fetal Monitor at the Hospital

when the nurse or attendants are not able to be in the room.

If you're getting Pitocin, you are going to have to be monitored. Pitocin has dangers associated with it, and of course labor has some dangers associated with it. The hospital has to monitor the baby to make sure that everything is going well. Some hospitals use Bluetooth monitors, which allow you to be upright and moving. If you are having a natural birth at the hospital without an epidural and without Pitocin, those are wonderful.

About 80 percent of my clients that go to the hospital get an epidural. Again, most of my clients are going in for non-progression and are looking at a Pitocin-induced remainder of the labor and birth, and at that point I definitely suggest an epidural so you can rest and dilate. This way you are more rested, and you may even be able to sleep. You want to have enough energy to push your sweet baby out and to bond with them after the birth.

If you're planning a hospital birth, induction and augmentation rates in the US are quite high, so this may also apply to you.

Epidural

An epidural is a type of anesthesia that involves injecting medication into the epidural space around the spinal cord. Epidurals are only done in a hospital setting. They are commonly used to provide pain relief during childbirth, but they can also be used for other procedures, such as c-sections, back surgery, cancer pain management, and for pain relief after surgery. An epidural works by blocking the transmission of pain signals from the nerves in the lower back to the brain. This allows the person to feel pressure, but not pain. Epidurals can be adjusted to provide different levels of pain relief, depending on the person's needs. The initial injection of the numbing medication prior to the epidural being administered can be briefly painful—a stick and a sting—but most women say that the pain is minimal. After that, you will only feel pressure and an occasional twinge-y feeling.

The epidural medication takes about 15 minutes to start working and can be left in place for up to 24 hours. You will have to lie flat on your back for a period of time after the epidural is placed so it can evenly distribute. If you move to your side too soon gravity can make the numbing medication drain to one side and you will not have adequate relief. You will also have a urinary catheter that stays in your bladder to empty it since you cannot feel anything. You may have some numbness or tingling in your legs after the epidural, but this usually goes away within a few hours.

The epidural rate for childbirth in the United States is 67 percent, although it is more likely between 70–80 percent in many areas and for some populations due to a number of factors including access to care. I believe it is important to be informed about the potential risks associated with the procedure, such as:

- Headache
- Low blood pressure
- Nausea and vomiting
- Numbness or tingling in the legs
- Infection
- Difficulty urinating

A risk that is not talked about near enough is that if the mother's blood pressure drops rapidly it can cause a serious drop in the baby's heart rate and lead to an emergency c-section. One of the ways the hospital tries to prevent this risk is by always making sure that the mother is super well hydrated with significant amounts of IV fluids. This helps to prevent the mother's blood pressure from dropping. Another issue to consider is that with an epidural you can only be in the bed because your legs no longer function. An epidural on its own can slow down labor, likely due to the numbing nature of the procedure and the effects it has on the nerves and nervous system. The fact that you are immobilized compounds this problem even more. If labor slows down too much this will lead to non-progression and an eventual c-section.

Scientific studies have shown it is incredibly important to be active and moving during labor.[158] When you get an epidural movement is off the table. Epidurals are very beneficial, as are inductions and even c-sections, when they are necessary. These can be lifesaving, but we should not be *starting* the labor and birth process with an induction and an epidural that can potentially end in a c-section.

Other risks from epidurals—about which birthing women are rarely, if ever, informed—include the fact that the medication in the epidural affects the baby and often makes newborns "floppy" at birth.[159] Epidurals can also result in a temperature rise in the mother; often doctors don't know whether that rise reflects an infection-induced fever or is simply a result of the epidural.[160] As a result, many newborns whose mothers have fevers at birth (10–15 percent) are given antibiotics, which have been associated with harmful alterations in babies' gut microbiomes.[161]

Other Methods of Pain Management

There are several types of pain relief available at the hospital and sometimes at birth centers that can be used before an epidural is resorted to. Some of these are mild sedatives. If it's really early in your labor, Stadol, Demerol, or Toradol can be used to take the edge off. Sometimes the early part of active labor can be very difficult, and these medications can aid you in coping and getting used to the sensations. They do not take all the pain away but will take the edge off and make you sleepy. This can be helpful if you need to rest or are laboring in the middle of the night. If you need pain management, the time to get it is in early labor or the earlier part of active labor. Something to consider is that these medications last several hours and if given too late in the process can cause the baby to be born very sleepy, unable to breathe easily, and less able to bond or breastfeed.

Nitrous oxide is another option for pain management within the hospital as well as in some birth centers. It is a gas that is administered by mask and is typically used at the dentist's office. The mother has to hold the mask to her face during the contraction so she is unable to inhale too much of the gas as her hand will drop and the mask will fall away. Women have spoken very highly of the effects of this, which are short lived but helpful. It's important to note that the mask is never tied to your head or you could get more than you and the baby are supposed to. This relief can be a blessing.

Very few midwives offer nitrous oxide at home. There may be a few, but not many. I do carry some pain medications, but I give them incredibly rarely and almost always for pre-labor or in very intense early labor.

I think it is so important to provide you with all of this information, including the risks and benefits, so you understand the different options available to you and your family. Everyone does not have to do it the same way. This is *your* ideal, perfect birth!

Caesarean Section (C-Section)

If the nurse administers Pitocin and after many hours there is not any progress, the doctor usually suggests a c-section, and I would agree. The main complications that would require a c-section are as follows.

- Failure to progress.
- Severe high blood pressure that can't be controlled by medication.
- Persistent malpresentation leading to arrest of labor.
- Fetal distress in a baby who will not respond favorably to any of the often-effective therapies.
- Unexplained bleeding.

 For a planned home birth, the partner and I both go into the operating room with the woman. For a planned hospital birth, your doula may or may not be admitted to join you if you have one, based on the hospital's policies, and your partner will most likely be encouraged to join you. The hospital staff boosts the epidural and then it takes about 10–15 minutes to get the baby out and another 30–40 minutes to repair the uterus and abdominal muscles before the mother is taken to the labor, delivery & recovery room (LDR) or a separate recovery room.

Most hospitals will allow the baby to come up into your arms behind the drapes they use for cleanliness so the mom can bond with her baby for a few moments before they go to the nursery. Once you've had some time to bond with your baby, it's good to go ahead and do the weighing measuring and initial newborn procedures while your incision is being repaired.

The partner goes to the nursery with the baby after it is born while you are being repaired, and then, as long as everything is fine after you have been briefly checked out, the partner and baby come back to the recovery room. We will initiate breastfeeding once everyone is back to the recovery room or back to the LDR.

Two to three hours after the birth you are transferred to the postpartum floor to a room and your partner and baby can stay with you. In my experience, hospitals are very supportive of rooming in and being together through the postpartum process. If the partner can't stay, you must have a friend or family member who can stay with you during c-section recovery.

The hospital that I transport to in Austin offers a family centered c-section, where we are able to have the baby stay with the mom and dad in the operating room without being transported to the nursery— as long as the baby is doing all right of course and there are no factors with the baby that would require other interventions. The baby can nurse unlimitedly if the mother is feeling up to it.

There is also a relatively new phenomenon called the *gentle cesarean*, in which either the surgical drapes are lowered, or they are made of clear plastic or have a clear plastic window sewn into them so the mother can watch the birth of her baby, who is then immediately placed into her arms, or she is allowed to reach down and

Robbie: When my 26-hour labor with my first child, during which I felt completely embodied, ended in a cesarean, I was beyond shocked at the sudden and total mind-body separation that I experienced when the epidural took effect. This separation was also visual: I could not even *see* the body that I could not feel. Being "awake and aware," I asked the obstetrician to *please* place the curtain blocking my view above my head so I could bear witness to the birth of my daughter, but this was in 1979—a time when such an idea was "beyond conception." I would have given anything to have a gentle cesarean like the ones described above!

pull her baby up to her chest. And just as in the "family-centered" cesarean described above, the mother can breastfeed for as long as she likes. In case you end up having a cesarean birth, or choose to schedule it, ask your hospital well in advance if this option is offered there, and if it isn't, you can serve as a change agent by informing your hospital about the gentle cesarean and asking them to implement it. You can find plenty of information about this on the internet.

While many obstetricians say that c-sections are extremely easy to perform, they are often challenging for the mother. Sometimes during the procedure, you might feel some nausea and can even experience some vomiting due to nerves being stimulated that make you very, very queasy. But as long as you're doing fine, the baby can nurse while the doctors are doing the repair, and then you, your partner, and your newborn baby can go back to the LDR to continue breastfeeding in a more comfortable environment. You may want to find out if your local hospitals offer this in case you end up with a c-section.

We'll talk about c-section recovery in *Volume II*.

When Are Interventions a Good Idea?

Let's talk for a moment about when some of these interventions are a good idea. I believe an induction or intervention is likely indicated if:

- You are past 42 Weeks and not having any impending signs of labor.
- When the baby is not thriving.

- If you have placental problems like placenta previa.
- There is not enough amniotic fluid (*oligohydramnios*).
- Your blood pressure is too high.

There are other situations that we could discuss where an induction is indicated, but these are the major ones to note. Your care provider will help you to identify these types of situations. I want to say that if you do have an induction, Pitocin can be a relentless climb and increasingly painful, and an epidural can bring relief.

If you are transported to the hospital from a home or birth center birth for non-progression of labor, nine times out of ten you are going to have to be augmented with Pitocin because the birth is not progressing as it should. This can also happen after laboring naturally in the hospital. There comes a point, sometimes, when you may need help. In these cases, I always recommend an epidural. Most of these women have been seriously laboring for many hours and they are very tired. The labor needs to be helped along and an epidural will allow them to sleep through the hours and hours of work and contractions they are still facing before they are dilated fully. It is important to remember that women in this situation still have to push the baby out and have the energy left for bonding and breastfeeding.

The Mindset to Adopt if You Transport

I have heard that in premodern times about 2–3 percent of moms and 2–3 percent of babies died in childbirth. I have about a 6–7 percent c-section rate for my clients and I believe that this is representative of everybody that would have died in ages past, without the lifesaving medical intervention we have access to now. In 1970, the c-section rate in the US was 5.5 percent.[162]

In ages past, women of childbearing age died primarily from one of four things (though there are certainly many other less likely complications that were deadly as well):

- High blood pressure.
- Hemorrhage.
- Postpartum infection.
- A too large a baby/baby that was in an undeliverable position.

These four things were responsible for the majority of the mortalities in childbirth, and now we have remedies for all of them. With good care there's less reason for maternal mortality in most instances.

If you have a planned home birth end up in the hospital, don't look at it as a failure or a really bad thing that has happened to you, look at it as if you are one of the lucky people who has benefited from the technology of birth instead of being oppressed by it. You are being saved by the miracle of modern medicine!

If you have a planned home birth and end up in the hospital, don't look at it as a failure or a really bad thing that has happened to you, look at it as if you are one of the lucky people who has benefited from the technology of birth instead of being oppressed by it. You are being saved by the miracle of modern medicine!

The technology that is overused now then becomes lifesaving and wonderful. I had two of my own planned home births end up in the hospital and I had to remember that this was part of my baby's perfect birth, it just included going to the hospital, which I hadn't planned.

Birth is a spiritual experience, even when it is complicated, and I want you to remember that your beautiful spiritual birth is happening, no matter where you are experiencing it. I always give my clients a home birth certificate with the baby's footprints on it. They had a home birth, they just had to go to the hospital to finish it up. Don't be afraid, take deep breaths, and remember that this is all just information to educate and inform you.

How Long You'll Be There

Most people stay in the hospital for one to two days following the birth, but it's possible you may not be released for three or four days. Please be prepared.

There will be a lot of hospital staff traipsing in and out of your room; I encourage you to limit personal visitors to the barest minimum until you return home, so you can get as much rest as possible during your stay at the hospital and spend as much time as possible with your baby.

What to Do in the Case of Sudden Childbirth

 I love to tell people, "You should be so lucky if your baby just falls out because it is just a snap!" It usually means everything is just perfect, but it can be disconcerting to the partners that the baby could come without their midwife on hand, or before they can make it to the birthing center or hospital. I have found that after partners hear about sudden childbirth, they are more diligent to make sure to call their midwife and make sure she's aware when labor starts.

Many years ago, I received a call from a father-to-be saying it was time for me to come, things were really happening. Contractions were four minutes apart and getting a lot stronger. I said I would head on out, and I reminded him of what to do, the things he had learned in my childbirth classes so he could be ready. I put my birth kit in the car, called the apprentices, and

headed out as fast as I could. This couple lived out in the country, and it was a good hour-long drive for me to get there.

I finally arrived and went down a long driveway in the woods. As I pulled around the corner, I could see the dad standing in the driveway, and I thought, *Well, I guess things aren't as far along as he thought.* I got out of the car and asked, "How are things going?"

He said, "Oh, I think we need to get everything in the house," and suddenly, from where I stood in the driveway, I could hear the mother and the tone of her vocalizations told me she was in a really serious way. I told the father what to grab and ran into the house. When I got to the mother, I could see the baby's head. I reached down and the baby fell out into my hands. This woman could have had her baby completely alone. It was not even two

---

Aleah: My first baby was born after less than five hours in labor and my second was born in about an hour-and-a-half. I do not wish a super quick labor on anyone. I don't wish an 18-hour labor or 24-, 36-, or 48-hour labor on anyone either. People say, "Oh, how lucky you are!" but having labor go that fast is like having a freight train hit you. I was completely and utterly in another world. I was not here. It was very hard to be present for it or to have any kind of enjoyment. There were no moments of anticipation like, "Oh, yes! The baby's coming!" No time for that moment of realization, no time to get comfortable with the idea that you're in labor and your baby's coming soon.

It was very hard for me, and I did not really get a chance to enact my birth plan or have much time to be supported by my partner or other support people because everything was so rushed. I have slightly jokingly told my husband that if we have another baby, I will likely sneeze them out and he will be employing what we learned for sudden childbirth in MariMikel's classes.

minutes after I got in the door before the baby was born.

In my heart, I felt that father had let his fear get the best of him. As a result, I strove to make my classes more educational to help the partners to better understand their role. Partners, you must stay by your woman's side. Don't go to another room, don't wait for your midwife in the driveway. Stay there and help her.

If the mother says that the baby is coming or she feels like pushing, this means that the baby is coming *fast*. Please try to remain calm. Birth is a natural occurrence. Most babies do not need any help and many non-professional people have caught babies. I definitely prefer for women to have someone experienced and knowledgeable on hand as your first option, but sometimes babies come very quickly.

Important Steps for the Partner to Take

 This section is primarily for my clients who are prepared for a home birth and whose labor is proceeding faster than anticipated. They have taken childbirth classes. They have birth equipment on hand, and I am on the phone with them, talking them through every step of the way as I am on the way to them.

While I prepare all my clients for a sudden childbirth, when it happens (which is not too often) it's because it's going so fast that no one can get there, and is often an indication that it's going to go well, but that is not always the case. If your baby is emerging suddenly, or if you as the partner can see that the baby is coming too fast to get anyone there or to make it to the hospital or the birth center, this is what you're going to do. Otherwise get help!

1. **First, call EMS (911)** and tell them there's a baby coming. They will have people come and help you and then take you to the hospital afterward.

   It's important that you call EMS. This is not in any way shape or form designed to encourage people to have their babies at home unattended. I have a lot of anxiety when I hear about unattended birth. In the almost 50 years that I have been catching babies, well over 3,000 births, I have saved many lives. That is because I am educated, skilled, equipped, experienced, and I have excellent backup. I don't say this to scare you, but to make sure that you are prepared. If there is a serious hemorrhage or the baby comes out stunned and unable to start breathing, you have to have skilled people with you to administer the anti-hemorrhage drugs and to help a baby that needs resuscitation.

2. Ensure that the mother is in a **safe place, preferably her bed**. Get the mother to lay down immediately. **Lay her on her left side**. Keep talking to her throughout the time you are setting up.

   When the mother is lying on her left side, the oxygen is increased to the baby somewhat. Lying down often takes the pressure of the head off of the cervix and will slow labor down a little bit. You are trying to buy time to let your care provider or EMS get to you. Make sure she is lying down.

3. **Call your midwife or your provider** and follow their instructions.

4. Quickly **get help from a friend, neighbor, or even a stranger.** I have flagged down a mail carrier before and entreated them to help me catch a baby. It is important to have a second person to help you. This person will be used only if necessary to call for further aid or as a second pair of hands if required.

5. **Unlock the entrance door!** (Please don't make your midwife break a window.)

6. **Start boiling scissors** (for cutting the cord) in a shallow pan with a small amount of water. Cover the scissors with at least ¾" of water. They must boil for twenty minutes; set a timer.

7. **Boil another pot of water** for hot packs and cleaning. Set a timer!

8. Bring **two bowls** into the bedroom, fill one halfway with hot water and reserve the other one to catch the placenta in.

9. **Wash your hands** thoroughly.

10. Make sure the **bedroom is quite warm** for the baby's arrival: 80–85°F. Set the thermostat higher. Sometimes you just need to close the AC vent in the birthing room. Bring in a portable source of heat if it's cold and you have time.

11. If you have planned for a home birth, **gather your birth supplies,** and place them on the bed. Open

them up and take everything out, placing all items within your reach, next to the mother in the bed. It is most important to have **gauze, gloves, and suction devices** in your immediate reach. Open the bulb syringe, gloves, and DeLee ahead of time. Get a bottle of **olive oil** as well. Use the empty box for garbage by folding the lid in. If you were not planning to have a home birth, gather what you can from this list.

12. Place a **chair next to the bed**, so you have a place to put the olive oil (with the lid on and ready) and the bowl with hot water. A chair will remain stable whereas the bed will not. Put six pieces of gauze into the hot water.

13. Put a **disposable underpad** beneath her bottom, plastic side down, and place a large, clean towels on top of it so the baby can come out onto this. The towel will absorb the amniotic fluid and keep it from going everywhere.

14. Also have a few **baby blankets** ready to dry the baby off immediately. After the baby is born you will dry them off, put the used blankets aside, then use a new, clean blanket to cover the baby on the mother's skin.

15. Wait for the mother to have an involuntary urge to push and check to see if you can see the baby's head. **If you can see the head**, don't have her push with too much extra effort. Put on gloves (or don't). **Massage the perineum** with a few

tablespoons of olive oil and **support the perineum** with hot gauze from the bowl of water. Make sure and let the baby come out and don't hold it back.

16. When the head is born, **wipe the face with gauze** and **check to see if the cord is around the neck**. If the cord is around the neck, loop it over the baby's head or slide it down the body as the baby comes out.

17. To **deliver the body,** wait for the next contraction, then pull the head down gently but firmly until the shoulder can be seen. Then lift up and out and the rest of the body will be born! The baby MUST come out soon after the head is born. (If the baby is not born in the next contraction, change the mother's position to hands and knees and try to move the baby's shoulder from behind the pubic bone.)

18. Once the baby is out, **put the baby on the mom's belly** with the head lower than the rest of the body.

19. Quickly and vigorously **rub the baby** with a baby blanket to dry them off and to also stimulate breathing. If they are not breathing, rub the spine vigorously, slap the feet, talk to them, and set an example for them by breathing very deeply.

20. You and the mom should also *call the baby*. Ask the spirit to choose to come into the body. Many midwives encourage the parents to do this. First, it does no harm, and second, it often works, and if it does, then

there is no need for further efforts to get the baby to breathe.

21. **If the baby does not breathe with stimulus**, cover their mouth and nose with your mouth, and breathe out just what is in your cheeks. The baby's head has to be tilted back a bit. Be careful not to put too much air pressure into the baby as this could damage the baby's lungs. Sometimes they are a bit in shock and the first breath requires a herculean effort on their part; they could need you to inflate their lungs for them to give them a boost.

If they aren't breathing within 60 seconds, call 911 or emergency services outside the US.

22. After respiration is established, put a **dry blanket, hat, and booties** on the baby to keep them warm.

23. Do not pull on the cord, and there is no need to cut the cord right away.

24. **Birth the placenta**. The placenta must be detached in order for it to be born. This can take 10-15 minutes or more. If the mother feels the placenta in her vagina or if she is feeling a contraction, have her try to push a little. If the placenta does not come in the next contraction, have her squat over a bowl to get the placenta out.

If you are working with a midwife, leave the placenta alone; don't do anything you don't have to do. If the placenta is obviously coming out, let it happen. Most of the time it is not going to come out until a skilled person helps it. It is a little trickier than it looks, and many times takes longer than you might think.

25. Keep the mother lying down and calm with the baby on her chest but **do not start breastfeeding before the placenta is born** or someone arrives to help. I have had women begin breastfeeding because the placenta was taking a while, and initiating breastfeeding clamped the uterus down around the placenta and we had to transport to the hospital because it would not come out. Most babies need a period of time after the birth to calm down from the pain in their face and body due to the big squeeze. They need that period of time before the placenta comes out to recover before they start breastfeeding.

26. After the placenta is out, **massage the mother's uterus** to help it clamp down. Most of the time the placenta detaches fairly quickly after the birth of the baby. Sometimes it can be a while. Leave it alone until somebody arrives.

If your baby comes really fast, it can be pretty scary for both the mom and the partner. I just want to encourage you that when birth happens this fast it is because everything is pretty perfect. I am not teaching you about sudden childbirth to scare you. As with this entire guidebook, I am sharing this information with the purpose of empowering you and easing your heart and mind. As always, relax, surrender, and breathe. You've got this! Don't forget to sit back and enjoy your baby. Birth is a natural and beautiful experience.

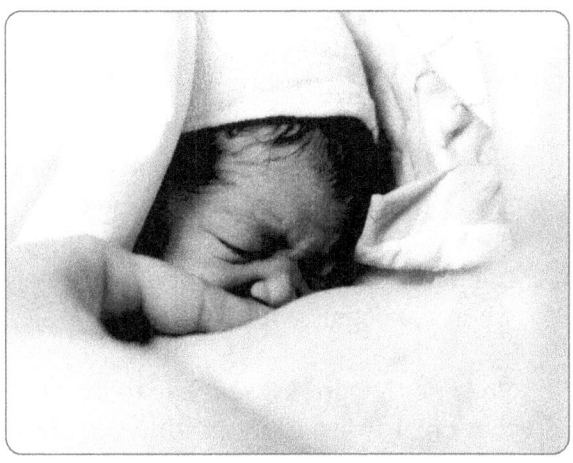

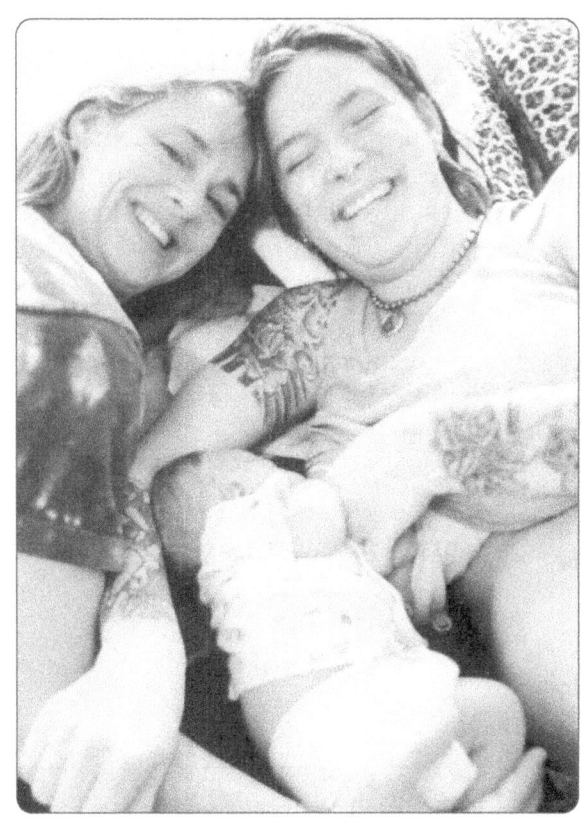

BEFORE I LEAVE YOU

Thank you for sharing your pregnancy journey with me. I truly hope I have offered some assistance, perspective, and understanding for you as you have traveled this path. I know that by reading this book you have the agency to have your own ideal, perfect birth.

I hope by now you have begun to have a deep appreciation for how very different your life becomes with the transformation that is catalyzed at conception and realized in birth. I fervently hope that the real message that has come through in this book is one about the astonishing beauty of the process, the creation of sacred space, the joy and mystical nature of new beginnings, and the profound transformation when life begins anew.

The one thought I would like to leave you with is that this is a spiritual process, one that creates sacredness within your heart, your life, and your family. A precious baby coming into your life is a new beginning and transformation on every level possible. Some of the changes you will be prepared for, but the truth is that there is so much more to come.

Most of us have never spent a whole lot of time around new humans. I deeply encourage you to prepare for your postpartum period well before you give birth. For decades my clients have been asking me to write a guidebook for them, so they have something to refer to when they have questions about their newborn, and so they have support at their fingertips for those first few months. *The Book of Birth Volume II: Your Postpartum Journey through the Fourth Trimester* is that guidebook. If you have found my guidance beneficial through your pregnancy, I urge you to prepare just as thoroughly for the time after your baby arrives. It's best for you to read it during the end of your pregnancy.

And now my dears, I have put absolutely everything helpful I could into these pages. The rest is up to you. I send you so much light and love as you walk your own path.

Blessings and light,

Marimikel Potter

PS—I almost forgot to invite you to sign up to get my newsletter. It's free to you, and chock full of great pregnancy tips and reminders. Plus, you'll be among the first to find out when my new books come out. Here's where you can sign up: https://sendfox.com/marimikelpotter

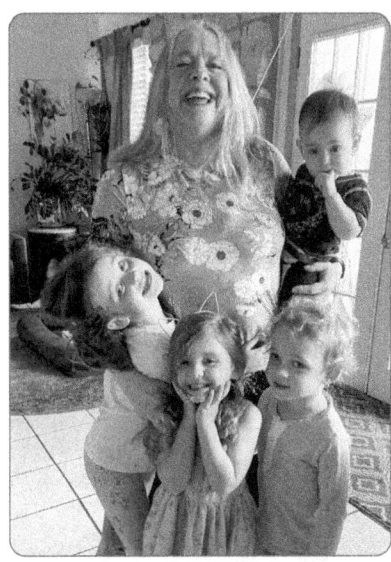

*MariMikel with Four of Her
Six Grandchildren*

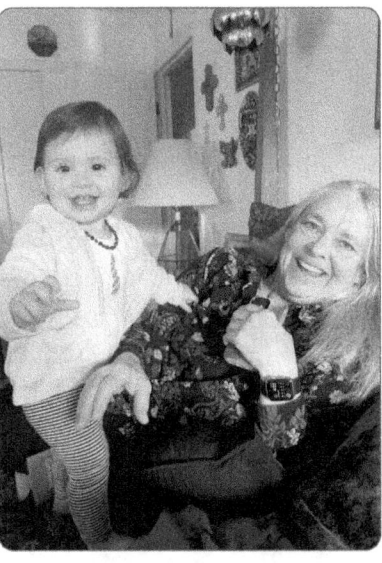

*MariMikel with
Granddaughter Téa*

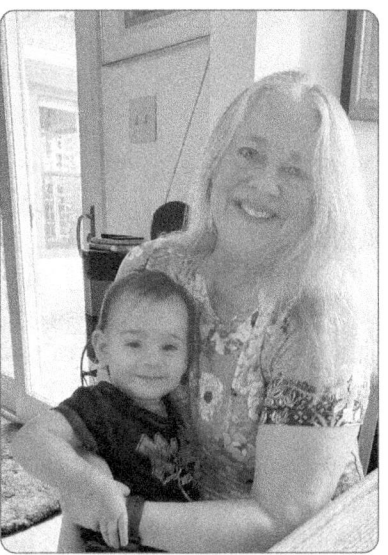

*MariMikel with
Granddaughter Ava*

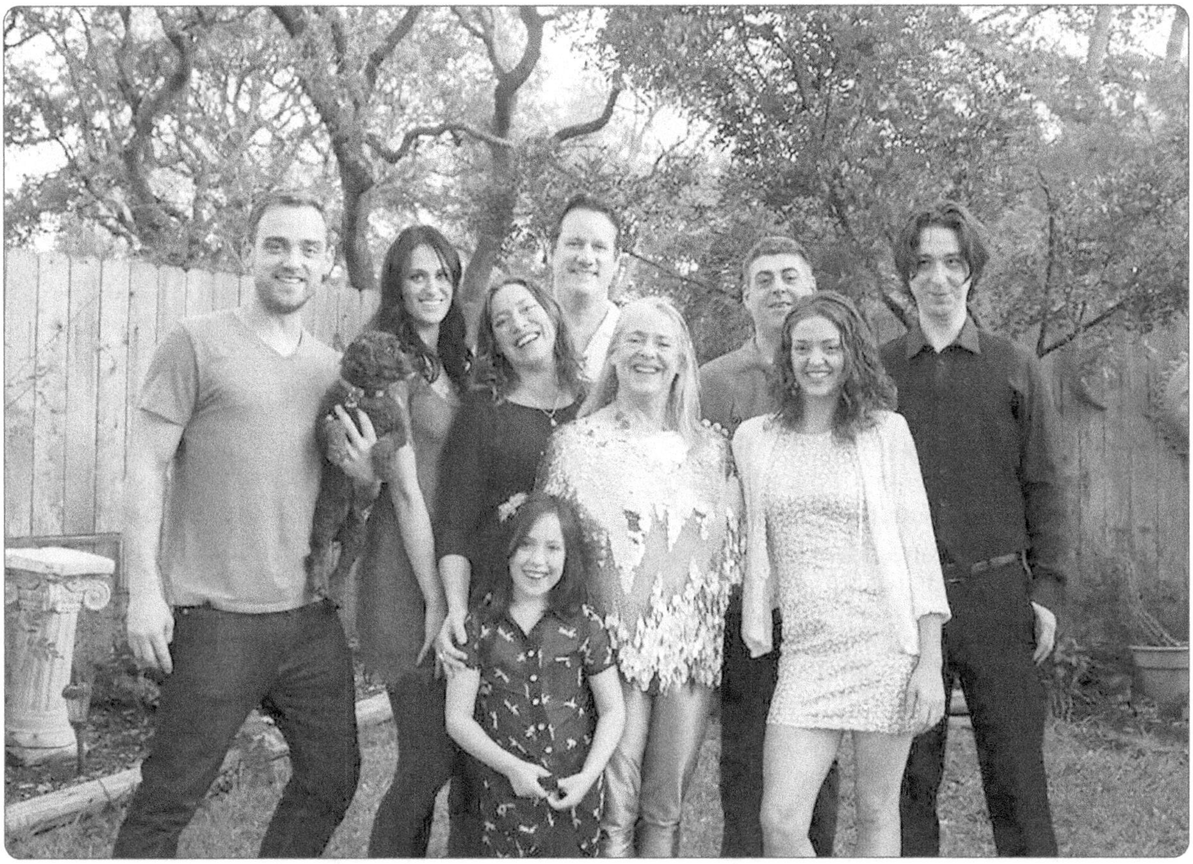

MariMikel with Her Children, Son- and Daughter-In-Law, and Granddaughter

EPILOGUE

What I think desperately needs to happen is that more women need to go into midwifery careers—both as certified nurse-midwives (CNMs) and as certified professional midwives (CPMs). We need lots more midwives. I can't stress this issue strongly enough. At this juncture—and it changes quite frequently—the US is 57th in the world in infant maternal mortality/morbidity. Uzbekistan and Romania have better statistics than the United States, and it's really a serious problem.

A lot of it is due to racial injustice. Women of Color are marginalized in the healthcare system and just given the dregs of decent care. We can completely transform these maternal statistics in a short period of time through midwifery care because the sorry standard of care in the US is simply not the way midwives practice—any of them. Instead, most US midwives practice what is internationally known as "the midwifery model of care." This deeply humanistic and holistic model stresses knowledge about how to best support the normal physiology of birth, how to identify risks during pregnancy, birth, and the postpartum period, and how best to handle them. It is all about compassion, relationships, and caring for the mother and her family.

If the idea of becoming a midwife appeals to you, I urge you to look to the following organizations to help explore and develop your career.

The Path to Midwifery as a Career

We need lots of CNMs to work in hospitals and lots more CPMs to care for women who are planning to give birth in their own homes. Some CNMs and CPMs work in freestanding birth centers, and a few CNMs also attend home births. Occasionally, CNMs and CPMs establish joint practices in which they work together.

The Path to Home Birth Midwifery (CPM)

A coalition of doctors, nurses, pediatricians, neonatologists, midwives, and others developed a training program for midwives. This program is run by the Midwife Education Accreditation Council (MEAC), which credentials midwifery programs for CPMs.

The Midwives Alliance of North America (MANA) is the umbrella organization supporting all types of midwives but has a bigger focus and membership in the non-nurse midwife group (who tend to be home birth midwives). I helped to create the pathway toward becoming a CPM, which was further developed by the North American Registry of Midwives (NARM).

When you have graduated from a credentialed midwifery program, you can sit for the NARM exams and be certified as a certified professional midwife. You must then maintain your license with continuing education. That's what I am, a certified professional midwife. Most of the states in the United States use the CPM process as their way of credentialing midwives who are non-nurse midwives.

The Path to Hospital-Based Midwifery (CNM)

A CNM, or hospital-based midwife, must pursue a master's degree in nursing with a specialization in midwifery, and then they can pursue a working relationship in a hospital.

The Path to Becoming a Doula

We also need lots more pregnancy and postpartum doulas. If this support role is appealing to you, please search for doula training programs in your area.

My Plea to You

If this path is calling to you, I urge you to explore it. It is such a fulfilling and fantastic career. Please join us. It is the calling of a lifetime and I have led a life full of blessings because of it.

ACKNOWLEDGEMENTS

This book would never have come into being without the encouragement and financial support I received from Christy and Jim Finnegan. Knowing how much I wanted to write a book, they loaned me the funds to hire the support I needed to get it off the ground. Without their enormous belief in my message and extremely generous financial support, this book might never have transitioned from dream to reality. I thank you both from the bottom of my heart.

I want to take this opportunity to acknowledge the amazing and wonderful team that brought this endeavor to life. I have talked for over 40 years about wanting to write a book about how to have a healthy pregnancy, birth, and baby. Two years ago, my incredible daughter Aleah said, "Mom, you have got to stop talking about it and do something. It's time."

As I tried to put my thoughts together, I had the horrifying realization that I was a good-to-great teacher and speaker but a really lousy writer. Aleah reminded me that she had a nannied for a wonderful woman and friend who was an author and editor, and who truly knew this book business and all about it like we did not. Aleah suggested we call her to ask for her help to find someone who could assist us. The magnificent Alyssa Archer responded to Aleah's questions by enthusiastically saying, "What about me? I want to do it!"

Our very first meeting was magical and we all three immediately knew this triumvirate was really, truly a thing of destiny and absolutely the perfect combination. Alyssa used her amazing skillset and decades of experience to take over 40 years of written and oral material and pull it all together into a cohesive form. Alyssa's patience and endurance through this intense and extensive project has been above and beyond the call of duty.

Aleah was able to harness her years of apprenticeship with me and help me to refine the huge amount of material that was within me and needed to be born. Aleah's skills as a master's level social worker and project manager were just what we needed to shepherd this huge project.

Their incredible dedication, commitment, expertise, and belief in the world changing potential of this book has brought my dream to fruition. I will forever and always be grateful for the deep connection that has bonded us and will not only last a lifetime but will also light our way as we continue into the next Volume of *The Book of Birth*.

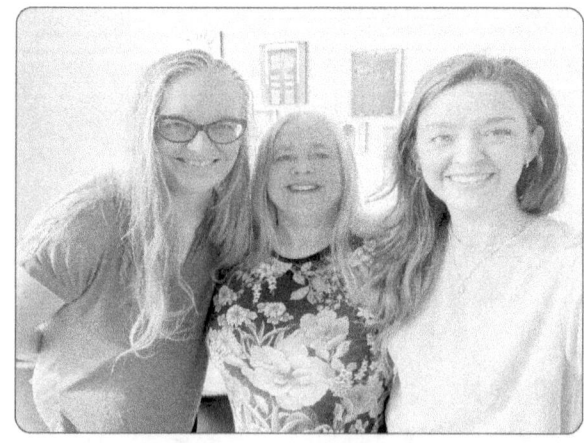

Alyssa, MariMikel, and Aleah

Thank you, thank you, thank you Aleah and Alyssa, from the bottom of my heart.

I often talk about how birth experiences are as unique as women are, and it's so helpful to be able to show that through the medium of story. Several women were courageous enough to share their very intimate birth stories with you in these pages, and I am grateful for their contributions. Thank you, Sarah, Penelope, Robbie, Justus, Sheryl, Monica, Aleah, and Juliana.

Pictures do tell a story of a thousand words, and I'm grateful to the women who allowed me to share their pregnancies and sometimes their very intimate birth experiences with you through their photos. Thank you, Aleah, Talitha, Robbie, Sheryl, Penelope, Monica, Sarah, and Olivia.

I called upon several excellent peers, clients, and friends to help me out by reading an early draft of this book and providing critical feedback. I want to thank Robbie Davis Floyd, Olivia P. Kramer, Hayley Raigosa, Faith Wallick, Raichel McDonald, Kersten Guarnaccia, Owen Gilbert, and Landon Shultz for your helpful critical reviews. Robbie especially went above and beyond and provided me with so much incredible feedback that helped to make this book more inclusive and more representative of different birth experiences. Many, many thanks.

Portions of the Breathing sections were contributed to heavily by my son, Deven, who teaches martial arts. Thank you, Deven!

I would like to thank my spiritual advisor, faithful friend, master prayer, and my minister of more than 40 years, Landon Shultz and his dear wife and my wonderful friend and singing companion, Kristin Shultz.

I would like to thank Dr. David Wagner, my chiropractor friend extraordinaire who has supported me physically, intellectually, and emotionally over many decades, and who contributed to the "Other Helpful Care Providers" section. David has been my chiropractor for over 20 years and has seen hundreds of my clients. His expertise, compassion, and intelligence has been incredible and amazing in my life, and my body is stronger for the chiropractic care that I have received from him. Thank you, David!

The portion of Appendix A about Grass-Fed Sources of Meat and Dairy was contributed to heavily by one of our Texas Hill Country ranchers, Olivia P. Kramer from Wild Herd Cattle + Kitchen. Thank you, Olivia!

I owe this book to the thousands of women and families that have trusted me to guide them through their pregnancies and births. I also want to acknowledge my incredible, wonderful children: Christian Horne, Talitha Green, Colin Chase, Aleah Ruiz, Deven Penn, and their amazing spouses. They and my six grandchildren are my reason for living. They are the impetus for my continued growth, work, service, and the source of joy on my life path.

I want to acknowledge those that have helped me so much in my life to be who I am and who helped me to get here today— my dearest friend Faith Wallick—she has been my bedrock, holding space for me in especially tumultuous times when the river of my emotions threatened to drown me.

I want to thank the midwives who have been so instrumental in my education and furthering as a midwife: Nikki Richardson, Allison Nash, Jane Goehring, Cathy Walker, Claire Bruno, Deborah Day, Julia Pirie, Mary Barnett, Michele Fitzgerald, and most recently Varshna Naramenchi. Rima Star and Robbie Davis Floyd have also been instrumental in my path. Without these women I would never have made it as a midwife.

I would also like to acknowledge St. David's Main hospital in Austin, Texas. This facility and the amazing nurses, doctors, and nurse midwives there have been a solid support for many decades. It has not always been a smooth road. But without them I could never have safely been a midwife. I have been educated, supported, encouraged, guided, and corrected, and my clients have received excellent care in their capable and loving hands. The doctors that have helped me the most in my path are the long departed and wonderful Dr. Milton Railey, Dr. Eldrid Kaplan, and Dr. Jonathan Buten, as well as Dr. Clive Polon, Dr. Jerry Hudson, Dr. David Ruiz, Dr. Robert Sorin, Dr. Mikal Love, Dr. David Berry, and a loving shoutout to the wonderful Dr. John Day.

There have been many, many more midwives and apprentices in my path that have helped me, educated me, and lifted me up. I thank each and every one of you and love you all.

There are many more people to thank and acknowledge; any omissions are my own error. I give each of you my love and appreciation.

Finally, dear reader, I am so grateful that you've chosen to spend your time with me in these pages. I love and appreciate you, and I wish you the very best on your journey toward your own ideal, perfect conception, pregnancy, and birth.

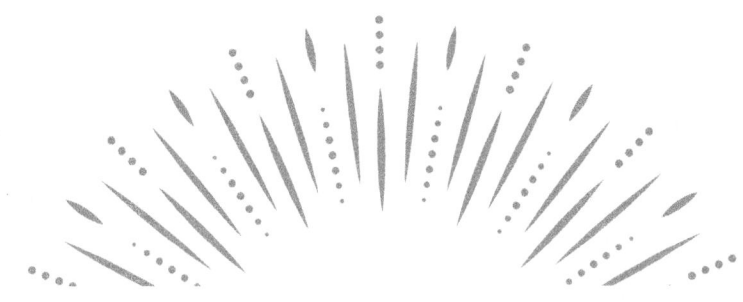

APPENDICES

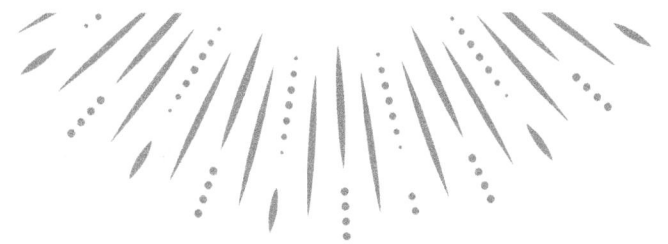

Appendix A: Product Recommendations & Vendors

Product Recommendations

I've got a few lists for you here of products I recommend you buy. For products where I don't have a brand preference, I have not specified one; any good brand will do. Where I do have a specific preference, I have stated it. This is not to say it's the only good brand, but it is one that I heartily recommend.

I also want you to know that I have limited these lists to include the things most pregnant women will need. You may have special needs, for special conditions. In those instances, I have left my recommendations in each specific related section in this book.

Make sure to give yourself time to look at all of your options for things you will need to purchase, and remember to have fun picking out all the items you will be using for yourself and your sweet baby over the next months and years!

Conception

Lubricants: ASTROGLIDE, K-Y True Feel Silicone Lubricant, K-Y Ultragel

Mattress topper—Tempur-Pedic

Menstrual pads—important to buy 100% cotton with no chemicals or PFAs!

Natural Medicine Chest Product Recommendations
These are some of the specific brands I use in my own natural medicine chest at home.

I am able to find most if not all of them in the natural section of my local grocery store. If you cannot find them or they are not available to you, I suggest looking at websites to determine whether the company producing the brand you are interested in ensures their products are what they say they are through third party verification and independent testing.

- Boiron Arnica tablets, gel and cream
- Boiron Oscillococcinum
- Gaia Oil of Oregano (liquid or capsules)
- Herb Pharm 4 Plant Part Blend Super Echinacea
- Herb Pharm Astragalus
- Nutribiotic Vegan Grapefruit Seed Extract Concentrate
- Sambucal Elderberry Syrup
- Sovereign Silver bio active Silver Hydrosol 10PPM

Probiotic—Garden of Life

Salt alternative—Gomasio

Snacks—Kind bars, Rx bars, Larabars, EPIC bars, Gluten-free crackers: Nut-Thins, Mary's Gone Crackers, or Simple Mills Almond flour crackers are all good products.

Vitamins, prenatal
While I recommend the vitamin regimen described in the Conscious Conception Nutrition Supplement section of this book,

if that's too much for you, try one of these (ranked from lowest to highest monthly cost). I've also included ideas for you to enhance the most egregious omissions from these multivitamins.

- Innate Baby and Me Multivitamin—supplement with calcium and magnesium.
- Perelel Prenatal Packs—supplement with probiotics in your first two trimesters.
- FullWell—supplement with iron.
- Needed Prenatal Multi—supplement with iron.
- Metagenics PlusOne Prenatal Packs—supplement with Vitamin D and iron.

Pregnancy

Belly support system/belly band—abdominal support band like the Loving Comfort Maternity support by CMO.

Ginger lozenges, suckers, or candied ginger for calming nauseated stomachs.

Protein powder: NaturesPlus SPIRU-TEIN

Vitamin E Oil for perineal massage

Birth

Check the Third Trimester equipment checklists for a complete birth supply list. The items that appear on this and the postpartum list are only the ones I have a brand preference for and strongly recommend.

Birthing pool—INTEX 57190EP Swim Center Inflatable Family Lounge Pool

Drinks/Electrolyte Replacement—Recharge

My clients buy a **home birth supply kit** from In His Hands birth supply (inhishands.com). If you are planning a home birth, work with your midwife to understand her preferred birth kit. I highly recommend this company, though, and you can order many of the things you'll need from them regardless of whether you are working with me or someone else. They carry the tinctures and herbal blends I suggest you buy, for example.

Postpartum

Check the Third Trimester equipment checklists for a complete postpartum supply list. The items that appear on this and the postpartum list are only the ones I have a brand preference for and strongly recommend.

Baby cream—Weleda brand

Breast pump—There are so many options out there these days, but here are some good options for hands-free, manual, and budget friendly pumps. I highly suggest you do research to find what is best for you. Keep in mind that your insurance will often pay for a pump so you can check with your insurance company first to see what they cover and/or if there are any restrictions.

- Spectra S2 Plus Electric Breast Milk Pump
- Evenflo Deluxe Advanced Double Electric Breast Pump
- Elvie Wearable Double Electric Breast Pump

- Momcozy Hands-Free Breast Pump
- Elvie Stride Breast Pump
- Spectra S1 Plus Electric Breast Pump
- Medela Harmony Manual Breast Pump
- Spectra 9 Plus Breast Pump
- Medela Pump In Style With MaxFlow
- Philips AVENT Double Electric Breast Pump

Diapers: Disposable
I have been told by many of my clients that Costco has great disposable diapers that are very affordable. Honest Brand, Pampers Pure, Coterie, Seventh Generation and Huggies Special Edition are also good options.

Diaper cream—Weleda diaper cream, Boudreaux's Butt Paste, and PINXAV.

Nipple cream—Lansinoh and Motherlove Nipple Creams are both great.

Nipple shields
What may work for one person may not always work for another, so this is another product that you may have to experiment with to find what is right for you. A few brand recommendations I have found to be useful to experiment with include Medela, Lansinoh, and Avent.

Nursing pillow—Boppy

Playpen—GRACO Deluxe or similar

Postpartum Soaking Container—I suggest getting a plastic underbed storage container that is at least 2'x2' and about 6" deep or you can also use a flat-bottomed baby bathtub.

Sitz Bath Herbs—This is for soaking your perineum after the birth, especially if you have a tear or stitches and is made by Wish Garden.

Snot suckers—the Nose Frida is a great option.

Tinctures—WishGarden makes an herbal tincture called "After Ease" that can help with cramping after the birth and during periods. They also make a tincture "Happy Duct" that can support milk production.

Toilet stool—Squatty Potty (or similar)

Wipes—water wipes, Seventh Generation, honest, and Kirkland Signature (Costco) are all good options.

Appendix B: Recipes and Tips

Tips for Scratch Cooking

Here are some general tips that I suggest applying to all of the following recipes, as well as to all your cooking and recipe preparations:

Ingredients Matter

Always look for good quality, whole ingredients. This is the most important thing you can do to enhance the quality of the food you are eating.

Buy organic ingredients as much as possible. The most important products to buy organic include:

- All of the fruits and veggies on the Dirty Dozen list.

- Berries—it's particularly hard to wash pesticides off of them.

- Meat, poultry, and dairy products—buy organic, 100 percent grass fed and/or pasture raised. See the Sources of Grass-Fed Meat and Dairy section, to follow, for more information and a list of suppliers. A great choice is to buy from a local farmers market or farmer when possible. If you buy any processed meats, like deli meat or sausages, make sure they are organic, minimally processed, with no nitrites or nitrates, and that no hormones or antibiotics are used on the animals.

Wash Your Produce

Wash all your fruits and vegetables with a veggie wash or with a vinegar water solution of 3 parts water to 1 part vinegar. You can use either white distilled vinegar or apple cider vinegar for this solution. Simply combine the vinegar and water in a clean bowl or spray bottle. Then, soak your produce in the solution, or spray it with the solution, and leave for 15-20 minutes. Be sure to rinse the produce thoroughly with plain water after soaking or spraying to remove any traces of vinegar.

Vinegar is especially effective for cleaning berries. This will help them to stay fresher for 2-3x longer than just washing with a veggie wash solution or plain water.

Buy a Kitchen Scale

Some of the portions in the following recipes are in weight, not volume. If you don't have one on hand already you can purchase a small kitchen scale to facilitate these measurements.

Cook Meat to Temperature

It is always best to use a meat thermometer to check the internal temperature when cooking meat to ensure that it is cooked to a safe temperature. The safe minimum internal cooking temperatures for different meats vary depending on the cut of meat and the desired doneness. Here are some general guidelines.

It is important to note that these are just general guidelines. The actual cooking time and temperature may vary depending on the thickness of the meat, the type of cooking method used, and your personal preference.

Protein	Temperature
MEAT Beef Veal Lamb Pork	145°F (63°C) for medium-rare 160°F (71°C) for medium 170°F (77°C) for well done
Ground Beef	160°F (71°C) for all doneness levels
POULTRY Chicken Turkey	165°F (74°C) for all parts of the bird, including the stuffing
FISH whole fish or fillets	145°F (63°C) flesh should be opaque and separate easily with a fork
SHELLFISH Shrimp Lobster Crab Scallops	145°F (63°C) flesh should be pearly or white and opaque
Clams Oysters Mussels	145°F (63°C) Steam until the shells open during cooking. If the shell doesn't open, don't eat that one.

Grass-Fed Meat and Dairy Labels and Sources

Many local groceries and supermarkets now carry grass-fed meat and dairy, but if you aren't able to vet a farmer's practices directly you need to be discerning of labels.

Dairy Standards

Organic standards require cows to be on pasture for a minimum amount of time per year. These are considered "grass-fed." If you want purely grass-fed dairy, you need to verify practices with a farmer or look for the "Certified Grass-Fed Organic" label. Many farms use the term "grass-fed," but it is not a well-regulated term in the US dairy industry.

About Grass-Fed Meat

A note on grass-fed meat labeling: USDA/ Food Safety and Inspection Service (FSIS) regulates the term "grass-fed" as an animal raising claim. The term "grass fed" on packaging must be approved by FSIS before a company slash farm uses the term on their packaging.

The term "grass-fed and grass-finished" and/or "100% grass fed" on a package means the animal was raised solely from forages (pasture, hay, silage, etc.) and have continuous access to pasture before slaughter.

Meat that solely has the term "grass fed" on the product means that the animal may have spent the final 20 percent of their life eating grain in order to fatten them up, and they are not 100 percent grass fed.

The grass-fed claim can either be verified by the farmer through a series of required documents or verified by an agricultural marketing service (AMS) auditor. That being said, in the US the verification via documentation is not directly audited by anyone on site, so knowing your farmer is always the best way to know the product!

Sources

While by no means comprehensive, this is a list of organizations that either offer grass-fed sources of meat and dairy or provide information to help you find these natural foods in your area. These are primarily for US residents. Hopefully you have access to fantastic, fresh, organic, pasture-raised meats and dairy in your area already or you have similar directories you can find online to help you if you live elsewhere.

Eatwild.com—Provides a state-by-state and Canadian directory of local pasture-raised food sources. Requires farmers listed in the directory to self-attest their ruminant animals (cows, sheep, goats) are 100 percent grass fed and finished.

Realmilk.com—Find raw milk near you with their map-driven directory. You will need to find out from the farm if the cows are minimally supplemented with grain or 100 percent grass-fed.

Localharvest.org—Helps you to find farmers and markets near you.

US Wellness Meats (https://grasslandbeef.com/)—Ships grass-fed, pasture-raised meat throughout the US.

Texasrealfood.com—Directory of Texas farms & ranches, farmers markets, and farm-to-table restaurants. If you don't live in Texas, look for a similar directory for your state, province, or region.

Localhens.com—Local Hens connects you to local farms, restaurants, outdoor markets, Community Supported Agriculture or CSAs (which provide a (usually) weekly share of a local farm's produce directly with you), producers, and grocery stores where you can find fresh, local foods.

Getrealchicken.com—Connects you with local poultry farmers raising their flocks on pasture.

American Grassfed Association (Americangrassfed.org)—Provides a map-driven directory of ranchers who pasture raise their herds.

List of Recipes

These are the recipes you will find in this section. Please note that if a recipe calls for a storebought soup to be added, my preference is Pacific brand.

1. Morning Smoothie
2. Mimi's Special Spinach
3. Breakfast Tacos
4. Egg Muffins
5. Migas
6. Tuna Salad
7. Mimi's Nut Butter
8. Aleah's Everyday Salad
9. Mimi's Pasta Salad
10. Shepherd's Pie
11. Mimi's Stir Fry
12. Chicken Fried Cutlets
13. Aleah's Rainbow Bowl
14. Venetian Stuffed Chicken
15. White Wine Sauce
16. Chicken Tikka Masala
17. Turkey Burgers
18. Mimi's Spaghetti
19. Garlic Lemon Chicken with Roasted Vegetables
20. Country Captain Chicken
21. Mimi's Soup Stock
22. Mimi's Chicken Soup
23. Mimi's Salad
24. Creamy Coconut Chicken Soup
25. King Ranch Casserole
26. Toodle Oodle Casserole
27. Mexican Casserole
28. Dr. Ray Peat's Raw Carrot Salad
29. Mimi's Fruit Salad
30. Avocado Pudding
31. Chia Seed Pudding
32. Pregnancy Tea

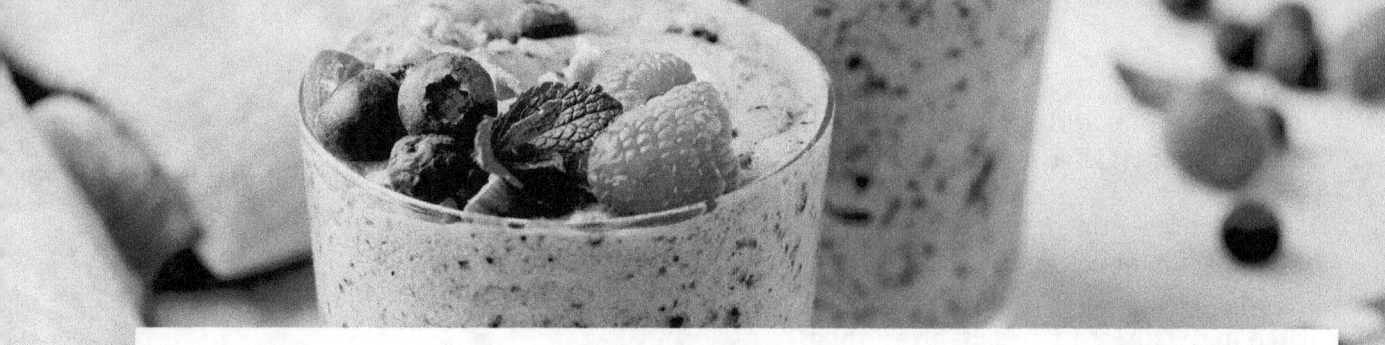

Morning Smoothie

Once you are pregnant, I would love for you to start your day with this delicious smoothie.

INGREDIENTS

Organic milk/milk substitute or coconut water

1 ½ cups ice and 1 ½ cups fresh fruit
OR
3 cups frozen fruit

1 banana

1 Tbsp melted coconut oil
1 scoop protein powder (I use SPIRU-TEIN vanilla flavored protein powder)

For an added nutritional boost, add a scoop of Green Vibrance. It's so good for you and delicious, too!
Include flax or chia seeds if you like.

DIRECTIONS

1. Mix all your liquid ingredients with ice and/or fresh or frozen fruit in the blender first, then, after they are fully combined, add your powders and the oil while the blender is still running. It is best to melt the oil before adding it to the smoothie so that it doesn't clump. Drink and enjoy!

Fruit can get expensive if you buy it fresh. Costco has an inexpensive brand of organic frozen fruit with blueberries, raspberries, and blackberries. It's difficult to wash pesticides off berries, so make sure to buy organic whether fresh or frozen. Other fruits like bananas and oranges that you peel are usually okay to buy non-organic. Check the dirty dozen list before buying conventional fruits.

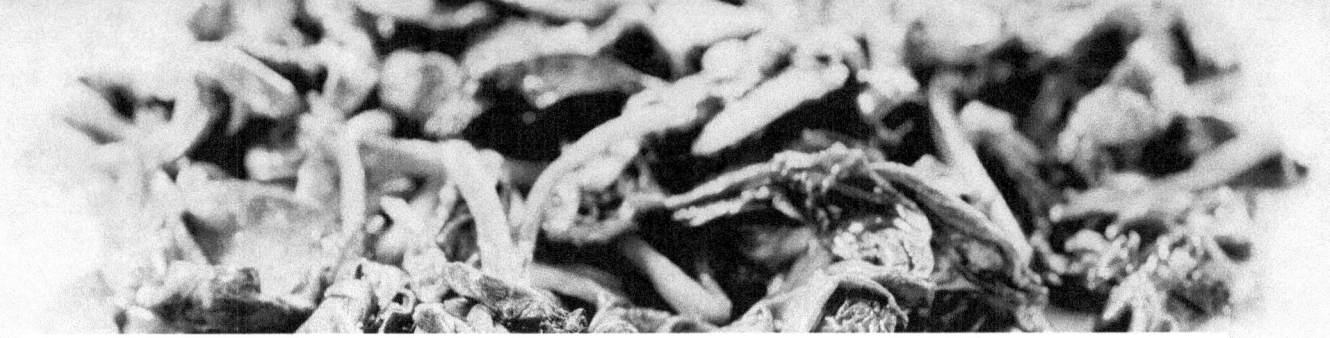

Mimi's Special Sauteed Spinach

You can use this as a wonderful omelet filling or as the base of a sandwich, taco, or tostada. You can also put chicken, beans, eggs, or cheese on top for a balanced meal.

INGREDIENTS

1 Tbsp avocado oil

1/2 cup carrot, finely diced

3/4 cup yellow onion, finely diced

1 lg clove garlic, minced

6 cups baby spinach, washed, dried, & roughly chopped

1/4 tsp salt

1/4 tsp pepper

1/4 tsp oregano

Optional—1 cup sliced, chopped mushrooms

DIRECTIONS

1. Heat the avocado oil on medium high heat until shimmering. First add the diced carrot and cook for two minutes, then add the yellow onion and cook for two minutes, stirring occasionally.
2. If you are going to add mushrooms add them now and cook for two more minutes or until they are brown and soft.
3. Add garlic and cook for an additional 30 seconds or until fragrant.
4. Add the spinach and spices and cook just until the spinach is wilted.
5. Move the mixture to a bowl to stop the spinach from continuing to cook in the pan.

Store the mixture in an air-tight container in the fridge.

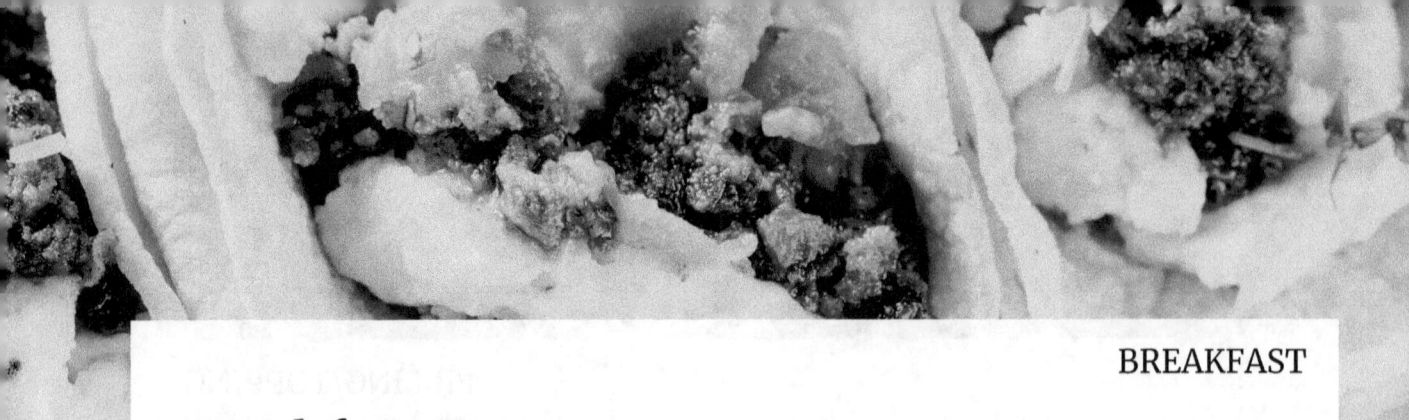

Breakfast Tacos

Breakfast tacos are a staple here in Texas, and I've heard that they aren't common in other parts of the country. Y'all are in for a treat if these are new to you. The combinations are endless; be creative until you find what you like. Breakfast tacos are essentially tacos made with egg as the main protein source. The key to good breakfast tacos is good quality corn tortillas. Find a brand with no chemicals like El Milagro. The other key to great breakfast tacos is adding good salsa!

INGREDIENTS

Corn tortillas

1/2 Tbsp butter

2 eggs per taco

Salt and pepper for seasoning

Plus your choice of:

Fried or roasted potatoes

Refried or whole black beans

Cooked, crumbled bacon

Chorizo or breakfast Sausage

Cheese

Avocado

Cilantro

Mushrooms, chopped

Mimi's Special Spinach

Tomato

White or red onion

Crumbled tofu fried in cumin and salt

Salsa

DIRECTIONS

1. Heat butter on med–low heat in a skillet.
2. Beat the eggs.
3. Cook the eggs low and slow, folding occasionally until cooked through, add salt and pepper halfway through cooking, then remove from the heat.
4. Warm up your tortillas in the pan.
5. Fill the tortillas with eggs and your toppings of choice.
6. You can make several at once (don't include ingredients that won't keep well), wrap in foil, and store in the fridge to reheat for breakfasts.

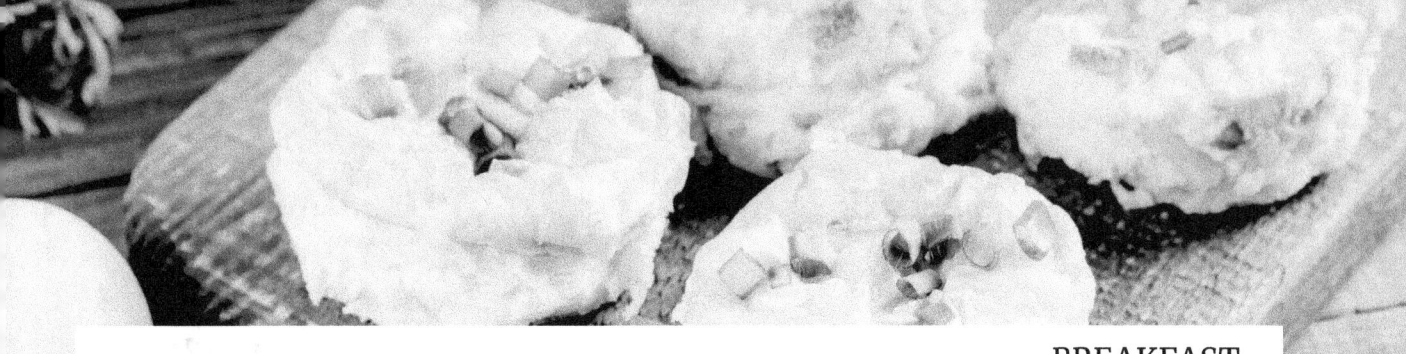

Egg Muffins

This is a fantastic, vegetable and protein-packed start to your day that you can easily make lots of in advance and freeze for later consumption.

INGREDIENTS

24 eggs

3 tsp salt

2 tsp pepper

Your choice of:

Sliced, chopped mushrooms

White or green onions, diced

Bell peppers, diced

Crumbled, cooked bacon

Cheddar or Swiss cheese

Spinach, Swiss chard, or kale

Tomato

Cilantro

Sausage

DIRECTIONS

1. Preheat the oven to 350 degrees F.
2. Line a 12-cup muffin tin with liners, or prepare the sides and bottom with butter or your choice of nonstick spray.
3. Beat the eggs, salt, and pepper. I use a stand mixer or hand mixer rather than doing this quantity by hand.
4. Fill each muffin cup 1/3 full with your ingredients of choice.
5. Fill the cup until 1/2 full with the beaten eggs.
6. Bake 15 - 20 minutes or until eggs are firm.

If freezing for later, first cool to room temperature. Then place on a baking sheet and wrap in plastic wrap before freezing for 24 hours. Then you can put the muffins into a gallon-size resealable plastic bag without fear that they will stick together.

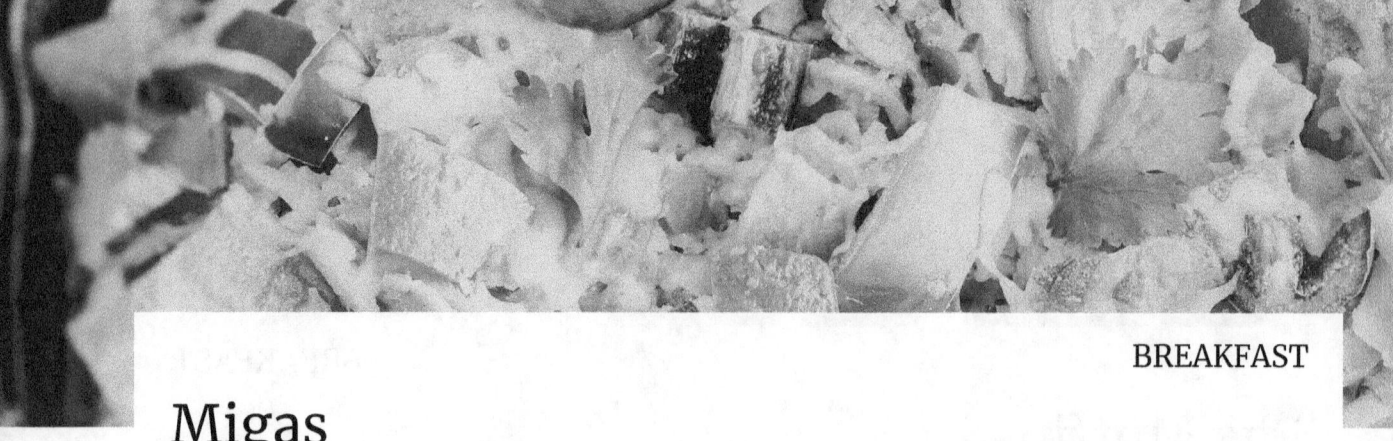

Migas

This is a dish you may not have in your area. It's common in Texas in our diners and Tex-Mex restaurants, and delivers a wonderful zing to your breakfast. I slice the fresh peppers and deseed them first, so that the dish is flavorful but not as spicy.

Be careful to not touch anything while you are handling the peppers and wash your hands thoroughly with soap and water immediately after-or wear gloves when you're working with them. Pepper burns are no joke. Depending on how hot you like it, feel free to experiment with leaving seeds in or using more or less to suit your taste

INGREDIENTS

1 Tbsp olive oil

4 large eggs, beaten with 1 Tbsp milk or water

4 Tbsp onion, finely diced

1/2 small tomato, diced

2 Tbsp pickled jalapeno or fresh jalapeno/serrano, diced

1 cup tortilla chips gently broken into bite sized pieces or corn tortilla strips lightly fried

3 Tbsp shredded cheddar cheese

DIRECTIONS

1. Heat olive oil in a skillet on medium high heat until shimmering.
2. Add onion and cook for 1 minute.
3. Add jalapeno/serrano and cook until soft, about 3-4 minutes.
4. Add tomato and cook an additional 2 minutes.
5. Add the chips, mix, then add the beaten eggs. Cook the mixture, stirring gently until the eggs are cooked, about 2-3 minutes. If you want to use your own corn tortillas instead of chips, cut 1-2 tortillas into 1/2 strips and lightly fry them in a pan with a few Tbsp of avocado oil for about 5 minutes or until golden brown and crispy and then add them in at this stage.
6. Add the cheese, mix quickly, then immediately remove from heat and serve.

Optional additions that are delicious include whole or refried beans on the side. Migas can also be eaten with tortillas or tortilla chips.

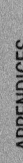

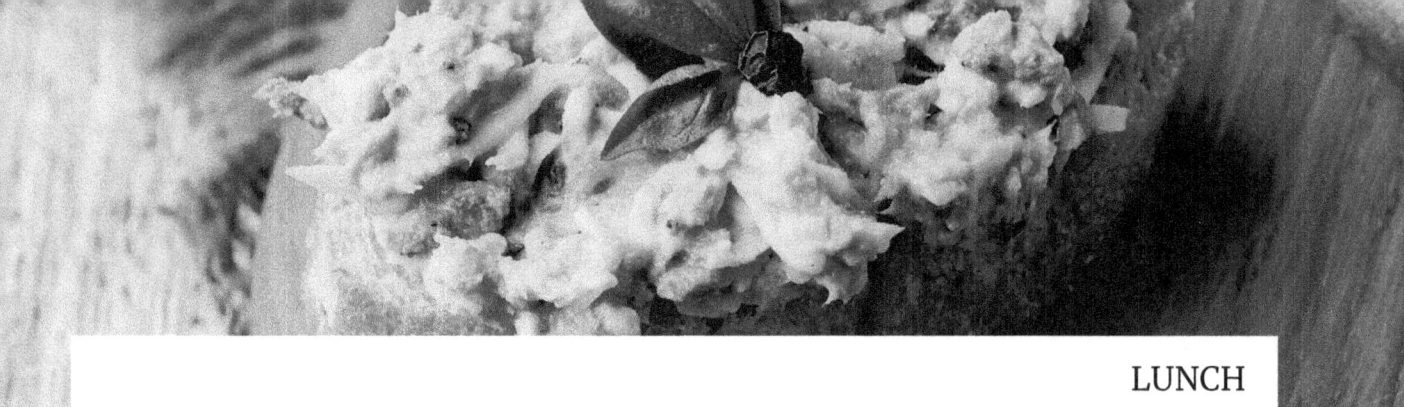

Tuna Salad

This is my take on a sandwich staple. Enjoy!

INGREDIENTS

2 cans Albacore tuna in water

1/3 small red onion, finely diced

1–2 stalks celery, finely diced

1 clove garlic, minced

1 cup grapes, quartered

1/2 cup avocado oil-based mayonnaise or substitute

1/2 tsp salt

Pepper for seasoning

DIRECTIONS

1. Drain the tuna well and put it in a mixing bowl.
2. Use a fork to break up all of the tuna into flakes.
3. Add all remaining ingredients to the mixing bowl and mix well. Add more mayonnaise if needed to get the right consistency for you.
4. Optional: add pecans or walnuts.

Serve on bread or with corn chips, crackers, cucumber slices, or over salad or a piece of lettuce for a lower calorie option. If you are avoiding grains you can also cradle this in an avocado boat or stuff it in the well of a few celery sticks.

I like to use one piece of bread with the tuna salad on top then add a piece of lettuce in place of the other piece of bread. You can also add avocado or tomato to the sandwich for a nice addition.

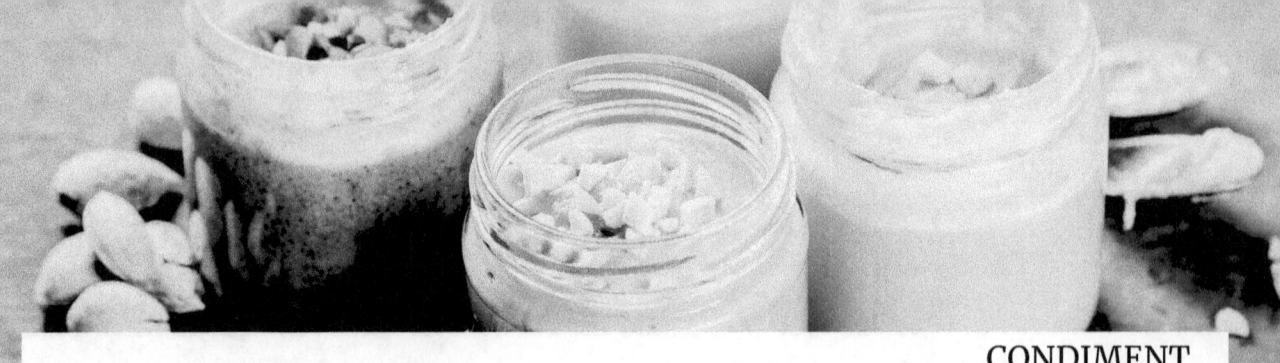

Mimi's Nut Butter

Plain peanut butter isn't the greatest for you, but pure nut butters can be stiflingly expensive. This blend adds nutrients to your peanut butter without breaking the bank.

INGREDIENTS

1/4 cup almond butter

1/4 cup cashew butter

1/4 cup tahini or sesame butter

1/4 cup smooth or crunchy peanut butter

DIRECTIONS

1. Mix the almond, cashew, and tahini or sesame butters together until well blended.
2. Add the nut butter blend to your peanut butter and mix well.
3. Use this in place of peanut or almond butter!

Check your grocer's bulk food section before buying in jars. You'll often find the best prices and freshest butters there.

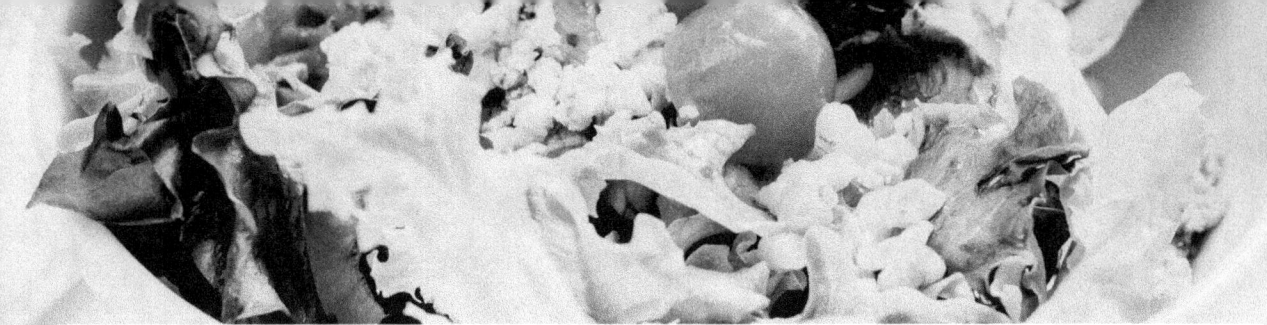

Aleah's Every Day Salad

Aleah eats this literally every day for lunch. The best part is, you can prep the base of the salad once and eat for the whole week adding whatever toppings you like daily.

INGREDIENTS

1 cup chopped romaine lettuce

1/2 cup chopped radicchio lettuce

1/4 cup sliced or shredded carrots

1/4 cup cherry tomatoes

1/4 avocado, cubed

2 - 4 Tbsp feta cheese, crumbled

1/4 cup sliced ham or chopped grilled chicken

2 Tbsp sprouted pumpkin seeds (or nuts of choice)

1-2 Tbsp Champagne vinaigrette

Optional:

1/8 cup shredded red cabbage

1/8 cup sliced baby Bella mushrooms

2 Tbsp sliced Kalamata olives

DIRECTIONS

1. Wash and dry the romaine and radicchio lettuce then slice into about 1/2-1" strips. Add the washed and sliced or grated carrots (and cabbage if you want) and mix all together.
2. Add the mushrooms if you like more veggies.
3. Slice the tomatoes in half and add to the salad.
4. Add the avocado.
5. Top with the ham or chicken, feta, pumpkin seeds, and the dressing and toss.
6. Add Kalamata olives on top for great flavor, unless you don't need extra calories. Olives are high in good fats.

I like to prepare a big base salad at the beginning of each week to keep in the fridge. Once I've done that, this is so easy to make daily as a healthy and delicious lunch.

If you do want to meal prep the large salad base in advance, I suggest using 1 big head of romaine lettuce, 1-2 heads of radicchio, 1-2 bags of pre-washed and sliced carrots, and 1/2 head of red or green cabbage to make it easy. Mix all together and keep in a large, air-tight container. Add your desired toppings each day and change it up to meet your taste buds in flavor town.

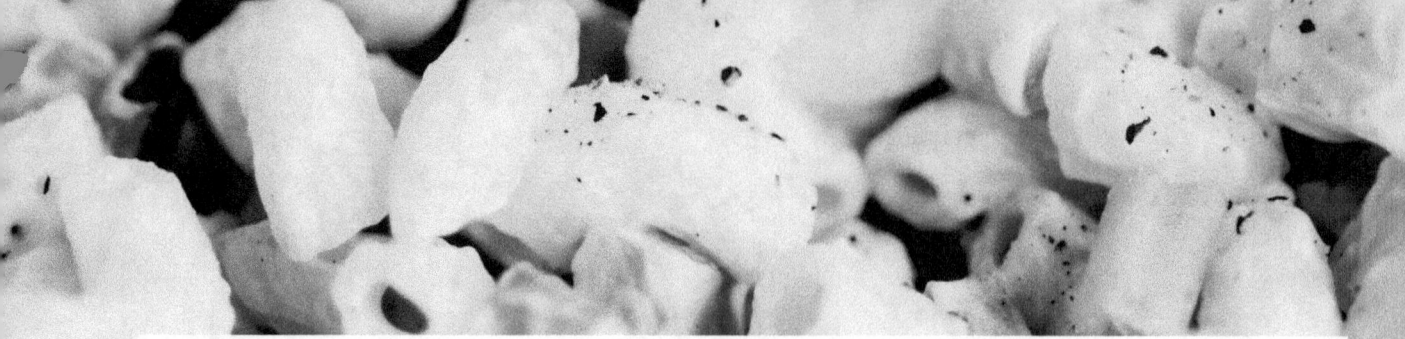

Mimi's Pasta Salad

This is excellent on its own for lunch, or it's fabulous to make and keep on hand to snack on or use as a side dish for dinner.

INGREDIENTS

8-ounces of small tubular or macaroni pasta

2 celery sticks, diced

1/3 red onion, diced

1/2 cup salad olives, chopped

1/4 cup capers

1/2 red bell pepper, diced

1/2 green bell pepper, diced

1/2-3/4 cup mayonnaise or substitute

1/4 tsp dried oregano

1/4 tsp dill

1 tsp apple cider vinegar

DIRECTIONS

1. Cook and drain the pasta to your desired level of firmness and set aside in a mixing bowl.
2. While the pasta cools, dice and prep all veggies and spices.
3. Mix all ingredients in a large mixing bowl with the pasta and enjoy!

Keep in an air-tight container in the fridge and enjoy leftovers cold as a side dish or snack.

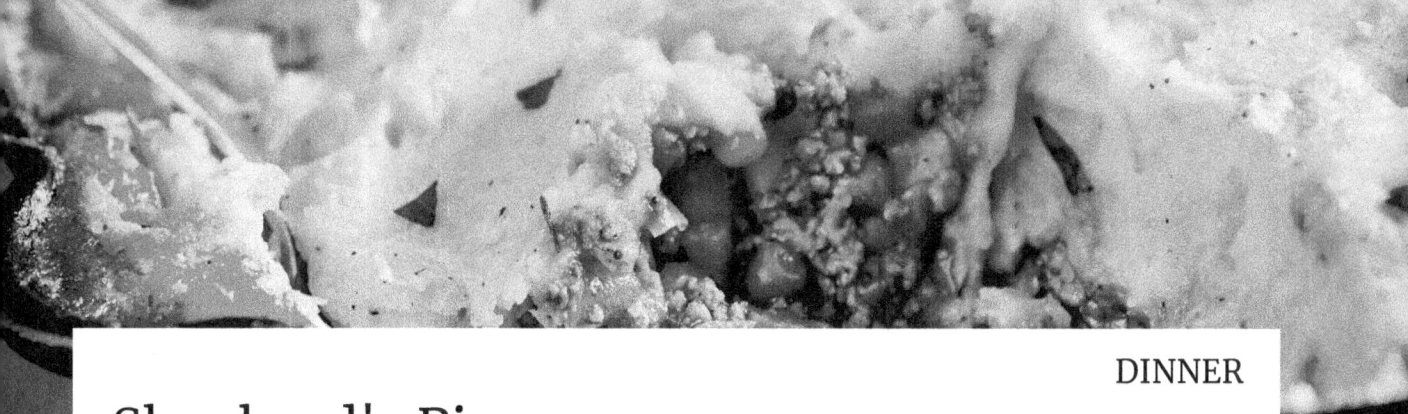

Shepherd's Pie

A hearty, savory fall or winter meal.

INGREDIENTS

2 Tbsp olive oil

1 lb ground meat of choice (I prefer turkey or chicken)

1 tsp salt

1 tsp ground fennel

1/2 tsp black pepper

1/8 tsp cayenne pepper

1 cup diced yellow or sweet onion

3 garlic cloves, minced

2 Tbsp tomato paste

1-2 Tbsp Worcestershire sauce

1 Tbsp all-purpose flour

1/4 cup water

3-4 lbs. Russet or yellow potatoes, cooked and mashed

2-3 zucchini cut into 1/2" slices and blanched

5-6 tomatoes on the vine, washed and sliced thick

1 cup shredded cheddar or grated parmesan cheese

Fresh parsley leaves for garnish

Optional:

1 cup frozen peas and diced carrots

DIRECTIONS

1. Preheat oven to 375 degrees F.
2. Heat oil in a medium skillet over medium heat. Add meat, breaking apart with a wooden spoon, until slightly browned and crumbly, about 5 minutes.
3. Add the spices, peas and carrots (optional), onion, garlic, tomato paste, and Worcestershire sauce to the skillet. Cook, stirring occasionally, until vegetables are slightly softened, about 5 minutes.
4. Sprinkle with flour; cook, stirring occasionally, until flour is absorbed and toasted, about 2 minutes.
5. Add water; stir to release brown bits. Reduce heat to medium low; cover and cook until mixture is saucy and vegetables are tender, about 5 minutes more.
6. Spoon mixture into an 11"x7" baking dish. Layer the blanched zucchini, then the sliced tomatoes, on top of the meat mixture. Top with mashed potatoes, spreading to cover in an even layer. Sprinkle with cheese.
7. Cook in oven until you can see the juices bubbling up along the edges from underneath the mashed potatoes and the cheese is golden brown, usually 30-45 minutes.

Garnish with parsley, if desired.

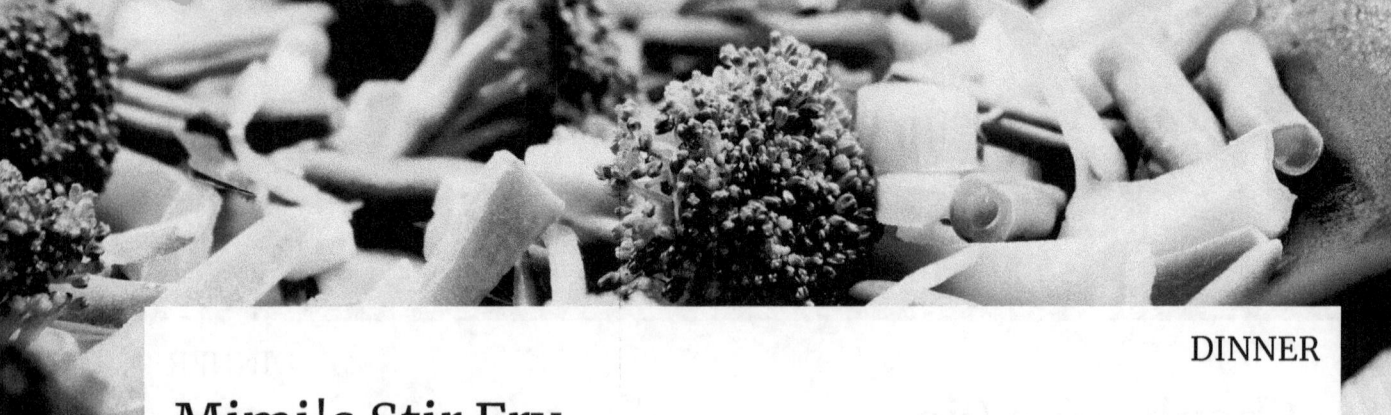

DINNER

Mimi's Stir Fry

While the ingredient list may look daunting, stir fry is easy and versatile. Use lots of veggies with tons of color to add beneficial phytonutrients. You'll find two styles of stir fry here to try: carrot and broccoli.

INGREDIENTS

CHOOSE ONE PROTEIN

1-1 ½ lbs chicken thighs

1-1 ½ lbs whole, peeled, veined, medium shrimp

1 lb firm tofu, cubed

MARINADE

1/4 cup soy sauce

1 ½ tsp fish sauce

2 tsp toasted sesame oil

2 garlic cloves, minced

3-4 Tbsp avocado oil

STIR FRY VEGETABLES

One large yellow or white onion, diced

2 large celery stalks, diced

2 large garlic cloves, minced

1/2 red bell pepper, moderately diced

1/2 yellow or orange bell pepper, moderately diced1

½ cup green beans cut into 1-1 ½" lengths

1 medium to large zucchini, moderately diced

(continued)

DIRECTIONS

1. Combine all marinade ingredients and add your chosen protein. It's great to use a gallon-size resealable plastic bag for this. Marinate chicken for 1-2 hours, shrimp for 15-30 minutes and tofu for 15 minutes. Gently manipulate the protein in the bag and turn it over halfway through.

2. While the protein marinates, prepare the veggies.

3. Sauté 1/2 cup of onion in vegetable oil at med-high heat, cook for 1-2 minutes, then add your protein (drain the marinade first). Cook chicken until 165 degrees F, shrimp until almost completely cooked, and tofu until slightly golden brown on the edges. Remove the protein from the heat to a bowl so it doesn't keep cooking.

4. **Carrot version**: In a gallon pot or wok, heat 2-3 Tbsp avocado oil on medium high heat until the oil is shimmering but not smoking. Put carrots in first and sauté for 2 minutes, then add onion, celery, bell peppers, green beans, kale, and sauce, and cook for 3 minutes. Next add the zucchini, spinach, mushrooms, and garlic and cook for an additional 2 minutes. Add the cooked protein back into the pot and cook for a few more minutes on lower heat. (continued)

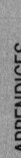

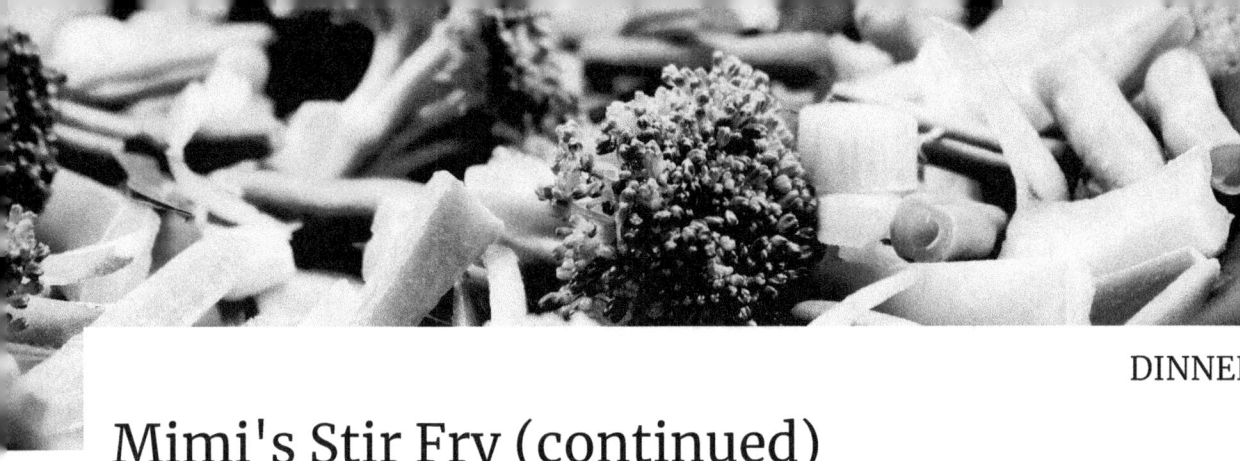

Mimi's Stir Fry (continued)

INGREDIENTS

1 cup white or baby Bella mushrooms, roughly chopped

ADDITIONAL VEGETABLES TO ADD
CARROT VERSION
2 carrots finely diced
2 cups chopped kale
2 cups roughly chopped baby spinach

BROCCOLI VERSION
1 head of broccoli, florets and stems, chopped
2 cups chopped kale
1 cup red cabbage finely sliced then chopped

SAUCE
Whisk together:
2 Tbsp soy sauce
1 Tbsp fish sauce
1 tsp oregano
2 minced garlic cloves
1 tsp thyme
 Optional: 1/2 tsp dried Thai chilies/red pepper flakes

Cooked Basmati or brown rice

DIRECTIONS

6. **Broccoli version:** In a gallon pot or wok heat 2-3 Tbsp avocado oil on medium high heat until the oil is shimmering but not smoking.

7. Add onions and cook for 1 minute, then add broccoli, broccoli stems, kale, and cabbage with the sauce and cook for 2 minutes.

8. Add celery, peppers, green beans, zucchini, mushrooms, and garlic then cook just until vegetables are tender.

Add the cooked protein back into the pot and cook for a few more minutes on lower heat.

Serve either version with 1-2 cups cooked brown or basmati rice.

I like to make enough to have leftovers, but know that brassicas like broccoli, cabbage, or kale don't do as well on day two.

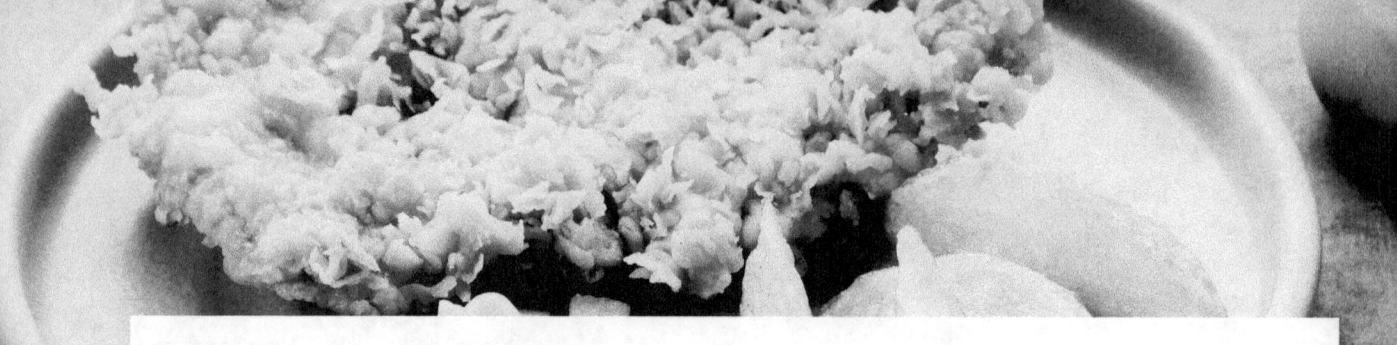

Chicken-Fried Cutlets

When you're in need of some Southern comfort food, there's nothing better than this. I love serving this with potatoes and steamed green beans or roasted vegetables.

INGREDIENTS

4 turkey cutlets or 2 chicken breasts split in half horizontally

Salt and pepper for seasoning

1/2 cup flour

2 eggs, beaten

1/2 cup fine bread crumbs or panko

1/4-1/3 cup avocado oil

1/2 tsp salt

1/2 tsp pepper

1 tsp Italian seasoning or herbs (oregano, basil, thyme, rosemary)

1 lemon, quartered

Optional: fresh parsley, washed and chopped

DIRECTIONS

1. Cover a cutting board with a full piece of plastic wrap or parchment paper. Put the meat on top, cover with another sheet, then pound with a mallet or heavy pan to flatten them to 1/4"-1/2" even thickness. A tortilla press is fantastic for this if you have one. This tenderizes the meat and helps it to cook faster and more evenly. Sprinkle the tenderized meat with salt and pepper.

2. Prepare three shallow dishes. These need to have sides, like small casserole dishes, and not be flat like plates. Put flour, salt, pepper, and Italian seasoning mixed together in one, eggs in the second, and breadcrumbs in the third.

3. Dredge each piece of meat first in the flour, then dip in the egg, and then cover with the breadcrumbs. Put the breaded meat on a plate until all are coated and ready for cooking.

4. Heat the avocado oil in a large, heavy skillet; cast iron is great. When the oil is very hot and glistening but not smoking, add the cutlets and cook for 1-1 ½ minutes per side before flipping. They should be golden brown. Turn 2-3 times to get the perfect golden-brown color being careful not to let them burn.

5. Drain cutlets on paper towels and blot the top to remove excess oil.

6. Serve with fresh lemon and parsley (optional).

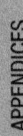

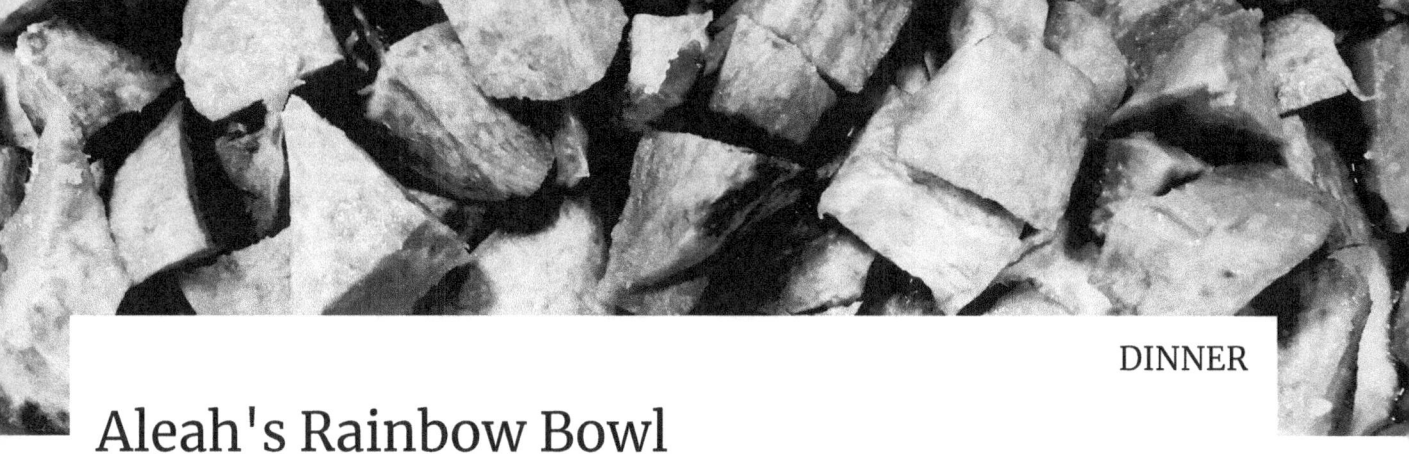

Aleah's Rainbow Bowl

One of my all-time favorites, this is packed with nutrients and so delicious and easy!

INGREDIENTS

1 lb ground chicken

1-2 cups cooked rice

1 sweet onion, diced

1 bunch kale, chopped

2 medium zucchinis quartered & sliced into 1/4-1/2" pieces

8 oz baby Bella mushrooms, quartered

2 large sweet potatoes peeled and cubed

1 large avocado, cubed

1 bunch of cilantro, chopped

3-4 Tbsp avocado oil

1 cup cherry tomatoes, chopped

2 cloves of garlic, minced

3 tsp chili powder

3 tsp garlic powder

1 tsp cumin

1 tsp coriander

1/2 tsp cayenne pepper

2 Tbsp curry powder

3 tsp salt

Pepper for seasoning

(continued)

DIRECTIONS

1. Preheat oven to 450 degrees F.
2. Wash and prep all vegetables .
3. Line a baking sheet with parchment paper.
4. Add the sweet potato into a bowl with 1 Tbsp of avocado oil, 1 tsp salt, 1 tsp garlic powder, 1 tsp chili powder, 1 Tbsp of curry powder, and some cracked pepper. Mix the ingredients gently until the potatoes are coated with the oil and seasoning, you can add a little more if needed, and transfer to the baking sheet. Bake for 25-30 minutes or until soft with crisp edges, flipping halfway through cooking.
5. While the potatoes are cooking, heat 1 Tbsp of the avocado oil in a large skillet or wok on medium high heat until shimmering.
6. Add half of the sweet onion and cook for 2-3 minutes.
7. Add the kale, half the garlic, and 1 tsp salt, and cook for 5-6 minutes, stirring frequently until done then remove from heat.
8. In another skillet, heat 1 Tbsp of avocado oil on medium high heat until shimmering. Add the rest of the sweet onion and cook for 2-3 minutes.

(continued)

Aleah's Rainbow Bowl (continued)

INGREDIENTS

Sauce:
8 oz sour cream
1 small pkg ranch powder
1 bunch of green onions or 1/4 cup red onions, diced
1/2 lemon, squeezed

DIRECTIONS

9. Add the ground meat and break up into small, bite size pieces. Cook for about 5 minutes then add the rest of the garlic, zucchini, mushrooms, and remaining spices.

10. Cook for another 5 minutes until the meat is fully cooked and the veggies are cooked but still firm.

11. Mix the sauce ingredients together in a small bowl. Sub plain Greek yogurt for the sour cream if you prefer.

12. Once all the rainbow bowl ingredients are prepared, use large bowls to layer with rice, kale, chicken veggie mix, sweet potatoes, avocado, rainbow sauce, and garnish with cilantro (optional).

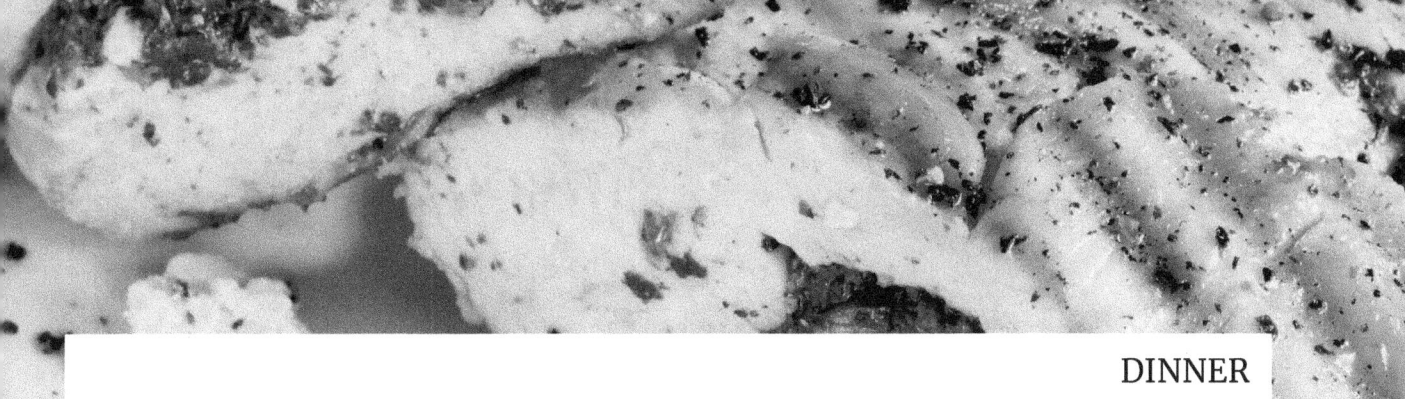

Venetian Stuffed Chicken

This one is a little tricky, but I know you can pull it off beautifully and everyone will exclaim at what a fabulous chef you are when you serve it!

INGREDIENTS

1/2 Tbsp of avocado or olive oil

4 large chicken breasts

6 cups baby spinach roughly chopped

1 white or sweet onion diced

1 large clove of garlic, minced

1 ounce prosciutto, chopped

4 small, very thinly shaved prosciutto slices for topping

8-oz feta, crumbled

4 oz mushrooms, chopped

4 slices of mozzarella or fontina cheese

1 cup chicken broth

1 cup dry white wine

DIRECTIONS

1. Preheat the oven to 350 degrees F.
2. Prepare the pockets for stuffing: Take the chicken breasts and cut each one straight down the middle on the top side of the breast stopping ½" from the bottom. Then, using a pairing knife, cut a 1-½" slit horizontally from the bottom of that first cut toward the outer edge of the breast. Again, don't cut all the way through. Then do this on the other side, toward the outer edge of the other side of the breast. Make sure you do not cut all the way through the chicken as you want the pocket to hold in all the juices and flavoring.
3. Heat the oil in a large skillet, then sauté the onion for 1 minute. Add prosciutto and cook for 2 minutes until it starts to get brown and crispy, then add the garlic and mushrooms and cook 3 minutes more.
4. Add the spinach and cook just until wilted.
5. Take the mixture out of the pan and put into a bowl, so it does not keep cooking. Once it cools to lukewarm, add the feta to your taste.
6. Stuff each chicken breast with as much filling as you can get into it. (continued)

Venetian Stuffed Chicken

DIRECTIONS, CONTINUED

7. Top with a slice of cheese and put a very thin slice of prosciutto on top of that.

8. Whisk the wine and broth together. Put the breasts in a glass baking dish and add the liquid. This will poach the chicken and be the base for a great sauce. Cook for approximately 20−25 minutes. Use a meat thermometer to check the chicken to make sure it hits 165 degrees F in the thickest part of the meat.

9. Once it's cooked, remove the chicken breast to a serving dish, and add the remaining poaching liquid to a saucepan. Add more chicken broth and wine to make about 2 cups and bring to a simmer.

Take a small jar and put 2 Tbsp of the wine and chicken broth liquid and 2 Tbsp cornstarch to the jar. Tighten the lid and shake very well until there are no lumps. Add this mixture back to the other simmering liquid and cook until thickened, usually about 5 minutes.

Pour the sauce over each chicken breast and serve. *Buon appetito!*

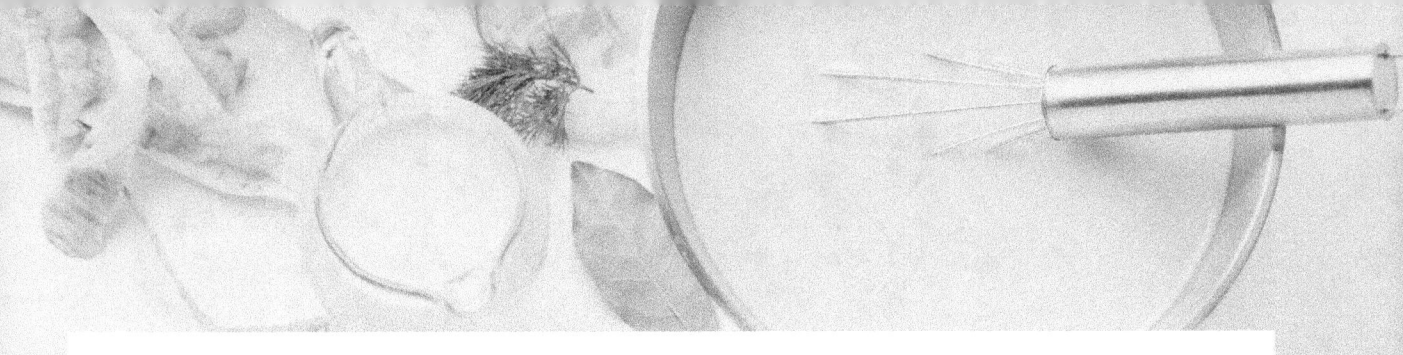

White Wine Sauce

Fantastic on any white meat or light fish, this simple sauce really jazzes up your meal.

INGREDIENTS

1/4 cup butter
1/4 cup unbleached, all-purpose flour
1/2 cup dry white wine
1/2 cup half & half
1/2 cup chicken broth

Optional:
1/4-1/3 cup grated parmesan, sharp cheddar, or nutritional yeast flakes for a vegan option.

DIRECTIONS

1. Melt the butter in a saucepan on low-med heat.
2. Add flour to the melted butter slowly, whisking in each portion before adding more.
3. Cook 2-3 minutes to remove the starchy taste of the flour.
4. Add the white wine, half & half, and chicken broth and simmer, stirring frequently for about 3-5 minutes until thickened.
5. Add salt and pepper to taste, about 1/4 tsp of each should do. A pinch of nutmeg is also a delicious addition to this sauce, especially in the fall and winter.
6. To make a cheese sauce, you can add 1/4-1/3 cup grated parmesan or sharp cheddar after the sauce has thickened or 1/4-1/3 cup nutritional yeast flakes if you want a dairy alternative. Add the cheese and continue to stir until it has melted.

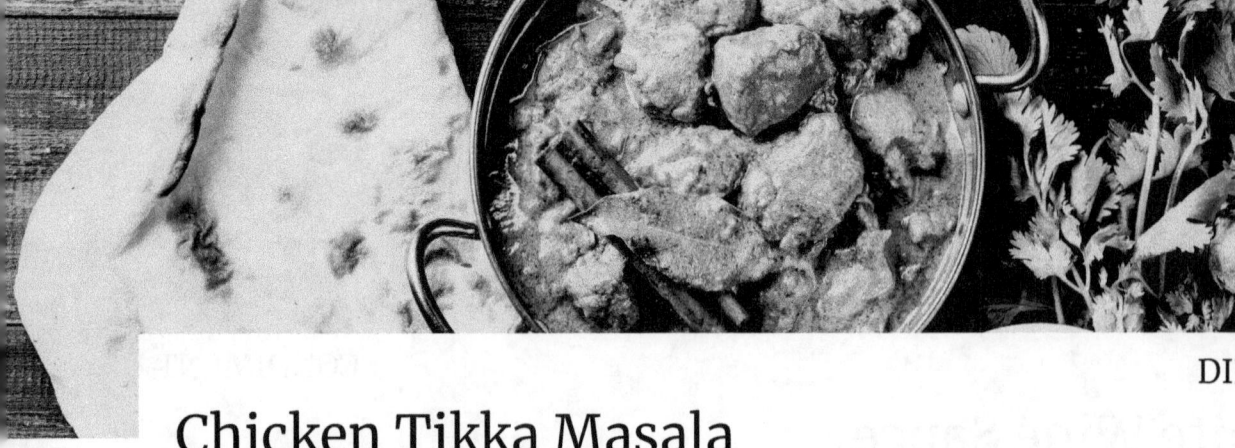

Chicken Tikka Masala

This delicious Indian stew is wonderful with butter or lemon rice and warm naan bread.

INGREDIENTS

28 oz boneless and skinless chicken thighs cut into bite-sized pieces

Marinade
1 cup plain yogurt
1 ½ Tbsp minced garlic
1 Tbsp grated ginger
2 tsp garam masala
1 tsp turmeric
1 tsp ground cumin
1 tsp Kashmiri chili (or 1/2 tsp ground red chili powder)
1 tsp salt

Sauce
2 Tbsp avocado oil
2 Tbsp butter
1 large sweet onion, finely diced
1 ½ Tbsp garlic finely grated
1 Tbsp ginger finely grated
1 ½ tsp garam masala
1 ½ tsp ground cumin
(continued)

DIRECTIONS

1. In a bowl, combine chicken with all of the ingredients for the chicken marinade; marinate for 30-60 minutes or overnight if time allows.
2. Heat oil in a large skillet or pot over medium-high heat. When sizzling, add chicken pieces in 2-3 batches, making sure not to crowd the pan. Fry until browned, about 3 minutes on each side. Set aside and cover to keep warm.
3. Melt the butter in the same pan. Fry the onions until soft (about 3 minutes) while scraping up any browned bits stuck on the bottom of the pan.
4. Add garlic and ginger and sauté for 30 seconds until fragrant, then add garam masala, cumin, turmeric and coriander. Fry for about 20 seconds until fragrant, while stirring occasionally.
5. Pour in the tomato sauce, chili powders, and salt. Let simmer for about 10-15 minutes, stirring occasionally until sauce thickens and becomes a deep red-brown color.
6. Stir the cream and sugar through the sauce.
7. Add the chicken and its juices back into the pan and cook for an additional 8-10 minutes until chicken is cooked through (165F) and the sauce is thick and bubbling. Add water to thin the sauce, if needed.

(continued)

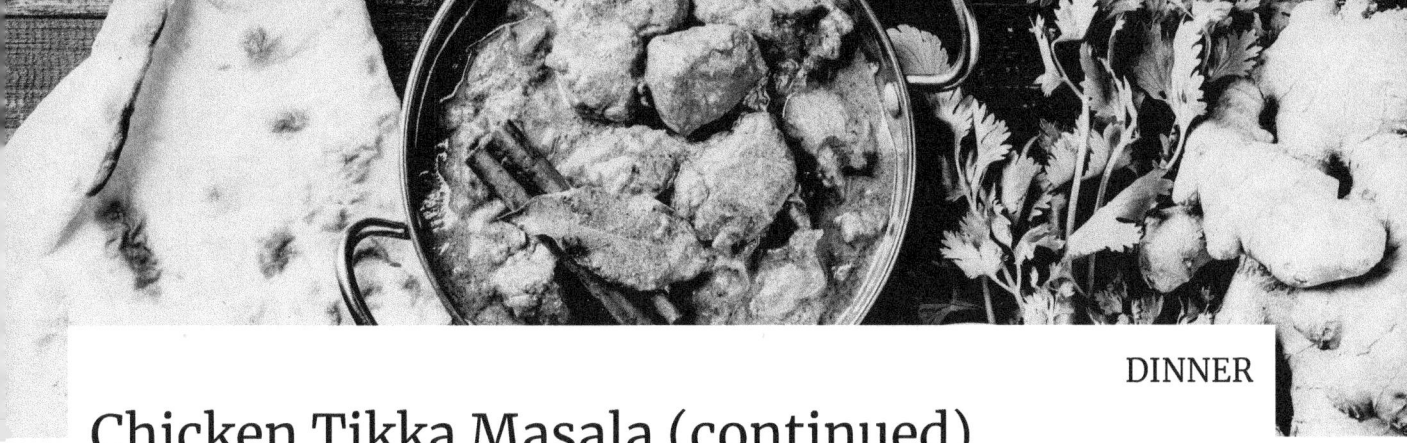

Chicken Tikka Masala (continued)

INGREDIENTS

1 tsp turmeric powder

1 tsp ground coriander

14 oz tomato sauce

1 tsp Kashmiri chili (optional for color and flavor)

1 tsp ground red chili powder (adjust to your heat preference)

1 tsp ground coriander

14 oz tomato sauce

1 tsp Kashmiri chili (optional)

1 tsp ground red chili powder (adjust to your heat preference)

1 tsp salt

1 ¼ cup heavy cream (or use evaporated milk for a lower fat content)

1 tsp brown sugar

1/4 cup water if needed

Optional

4 Tbsp chopped fresh cilantro to garnish

DIRECTIONS

Garnish with cilantro (optional). and serve on top of rice.

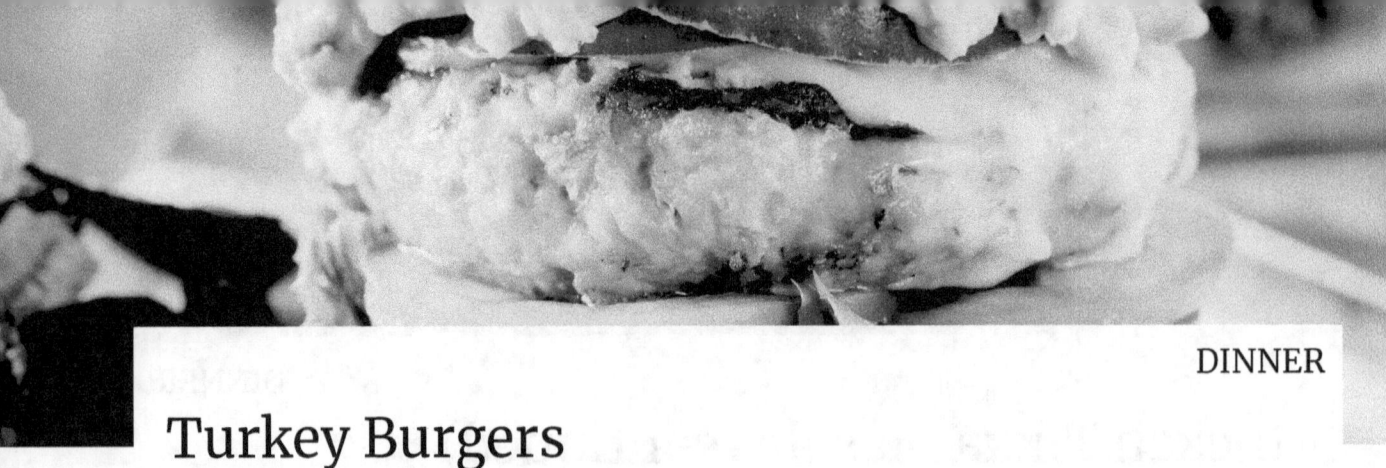

Turkey Burgers

The secret to a great turkey burger is in the Worcestershire sauce. Give these a try and see if you don't agree!

INGREDIENTS

2 lbs ground turkey thighs

1 small-medium yellow onion, finely diced

1/4 cup fine bread crumbs

2 eggs, lightly beaten

3 Tbsp olive oil

1 tsp garlic powder

1 tsp oregano

2 tsp salt

1 tsp pepper

1/4 cup Worcestershire sauce

DIRECTIONS

1. Mix all the ingredients together with your hands.
2. Form the meat into 8-10 patties. Preheat an oiled skillet to med-high heat.
3. Sear on both sides and cook thoroughly, about 4 minutes on each side.
4. Serve on a whole wheat or gluten free bun or on top of a piece of lettuce for a lower calorie /carb option.
5. I add mayonnaise, mustard, red onion, lettuce, tomato, and occasionally sliced cheese or avocado to my burgers.

If you don't want to cook all of them at once, they freeze very well. Put wax paper underneath the burgers and in between them and store in a gallon-size resealable freezer bag, then freeze and use later.

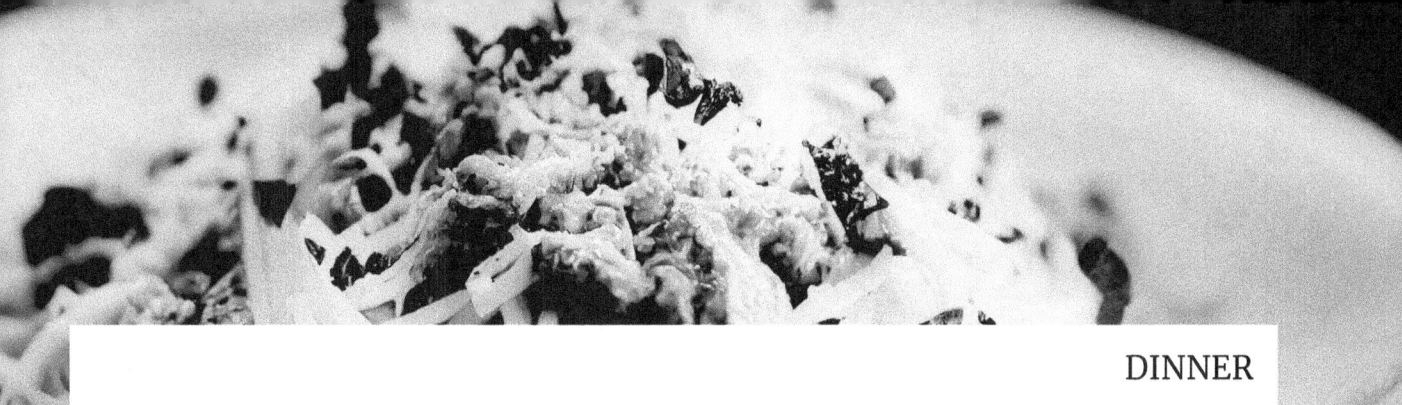

MiMi's Spaghetti

This is my take on a classic. It's already full of great vegetables and nutrients, but if you want to make it even better, consider adding ripe black olives, artichoke hearts. and/or 2 cups spinach, rough chopped or 2 cups kale, chopped.

INGREDIENTS

1 lb ground chicken or turkey

1/2 small yellow onion, diced

3 Tbsp olive oil

3 cloves garlic, minced

1 large carrot, finely diced

2–3" fennel stalk, sliced and chopped

2 large stalks of celery, diced

1 small red bell pepper, diced

1 small yellow or orange bell pepper, diced

1 cup green beans, chopped

1 medium zucchini, diced

4 oz of white or baby Bella mushrooms, sliced

4 cans tomato sauce

2 cans tomato paste

1 lg can San Marzano tomatoes

1 ½ tsp salt

2 tsp pepper

2 Tbsp oregano

4 Tbsp basil

1/2 tsp rosemary

(continued)

DIRECTIONS

1. Prepare all vegetables as directed.
2. Heat olive oil in a 1 gallon pot then add 1/2 small yellow onion and cook 1 minute over med heat. Add the ground meat. Break up the meat while it's cooking with the sharp edge of a spatula. Cook until the pink is gone, but don't overdo it, as it will continue to cook once you add the remaining ingredients. Remove the meat from the pot and return the pot to the stove for the next step.
3. Add 1 Tbsp olive oil and heat on med-high heat.
4. Add the diced carrot and cook 1-2 minutes.
5. Add fennel, celery, bell peppers, and green beans and cook 4 minutes, stirring occasionally.
6. Add the zucchini, mushrooms, and spices and cook for another 4 minutes.

(continued)

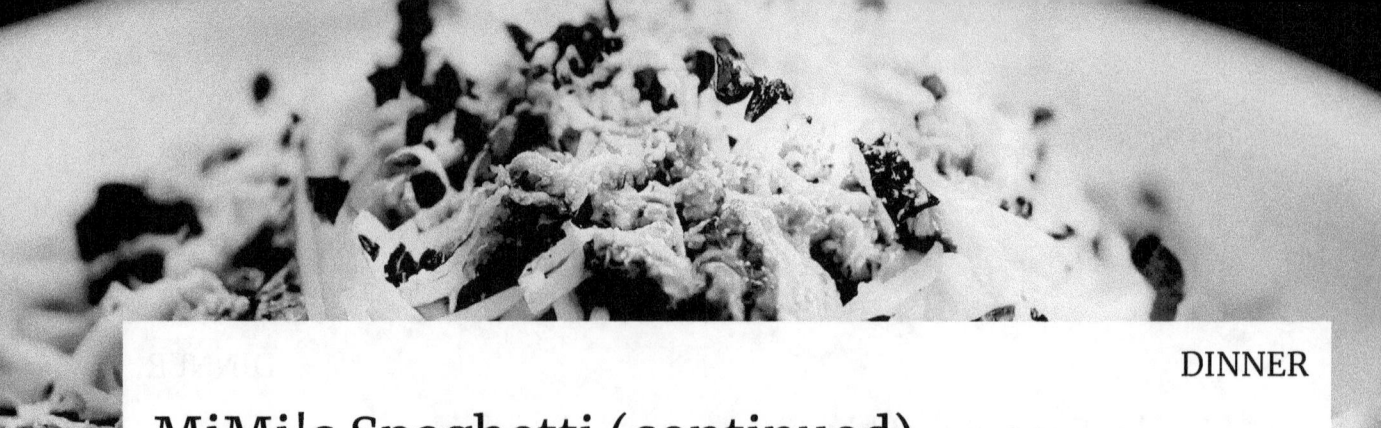

MiMi's Spaghetti (continued)

INGREDIENTS

1/2 tsp rosemary

1/2 tsp thyme

1 tsp ground fennel seed

2 Tbsp brown sugar

1 package Italian or GF spaghetti

Shredded or grated Parmesan

DIRECTIONS

7. Add the tomato sauce, paste, and the can of San Marzano Italian tomatoes. I suggest putting the San Marzano tomatoes in a separate bowl first and squeezing them with your hands to break them up, do not drain, use all the juice from the can and the tomatoes and add to your sauce. Add your meat and meat juice back in and cook the entire mixture for 20–30 minutes on low-med heat, stirring occasionally.

8. Boil 2 quarts of water in a large pot on the stove and cook your spaghetti according to the package or to your preference.

9. Once the pasta is cooked, drain and serve smothered with sauce and a sprinkling of parmesan on top.

If you are going to eat all the spaghetti that night, you can mix the pasta with the sauce after the pasta is cooked, but if you are planning on saving it, I suggest adding a small amount of olive oil to the cooked pasta and storing the sauce separately.

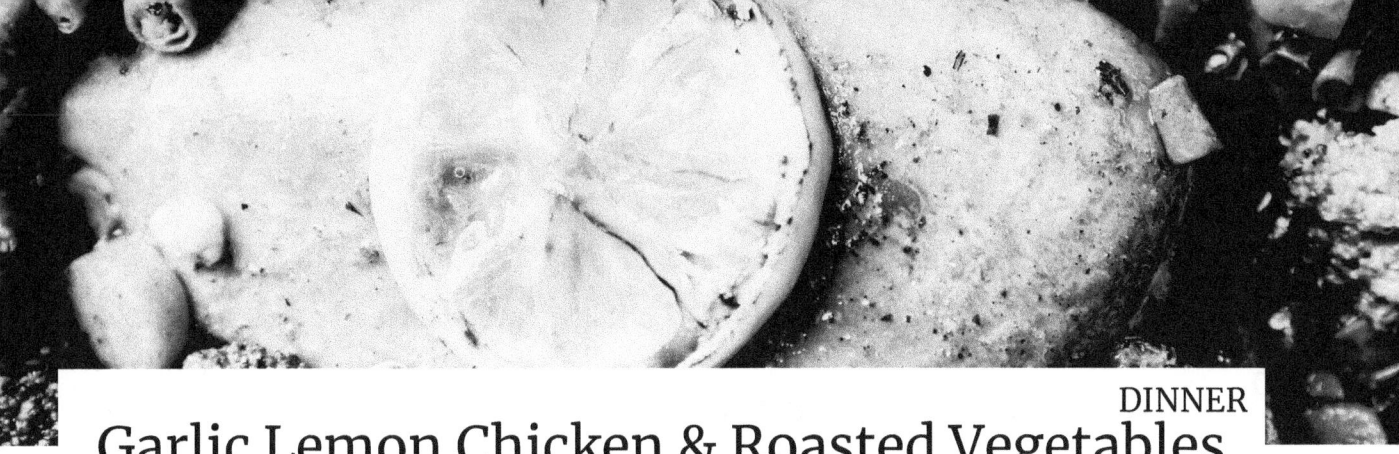

Garlic Lemon Chicken & Roasted Vegetables

An easy and delicious dish great for any season.

INGREDIENTS

4 boneless, skinless
chicken breasts
4 cloves garlic, minced
1/4 cup olive oil
Juice and zest of 1 lemon
1 Tbsp chopped fresh
thyme
1/2 tsp salt
1/4 tsp pepper

2 - 4 cups in season
vegetables
2 Tbsp avocado oil
2 tsp balsamic vinegar
Salt and pepper for
seasoning

DIRECTIONS

1. Use a microplane zester or the smallest grating option on a cheese grater to zest the peel of a clean lemon.
2. To make the juice, first roll your zested lemon on a flat surface to help release the juice from the pulp. Cut the lemon in half and squeeze the juice into a bowl. You can either squeeze through a sieve or remove any seeds by hand.
3. In a large bowl, whisk together garlic, olive oil, lemon juice and zest, thyme, salt, and pepper.
4. Add the chicken breasts to the bowl and coat with the marinade.
5. Cover the marinating chicken and refrigerate 30 mins–4 hrs.
6. Preheat oven to 400 degrees F.
7. Chop veggies into chunks and put them in a bowl, add oil, vinegar, salt and pepper to taste, and toss to cover, then arrange in one layer on a baking sheet.
8. Put the veggies in the oven for 20-30 minutes.
9. Preheat grill (or skillet) to medium–high heat.
10. Discard the marinade and place the chicken on the grill. Cook for 6-8 minutes on each side or until 165 degrees F. When the chicken is fully cooked, if you cut it, the juice will come out clear. If it's still pink, it's not done.

Serve together as a complete meal or add a starch like rice, mashed potatoes, or a nice, crusty bread.

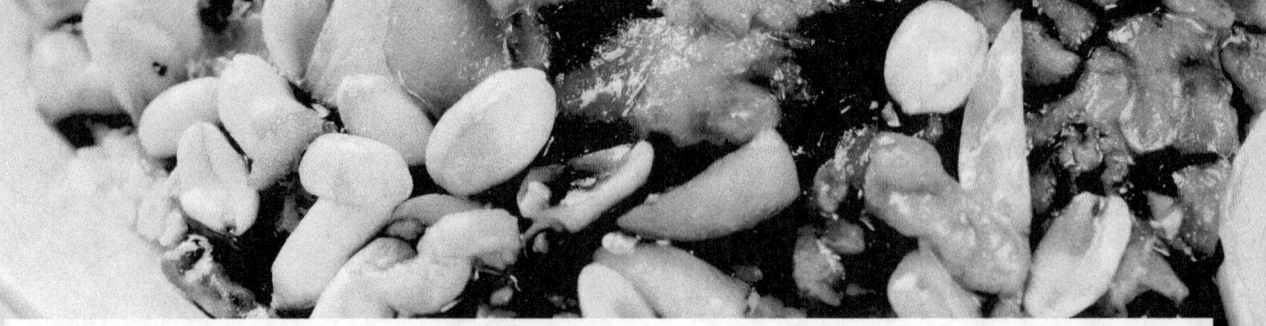

Country Captain Chicken

This is excellent served over rice. It's an easy, two-dish recipe (fewer dirty dishes) that is a delightful dance of flavors on your palate and extremely healthy to boot!

INGREDIENTS

6 slices bacon

4 chicken thighs

Salt and pepper for seasoning

2 large white onions

1/4 cup raisins

1/2 cup cashews

2 Tbsp garlic, minced

2 cups chicken broth

2 Tbsp curry powder

DIRECTIONS

1. Preheat oven to 350 degrees F.
2. Place the bacon in a large, cold skillet and cook on med-high heat until the bacon is crispy.
3. Remove the bacon to a paper towel-lined plate, leaving the bacon grease in the pan.
4. Cook the chicken thighs 4 minutes per side in the bacon grease. Place them so they're not crowded and don't mess with them.
5. Remove the thighs to a small glass baking dish.
6. Add the onions to the skillet and cook for 4 minutes.
7. Add the cashews and cook for 1 minute.
8. Add the raisins and cook until the onions are translucent and the cashews are slightly soft.
9. Add the garlic and cook for 30 seconds longer.
10. Cover the chicken with this mixture and return the skillet to the stove.
11. Add the chicken broth and curry powder to the skillet, using a wooden spoon to scrape up the browned bits from the bottom of the pan.
12. Cook for 3-5 minutes, until slightly thickened, then pour it all over your chicken and onion mixture.
13. Tightly cover with foil and bake for 45 minutes or until the chicken registers 165 degrees F at the thickest part.
14. Chop the bacon while the chicken dish cooks.
15. Serve on top of rice with a generous portion of sauce and a sprinkling of bacon on top.

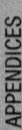

Mimi's Soup Stock

Store bought stock is always an option, but they often come loaded with preservatives and too much salt. This is a great way to use up roasted chicken carcasses and vegetables.

INGREDIENTS

2 roasted chicken carcasses
 (I freeze rotisserie chickens
as I buy them and then use
them for this recipe)
1 large onion, roughly
chopped
2 large carrots, roughly
chopped
4 stalks of celery, roughly
chopped
4 bay leaves
2 Tbsp salt
2 Tbsp black pepper
2 Tbsp oregano
2 Tbsp apple cider vinegar
(This helps to release all the
collagen and minerals from
the bones and increases the
nutritional content of the
stock)
3 cups dry white wine
(All the alcohol boils off as
you simmer)

DIRECTIONS

1. Place the chicken carcasses in a large deep soup pot and cover with 2-3 gallons of filtered water.
2. Add all ingredients to the pot.
3. Bring the mixture to a boil then reduce heat to simmer for 3-8 hours, the longer the better.
4. Strain the broth and then skim with a fine mesh sieve or strain through cheese cloth then let cool.
5. Freeze or use immediately as a base for chicken soup.

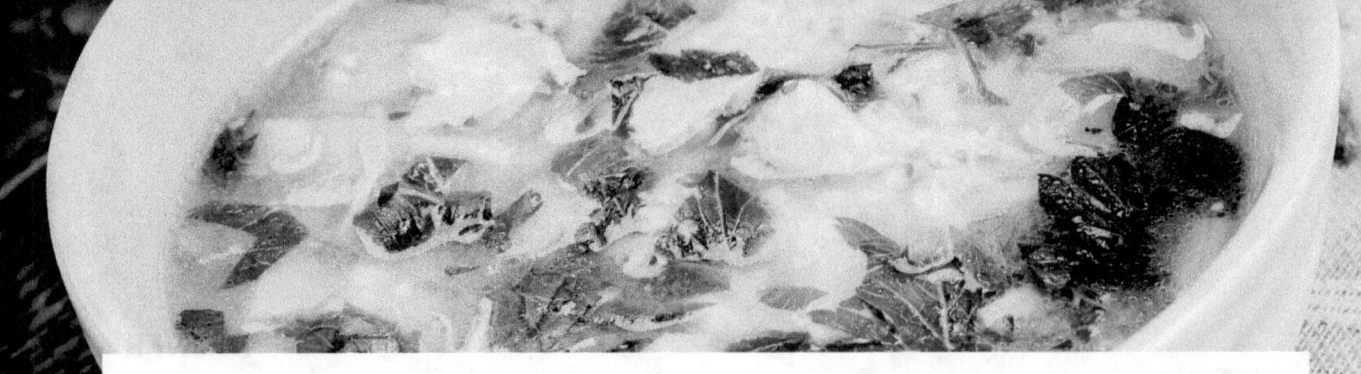

Mimi's Chicken Soup

This is another recipe that tastes like home. Perfect for a cool, fall or winter evening.

INGREDIENTS

3 large carrots, peeled and thinly sliced

1 small fennel, sliced thin and roughly chopped

1 large yellow or sweet onion, diced

3 stalks of celery, cut on the diagonal

1-2 cups potatoes, cut into 1/2" pieces or use small red, white, or fingerling potatoes cut in 1/2

1/2 lb kale, sliced from the stem and chopped

1/2 red bell pepper, diced

1/2 yellow bell pepper, diced

Shredded meat from 1 rotisserie chicken or 6 chicken thighs cooked then chopped or shredded

2 zucchini, sliced in half lengthwise then cut into 1/2" half-moon slices

1 cup whole baby Bella or Shitake mushrooms, quartered

3-4 quarts Mimi's Chicken Stock (or store-bought)

1/2 cup dry white wine (e.g., Sauvignon Blanc or Pinot Grigio)

DIRECTIONS

1. Bring the stock to a simmer then add carrots and cook for 2-3 minutes.
2. Add the fennel, onion, and celery and cook for 5 minutes.
3. Add potatoes, kale, peppers, chicken, spices and cook for 10 minutes.
4. Lastly, add the zucchini and mushrooms, fresh herbs and any of the optional additions. Cook for another 5-10 minutes or until the zucchini is barely tender. Serve immediately (it will continue to cook and you don't want the zucchini to turn to slop)

Serve with warm, crusty bread.

Ingredients, Continued

1/2 bunch Italian parsley, chopped

2 Tbsp oregano

1 Tbsp thyme

1-2 Tbsp salt

1 ½ Tbsp pepper

Optional: 1 bunch cilantro, chopped

1 can white, black, or red beans, drained

1/2 - 1 cup cooked rice, quinoa, or pasta

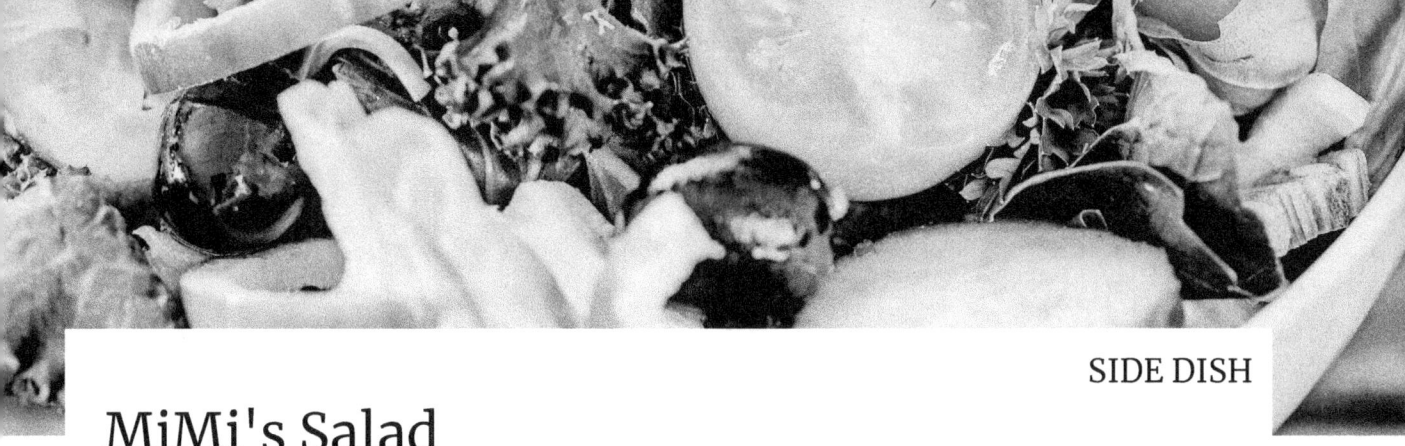

MiMi's Salad

This is excellent on its own for lunch, or it's wonderful to make and keep on hand to snack on or use as a side dish for dinner.

INGREDIENTS

1/2 lb fresh baby spinach

1/2 lb leafy lettuce torn into moderate-sized pieces

1 bunch radishes, sliced

2 stalks celery sliced on the diagonal

1 large carrot, peeled then grated

1 small-medium beet, grated

3/4 cup green cabbage, finely shaved

3/4 cup red cabbage, finely shaved

3/4 cup fresh mushrooms, sliced

Optional additions:

Good quality deli meats

Cheeses like feta, blue, or Cheddar

Tofu or tempeh

Hearts of palm, artichoke hearts, capers or olives

Sprouted raw sunflower or pumpkin seeds

Hemp hearts

Toasted ground sesame seeds

Tomatoes

Salad dressing of choice

DIRECTIONS

1. Wash and prepare all vegetables.
2. Peel then grate the beet onto a plate separately and let it sit to dry for 15 - 30 minutes so it does not dye the salad pink—or skip the waiting period if you want a Barbie salad!
3. Mix all veggies together and put into a large bowl or Tupperware with a tight-fitting lid. This will last for 5 - 7 days and will make multiple servings. You may want to add the mushrooms daily as they can get slimy by day 7. Eat it regularly to help ensure you are getting a great portion of vegetables in each day.

I have many different salad dressings that I use and even mix together to create different flavor profiles based on what I am craving. One of my favorite options is to mix 1 Tbsp vinaigrette with 1 Tbsp creamy dressing like blue cheese or buttermilk ranch. Experiment and get creative!

Creamy Coconut Chicken Soup

This is a template to design a creamy coconut soup you love. This soup is art and you are the artist! Every time I make this, someone asks for the recipe. Enjoy with naan!

INGREDIENTS

2 lbs cubed chicken thighs or breasts or shelled shrimp

2 cans full fat coconut milk

Salt for seasoning

2 Tbsp coconut oil

1 white or sweet onion, diced

2 stalks celery, diced

2 tsp minced garlic

1 ½ cups cubed butternut squash (or any other winter squash, sweet potato, cauliflower, turnips, parsnips …)

4 cups chicken broth

1 ½ tsp salt

1 tsp ground pepper

2 Tbsp curry powder

Pinch of nutmeg

1 tsp ginger

8-10 white mushrooms, stalks removed, quartered

Optional:

2 cup chopped kale

1 bunch of cilantro, chopped for topping

Any other veggies you like!

DIRECTIONS

1. Heat 1 Tbsp of the coconut oil in a large skillet on medium high heat then add the chicken, coconut milk, and salt to taste and bring to a boil, then turn to low and simmer for about 15-20 minutes (10 minutes for shrimp).

2. Sauté the onion and celery in a second large pot in the remaining coconut oil until translucent. Add minced garlic and cook for a few more minutes.

3. Meanwhile, cut open the butternut squash, scrape out the seeds, and cut flesh into 1" cubes. Costco sometimes has packages of organic butternut squash already cubed, which can be a great time saver.

4. Pour in 4 cups of chicken broth and the cubed squash when the onions and celery are ready. Add all the seasoning in. This is where you can add any other vegetables you like!

5. Simmer with the lid on until the squash is soft (you can easily pierce it with a fork), about 15 minutes.

6. Carefully blend the cooked squash with the broth and veggies until creamy and smooth. It's best to use an immersion blender, but a stand blender will work.

7. Add the meat/coconut mix to the vegetable puree.

8. Add the mushrooms and simmer for 5-20 minutes more or keep it warm until you're ready to eat. If you need a bit more fat, you can drizzle coconut milk in your bowl. Garnish with cilantro or other herbs and enjoy!

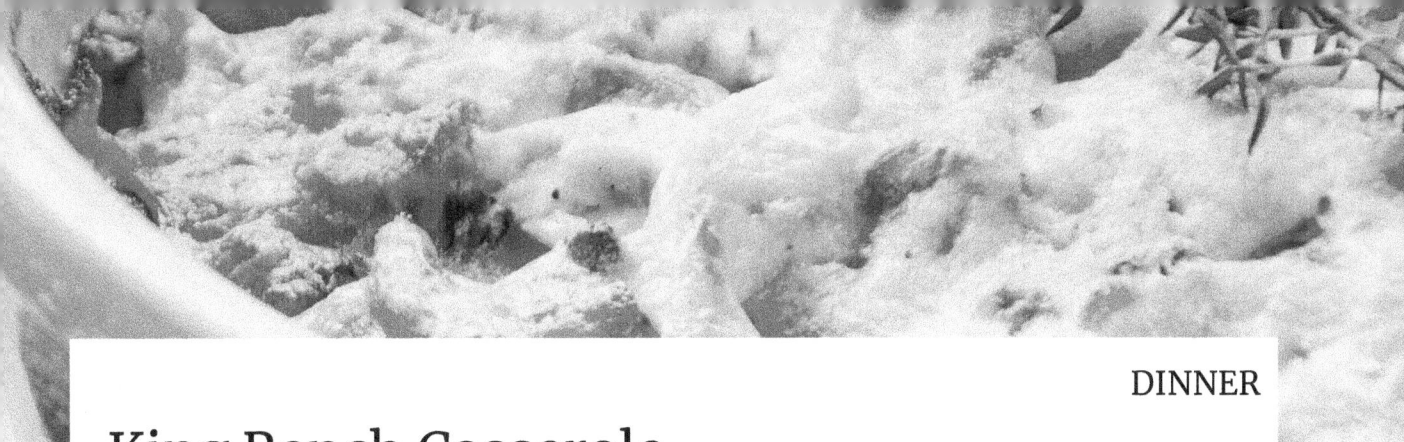

King Ranch Casserole

This is easy to make and easy to enjoy. This dish is as good as the ingredients going in, so use good corn tortillas without preservatives. You can order them online if need be.

INGREDIENTS

1 Tbsp avocado oil

15 corn tortillas, quartered or cut into strips

Meat from 1 rotisserie chicken, shredded (about 3 lbs)

1 can condensed cream of mushroom soup

1 can cream of chicken soup

1 can diced tomatoes and chilis

2 ribs of celery, diced

1 large white onion, diced

1 large red bell pepper, diced

1 large yellow or orange bell pepper, diced

2 cups organic sour cream

8 ozs sharp cheddar cheese, shredded

1 small can of poblano peppers (optional)

3 tsp ground cumin

1 tsp ancho chili powder

2 tsp oregano

1 ½ tsp chipotle chili powder

1/2 tsp salt

DIRECTIONS

1. Preheat oven to 350 degrees F.
2. Sauté the veggies together for 3-4 minutes in oil (you don't need to cook more than this as they will continue to cook in the oven).
3. Mix together the sauteed veggies, soup, diced tomatoes and chilies or Rotel, sour cream, and all the herbs.
4. In a large, greased baking dish layer 1/3 of the tortillas on the bottom of the pan, then 1/3 the sauce, 1/3 of the chicken, then 1/3 the cheese.
5. Next repeat this layering 2 more times until you have used all the ingredients and finish with cheese on top.
6. Bake for 45 minutes or until bubbling and golden brown.

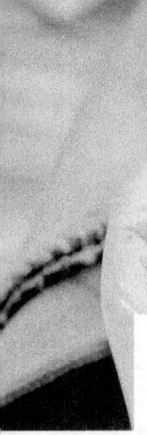

Toodle Oodle Casserole

The quintessential definition of home cooking. This tastes like mom made it. And it's so good for you. I call it the Toodle Oodle Casserole because it's gone before you know it.

INGREDIENTS

4 cans water packed albacore tuna (unsalted)

2 cans condensed cream of mushroom soup

1 can condensed cream of celery or cream of chicken soup

2-3 cups sharp cheddar, grated

7.5 ozs green salad olives with pimentos

1 large carrot, peeled and diced

1-2 stalks of celery, diced

1 medium yellow or sweet onion, diced

1/2 large red bell pepper, diced

1/2 large yellow/orange bell pepper, diced

1 medium-large zucchini, diced

8 oz white or baby Bella mushrooms, chopped

2 Tbsp olive oil

1 lb Italian elbow macaroni

DIRECTIONS

1. Preheat oven to 375 degrees F.
2. Prepare all vegetables as directed.
3. Heat olive oil in a 1 gallon pot. Add the diced carrot, cook 1-2 minutes over medium heat.
4. Add celery, onion, and bell peppers and cook for 3 minutes.
5. Add zucchini, cook for 2-3 more minutes.
6. While your veggies are cooking boil water for pasta (2 quarts in a large pot, add 1 tsp salt once boiling).
7. Drain and then break up tuna with a fork into a large bowl.
8. Add both soups to the tuna.
9. Cook pasta, drain well and cool for 2 minutes, then add to the tuna and soup and mix together.
10. Once all veggies are cooked add those to the pasta mix and add 1/3-1/2 of the cheese, then mix together well.
11. Put the mixture in a greased 9"x13" baking pan. Add the remaining cheese to the top.
12. Bake for 30-45 minutes or until bubbling and cheese is browning.

Serve hot and keep leftovers in the fridge for lunch the next day.

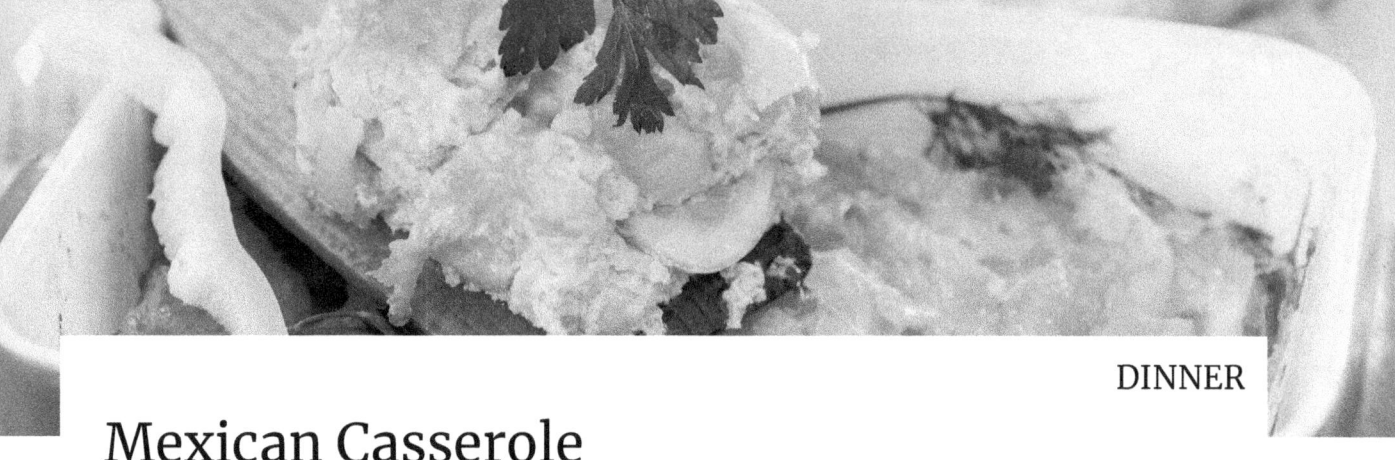

Mexican Casserole

This is a great way to up your protein. You can get creative with this one and load it with expiring vegetables from your vegetable drawer, too. It's a great "clean-your-fridge" dish.

INGREDIENTS

1 Tbsp butter

2 11-oz cans whole hatch green chilis

1 lb Jack cheese, shredded

1 bunch cilantro, chopped (optional)

1 cup red or green salsa

8 ozs whole white or baby Bella mushrooms, stemmed

12-16 eggs

Optional extras:

Artichoke hearts

Black olives

Cooked zucchini or yellow squash

DIRECTIONS

1. Preheat oven to 350 degrees F.
2. Prepare a 9"x13" casserole dish by spreading the butter all over the inside of the dish.
3. Layer the chilis from one can (drained) on the bottom of the dish.
4. On top of that place a layer of button mushrooms and any other vegetables you'd like.
5. Add a thin layer of cheese and a sprinkling of cilantro.
6. Repeat until all ingredients except for the eggs, salsa, half of the cheese, and half of the cilantro are used up.
7. Beat all eggs together in a stand mixer (or whisk vigorously) for 1 minute (to incorporate lots of air and make them fluffy).
8. Stir the salsa into the eggs.
9. Pour the eggs over the ingredients in the baking dish.
10. Bake for 30 minutes, then add the remaining cheese and cook for an additional 15 minutes or until the eggs are cooked through.
11. Sprinkle with cilantro on top (optional) and serve with rice.

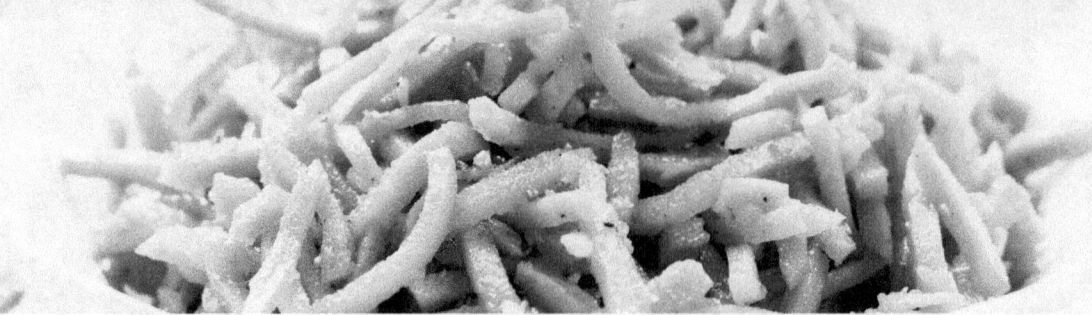

Dr. Ray Peat's Raw Carrot Salad

This is an excellent snack to eat daily. It provides essential fats and vitamins like beta carotene, and the raw carrot acts as an estrogen-binder, which is great in our phytoestrogen-rich environment. Regularly consumed, it will help to lower metabolic stress.

INGREDIENTS

1 medium carrot, grated

1/2 Tbsp coconut oil

1/2 tsp of your favorite vinegar

Salt for seasoning

DIRECTIONS

1. Combine all ingredients.
2. Enjoy!

I like to make this one in bulk, multiplying everything by 7 to have enough on hand for a week. I prepare the carrots and store them in water in the fridge. Then I prepare the dressing and store it separately, in a mason jar with a lid, at room temperature. When I want to eat some of this, I take a serving of carrot, mix with the dressing and voila! You can add other things to this to change it up, like raisins or nuts.

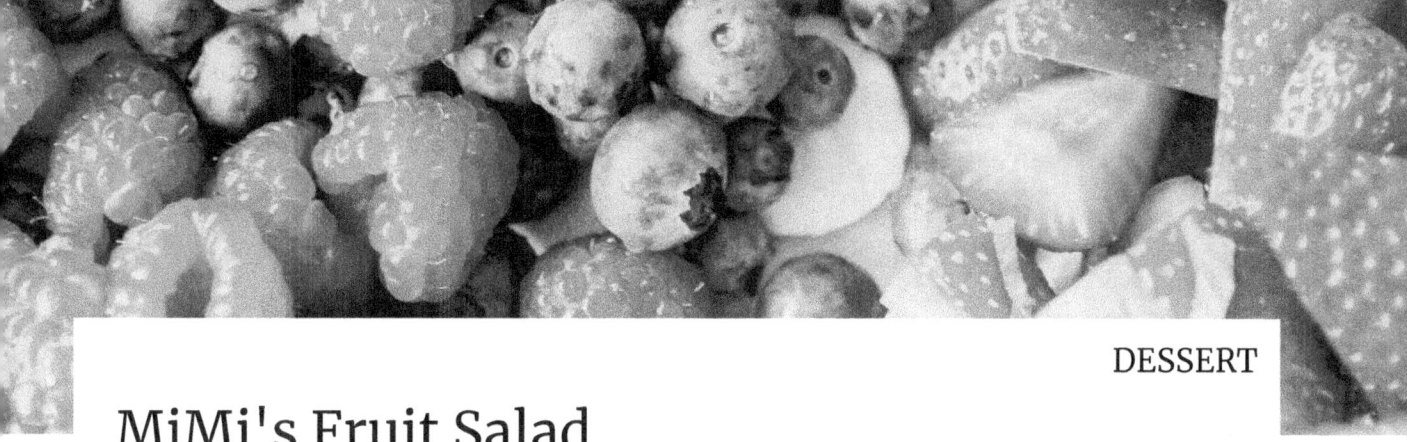

MiMi's Fruit Salad

This is excellent on its own for lunch, or it's fabulous to make and keep on hand to snack on or use as a side dish for dinner.

INGREDIENTS

1 small Gala apple, diced

1 small ripe pear, diced

1 ½ lb ripe strawberries, sliced or quartered

1 cup blueberries

1 cup raspberries

1 small ripe mango, diced

1 cup grapes, halved

1 small banana

Optional in-season fruit:

1 ripe peach

1/2 lb cherries, pitted and halved

*Only add bananas when serving

*You can get creative with other additional fruits that are in season or that you like!

DIRECTIONS

1. Stir the fruits together in a large bowl and enjoy!

Store in the fridge and eat within 3 days.

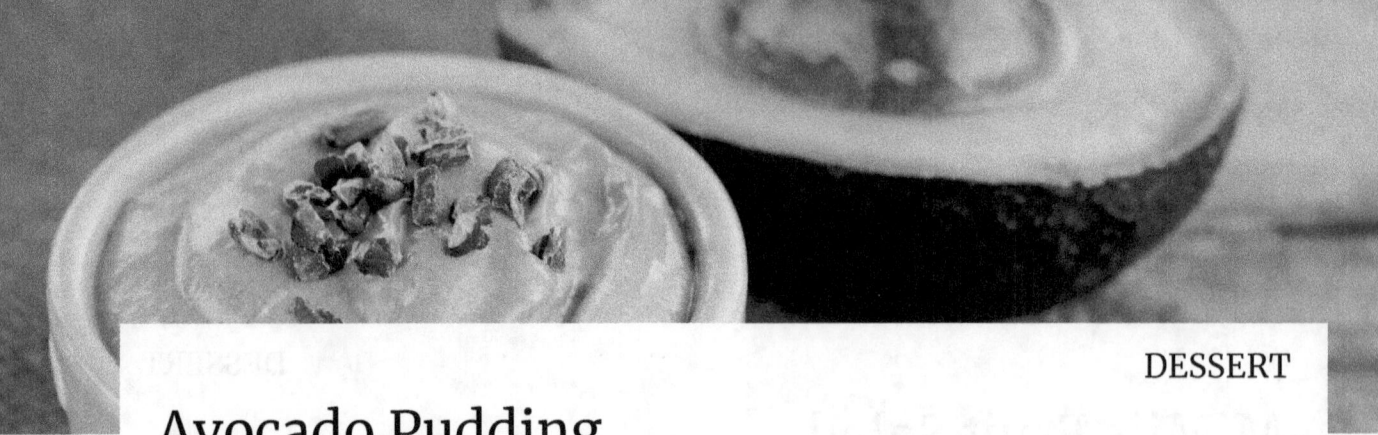

Avocado Pudding

Remember this dish when your baby is a toddler and refuses to eat anything green. It's a delicious and healthy dish that makes for an easy, healthy treat.

INGREDIENTS

Flesh from 4 ripe avocados

1/4 cup maple syrup, honey, or agave syrup

1/2 cup heavy cream

1/2 cup cocoa powder

Whipped cream for topping

DIRECTIONS

1. Place all ingredients except the whipped cream in a food processor or blender and blend on high speed until smooth and creamy. The mixture will resemble a creamy chocolate pudding and take on a glistening texture.
2. Chill in the fridge for a few hours before eating.
3. Top with whipped cream and serve!

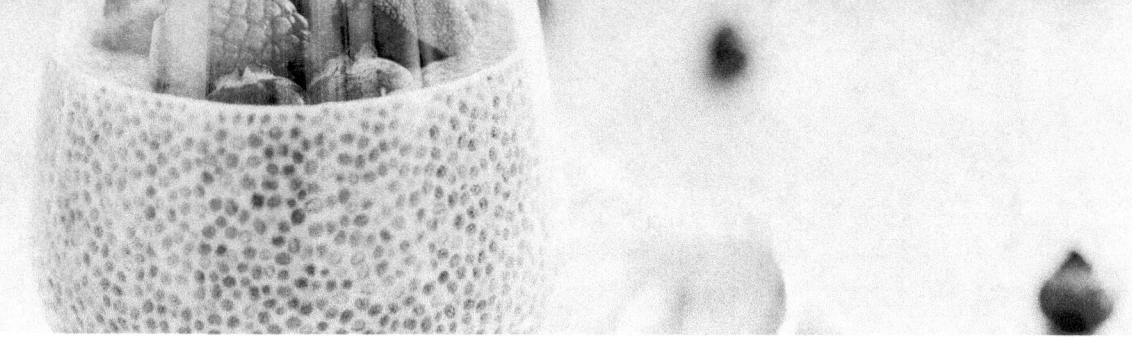

Chia Seed Pudding

This is an easy and light dish to keep on hand. You can use any dairy-free milk you like. Milk of Macadamia is one of my favorites. Use 6 Tbsp chia seeds for a thinner pudding, 8 Tbsp if you like it thick.

INGREDIENTS

2 cups dairy-free milk

6–8 Tbsp chia seeds

1/4-1/2 tsp cinnamon

1 Tbsp maple syrup

2 tsp vanilla extract

Optional Additions

Drizzle of maple syrup on top

1/4 cup of any fruit: raspberries, strawberries, and blueberries are my favorites

1–2 Tbsp chopped walnuts or pecans

DIRECTIONS

1. Stir together your chia seeds and milk in a bowl or storage container.
2. Once the chia pudding mixture is well combined, add cinnamon, maple syrup, and vanilla and stir well.
3. Cover and place in fridge for 2 hours or overnight.
4. When ready, the pudding should be nice and thick. If it is not thick enough, you can stir in more chia seeds and give it a little more time in the fridge. You'll learn what works for you over time.
5. Drizzle maple syrup on top, add fruit, and nuts (optional), and enjoy.

Eat this as part of your breakfast, for a nutrient-packed snack, or as a healthy desert option.

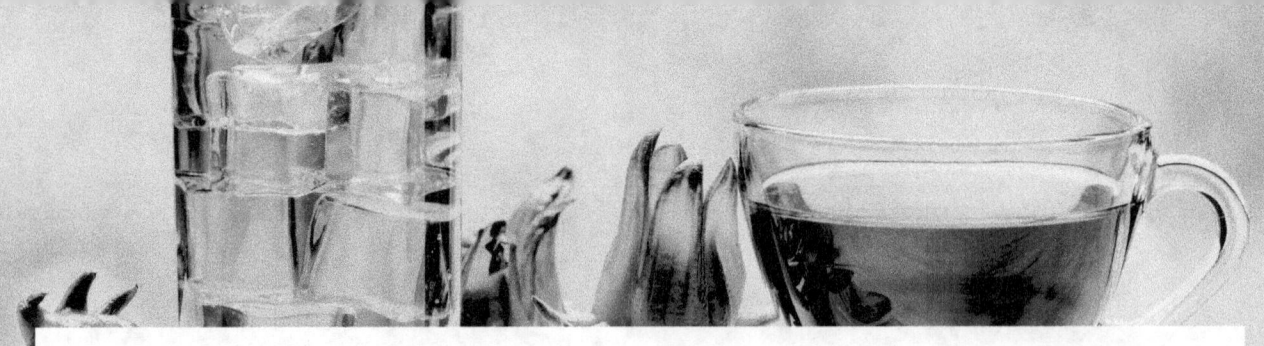

Pregnancy Tea

I have included a recipe below for Pregnancy Tea that you can consume iced or hot 2-3 times per day throughout your pregnancy. Red Raspberry leaf and pregnancy teas both tone the uterus and nothing here will harm you or your baby. Drinking a few cups a day will contribute to your gestational health and help lessen your pain and bleeding during birth. Keep some on hand in the fridge and drink it often throughout your pregnancy as well as postpartum to help build a healthy supply of milk!

INGREDIENTS

Red Raspberry Leaf

Contains vitamins A, B, and E, as well as calcium, phosphorous, iron, and is an acid neutralizer.

Stinging Nettles

Stinging nettles is a blood cleansing and blood building herb with high iron content. It is very nourishing to the kidneys and liver and will help relieve (or prevent altogether) vascular problems common during pregnancy. It also helps build a good milk supply.

DIRECTIONS

1. Combine 1-part red raspberry leaf to 1-part stinging nettles.
2. Add some or all the optional herbs if desired.
3. A general rule of thumb is 1 Tbsp of herb to 1 cup water.
4. Place herbs in a non-metal container, preferably a half gallon mason jar, and cover the herbs with almost boiling water then cap tightly.
5. Let this steep for 4-6 hours. Pour mixture through a strainer and discard the herbs.

The tea will keep for up to 4 days if refrigerated. A small amount of fruit juice (grape, apple, raspberry) can be added as a sweetener if you like. There is no right or wrong way to make the tea. Experiment and find a mixture that works for you!

Add any of the following for variety:

Alfalfa: Contains vitamins A, B12, D, and E, calcium, and phosphorous. Great for the milk supply.

Rose Hip: Contains the entire vitamin C complex. Good for vascular problems (hemorrhoids and varicose veins) and to boost the immune system. Recommended for Rh negative women for fighting off infections.

Spearmint: Soothing to the stomach, helps digestion, and lends a pleasant taste to the mixture. A little goes a long way. If you are taking homeopathic remedies, leave the spearmint out while the remedies are still active as spearmint contradicts some homeopathic remedies.

Red Clover: This blood purifying herb is especially good during acute illness and for high blood pressure.

Appendix C: Medical Questionnaire

This questionnaire is the one I provide to my clients to both inform me as their care provider and to help them to understand their own birth stories.

Your provider will likely have their own questionnaire for you to use; I include this here by way of example.

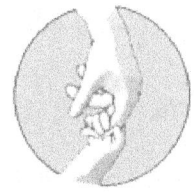

NEW LIFE BIRTH SERVICES

NAME: _____

MATERNAL FAMILY MEDICAL HISTORY

	Client's Father	Client's Mother	Client's Sibling	Paternal Relative	Maternal Relative	Outcomes/Details
Allergies						
Cancer						
Congenital Abnormalities						
Diabetes (age at onset)						
Drug or alcohol problems						
Seizure Disorders						

	Client's Father	Client's Mother	Client's Sibling	Paternal Relative	Maternal Relative	Outcomes/Details
High blood pressure						
Heart disease						
Kidney disease						
TB						
High/low birth weight						
Twins						
Stroke						
Other						

CLIENT'S MOTHER'S OBSTETRICAL HISTORY (MATERNAL):

Number of Pregnancies

Births

Miscarriages

Hospital births

Breech births

Cesarean births

Approximate weights

Other

Complications of pregnancy, labor, or delivery (prolonged labor, hemorrhage, etc.) or postpartum

_____

_____

_____

Attitude toward childbirth _____

Number of babies breastfed? _____ Difficulties _____

Were you breastfed? _____ How long? _____

Did your mother take diethylstilbestrol (DES) during the pregnancy leading to your birth?

_____

Did anyone significant die or did your mother experience severe trauma while she was pregnant with you, or before you were one year old?

_____

_____

Your sister's obstetrical history

_____

Please briefly describe your own birth

_____

_____

_____

Describe your relationship with your mom and dad

_____

_____

_____

PATERNAL FAMILY MEDICAL HISTORY

	Client's Father	Client's Mother	Client's Sibling	Paternal Relative	Maternal Relative	Outcomes/Details
Allergies						
Cancer						
Congenital Abnormalities						
Diabetes (age at onset)						
Drug or alcohol problems						
Seizure Disorders						
High blood pressure						
Heart disease						
Kidney disease						
TB						
High/low birth weight						
Twins						
Stroke						
Other						

CLIENT'S MOTHER'S OBSTETRICAL HISTORY (PATERNAL):

Number of Pregnancies _____

Births _____

Miscarriages _____

Hospital births _____

Breech births _____

Cesarean births _____

Approximate weights _____

Other _____

Complications of pregnancy, labor, or delivery (prolonged labor, hemorrhage, etc.) or postpartum

_____

_____

_____

Attitude toward childbirth _____

Number of babies breastfed? _____ Difficulties _____

Were you breastfed? _____ How long? _____

Did your mother take diethylstilbestrol (DES) during the pregnancy leading to your birth?

_____

Did anyone significant die or did your mother experience severe trauma while she was pregnant with you, or before you were one year old?

_____

_____

Your sister's obstetrical history

_____

Please briefly describe your own birth

_____

_____

_____

_____

Describe your relationship with your mom and dad

_____

_____

_____

_____

Appendix D: Resources for Miscarriage and Grief

Twenty-five percent of women—yes, at least one out of every four—experience a pregnancy or infant loss. Women around the world carry this grief their entire lives. These are some resources and groups available to help you feel not so alone if you are facing grief and loss. I encourage you to find community to help you through this.

stillbirthday: A robust resource regarding pregnancy loss for both parents and birth professionals. They can connect you with bereavement doulas who can help you through the stages of grief. www. stillbirthday.com

Now I Lay Me Down to Sleep: Provides photography services for stillbirth and infant loss. www.nowilaymedowntosleep. org

Compassionate Friends: Provides in-person support groups for bereaved parents. www.compassionatefriends.org

Loss Doulas International: Certifies doulas to support during miscarriage or stillbirth and afterwards. www. lossdoulasinternational.com

Still Standing Magazine: A resource for parents. https://stillstandingmag.com/

SHARE Pregnancy & Infant Loss Support: Offers support groups and resources for families surviving a loss. https://nationalshare.org/

March of Dimes Offers supportive guidance on the website. https://www.marchofdimes.org/find-support/topics/miscarriage-loss-and-grief

Miscarriage Matters, Inc.: This is a solid compilation of resources for you to explore. You may find local groups that you can meet with in person. mymiscarriagematters.org

Suicide Prevention: If you are feeling like you want to follow your child, please contact the National Suicide Prevention Lifeline: 800-273-8255.

I highly encourage you to find support, so you are not alone during periods of grief and loss. If you are outside of the United States, some of these resources may not be available to you. Look for resources in your area by searching the internet to find support through local mental health organizations and support groups.

Appendix E: Organizations

Midwives

Midwives Alliance of North America (MANA)

www.mana.org

North American Registry of Midwives (NARM)

https://narm.org/

Midwifery Education Accreditation Counsel (MEAC)

https://www.meacschools.org/

American College of Nurse Midwives (ACNM)

http://www.midwife.org/

Doulas

Doulas of North America (DONA)

www.dona.org

Breastfeeding Support

La Leche League

https://www.llli.org/

Cord Blood Banking

Private

The Cord Blood Registry

www.cordblood.com/

Viacord

Offers public and private banking.
https://www.viacord.com/

Americord

https://www.americordblood.com/

AlphaCord

https://www.alphacord.com/

Public

Be the Match

https://bethematch.org/

Viacord

https://www.viacord.com/

You may also find more local public banks in places with larger populations, like New York, California, and Texas.

USDA Food Recall Information

The USDA recommends that consumers check the USDA's Food Safety and Inspection Service website for the latest recall information.

If you have any questions or concerns about a meat or poultry product, you can contact the USDA's Meat and Poultry Hotline at 1-888-MPHOTLINE (1-888-674-6854).

Appendix F: Book Recommendations

Conscious Conception

The Book of Birth Volume I: A Sevenfold Approach to Your Ideal, Perfect Conception, Pregnancy, and Birth by MariMikel Potter, CPM, LM, RN-BSN

Burnout: The Secret to Unlocking the Stress Cycle by Emily Nagoski and Amelia Nagoski

Come As You Are: Revised and Updated: The Surprising New Science That Will Transform Your Sex Life by Emily Nagoski

It Starts With the Egg, Getting Pregnant with PCOS by Rebecca Fett

The Infertility Cure by Randine Lewis

Making Babies by Jill Blakeway and Sami David

Taking Charge of Your Fertility, 20th Anniversary Edition: The Definitive Guide to Natural Birth Control, Pregnancy Achievement, and Reproductive Health by Toni Wechsler

Pregnancy

The Book of Birth Volume I: A Sevenfold Approach to Your Ideal, Perfect Conception, Pregnancy, and Birth by MariMikel Potter, CPM, LM, RN-BSN

Birth Matters: A Midwife's Manifesta by Ina May Gaskin

Gentle Birth Choices by Barbara Harper R.N.

Ina May's Guide to Childbirth by Ina May Gaskin

Mind Over Labor by Carl Jones

Spiritual Midwifery by Ina May Gaskin

The Expectant Father by Armin A. Brott and Jennifer Ash Ruddick

Parenting

Infancy

The Book of Birth Volume II: Your Postpartum Journey through the Fourth Trimester by MariMikel Potter, CPM, LM, RN-BSN

Circumcision: The Hidden Trauma by Ronald Goldman

Infant Massage: A Handbook for Loving Parents by Vimala McClure

Your Amazing Newborn by Marshall H. Klaus, MD & Phyllis H. Klaus, C.S.W., M.Ed.

General

The Absorbent Mind by Dr. Maria Montessori

The Attachment Parenting Book: A Commonsense Guide to Understanding and Nurturing Your Baby (Sears Parenting Library) by William Sears MD, Martha Sears

The Happiest Baby On the Block by Harvey Karp, M.D.

How to Talk So Kids Will Listen and Listen So Kids Will Talk by Adele Faber and Elaine Mazlish

The Mind of Your Newborn Baby by David Chamberlain

The Sears Baby Book, Revised Edition: Everything You Need to Know About Your Baby from Birth to Age Two by William Sears MD, Martha Sears, RN, Robert W. Sears, MD, and James Sears, MD

The Secret Life of the Unborn Child by Thomas Verney, M.D., with John Kelly

The Wonder Weeks, A Stress-Free Guide to Your Baby's Behavior by Hetty van de Ritj, PhD, Frans X. Plooij, PhD, and Xavier Plas-Plooij

Whole Brained Child by Daniel J. Siegel, M.D. and Tina Payne Bryson, Ph.D

Breastfeeding
Ina May's Guide to Breastfeeding by Ina May Gaskin

The Womanly Art of Breastfeeding by Diane Wiessinger, Diana West, et al

Co-Sleeping
Safe Infant Sleep: Expert Answers to Your Cosleeping Questions by James J. McKenna Ph.D.

Nutrition and Cookbooks
Food Combining Made Easy by Herbert M. Shelton

The Joy of Cooking by Irma S. Rombauer

Nourishing Traditions by Sally Fallon

Real Food for Pregnancy by Lily Nichols

Well Fed, Well Fed 2, and *Well Fed Weeknights* by Melissa Joulwan.

These are wonderful guides to excellent dishes from a wide spectrum of cuisines, and they will help you to cut down on wheat consumption, up your veggie intake, and manage your meal planning and grocery shopping.

Vegetarian Cookbooks
The Moosewood Cookbook by Mollie Katzen

The New Enchanted Broccoli Forest by Mollie Katzen

The New Farm Vegetarian Cookbook by Louise Hagler and Dorothy R. Bates

The Vegetarian Epicure by Anna Thomas

Other
Atomic Habits by James Clear

Adrenal Thyroid Revolution by Aviva Romm M.D.

All Creatures Great and Small by James Herriot

A Course in Miracles by Foundation for Inner Peace

Breath by James Nestor

Evolutions End, Magical Child, Magical Child Revisited, and *Crack in The Cosmic Egg* by Joseph C. Pearce

Homeopathic Medicine for Women by Trevor Smith, M.D.

Out of Print but Worth Locating

These are books I have long cherished but are no longer in print, and so may be more difficult to find.

Birth Reborn by Michel Odent

The Blessingway by Veronika Sophia Robinson

Breastfeeding Your Baby by Sheila Kitzinger

Circumcision: An American Health Fallacy by Edward Wallerstein

Cucina Amore by Nick Sellino

The Family Bed by Tine Thevenin

Immaculate Deception II: Myth Magic and Birth by Suzanne Arms

Macrobiotic Pregnancy and Care of the Newborn by Michio and Aveline Kushi

Making Love During Pregnancy by Elisabeth Bing and Libby Colman

Parenting Begins Before Conception by Carista Luminare-Rosen

The Silent Knife: Cesarean Prevention & Vaginal Birth After Cesarean by Nancy Wainer Cohen & Lois J. Estner

The Year After Childbirth by Sheila Kitzinger

UNTOUCHED: The Need for Genuine Affection in an Impersonal World by Mariana Caplan

Appendix G: Tracking Contractions

TIMING CONTRACTIONS

Time Contraction Starts			Time Contraction Ends		
Hour	Minute	Second	Hour	Minute	Second
:	:		:	:	
:	:		:	:	
:	:		:	:	
:	:		:	:	
:	:		:	:	
:	:		:	:	
:	:		:	:	
:	:		:	:	
:	:		:	:	
:	:		:	:	
:	:		:	:	
:	:		:	:	
:	:		:	:	

GLOSSARY

4-hour Rule—MariMikel's rule: In the final weeks of your pregnancy, do not attempt to take on projects that last for more than four hours and take a significant break at the two-hour mark.

A

Abdominal—Relating to the abdomen, which is the area between the chest and the pelvis that contains the stomach, intestines, liver, and other organs.

Abscess—A localized collection of pus within a tissue or organ, usually caused by an infection. It often appears as a swollen, painful, and inflamed area.

Abstinence—The act of refraining from partaking in a particular activity or substance, like sex, alcohol, or drugs.

Acidophilus— A type of live bacteria that is found in the digestive system. Acidophilus is often taken as a supplement to help improve digestion and gut health.

Acknowledgment of Paternity (AOP)—A legal document signed by a father who is not married to the mother in order to establish his paternity. This allows him to be named on the birth certificate. If you are married, no AOP is needed. The signing of the AOP confirms that he is the biological and legal father of a child with the rights and responsibilities that conveys.

Active Labor—The phase of childbirth in which the cervix is dilating from 4−7 centimeters, and contractions become stronger and more frequent, leading to the delivery of the baby.

Algae oil—A supplemental source of omega-3 fatty acids.

Amylase—An enzyme that breaks down starch into sugar. Amylase is found in saliva and pancreatic juice, and it plays a role in digestion.

Analgesia—The absence of pain. Analgesia can be achieved through medication, such as over-the-counter pain relievers or prescription painkillers. It can also be achieved through non-medication methods, such as acupuncture or massage therapy.

Anencephaly—A severe birth defect in which the baby is born without parts of the brain and skull. It is a life-threatening condition.

Anesthesia—The use of medication to prevent pain or induce unconsciousness during medical procedures or surgery.

Anterior fontanel—A soft spot on the baby's skull where the skull bones have not yet fused. It is located at the front of the head and is usually present until around 18-24 months of age.

Antibodies—Proteins produced by the immune system in response to the presence of foreign substances (antigens) such as bacteria, viruses, or other pathogens. Antibodies help the body recognize and fight off these invaders.

Areola—The pigmented area of skin surrounding the nipple on the breast. It may vary in color and size among individuals.

Astragalus—An herbaceous plant belonging to the Fabaceae family. It is commonly used in traditional Chinese medicine and other herbal practices. The root of the astragalus plant is particularly prized for its potential medicinal properties. It is often used as an adaptogen, which means it may help the body adapt to stress and support overall well-being. Astragalus is also believed to have immune-enhancing properties and is used to support immune system function. It is available in various forms, including teas, tinctures, and capsules.

Asynclitic—A term used to describe a baby's position in the uterus in which the fetal head is not aligned with the center of the mother's pelvis. Asynclitism is a common occurrence during pregnancy, and it usually does not cause any problems. However, in some cases, it can lead to a difficult labor and delivery.

Augmentation—Refers to the medical intervention used to enhance or accelerate the progress of labor when it has slowed or stalled. It involves interventions aimed at increasing the frequency, duration, or strength of uterine contractions to promote efficient cervical dilation and progress toward childbirth.

B

Barrier method—A type of contraception that uses a physical barrier to prevent sperm from fertilizing an egg. Barrier methods include condoms, diaphragms, and cervical caps.

Bilirubin—A yellow pigment produced by the breakdown of red blood cells in the liver. Elevated levels of bilirubin can cause jaundice, a condition characterized by yellowing of the skin and eyes.

Bioflavonoid—A type of plant compound that has antioxidant and anti-inflammatory properties. Bioflavonoids are often taken as a supplement to improve cardiovascular health, reduce the risk of cancer, and boost the immune system.

Birth canal—The passageway through which the baby travels during childbirth. It includes the cervix, vagina, and vulva.

Birth certificate—A legal document issued by the government to record the details of a person's birth, including their name, date of birth, place of birth, and parents' names.

Bloody show—A discharge of blood-tinged mucus from the vagina that can occur during late pregnancy or the early stages of labor. It is often a sign that the cervix is dilating, and the body is preparing for childbirth.

Borage—A plant with bright blue flowers that is often used for medicinal purposes.

Brassica—A genus of plants that includes various cruciferous vegetables such as broccoli, cabbage, kale, and Brussels sprouts.

Breastfeeding—The act of feeding an infant with breast milk produced by the mother. Breast milk provides essential nutrients and antibodies, promoting the baby's health and development.

Bromine—A chemical element that is found in the Earth's crust and oceans. Bromine is used in a variety of industrial and commercial applications, such as the production of flame retardants, pesticides, and pharmaceuticals.

C

Carbohydrates, complex—Complex carbohydrates consist of longer chains of sugar molecules and are often found in whole grains, legumes, vegetables, and fruits. They take longer to digest due to their complex structure, providing a more sustained release of energy and a slower increase in blood sugar levels. Complex carbohydrates are typically higher in fiber, vitamins, and minerals compared to simple carbohydrates. They offer more nutritional value and can help maintain stable energy levels throughout the day. Examples of complex carbohydrates include whole wheat bread, brown rice, oats, quinoa, lentils, and starchy vegetables like sweet potatoes.

Carbohydrates, simple—Simple carbohydrates, also known as simple sugars, are composed of one or two sugar molecules. They are quickly digested and absorbed into the bloodstream, leading to a rapid increase in blood sugar levels. Common sources of simple carbohydrates include table sugar (sucrose), fruit juices, honey, candy, and desserts. Consuming excessive amounts of simple carbohydrates, especially from refined sources, can contribute to blood sugar spikes, energy crashes, and potential long-term health issues if consumed in excess.

Carbs/carbohydrates—One of the three main macronutrients found in food, along with proteins and fats. Carbohydrates are a primary source of energy for the body and are commonly found in grains, fruits, vegetables, and dairy products. Carbohydrates can be simple or complex.

Carcinogenic—Refers to substances or agents that have the potential to cause cancer or increase the risk of developing cancer when exposed to or consumed over time.

Cardiopulmonary Resuscitation (CPR)—An emergency procedure performed to restore blood circulation and breathing in someone who is experiencing cardiac arrest or respiratory failure. CPR involves chest compressions and rescue breaths.

CDC—The Centers for Disease Control and Prevention, a national public health agency in the United States. The CDC is responsible for protecting public health and safety through the control and prevention of diseases, injuries, and disabilities.

Cervical cap—A small, flexible device made of silicone that is inserted into the vagina and placed over the cervix to prevent pregnancy. It acts as a barrier method of contraception.

Cervix—The lower, narrow part of the uterus (womb) that connects to the vagina. During childbirth, the cervix dilates to allow the passage of the baby from the uterus to the birth canal.

Cesarean section (c-section)—A surgical procedure in which a baby is delivered through an incision made in the mother's abdomen and uterus. C-sections are performed when vaginal delivery is not possible or deemed unsafe.

Chelate/chelation—refers to a process of binding a mineral to an amino acid or organic acid to protect it from stomach acid and improve its absorption.

Chi—In traditional Chinese medicine, "chi" (or "qi") refers to the vital energy or life force that flows throughout the body. It is believed to be essential for health and well-being and is often manipulated through practices such as acupuncture or tai chi.

Chlamydia—A sexually transmitted infection (STI) caused by the bacteria Chlamydia trachomatis. Chlamydia can infect both men and women, and it can cause a variety of symptoms, including pain during urination, unusual vaginal discharge, and pelvic pain. It can also have no symptoms at all.

Colic—A condition characterized by severe, often fluctuating, abdominal pain in infants. Colic is usually temporary and often occurs in otherwise healthy babies.

Colostrum—The thick, yellowish fluid that is produced by the breasts during pregnancy and in the first few days after childbirth. Colostrum is rich in antibodies and provides essential nutrients for the newborn.

Comfrey—A plant with hairy leaves and bell-shaped flowers that has been traditionally used for medicinal purposes. It is known for its potential healing properties, particularly in the form of topical applications. Used for bruises, sprains, torn ligaments and muscles, and broken bones.

Compartmentalization—A defense mechanism in which a person mentally separates conflicting thoughts, feelings, or beliefs into distinct compartments or categories to reduce cognitive dissonance. It allows individuals to keep contradictory aspects of their lives or themselves separate and avoid psychological discomfort.

Contraindicated—A medical term that means something is not recommended or safe to do. For example, certain medications may be contraindicated for people with certain medical conditions.

Cord, clamping—The act of clamping the umbilical cord after childbirth.

Cord, cutting—The act of cutting the umbilical cord, which connects the baby to the placenta in the womb.

Coronavirus—A family of viruses that can cause illness in humans and animals. Examples of coronaviruses include the common cold and more severe respiratory illnesses such as severe acute respiratory syndrome (SARS) and Middle East respiratory syndrome (MERS).

COVID-19—Short for "coronavirus disease 2019," COVID-19 is an infectious disease caused by the SARS-CoV-2 virus. It primarily affects the respiratory system and can cause a range of symptoms from mild to severe.

CPR—Abbreviation for Cardiopulmonary Resuscitation, as mentioned earlier. It is an emergency procedure performed to restore blood circulation and breathing in cases of cardiac arrest or respiratory failure.

Cradle cap—A skin condition that affects babies and toddlers. Cradle cap is characterized by scaly, crusty patches on the scalp. It can be helped or prevented by brushing the baby's head regularly.

C-Section—See Cesarean Section.

D

Defense mechanism—A psychological strategy or coping mechanism that individuals unconsciously use to protect themselves from anxiety, emotional distress, or threatening thoughts or feelings.

DeLee—The DeLee suction apparatus is a handheld device that is used to remove mucus, fluid, or blood from the baby's airways. It is named after John DeLee, an American obstetrician who developed it in the early 1900s. It consists of a tube that goes into the baby's esophagus, a mucus trap, and a tube with a mouthpiece that the professional uses to create suction.

Denial—A defense mechanism in which a person refuses to acknowledge or accept the reality of a distressing or anxiety-provoking situation, thought, or feeling. It can involve blocking out information, minimizing the significance of events, or simply refusing to believe or face the truth.

Depo Provera—A brand name for the contraceptive injection that contains the hormone progestin. Depo Provera is administered every three months to prevent pregnancy.

Diaphragm—A barrier contraceptive device made of flexible silicone that is inserted into the vagina to cover the cervix and prevent sperm from entering the uterus. It is used as a form of birth control.

Dilation—The process of the cervix opening or widening in preparation for childbirth. It is measured in centimeters and is an essential part of the birth process.

DNA methylation—A process that adds a methyl group to DNA, which can alter gene expression. DNA methylation is a normal process that occurs in all cells, but it can also be involved in the development of diseases such as cancer.

Ducts—Tubes or channels that carry fluids within the body. In the context of breastfeeding, ducts refer to the milk ducts in the breasts that transport milk from the milk-producing glands (lobules) to the nipple.

Due date—A date set 40 weeks after your last menstrual period started, considered full term.

Due range—A three-week range during which your baby will most likely be born.

E

e. Coli—A type of bacteria that is commonly found in the intestines of humans and animals. Most strains of E. coli are harmless, but some strains can cause food poisoning.

Early labor—The initial phase of labor from 1–4 centimeters, characterized by the onset of regular contractions and the gradual dilation and effacement of the cervix. Early labor is usually the longest phase of labor.

Echinacea—A group of flowering plants native to North America. Echinacea is commonly used as an herbal remedy believed to boost the immune system and alleviate symptoms of the common cold and other respiratory infections.

Effaced/effacement—The thinning and shortening of the cervix during pregnancy and labor. Effacement is measured in percentages and indicates the progress of cervical preparation for childbirth.

Engorgement—The condition in which the breasts become overly full, swollen, and uncomfortable due to an increased blood flow and milk production. Engorgement commonly occurs in the early days after childbirth or when breastfeeding is established.

Epigenetics—The study of how changes in gene expression can occur without changes in the DNA sequence itself. Epigenetic changes can be caused by environmental factors such as diet, lifestyle, and exposure to toxins.

Episiotomy—A surgical incision made in the perineum (the area between the vagina and anus) during childbirth to enlarge the vaginal opening.

Esophagus—The muscular tube connecting the throat (pharynx) to the stomach. The esophagus is responsible for transporting food and liquids from the mouth to the stomach through peristaltic contractions.

F

Fatty acid— A type of lipid that is made up of a long chain of carbon atoms with hydrogen atoms attached. Fatty acids are an important source of energy for the body, and they also play a role in cell signaling and other important functions.

Fight or flight response—A physiological response triggered in the body in response to stress or danger. It prepares the body for action by increasing heart rate, blood pressure, and adrenaline release, enabling a person to either confront the threat or flee from it.

Fistulas— An abnormal connection between two organs or body cavities. Fistulas can develop anywhere in the body, but they are most common in the digestive and urinary systems.

Flexion—A specific positioning of the baby's head during labor and childbirth. It occurs when the baby's head is bent forward, with the chin tucked into the chest. Flexion of the baby's head allows for the smallest diameter of the head to enter and pass through the birth canal, facilitating the process of vaginal delivery.

Frenulum—A small fold of tissue or muscle that helps attach and restrict the movement of certain body parts. For example, the lingual frenulum connects the underside of the tongue to the floor of the mouth.

G

Galactagogue—A substance or medication that promotes the production and flow of breast milk. Galactagogues can be herbal remedies, pharmaceuticals, or certain foods.

Gamma linoleic acid (GLA)—An omega-6 fatty acid found in certain plant-based oils, such as evening primrose oil and borage oil. GLA is believed to have anti-inflammatory properties and is sometimes used as a dietary supplement.

Gestate (v.)—To develop in the womb, from conception to birth.

Gestation (n.)—The period of time during which an embryo or fetus develops in the womb.

GLA—see Gamma linoleic acid.

Gluten—A protein found in wheat, rye, and barley. Gluten is responsible for the elastic texture of bread and other baked goods. However, gluten can cause problems for people with celiac disease or gluten intolerance.

Glutes—Short for gluteal muscles, also known as the buttock muscles. The glutes are a group of large muscles in the buttocks that provide stability, support, and movement to the hips.

Glycemic index—A measure of how quickly a food raises blood sugar levels. Foods with a high glycemic index can cause blood sugar levels to spike and then crash quickly, which can lead to hunger, fatigue, and other problems. Foods with a low glycemic index raise blood sugar levels more slowly and steadily, which can help to promote overall health and well-being.

Gonorrhea—A sexually transmitted infection (STI) caused by the bacteria Neisseria gonorrhoeae. Gonorrhea can infect both men and women, and it can cause a variety of symptoms, including pain during urination, unusual vaginal discharge, and pelvic pain.

H

Heart tones—The sounds of the baby's heartbeat heard during pregnancy using a device called a Doppler or a stethoscope. Monitoring heart tones helps assess the baby's well-being during prenatal visits.

Hesperidin—A bioflavonoid found in citrus fruits. Hesperidin has antioxidant and anti-inflammatory properties, and it is sometimes used as a dietary supplement to improve cardiovascular health, reduce the risk of cancer, and boost the immune system.

Hib—Short for Haemophilus influenzae type b, a bacterium that can cause severe infections, particularly in infants and young children. The Hib vaccine helps protect against these infections.

Homeopathy—A system of alternative medicine developed in the late 18th century by Samuel Hahnemann. It is based on the principle of "like cures like," which means that a substance that can cause symptoms in a healthy person can be used to treat similar symptoms in a sick person. Homeopathic remedies are prepared from natural substances, such as plants, minerals, or animal products, which are diluted and succussed (shaken vigorously). The dilution process is believed to enhance the healing properties of the substance while minimizing any potential toxic effects. Homeopathic treatments are individualized and tailored to the specific symptoms and characteristics of the patient.

Hormone—Chemical substances produced by the endocrine glands in the body. Hormones act as messengers, regulating various physiological processes and influencing growth, development, metabolism, mood, and reproduction.

I

Immune system—The body's complex network of organs, tissues, cells, and molecules that work together to defend against harmful pathogens (such as bacteria, viruses, and parasites) and protect the body from infections and diseases.

Immunization—The process of administering vaccines to stimulate the immune system's response to specific pathogens, thus providing protection against infectious diseases.

In-vitro Fertilization (IVF)—A fertility treatment in which eggs are fertilized by sperm outside of the body. The fertilized eggs are then transferred to the uterus, where they can implant and grow into a baby.

Induce—In the context of childbirth, the medical intervention or administration of medications to initiate or speed up labor contractions when they have not started spontaneously or are progressing slowly.

Infection—The invasion and multiplication of harmful microorganisms, such as bacteria, viruses, fungi, or parasites, in the body. Infections can lead to various symptoms and may require medical treatment.

Innervate—To supply with nerves.

Intellectualization—A defense mechanism in which a person excessively relies on abstract thinking, reasoning, or analysis to detach themselves emotionally from distressing or threatening situations. It involves distancing oneself from emotions and focusing on cognitive aspects to gain a sense of control or mastery.

Intrauterine insemination (IUI)—A fertility treatment in which sperm is injected directly into the uterus. This can be done to increase the chances of conception, especially in couples with certain fertility problems.

Isometric (exercises)—A type of exercise in which the muscles are contracted against a resistance, but there is no movement of the joints.

IUI—See Intrauterine insemination.

IVF—See In-vitro fertilization.

J

Jaundice—A condition characterized by yellowing of the skin, eyes, and mucous membranes due to elevated levels of bilirubin in the bloodstream. Jaundice can be a sign of various underlying health conditions, but is common in newborns.

K

Kick count—The monitoring and tracking of fetal movements, specifically the counting of a certain number of kicks or movements within a specified period. Kick counts are often used as an indicator of fetal well-being during pregnancy.

L

Labia—The folds of skin that surround the vulva, the external opening of the female reproductive organs.

Laceration—A tear in the skin or flesh.

Latching on—Refers to the process of a breastfeeding baby attaching to the breast and properly taking the nipple and areola into their mouth to nurse effectively.

Lead—A toxic heavy metal that can be found in the environment, including water, soil, and certain products. Lead exposure can have harmful effects on the body, especially on the nervous system.

Legume—A type of plant that belongs to the family Fabaceae, which includes beans, lentils, peas, and peanuts.

Letting down/Let down—In the context of breastfeeding, the release of milk from the milk ducts in the breast in response to the baby's suckling or to the stimulation of the breasts.

Limbic system—A complex network of structures in the brain, including the hypothalamus, amygdala, and hippocampus, involved in regulating emotions, behavior, memory, and the autonomic nervous system.

M

Mastitis—An infection of the breast tissue that results in breast inflammation, pain, swelling, and redness. Mastitis commonly occurs in breastfeeding women and is often caused by bacterial infection.

Measles—See Rubeola.

Measles, German—See Rubella.

Meconium—The thick, sticky, greenish-black substance that forms the first bowel movement of a newborn baby.

Medicine spoon—A small utensil or device used to measure and administer fluids or liquid medications in precise amounts, typically for infants and young children.

Menstrual cycle—The recurring process that occurs in the female reproductive system, typically lasting about 28 days, in which the uterus prepares for pregnancy. The menstrual cycle involves changes in hormone levels, the development and release of an egg (ovulation), and the shedding of the uterine lining during menstruation.

Menstruation—The process in which the lining of the uterus is shed through the vagina. Menstruation, commonly referred to as a period, typically occurs in women of reproductive age as part of the menstrual cycle.

Mercury—A heavy metal that can be found in various forms, including liquid, and is toxic to humans. Exposure to mercury can occur through contaminated food, certain medical treatments, or environmental sources.

Midwife—a trained health professional who provides care to women during pregnancy, labor, and the postpartum period. Midwives can deliver babies at birth centers or at home, and many can also deliver babies at a hospital. CPMs typically attend home births; CNMs usually attend hospital births. Either can work at a freestanding birth center.

Mucus Plug—A protective barrier of thick mucus that forms in the cervix during pregnancy, sealing the cervical opening to help prevent the entry of bacteria into the uterus. The mucus plug is typically expelled as a sign that labor is approaching.

Mumps—A contagious viral infection characterized by swelling and tenderness of the salivary glands, located near the jaw. Mumps can also cause other symptoms such as fever, headache, and muscle aches.

Myelin sheath—A protective fatty layer that insulates nerve fibers and helps to speed the transmission of nerve impulses.

N

NICU—Neonatal intensive care unit, a specialized hospital unit for the care of sick and premature newborn babies.

Nosocomial infection—Also known as a hospital-acquired infection (HAI) or healthcare-associated infection (HCAI), is an infection that is acquired while receiving medical care. Nosocomial infections are not present nor incubating at the time of admission to a hospital or other healthcare facility. They can develop during hospitalization, during a healthcare procedure, or after discharge from the hospital.

Nuchal hand—A condition in which a fetus's hand is positioned near or over its neck. Nuchal hand is usually harmless and does not require any treatment.

Nursing Bra—A specialized bra designed for breastfeeding mothers that provides easy access to the breasts for nursing. Nursing bras often have features such as clasps or flaps that allow for discreet breastfeeding.

Nursing—The act of feeding a baby with breast milk directly from the breast. Nursing provides essential nutrition and offers various health benefits for both the baby and the mother.

O

Occiput—The back of the head or the posterior part of the skull.

Occiput anterior position—A term used in obstetrics to describe the position of the baby's head during childbirth. In the occiput anterior position, the baby's face is facing downward, with the occiput (back of the head) positioned toward the front of the mother's pelvis (the pubic bone).

Omega-3 fatty acid—A type of polyunsaturated fatty acid that is found in oily fish, such as salmon, tuna, and mackerel. Omega-3 fatty acids have many health benefits, including reducing inflammation, improving heart health, and supporting brain development.

Omega-6 fatty acid—A type of polyunsaturated fatty acid that is found in vegetable oils, such as soybean oil, corn oil, and sunflower oil. Omega-6 fatty acids are also important for health, but they should be consumed in moderation, as too much omega-6 can promote inflammation.

Omega-9 fatty acid—A type of monounsaturated fatty acid that is found in olive oil, avocados, and nuts. Omega-9 fatty acids are considered to be healthy fats and can help to lower cholesterol levels and improve heart health.

Oocyte—An egg cell.

Os—Short for "ostium," os refers to an opening or orifice in the body. In the context of childbirth, os commonly refers to the cervical os, which is the opening of the cervix.

Ossification—The process of bone formation, in which soft tissues gradually harden and turn into bone. Ossification is an essential part of skeletal development and occurs throughout a person's life.

Oxytocin—A hormone produced by the hypothalamus and released by the pituitary gland. Oxytocin plays a crucial role in various reproductive processes, including labor and childbirth, milk letdown during breastfeeding, and the bonding between individuals.

P

Paci—see Pacifier.

Pacifier—A nipple-like device made of plastic or rubber that is given to infants to suck on for comfort. Pacifiers are also known as soothers, binkies, or dummies.

Pathogen— A microorganism that can cause disease. Pathogens can include bacteria, viruses, fungi, and parasites.

Perineal—Relating to the perineum.

Perineum—The area of skin and muscle located between the vagina and the anus in females, or between the scrotum and the anus in males.

Period—Also known as menstruation or menstrual period, it refers to the regular shedding of the uterine lining that occurs in women of reproductive age as part of the menstrual cycle.

Peristalsis—refers to the coordinated muscular contractions that occur in the digestive tract to propel food and fluids through the gastrointestinal system. It is a rhythmic wave-like movement that helps move contents along the digestive tract, from the esophagus to the stomach, small intestine, and large intestine. It is an essential physiological process that ensures the smooth movement of food and waste through the digestive system, allowing for effective digestion and elimination.

Peritonitis—Inflammation of the peritoneum, the thin tissue lining the abdominal cavity. It is typically caused by infection or other underlying conditions.

Pertussis—Also known as whooping cough, it is a highly contagious respiratory infection caused by the bacterium Bordetella pertussis. Pertussis is characterized by severe coughing fits and a distinctive "whooping" sound during inhalation.

pH—A measurement of the acidity or alkalinity of a substance, indicating its level of acidity (pH less than 7), neutrality (pH of 7), or alkalinity (pH greater than 7). In the context of the body, pH levels can be important for various biological processes.

Pituitary—The pituitary gland is a small, pea-sized gland located at the base of the brain. It is often referred to as the "master gland" because it produces and releases various hormones that regulate many bodily functions and control other endocrine glands.

Placenta—An organ that develops during pregnancy and is attached to the uterine wall. The placenta facilitates the exchange of nutrients, oxygen, and waste products between the mother and the developing baby.

Placenta prints—A form of artwork created by applying ink or paint to the surface of the placenta and then pressing it onto paper or fabric. Placenta prints are a unique and symbolic way for some individuals to commemorate the birth of their child.

Placental abruption—A condition in which the placenta separates from the wall of the uterus before the baby is born. Placental abruption can be a serious condition for both the mother and the baby.

Placental accreta—A condition in which the placenta attaches too deeply to the wall of the uterus. Placental accreta can make it difficult or dangerous to deliver the baby.

Placental percreta— A rare condition in which the placenta invades the muscles of the uterus. Placental percreta can be life-threatening for the mother.

PMS—See Premenstrual Syndrome.

Posterior fontanel—A soft spot on the baby's skull where the skull bones have not yet fused. The posterior fontanel is located at the back of the head and usually closes within a few months after birth.

Postpartum— The period of time following childbirth, typically lasting a few to several months, during which a woman's body undergoes various physical and emotional adjustments and recovery.

Poultice— A soft, moist mass of material that is applied to the skin to reduce inflammation or pain. Poultices can be made from a variety of substances, such as herbs, clay, or bread.

Prabhā—a Sanskrit word that translates to "radiance" or "splendor." In various spiritual traditions, including Hinduism and Buddhism, "Prabha" is used to describe the divine or luminous radiance associated with spiritual enlightenment or higher consciousness.

Prana—In certain spiritual traditions, prana refers to the life force or vital energy that permeates all living beings. It is believed to be responsible for sustaining physical and spiritual well-being.

Prebiotics—Prebiotics are non-digestible food ingredients that promote the growth of good bacteria in the gut. Good sources of prebiotics include onions, garlic, asparagus, and bananas.

Preeclampsia—A pregnancy complication characterized by high blood pressure and protein in the urine. Preeclampsia can develop after 20 weeks of pregnancy, and it can lead to serious health problems for both the mother and the baby.

Pregnancy brain—Commonly referred to as "momnesia" or "baby brain," it is a term used to describe temporary cognitive changes or forgetfulness that some pregnant individuals experience.

Pregnancy—The state of carrying a developing fetus in the womb. Pregnancy begins with conception and typically lasts until childbirth.

Pregnant—The condition of being with child or expecting a baby.

Pre-labor—also known as the "latent phase" of labor. The woman will eventually be in real labor but is not actively dilating yet.

Premature—Refers to a baby born before completing the full term of pregnancy, usually before 37 weeks of gestation.

Premenstrual Syndrome—A combination of physical, emotional, and psychological symptoms that occur in the days or weeks leading up to the menstrual period.

Probiotic—A live microorganism that is similar to the beneficial bacteria that naturally live in the human body. Probiotics are often taken as a supplement to improve gut health and digestion.

Prodromal symptoms—Early warning signs or symptoms that precede the onset of a particular condition or illness.

Prolapse—A condition in which an organ or body part slips out of place. Prolapse can affect any organ in the body, but it is most common in the pelvic region, including the uterus, bladder, and rectum.

Projection—A defense mechanism in which an individual attributes their own unacceptable or unwanted thoughts, feelings, or characteristics onto someone else. They may project their own anxieties, fears, or desires onto another person, often in a way that distorts or misinterprets the other person's actions or intentions.

Protease—An enzyme that breaks down proteins. Proteases are essential for digestion, but they can also be used to treat certain medical conditions, such as inflammation and blood clots.

Provitamin—A substance that can be converted into a vitamin in the body. For example, beta-carotene is a provitamin for vitamin A.

Pushing—The process of using abdominal muscles to exert downward pressure during the second stage of the birth process to help the baby move through the birth canal and be born.

R

Rationalization—A defense mechanism in which a person creates logical or plausible explanations or justifications for their thoughts, feelings, or behaviors to protect themselves from anxiety or guilt. It involves reinterpreting or reframing events or situations in a way that preserves self-esteem or relieves internal conflict.

RBCs—See Red blood cells.

Reaction formation—A defense mechanism in which a person unconsciously behaves in a manner that is the opposite of their true feelings or desires. For example, expressing exaggerated friendliness toward someone they actually dislike or displaying moralistic attitudes as a defense against their own forbidden impulses.

Red blood cells—Blood cells that are responsible for carrying oxygen from the lungs to the body's tissues and removing carbon dioxide. Red blood cells contain a protein called hemoglobin, which gives them their red color.

Reflex—An involuntary and automatic response or movement triggered by a specific stimulus. Reflexes can be protective or serve specific functions, such as the sucking reflex in newborns.

Regression—A defense mechanism in which a person reverts to earlier, more childlike patterns of behavior or coping strategies. It may involve displaying behaviors that were characteristic of an earlier developmental stage in response to stressful or challenging situations.

Relaxin—A hormone produced during pregnancy that helps relax and soften the ligaments and tissues in the pelvic area, preparing the body for childbirth.

Remedy—A treatment or solution intended to relieve or cure a health condition or alleviate symptoms. Remedies can be natural, herbal, pharmaceutical, or based on traditional practices.

Repression—A defense mechanism involving the unconscious exclusion or forgetting of distressing thoughts, memories, or impulses from conscious awareness. Repressed material is pushed into the unconscious mind, potentially leading to later psychological symptoms or manifestations.

Ripening (of the cervix)—The process by which the cervix gradually becomes softer, thinner, and more dilated in preparation for childbirth.

Rooting—A reflexive movement in newborns characterized by turning the head and opening the mouth in response to touch or stimulation near the mouth or cheek. Rooting helps infants find the breast for feeding.

Rubella—Also known as German measles, Rubella is caused by the rubella virus. It is a less severe viral infection compared to rubeola but can still pose risks, particularly for pregnant women. Rubella is typically characterized by a mild fever, swollen lymph nodes, and a rash that starts on the face and spreads to the body. The infection is of particular concern during pregnancy as it can cause birth defects and other complications. Vaccination with the MMR vaccine provides protection against rubella.

Rubeola—Commonly known as measles, rubeola is caused by the measles virus (MeV). It is a highly contagious respiratory infection characterized by fever, cough, runny nose, red and watery eyes (conjunctivitis), and a distinctive rash that starts on the face and spreads to the rest of the body. Measles can cause severe complications, especially in young children and individuals with weakened immune systems. Vaccination with the measles, mumps, and rubella (MMR) vaccine is an effective preventive measure against rubeola.

Rutin—Rutin is a flavonoid, which is a type of plant compound with antioxidant and anti-inflammatory properties. They are found in a variety of fruits and vegetables, including citrus fruits, berries, buckwheat, and asparagus.

S

SIDS—See Sudden Infant Death Syndrome.

Social security number—A unique identification number issued by the government in some countries, such as the United States, to track individuals for social security benefits and taxation purposes.

Softening of the cervix—The process by which the cervix becomes softer and more pliable in preparation for childbirth.

Softening of the cervix is an early sign of labor approaching.

Sonogram—a medical imaging technique that uses sound waves to create pictures of structures inside the body. Also known as ultrasound.

Spina bifida—A birth defect that occurs when the neural tube, which develops into the spinal cord and spine, does not fully close during fetal development. Spina bifida can lead to varying degrees of physical and neurological disabilities.

Stitches—Sutures or medical thread used to close a surgical incision or repair a tear, such as an episiotomy or perineal tear that may occur during childbirth.

Sublimation—A defense mechanism in which unacceptable or socially undesirable impulses or urges are channeled or redirected into socially acceptable and constructive behaviors. For example, channeling aggressive impulses into playing a competitive sport or using artistic expression to channel emotional energy.

Sudden Infant Death Syndrome (SIDS)—The sudden and unexplained death of an otherwise healthy infant, typically during sleep. SIDS is a rare occurrence, and its exact cause is still unknown. Research is ongoing, however, at the time of this writing, researchers believe that it is caused by a combination of factors, including:

- **Brain development abnormalities**: Some babies who die of SIDS may have abnormalities in the part of the brain that controls breathing and waking up from sleep.

- **Environmental factors:** Certain environmental factors, such as sleeping on the stomach or side, sleeping on a soft surface, or sharing a bed with parents or siblings, can increase the risk of SIDS.

- **Genetic factors:** There may be some genetic factors that make babies more susceptible to SIDS.

Synaptic connection—The connection formed between nerve cells (neurons) in the brain through synapses. Synaptic connections enable the transmission of signals and communication between neurons.

T

Talc/talcum powder—A soft mineral composed of magnesium, silicon, and oxygen, often used in cosmetic and personal care products. Talc can also refer to talcum powder, which is made from talc and used for various purposes. Talcum powder has been identified as a potential source of exposure to asbestos fibers, which are known to be carcinogenic. Asbestos contamination in talc products can occur due to the proximity of talc deposits to asbestos-containing minerals in the earth.

Tearing—In the context of childbirth, tearing refers to the occurrence of small to significant skin lacerations or tears in the perineum or vaginal area during delivery.

Ten centimeters—Referring to the measurement of cervical dilation during labor. When the cervix has dilated to 10 centimeters, it is considered fully dilated, indicating that the second stage of labor, pushing, can begin.

Thrush—A fungal infection caused by the overgrowth of Candida yeast. Thrush can occur in the mouth (oral thrush) or in other areas of the body and is characterized by white patches, discomfort, and itching.

Tincture—A concentrated liquid extract derived from herbs or plants, often preserved in alcohol or a solvent. Tinctures are commonly used in herbal medicine.

Tocopherols—A type of Vitamin E compound. Tocopherols are antioxidants that help to protect cells from damage. They are found in a variety of foods, including nuts, seeds, vegetable oils, and leafy green vegetables.

Tocotrienol—Another type of Vitamin E compound. Tocotrienols have similar antioxidant properties to tocopherols, but they may also have additional health benefits, such as reducing inflammation and cholesterol levels. Tocotrienols are found in some plant oils, such as rice bran oil and palm oil.

Transference—A defense mechanism in which a person redirects their feelings, desires, or unresolved conflicts from past relationships onto a different person in the present. It often occurs in therapeutic relationships, where the patient may transfer feelings, they have for significant others onto the therapist.

Transition—The final phase of the first stage of labor, just before the second stage (pushing) begins. Transition is characterized by strong and frequent contractions and often involves a shift in the cervix from around 7 centimeters to 10 centimeters dilation.

Triglyceride—A type of fat that is stored in the body's fat cells. Triglycerides are the main source of energy for the body. However, high levels of triglycerides in the blood can increase the risk of heart disease and other health problems.

U

Ultrasound—a medical imaging technique that uses sound waves to create pictures of structures inside the body. Also known as sonogram.

Uterus—A hollow, muscular organ in the female reproductive system where a fertilized egg implants and develops into a fetus during pregnancy. The uterus contracts during pregnancy and the birth process to facilitate childbirth.

V

Vaccine—A substance that stimulates the immune system to produce an acquired immunity to a specific disease, usually by introducing a weakened or inactivated form of the pathogen or its antigens. Vaccines help prevent and control infectious diseases.

Vagina—A muscular canal in the female reproductive system that connects the uterus to the external opening. The vagina serves as the birth canal during childbirth and is also involved in sexual intercourse.

Valtrex—An antiviral medication often prescribed to prevent or reduce the duration of a herpes outbreak.

VBAC—Vaginal Birth After Cesarean section. It refers to the process of giving birth vaginally after a previous delivery by c-section.

Vernix—A creamy, white, waxy substance that covers a baby's skin while in the womb. Vernix protects the baby's skin from amniotic fluid and assists in regulating body temperature.

W

Warm up labor—A practice period of contractions that can happen from a few days to a few weeks before labor. Sometimes known as "false labor."

Weaning—The process of gradually introducing solid foods and reducing or ceasing breastfeeding or bottle-feeding as a baby transitions to consuming a more varied diet.

Whooping cough—see "Pertussis."

Witch hazel—A plant-based remedy derived from the leaves and bark of the witch hazel shrub. Witch hazel extract is commonly used topically for its astringent and soothing properties.

Womb—Another term for the uterus, the organ in which a fetus develops during pregnancy.

X

Xylocaine—A brand name for lidocaine, a local anesthetic medication that is used to numb a specific area of the body for medical procedures or to relieve pain.

Xyphoid process—A small extension at the lower end of the sternum (breastbone) made of cartilage. It serves as an attachment site for some abdominal muscles.

Y

Yeast— A type of fungus that can cause infections in humans, such as vaginal yeast infections or oral thrush.

Yellow dock—A perennial herb with yellow roots that has been used in traditional medicine for its potential therapeutic properties, such as supporting digestion and detoxification.

Z

Zinc—A mineral that is essential for various physiological processes in the body, including immune function, cell growth and repair, and enzyme activity. Zinc is found in many foods and is often taken as a dietary supplement.

CREDITS

Cover Design
Megan Zvezda (Om Girl Marketing) and Alyssa Archer

Interior Design
Marites Bautista

Editing
Alyssa Archer and Robbie Davis Floyd

Photo and Illustration Credits

Image	Photographer/ Artist	Title	Source
RECURRING IMAGES			
Nourishment banner	@yulianny	Balanced Diet	depositphotos
Hydration banner	@robertsrob	Water	depositphotos
Movement banner	@photobac	Young Pregnant Woman Under Water	depositphotos
Emotional/Spiritual banner	@anyaberkut	Woman practicing yoga on the beach	depositphotos
Knowledge banner	@dedivan1923	Girl having a break with a cup of fresh ...	depositphotos
Rest banner	@grandfailure	Night scenery of young woman looking at the fallen moon ...	depositphotos
Joy banner	@puhhha	Freedom, enjoyment	depositphotos
Partner icon	@mrrashad	Maternity (2) .50. Glyph	Canva Pro
Feet in Hands line art	@zitusia	Hands holding baby foot	depositphotos
INTRODUCTION			
Dedication page graphic	@katyasuresh	Baby in mother womb during pregnancy	depositphotos
Mind body spirit line art	@Vectortradition	Triquetra Triangular Figure	Canva Pro
Aleah and MariMikel	@Aleah Ruiz	Aleah and MariMikel	Aleah Ruiz
All other photos in the Introduction	@New Life Birth Services	Various	MariMikel Potter

Image	Photographer/ Artist	Title	Source
CONSCIOUS CONCEPTION			
Line art, woman	@Anmark	Vector woman	Canva Pro
Carbs	@yulka3ice	Healthy products	Canva Pro
Seafood	@Artimas	Fresh Seafood Variety on Ice	Canva Pro
Poultry	@nitrub	Fresh chicken meat	Canva Pro
Meat	@bit245	Meat	Canva Pro
Line art journaling	@ngupakarti	Continuous one line drawing of a young woman ...	depositphotos
Abdominal massage	@Creative Credit	Young woman receiving abdominal massage	Canva Pro
Fertilization	@annyart	Female egg structure	depositphotos
Gastrulation	@VectorMine	Gastrulation stages as early embryo ...	depositphotos
5 week old embryo	@lookaround	Human fetus with internal organs ...	depositphotos
Conception first week	@megija	Embryo development. Secondary ...	depositphotos
FIRST TRIMESTER			
Introduction line art	@Iuliia	Woman Boy Silhouette Line ...	Iuliia's Images/Canva Pro
Morning smoothie	@VeselovaElena	Fresh mixed berry smoothie	Canva Pro
Penelope at ACL	@penelopegreene	Penelope at ACL	Penelope Greene
Pregnancy tea	@efired	Magenta Hibiscus Tea	Canva Pro
Couple silhouette	@Aleah Ruiz	Aleah and Frankie	Aleah Ruiz
i have been a thousand...	@Eriks Cistovs	Woman standing on Flower ...	Pexels/Canva Pro
Due date calendar	@pixelshot	3137275-0.jpg	Canva Pro
4-40 weeks gestation	@dr_OX	Growth of a human fetus in weeks	depositphotos
Stages of human fetal development	@AlexanderPokusay	Stages of human fetal development	depositphotos
Child's pose	@hamlet_ggl	A dark-skinned girl performs the yoga ...	depositphotos
Hospital environment	@SiimpleFoto	Nurses Inspecting Fetal Monitor	depositphotos
Ultrasound	@YsaL	Foetus ultrasound	Getty Images/Canva Pro
Birth center environment	@Science Photo Library	Birthing centre room	Canva Pro
Aleah in the tub	@Aleah Ruiz	Aleah in the tub	Aleah Ruiz
Robbie laboring	@Robbie Davis Floyd	Robbie Laboring	Robbie Davis Floyd
Aleah's indomitable spirit	@Aleah Ruiz	Aleah's indomitable spirit	Aleah Ruiz
Pool birth	@jbrown777	Happy Mom With Newborn	depositphotos
MariMikel with a client	@New Life Birth Services	MM with a client	MariMikel Potter

Image	Photographer/ Artist	Title	Source
Tackle boxes	@New Life Birth Services	MM's tackle boxes	MariMikel Potter
C-section incisions	@nnfotograf	Types of incisions in cesarean ...	depositphotos
Pregnant with cat	@pixelshot	Pregnant Woman with Cat ...	Canva Pro
Picnic	@Harbucks	Happy young friends group	Getty Images/Canva Pro
Game night	@Mladen Zivkovic	Happy girls playing board games	Getty Images Signature/ Canva Pro
SECOND TRIMESTER			
Intro Line Art	@Jirawan	Pregnant Woman Line Art	Canva Pro
Kerry Yoga	@Kerry Case	Kerry doing yoga while pregnant	Kerry Case
Baby Bump	@Kerry Case	Baby bump	Kerry Case
Aleah Radiant	@Aleah Ruiz	Aleah moments after birth	Aleah Ruiz
Baby Bump 2	@Lina Vanessa Merchán Jimenez	Portrait of Pregnant Woman	Diversifylens/Canva Pro
2T Development	@blueringmedia	Pregnatn fetus anatomy diagram	depositphotos
Placental structure	@Sakkura	Placental structure and circulation	depositphotos
Pelvic Floor Location	@Vectormine	Pelvic floor muscles...	depositphotos
Pelvic floor muscles	@Molotoka	Exercises to strengthen the muscle ...	depositphotos
Stages of Uterine Prolapse	@nnfotograf	Stages of uterine prolapse ...	depositphotos
Umbilical cord	@New Life Birth Services	Umbilical cord	MariMikel Potter
Check your body posture	@elenabs	Correct walking and running posture	depositphotos
Douche apparatus	@The Flents Store	Flents Douche and Enema Combination Kit for Men and Women, Large Capacity, Multipurpose Cleaning System, Made with Comfortable Material	The Flents Store
Acupuncture	@AndreyPopov	Man Getting Acupuncture ...	Getty Images Pro/Canva Pro
Robbie in labor, midwife	@RobbieDavisFloyd	Robbie Laboring	Robbie Davis Floyd
Hydrotherapy	a.dl	Woman Enjoying Indoor Pool	Canva Pro
2T Yoga	@Kerry Case	2T Yoga	Kerry Case
Penelope day trip	@penelopegreene	Penelope day trip	Penelope Greene
Glamping	@FRIMU EUGEN	Tent at Glamping, Night	Frimufilms/Canva Pro
Placenta Print	@Alyssa Archer	Aleah's Placenta Print	Alyssa Archer
Sun Your Belly	@Aleah Ruiz	Sun Your Belly	Aleah Ruiz
Babymoon	@Aleah Ruiz	Babymoon	Aleah Ruiz

Image	Photographer/ Artist	Title	Source
THIRD TRIMESTER			
Intro line art	@Saga Design Studio	Minimal Monoline pregnant woman	Saga Design Studio/ Canva Pro
Brassicas	@ThitareeSarmkasat	Cruciferous vegetables	Getty Images Pro/ Canva Pro
Pregnant Woman Squatting	@damicographics	Pregnant woman practices ...	Getty Images/ Canva Pro
Practicing Relaxation	@Wavebreakmedia	Pregnant woman getting ...	Getty Images/ Canva Pro
Robbie Floating in Labor	@RobbieDavisFloyd	Robbie Laboring	Robbie Davis Floyd
Visualizing in Nature	@Diego Cervo	Pregnant Woman Relaxing	Canva Pro
Sibling preparation	@Aleah Ruiz	Ava, Téa, and MariMikel	Aleah Ruiz
Sibling Preparpation Classes	@New Life Birth Services	Teaching Sibling Preparation Classes	MariMikel Potter
Full term in utero	@fighting fear	Normal Pregnant female anatomy	depositphotos
Belly Support System	@mykolasosiukin	Pregnant Woman in Under...	Canva Pro
MM teaching childbirth classes	@New Life Birth Services	Teaching Birth Preparation Classes	MariMikel Potter
Safe Place	@Aleah Ruiz	Ava's playstation	Aleah Ruiz
Modern cloth diapers	@Aurora uribe	Twin babies girls with ecolo ...	Getty Images/Canva Pro
Intex Pool	@intex	Intex Pool	Intex
Co Sleeper	@lauren@integrity brandmanagement.com	Side view of charming new ...	depositphotos
Infant seat	@Sementsova321	Side view of charming new ...	depositphotos
Engagement	@vitalio333	Countour Vector Outline ...	depositphotos
LOA	bearsky23@yahoo.com	Left Occiput Anterior	depositphotos
LOP	bearsky23@yahoo.com	Left Occiput Posterior	depositphotos
ROA	bearsky23@yahoo.com	Left Occiput Anterior	depositphotos
ROP	bearsky23@yahoo.com	Left Occiput Posterior	depositphotos
Table position	@robuart	Birth position for childbirth labor	depositphotos
Baby's positioning	@Betty 1994	Latin arabian brown skin baby Diff ..	depositphotos
Pack and Play	@Graco	Graco Pack 'n-Play Dome LX-Playard	The Graco Store
Nipple Shield	@BespaliyA	Contact nipple shield ...	depositphotos
Pelvic Stations	bearsky23@yahoo.com	Child in womb ...	depositphotos

Image	Photographer/Artist	Title	Source
Effacement and dilation	@Betty 1994	Cervical effacement and dilation	depositphotos
Intimacy in the 3rd trimester	@unknown	User-uploaded content	Canva Pro
The Starry Night by Vincent Van Gogh	@public domain	The Starry Night by Vincent Van Gogh	Rawpixel
Meditate pray connect	@Lolostock	Pregnant Woman Meditating	Canva Pro
Area Broken by Perpendiculars	@public domain	Area Broken by Perpendiculars by Joseph Schillenger	Rawpixel
Enjoying a day at the river 3T	@Wild Herd Cattle + Kitchen	River day in the third trimester	Olivia P. Kramer
THE BIRTH PROCESS			
Intro line art	@yanaillustrator @gmail.com	Continuous one line of pregnant ...	depositphotos
Triple Goddess	@robin_ph	Spiral goddess of fertility and triple ...	depositphotos
MariMikel and Aleah attending a birth	@Talitha Green	Talitha in labor	Talitha Green
Robbie in the pool	@Robbie Davis Floyd	Hot tub #1	Robbie Davis Floyd
Full term pregnancy	@drspix	Pregnant woman at the beach	depositphotos
Stages and phases of the birth process	@udaix	Stages of Labor and Birth in ...	depositphotos
Summary of the birth process	bearsky23@yahoo.com	Baby Fetus in Pregnant Woman ...	depositphotos
Talitha in labor	@Talitha Green	Talitha in labor	Talitha Green
Positions for Labor	@leremy	Childbirth labor positions and ...	depositphotos
Partner support	@New Life Birth Services	Partner support	MariMikel Potter
Labor support	@Aleah Ruiz	Labor support	Aleah Ruiz
Robbie laboring in water	@Robbie Davis Floyd	Hot tub #2	Robbie Davis Floyd
Helping to squat	@New Life Birth Services	Helping to squat	MariMikel Potter
Pushing	@Talitha Green	Pushing	Talitha Green
Crowning	@New Life Birth Services	Crowning	MariMikel Potter
Head is emerging	@New Life Birth Services	Head is emerging	MariMikel Potter
Turning the shoulders	@New Life Birth Services	Turning the shoulders	MariMikel Potter
Head emerges fully	@New Life Birth Services	Head emerges fully	MariMikel Potter
Supporting baby	@New Life Birth Services	Supporting baby	MariMikel Potter
Baby emerges	@New Life Birth Services	Baby emerges	MariMikel Potter

Image	Photographer/ Artist	Title	Source
Moments after birth	@New Life Birth Services	Moments after birth	MariMikel Potter
Conehead baby	@Aleah Ruiz	New baby	Aleah Ruiz
Skin to skin	@Aleah Ruiz	Skin to skin	Aleah Ruiz
Baby arrives	@Talitha Green	Baby arrives	Talitha Green
Family of four	@Talitha Green	Family of four	Talitha Green
Sarah's Little Boy	@Sarah Copper	Sarah's Little Boy	Sarah Copper
Sarah with her newborn	@Sarah Copper	Sarah with her newborn	Sarah Copper
Penelope's first born moments after birth	@Penelope Greene	Penelope's first born moments after birth	Penelope Greene
Penelope's first born in the minutes after birth	@Penelope Greene	Penelope's first born in the minutes after birth	Penelope Greene
Penelope's second child	@Penelope Greene	Penelope's second child	Penelope Greene
Penelope's third child	@Penelope Greene	Penelope's third child	Penelope Greene
Juliana 1	@Juliana Flores	Laboring at the Birth Center	Juliana Flores
Juliana 2	@Juliana Flores	Our Baby Is Here!	Juliana Flores
Monica 1	@Monica Munoz	Birth Center Team	Monica Munoz
Monica 2	@Monica Munoz	Monica 2	Monica Munoz
Monica 3	@Monica Munoz	Monica 3	Monica Munoz
Aleah 1	@Aleah Ruiz	Aleah 1	Aleah Ruiz
Aleah 2	@Aleah Ruiz	Aleah 2	Aleah Ruiz
Aleah 3	@Aleah Ruiz	Aleah 3	Aleah Ruiz
Aleah's family	@Aleah Ruiz	Aleah's family	Aleah Ruiz
Newborn picture 1	@New Life Birth Services	Client picture	MariMikel Potter
Newborn picture 2	@New Life Birth Services	Client picture	MariMikel Potter
Newborn picture 3	@New Life Birth Services	Client picture	MariMikel Potter
Newborn picture 4	@New Life Birth Services	Client picture	MariMikel Potter
Newborn picture 5	@New Life Birth Services	Client picture	MariMikel Potter
Newborn picture 6	@New Life Birth Services	Client picture	MariMikel Potter
Newborn picture 7	@New Life Birth Services	Client picture	MariMikel Potter
Ultrasound	@Wavebreakmedia	Pregnant woman undergoin...	Getty Images/ Canva Pro
Parents and baby line art	@galynatymonko	One continuous monoline si...	Canva Pro
Fetal monitoring	@joruba75	Pregnancy examination	depositphotos

Image	Photographer/ Artist	Title	Source
Newborn picture 8	@New Life Birth Services	Client picture	MariMikel Potter
Newborn picture 9	@New Life Birth Services	Client picture	MariMikel Potter
BEFORE I LEAVE YOU			
MariMikel with Four of Her Six ...	@New Life Birth Services	Family picture	MariMikel Potter
MariMikel with Her Children ...	@New Life Birth Services	Family picture	MariMikel Potter
MariMikel with Granddaughter Téa	@New Life Birth Services	Family picture	MariMikel Potter
MariMikel with Granddaughter Ava	@New Life Birth Services	Family picture	MariMikel Potter
ACKNOWLEDGEMENTS			
Alyssa, MariMikel, and Aleah	@Aleah Ruiz	Retreat photo	Aleah Ruiz
APPENDICES			
Morning Smoothie	@VeselovaElena	Fresh mixed berry smoothie	Canva Pro
Mimi's Special Spinach	@SherSor	Garlic sauteed spinach	Getty Images/Canva Pro
Breakfast Tacos	@bhofack2	Homemade Chorizo Breakfast Tacos	Getty Images/Canva Pro
Egg Muffins	@Qwart	Egg bites, omelet muffin	Getty Images/Canva Pro
Migas	@IslandLeigh	Tex-Mex Migas	Getty Images/Canva Pro
Tuna Salad	@Yuliya Furman	Canapes with Tuna Salad	Canva Pro
Mimi's Nut Butter	@oleksandranaumenko	Selection of Nut Butters	Canva Pro
Aleah's Everyday Salad	@Tonelson	California garden salad	Getty Images/Canva Pro
Mimi's Pasta Salad	@SondraP	Pasta salad	Getty Images Signature/ Canva Pro
Shepherd's Pie	@rudisill	Shepherd's Pie	Getty Images Signature/ Canva Pro
Mimi's Stir Fry	@kajakiki	Vegetable Stir Fry	Getty Images Signature/ Canva Pro
Chicken Fried Cutlets	@Tyas Indayanti	Crispy chicken Steak	Canva Pro
Aleah's Rainbow Bowl	@davidf	Roast Sweet Potato ...	Getty Images Signature / Canva Pro
Venetian Stuffed Chicken	@robynmac	Stuffed Chicken Breasts	Getty Images/Canva Pro
White Wine Sauce	@jmattisson	White wine sauce	Getty Images/Canva Pro

Image	Photographer/Artist	Title	Source
Chicken Tikka Masala	@Lisovskaya	Chicken tikka masala	Getty Images Pro/Canva Pro
Turkey Burgers	@bhofack2	Homemade Healthy Turkey ...	Getty Images Pro/Canva Pro
Mimi's Spaghetti	@Hansuan_Fabregas	7517639.jpg	pixabay/Canva Pro
Garlic Lemon Chicken with Roasted Vegetables	@pixelshot	Delicious Chicken Breast with lemon and vegetables	Canva Pro
Country Captain Chicken	@Tonelson	Kung pao chicken	Canva Pro
Mimi's Soup Stock	@AtnoYdur	Chicken stock soup	Getty Images/Canva Pro
Mimi's Chicken Soup	@Elena Photo	Chicken Soup with Rice and ...	Canva Pro
Mimi's Salad	@DAPA Images	Fresh Garden Salad	Canva Pro
Creamy Coconut Chicken Soup	@Nungning20	Butternut squash soup	Getty Images/Canva Pro
King Ranch Casserole	@gwenael le vot	Creamy chicken and potato	Getty Images/Canva Pro
Toodle Oodle Casserole	@EzumeImages	Macaroni Tuna Casserole	Getty Images/Canva Pro
Mexican Casserole	@peredniankina	Zucchini casserole	Getty Images/Canva Pro
Dr. Ray Peat's Raw Carrot Salad	@YelenaYemchuk	Salad with fresh raw carrot ...	Getty Images/Canva Pro
Mimi's Fruit Salad	@dan_kaplan	Fruit Salad	Getty Images/Canva Pro
Avocado Pudding	@AmaliaEka	Avocado chocolate pudding	Getty Images/Canva Pro
Chia Seed Pudding	@Jasmina81	Healthy chia pudding	Getty Images/Canva Pro
Pregnancy tea	@efired	Magenta Hibiscus Tea	Canva Pro

CREDITS

ENDNOTES

INTRODUCTION

[1] You can find more about my practice on my website if you like. http://www.newlifebirthservices.com/

[2] Centers for Disease Control and Prevention. (2021). *Births: Final Data for 2021, table 17* [PDF—1 MB]. https://www.cdc.gov/nchs/data/nvsr/nvsr71/nvsr71_01_tables.pdf#table17

[3] Centers for Disease Control and Prevention. (2022, March 1). *Racial and ethnic disparities in maternal and infant health.* Retrieved from https://www.cdc.gov/nchs/products/databriefs/db391.htm

CONSCIOUS CONCEPTION

[4] Cassidy, J., & Shaver, P. R. (2016). Attachment theory and research: Core concepts, measures, and interventions. In J. Cassidy & P. R. Shaver (Eds.), *Handbook of Attachment: Theory, Research, and Clinical Applications* (3rd ed., pp. 4-24). Guilford Press.

[5] Center for Food Safety. (2019, May 2). *Over 3,500 chemicals have not been tested for safety by the FDA.* https://www.centerforfoodsafety.org/press-releases/5845/over-3500-chemicals-have-not-been-tested-for-safety-by-the-fda

[6] Grandjean, P., & Landrigan, P. J. (2006). Developmental neurotoxicity of industrial chemicals. *The Lancet,* 368(9553), 2167-2178. https://doi.org/10.1016/S0140-6736(06)69665-7

Batool, Z., Sadir, S., & Liaquat, L. (2019). Impact of food additives on human health: A review study. *Journal of Chemistry,* 2019, 1-9. https://doi.org/10.1155/2019/3074241

Hao, Y., Wu, Q., Zhang, J., Zhou, X., & Feng, C. (2021). The effects of food preservatives and additives on human health: A review. *Journal of Food Quality,* 2021, 1-10. https://doi.org/10.1155/2021/9950272

[7] Greenfield, N. (2023, August 26). *The Smart Seafood Buying Guide: Five ways to ensure the fish you eat is healthy for you and for the environment.* Retrieved September 18, 2023, from https://www.nrdc.org/stories/smart-seafood-buying-guide

Environmental Protection Agency & Food and Drug Administration. (2023, January 24). *EPA and FDA advice about eating fish for those who might become or are pregnant or breastfeeding and children ages 1–11 years.* Retrieved from https://www.epa.gov/fish-tech/epa-fda-advice-about-eating-fish-and-shellfish

[8] Tilman, D., & Pimentel, M. (2014). Sustainability of meat-based and plant-based diets and the environment: A review. *Science, 343*(6170), 1212576.

[9] Wood, J. D., Enser, M., Fisher, A. V., Nute, G. R., Sheard, P. R., Richardson, R. I., Hughes, S. I., & Whittington, F. M. (2004). Fatty acid composition of meat from steers offered diets containing contrasting proportions of red meat and white meat silages. *Animal Science, 79*(4), 495-503.

[10] Smith, J. (2019). Glyphosate: Unsafe on any plate. *Journal of Environmental Protection, 10*(03), 297-317.

[11] Albert, C. M., Cook, N. R., Manson, J. E., Buring, J. E., & Hu, F. B. (2011). Intake of phytoestrogens and risk of heart failure in women. *Circulation: Heart Failure, 4*(1), 72-78.

Messina, M., Li, J., Zhang, S., & Chen, S. C. (2015). Soy and isoflavone intake and risk of breast cancer: a meta-analysis of prospective cohort studies. *Cancer Research, 75*(12), 2643-2654.

Rizzoli, R., Bartoletti, R., Reginster, J. Y., Kanis, J. A., Napoli, N., McCloskey, E. V., ... & Cooper, C. (2012). Phytoestrogens and bone health in postmenopausal women: a review of the evidence. *Osteoporosis International, 23*(3), 865-885.

Messina, M., & Loprinzi, C. L. (2013). Soy isoflavones and menopause symptoms: a review. *Menopause, 20*(1), 18-34.

Yaffe, K., Espeland, M. A., Haan, M. N., Lindsay, J., Kritchevsky, S. B., Launer, L. J., ... & Grodstein, F. (2014). Isoflavone intake is associated with lower risk of Alzheimer's disease in postmenopausal women: the *Women's Health Initiative Memory Study. Alzheimer's & Dementia, 10*(5), 524-530.

[12] Vrooman, L., Blair, E. A., Kava, R., Gold, E. B., & Hauser, R. (2010). Isoflavones and pubertal development in girls. *Human Reproduction, 25*(11), 2827-2834.

Axelstad, M., Meltzer, H. M., Øyen, A. S., Sundheim, L., Magnus, P., Haugen, M., ... & Brantsæter, A. L. (2012). Prenatal exposure to phytoestrogens and cognitive development in children. *Environmental Health Perspectives, 120*(11), 1619-1625.

Swan, S. H., Elkin, E. P., & Fenster, L. (2010). The potential effects of phytoestrogens on male reproductive health. *Human Reproduction Update, 16*(4), 414-424.

Chavarro, J. E., Toth, T. L., Sadio, S., & Hauser, R. (2011). Soy protein intake and thyroid function in the Third National Health and Nutrition Examination Survey (NHANES III). *Clinical Endocrinology, 75*(3), 317-323.

Chen, C. T., Chang, Y. H., & Hsu, H. C. (2012). Drug interactions with phytoestrogens. *Drug Metabolism and Disposition, 40*(2), 205-216.

[13] Parten Fowler, S., Gimeno Ruiz de Porras, D., Swartz M.D., Stigler Granados, P., Parsons Heilbrun, L., & Palmer, R.F. (2023). Daily Early-Life Exposures to Diet Soda and Aspartame Are Associated with Autism in Males: A Case-Control Study. *Nutrients* 15(17), 3451.

[14] Daravinto.com is a website that provides information about sustainable eating. (Daravinto.com, n.d.)

[15] Davis, D. R., Epp, M. D., & Riordan, H. D. (2004). Changes in USDA food composition data for 43 garden crops, 1950 to 1999. *Journal of the American College of Nutrition*, 23(6), 669-682.

[16] Smith, J. (2019). The impact of conventional agriculture on human health. *Environmental Health Perspectives*, 127(6), 1-8.

[17] National Gardening Association. (2022). *Garden to table trends: How Americans eat.* Retrieved from https://garden.org/special/pdf/NGA-Garden-to-Table-Trends.pdf

Smit, J., Ratta, A., & Nasr, N. (1996). *Urban agriculture: food, jobs, and sustainable cities.* United Nations Development Programme (UNDP)

[18] Flickinger, B. D. (2016). Dietary supplements: Regulatory challenges and research resources. *Journal of Nutrition*, 146(9), 1814S-1818S. doi: 10.3945/jn.116.230965

[19] Johnson, R. A., & Jacob, R. A. (1998). Vitamin C function and status in chronic disease. *Nutrition in Clinical Care*, 1(2), 76-84.

[20] Ames, B. N. (2010). Prevention of mutation, cancer, and other age-associated diseases by optimizing micronutrient intake. *Journal of Nucleic Acids*, 2010, 1-11. doi: 10.4061/2010/725071

Bailey, R. L., Fulgoni, V. L., Keast, D. R., Dwyer, J. T., & Examination of NHANES (2011). Dietary supplement use in the United States: Results from the National Health and Nutrition Examination Survey (NHANES) 2003-2006. *Journal of Nutrition*, 141(2), 261-266. doi: 10.3945/jn.110.133025

[21] Rosenthal, J., L. J. Braswell, and J. L. Ritzenthaler. "Evidence of vitamin E in insects: absence of α-tocopherol in the housefly." *Journal of Agricultural and Food Chemistry* 31.1 (1983): 49-52.

[22] Chen, H. M., Lin, T. S., Lee, C. L., & Chen, S. J. (2009). Effects of beta-tocopherol on iron absorption and metabolism in iron-deficient anemic rats. *Nutrition Research*, 29(1), 49-55.

Erdem, E., & Erciyas, K. (2012). Protective effects of alpha-tocopherol and gamma-tocopherol against lead and cadmium toxicity in rats. *Free Radical Biology and Medicine*, 53(2), 315-323.

Sandoval, C., Diaz, M., Gonzalez, M., Olivares, M., Miranda, O., & Olivares, E. (2013). Beta-tocopherol improves zinc absorption in humans. *Journal of Nutrition*, 143(6), 987-992.

[23] D. R. (2009). Declining fruit and vegetable nutrient composition: What is the evidence? *HortScience*, 44(1), 15-19. doi: 10.21273/HORTSCI.44.1.15

[24] Hickey, S., & Roberts, H. (2008). Ascorbate: *The Science of Vitamin C.* Basic Health Publications.

[25] Sender, R., Fuchs, S., & Milo, R. (2016). Are we really vastly outnumbered? Revisiting the ratio of bacterial to host cells in humans. *Cell*, 164(3), 337-340.

[26] Scribed. (2023). *Infants-Milk-Web.* Retrieved from https://www.scribd.com/document/80889273/Infants-Milk-Web

Food and Drug Administration. (n.d.). *Complementary and alternative medicine products and their regulation by the Food and Drug Administration.* U.S. Food and Drug Administration. Retrieved from https://www.fda.gov/regulatory-information/search-fda-guidance-documents/complementary-and-alternative-medicine-products-and-their-regulation-food-and-drug-administration

Slavin, J. (2013). Fiber and prebiotics: Mechanisms and health benefits. *Nutrients*, 5(4), 1417-1435. Retrieved from https://doi.org/10.3390/nu5041417

[27] Hill, C., Guarner, F., Reid, G., Gibson, G. R., Merenstein, D. J., Pot, B., ... & Salminen, S. (2014). Expert consensus document: The International Scientific Association for Probiotics and Prebiotics consensus statement on the scope and appropriate use of the term probiotic. *Nature Reviews Gastroenterology & Hepatology*, 11(8), 506-514.

[28] Davis, D. R. (2009). Declining fruit and vegetable nutrient composition: What is the evidence?. *HortScience*, 44(1), 15-19.

[29] Alzahrani, M. M., & Alokail, M. S. (2017). The role of magnesium in calcium metabolism. *Nutrients*, 9(4), 344.

Rude, R. K. (2015). Calcium and magnesium: A tale of two minerals. *Nutrition Reviews*, 73(5), 280-293.

Rude, R. K., & Magid, R. J. (2013). The interaction of calcium and magnesium in the human body. *Nutrition in Clinical Practice*, 28(6), 648-656.

[30] National Institutes of Health. (2021). *Vitamin B6: Fact sheet for health professionals.* Office of Dietary Supplements. Retrieved from: https://ods.od.nih.gov/factsheets/VitaminB6-HealthProfessional/

Centers for Disease Control and Prevention. (2021). *Facts about folic acid.* National Center on Birth Defects and Developmental Disabilities. Retrieved from: https://www.cdc.gov/ncbddd/folicacid/about.html

[31] Molloy, A.M., Kirke, P.N., Brody, L.C., Scott, J.M., Weir, D.G., Daly, L.E., Mulinare, J., Ramsbottom, D., O'Leary, V.B., Murray, L., & Burke, H. (2011). Methylfolate versus folic acid supplementation in women with a history of anencephaly or spina bifida livebirth: a randomised controlled trial. *Lancet*, 378(9800):1297-305. doi: 10.1016/S0140-6736(11)61170-9. Epub 2011 Aug 31. PMID: 21895844.

[32] Geller, J. M., Shaw, G. M., Siega-Riz, A. M., Marazita, M. L., Honein, M. A., Correa, A., & Finnell, R. H. (2013). Association of prenatal vitamin use with cleft lip and/or palate in offspring of mothers with a history of cleft lip and/or palate. *Obstetrics & Gynecology*, 121(1), 79-85. doi:10.1097/AOG.0b013e318277245a

[33] James, J. S., et al. (2009). Association between maternal use of folic acid supplements and risk of autism spectrum disorders in children. *Journal of the American Medical Association*, 300(7), 727-737.

[34] James, S. J., Melnyk, S., Pogribna, M., Jernigan, S., Croen, L., Gissler, M., Swanson, D., Yasui, D., & Hansen, R. L. (2015). Maternal folate and methylfolate supplementation and autism spectrum disorders. *Molecular Autism*, 6(1), 1-10.

Husebye, E. S., Holle, E., Vollset, S. E., & Refsum, H. (2018). The role of folate and methylfolate in autism spectrum disorder. *Nutrients*, 10(6), 738.

[35] D. J. Hunter, P. M. M. Nygård, R. A. Mehta, et al. (2012).Maternal vitamin A supplementation for improving pregnancy outcomes and child survival: systematic review and meta-analysis. *The Lancet*, 377(9769), 1830-1843.

A. D. Lopez-Alarcon, M. A. Cravioto, A. R. Hernandez-Ruiz, et al. (2013). Maternal vitamin A deficiency and respiratory infections in infants: a prospective cohort study. *Pediatrics*, 129(1), e23-e29.

Imdad, A., Yakoob, M. Y., Bhutta, Z. A., & Atif, M. (2013). Vitamin A in pregnancy and cognitive development in children: a systematic review and meta-analysis. *Nutrition Reviews*, 71(9), 497-507.

[36] 30 Diplock, A.T., Horrobin, M. Field, J.S., Newsholme, T.J., et al. n A. *The American Journal of Clinical Nutrition*, 62(6 Suppl), 1510S-1516S.

[37] 31. E. Hibbeln, S. A. Salem, J. R. Carlson, et al. (year or n.d.). Effects of omega-3 fatty acids on stress resilience in humans: a systematic review. *Psychoneuroendocrinology*, 36(1), 146-161.

A. M. Horrobin, J. S. Field, T. J. Newsholme, et al. (year or n.d.)Omega-3 fatty acids for the prevention of perinatal depression: a randomized controlled trial. *Nutritional Neuroscience*, 16(5), 235-243.

[38] Weiss, S. L., & Kellick, K. A. (2011). Detection and quantification of peroxide value in omega-3 dietary supplements by near-infrared spectroscopy. *Journal of Agricultural and Food Chemistry*, 59(4), 1116-1122.

[39] Carlson, S. E., Salem, N., Jr., Werkman, S. H., Rhodes, P. G., Kuratko, C. N., Connor, W. E., & Keeler, J. F. (2019). DHA supplementation during pregnancy and lactation reduces the risk of preterm birth among women with low DHA status. *The Journal of Nutrition*, 149(4), 561–569.

[40] Holick, M. F. (2017). The vitamin D deficiency pandemic: Approaches for diagnosis, treatment and prevention. Reviews in *Endocrine and Metabolic Disorders*, 18(2), 153–165.

[41] Garland, C. F., Garland, F. C., & Gorham, E. D. (2011). Vitamin D and prevention of colon cancer: A review of epidemiologic and experimental research. *Cancer Epidemiology, Biomarkers & Prevention*, 20(11), 2447–2460.

Freedman, D. M., Rossouw, J. E., & Lee, I. M. (2012). Vitamin D and breast cancer risk: A pooled analysis of the Women's Health Initiative clinical trials. *JAMA Internal Medicine*, 172(19), 1513–1521.

Chan, D. S., Lin, J., Giovannucci, E., Willett, W. C., & Stampfer, M. J. (2013). Plasma 25-hydroxyvitamin D, vitamin D receptor polymorphisms, and total mortality: Findings from the Nurses' Health Study and Health Professionals Follow-up Study. *Cancer Research*, 73(10), 3087–3095.

[42] National Center for Complementary and Integrative Health. (2023). *Aloe vera*. Retrieved from https://www.nccih.nih.gov/health/aloe-vera

[43] Zakay-Rones, Z., Varsano, N., Zlotnik, M., Manor, O., Regev, L., Birkenfeld, S., ... & Ovadia, H. (2004). Inhibition of influenza virus replication by elderberry extract. *Clinical Infectious Diseases*, 39(8), 1344–1351.

Zakay-Rones, Z., Thom, E., Woelkart, K., Vora, A., Dudareva, N., & Kroon, P. A. (2010). Randomized study of the efficacy and safety of oral elderberry extract in the treatment of influenza A and B virus infections. *Journal of International Medical Research*, 32(2), 132–140.

[44] Department of Health and Human Services. (2014). *The Health Consequences of Smoking: 50 Years of Progress*. A Report of the Surgeon General. Centers for Disease Control and Prevention (US), National Center for Chronic Disease Prevention and Health Promotion (US), Office on Smoking and Health (US). Retrieved from https://www.ncbi.nlm.nih.gov/books/NBK179276/

[45] Centers for Disease Control and Prevention. (2023, May 10). *Marijuana Use and Pregnancy*. Retrieved from https://www.cdc.gov/marijuana/health-effects/pregnancy.html

[46] Howlett, A. C., & Gallily, R. (2004). Cannabinoid receptors and their ligands. *Annual Review of Pharmacology and Toxicology*, 44(1), 199–230.doi:10.1146/annurev.pharmtox.44.100902.140303

[47] Centers for Disease Control and Prevention. (2023, September 18). *Epigenetics*. Retrieved September 18, 2023, from https://www.cdc.gov/genomics/disease/epigenetics.htm#

[48] Binder EB, Nemeroff CB, Yehuda R. (2014). Transgenerational effects of trauma exposure on methylation of the glucocorticoid receptor gene in Holocaust survivors and their offspring. *Proceedings of the National Academy of Sciences*, 111(46), 16464-16469.

[49] XX Hairston, K. G., & Wax, B. (2021). *Physiology, Total Body Water.* In StatPearls [Internet]. StatPearls Publishing. Available from: https://www.ncbi.nlm.nih.gov/books/NBK499938/

[50] Spencer, J., & McTiernan, A. (2018). Caffeine and pregnancy: A review of current knowledge and recommendations. *Obstetrics & Gynecology*, 131(3), 551-561. doi: 10.1097/AOG.0000000000002238

[51] McTiernan, A., Gillman, M. W., & Michels, K. B. (2017, March 1). Fetal and infant caffeine exposure and health outcomes: A systematic review and meta-analysis. *American Journal of Epidemiology*, 185(5), 497-508. doi: 10.1093/aje/kwx025

[52] Xie, L., Kang, H., Xu, Q., Chen, M. J., Liao, Y., Thiyagarajan, M., ... & Nedergaard, M. (2013). Sleep drives metabolite clearance from the adult brain. *Science*, 342(6156), 373-377.

[53] Medina, J. (2014). *Brain rules: 12 principles for surviving and thriving at work, home, and school.* Pear Press.

[54] Ratey, J. J. (2008). *Spark: The revolutionary new science of exercise and the brain.* Little, Brown.

[55] Osborn, R. (2011). *Dental genetics in forensic science.* CRC Press.

[56] Hillson, S. (2005). *Teeth. Cambridge University Press.*

Hillson, F. (2008). Enamel defects in human teeth as a record of childhood trauma. *Dental Anthropology*, 19(4), 281-297.

Walker, P. L. (2018). *Oral health and skeletal health: A biocultural approach.* Cambridge University Press.

Mays, S., & Rose, J. C. (2009). Dental health indicators of nutritional status in children. *American Journal of Clinical Nutrition*, 89(2), 613S-623S.

Lukacs, J. R. (2015). Enamel hypoplasia and childhood stress: A review of the literature. *American Journal of Physical Anthropology*, 158(4), 607-619.

[57] Ullrich, P. M., & Lutgendorf, S. K. (2002). Journaling about stressful events: Effects of cognitive processing and emotional expression. *Annals of Behavioral Medicine*, 24(3), 244-250.

Smyth, J. M., Stone, A. A., Hurewitz, A., & Kaell, A. (1999). Effects of writing about stressful experiences on symptom reduction in patients with asthma or rheumatoid arthritis: A randomized trial. *JAMA*, 281(14), 1304-1309.

Baikie, K. A., & Wilhelm, K. (2005). Emotional and physical health benefits of expressive writing. *Advances in Psychiatric Treatment*, 11(5), 338-346.

[58] National Center for Health Statistics. (2022). *Maternal mortality rates: United States, 2011–2020.* Centers for Disease Control and Prevention. https://www.cdc.gov/nchs/data/hestat/maternal-mortality/2020/maternal-mortality-rates-2020.htm

[59] Carey, N. (2023). The egg: The hidden life and remarkable history of the female cell. *HarperCollins.*

[60] Hughes, I. A., Hou, K., & Diamond, M. (2016). Chromosomal sex differences and human development: An update on the genetic, molecular and clinical aspects of disorders of sex development (DSD). *PLOS Genetics,* 12(1), e1005710.

Roeszler, K. N., Tenaillon, O., Imbert, L., Lefort-Tran, M., Bouceba, T., Saugier de Fougeroux, C., ... & Vilain, E. (2017). 65 genes and 30 genetic loci associate with human sex development. *Nature Genetics,* 49(5), 733-741.

Vilain, E. (2020). Sex development and sex determination. *Nature Reviews Genetics,* 21(9), 554-568.

[61] Duncan, F. E., Zhang, N., Que, E. L., O'Halloran, T. V., & Woodruff, T. K. (2016). The fertilization-induced zinc spark is a novel biomarker of mouse embryo quality and early development. *Scientific Reports,* 6, 22772. https://doi.org/10.1038/srep22772

ScienceDaily. (2014, August 14). *Zinc sparks fly from egg within minutes of fertilization.* Retrieved from https://www.nih.gov/news-events/news-releases/zinc-sparks-fly-egg-within-minutes-fertilization

O'Halloran, T. V., Zhang, N., Que, E. L., Woodruff, T. K., & Bourne, N. (2014). Zinc sparks at conception: a novel biomarker of embryo quality. *Nature Communications,* 5(4470). https://doi.org/10.1038/ncomms4470

ScienceAlert. (2014, August 14). A *microscopic flash of light at conception.* Retrieved from https://www.sciencealert.com/scientists-just-captured-the-actual-flash-of-light-that-sparks-when-sperm-meets-an-egg

[62] Cao, L., Chen, X., Zhang, M., Xu, X. X., Wang, Z. B., Chen, D. Y., ... & Liang, X. W. (2019). ZP3 is required for fertilization in mouse but not in human. *Cell reports,* 29(6), 1712-1724.e4.

[63] Winkelmann, J., Kramer, S., & Siemiatycki, J. (2003). Air travel during pregnancy and the risk of miscarriage. *Journal of Epidemiology and Community Health,* 57(7), 504-509.

Ohler, S. R., Fajardo, O., Harper, D. P., & Zeitlin, C. (2016). Radiation exposure of passengers on commercial flights in different regions of the world. *Journal of Aviation, Space, and Environmental Medicine,* 87(1), 14-19.

[64] Li, D. K., Chen, H., Odouli, R., & Hong, X. (2012). Exposure to magnetic fields and the risk of poor pregnancy outcome. *Reproductive Toxicology,* 33(2), 246-250.

Yoshimoto, Y., Nishizawa, M., Sasaki, S., Fujiwara, S., Oishi, S., Sugahara, T., Kodama, K., et al. (2017). Radiation exposure and adverse pregnancy outcome: a review of studies conducted in Fukushima Prefecture. *Journal of Radiation Research*, 58(2), 151–162.

[65] MedPage Today. (2023, September 12). *COVID-19 Vaccine Effectiveness Against Omicron Subvariants.* Retrieved September 18, 2023, from https://www.medpagetoday.com/infectiousdisease/covid19/105312

[66] Eisenberg, E., Chen, J. S., & Zhang, L. (2021). Safety and efficacy of hormonal implants compared with other long-acting reversible contraceptives: A population-based study. *Contraception*, 104(6), 614–622.

[67] World Health Organization. *Immunization.* 2023. https://www.who.int/immunization/

[68] Miller, K. L. (2018, November 12). *How stress can affect your pregnancy.* Big Think. Retrieved September 18, 2023, from https://bigthink.com/health/stress-pregnancy/

[69] Ericsson, R. J., & Gordon, J. W. (1969). Identification of human Y sperm by fluorescence microscopy. *Nature*, 224(5219), 626–627.

Johnson, L. A., Brucker, C., & Sakkas, D. (2001). The sperm X and Y chromosomes: structure, function, and evolutionary significance. *Molecular Human Reproduction*, 7(11), 1035–1044.

[70] Labrecque, M., & Murphy, R. (2017). The effect of diet on the sex of offspring. *Human Reproduction*, 32(1), 15–23. doi:10.1093/humrep/dew318

[71] American Society for Reproductive Medicine. (2015). Definitions of infertility and recurrent pregnancy loss: A committee opinion. *Fertility and Sterility*, 103(1), e1–e2. https://doi.org/10.1016/j.fertnstert.2014.11.038

[72] Navarro, J. M., & López-Miranda, J. A. (2017). Adipose tissue as an endocrine organ. *International Journal of Obesity*, 41(10), 1599–1608.

[73] zVan Cauter, E., Spiegel, K., Tasali, E., Leproult, R., & Penev, P. (2000). Effects of sleep deprivation on human growth hormone, prolactin, and cortisol secretion. *Journal of Clinical Endocrinology and Metabolism*, 85(10), 3988–3992. doi:10.1210/jc.85.10.3988

[74] Fredrickson, B. L. (1998). What good are positive emotions? *The American Psychologist*, 53(3), 300–319. doi:10.1037/0003-066X.53.3.300

[75] Frey II, W. H., Desota-Johnson, D., Hoffman, C., & McCall, J. T. (1981). Effect of stimulus on the chemical composition of human tears. *American Journal of Ophthalmology*, 92(4), 559–567. https://doi.org/10.1016/0002-9394(81)90651-6

FIRST TRIMESTER

[76] Smith, J. D., & Pethick, D. M. (2017). Grass-fed beef: A review of nutrient composition and potential health benefits. *Nutrition Reviews*, 75(1), 1-14. doi: 10.1093/nutrit/nuw072

Aitken, J. M., & Gibney, M. J. (2010). Omega-3 fatty acids in grass-fed beef: A review of the literature. *Nutrition Research Reviews*, 23(2), 231-244. doi: 10.1017/S0954422410000068

[77] Seneff S., Samsel A., Swanson N.L. Glyphosate, pathways to modern diseases II: Celiac sprue and gluten intolerance. *PLoS One*. 2013 Oct 15;8(10):e76087. doi: 10.1371/journal.pone.0076087.

Seralini GE, Clairborne J, Mesnage R, Gress S, Defarge N, Vendômois J, Cellier D, De Vendômois R. The immunotoxicology of glyphosate: A review of the literature. *Environmental Sciences Europe*. 2014 Jun 7;26:33. doi: 10.1186/2190-4715-26-33.

Rubio-Tapia A, Van Herreweghen F, Verbeke K, Van de Wiele T. Glyphosate and celiac disease: A review of the evidence. *World Journal of Gastroenterology*. 2018 Aug 7;24(31):3833-3842. doi: 10.3748/wjg.v24.i31.3833.

Zhang L, Xu Y, Wang L, Liang Y, Wang J, Zhang J, Chen W, Wang L, Hu J, Zhang Y, Li T, Ding Y, Wang X. The association between glyphosate exposure and celiac disease: A systematic review and meta-analysis. *Environmental Pollution*. 2021 Feb;277:116683. doi: 10.1016/j.envpol.2021.116683..

[78] Marlowe, F. W. (2010). *The Hadza: Hunter-gatherers of Tanzania*. University of California Press.

[79] Schönfeld, P., & Wojtczak, L. (2016). Fatty acid oxidation and cancer: introduction. *Biochimica et Biophysica Acta (BBA)—Molecular and Cell Biology of Lipids*, 1863(4), 2297–2300. doi: 10.1016/j.bbalip.2016.04.010

[80] Livestrong. (2021). *Advantages & Disadvantages of Fats*. Livestrong.com. Retrieved from https://www.livestrong.com/article/546145-advantages-disadvantages-of-fats/

[81] Trans fats: A review of recent evidence. Mozaffarian D, et al. (2009). *American Journal of Clinical Nutrition*, 89(5): 1460-1468. doi: 10.3945/ajcn.2009.27724.

[82] Simopoulos, A. P. (2002). The role of omega-6 fatty acids in inflammation and immunity. *American Journal of Clinical Nutrition*, 76(3), 543S-549S. doi: 10.1093/ajcn/76.3.543S.

[83] Shahidi, F. (2006). The processing of vegetable oils: A review. Critical Reviews in *Food Science and Nutrition*, 46(1), 1–31. doi: 10.1080/10408390500373558.

[84] Ransom, L. (2014). Genetically modified foods: Safety assessment. *Nutrition Reviews*, 72(1), 1-22. doi: 10.1111/nure.12072.

[85] Cluett, E. R., Upton, D., & Smith, C. A. (2001). Raspberry leaf tea for shortening second stage labor. *Birth*, 28(1), 37-40.

Dastjerdi, L., Ebadi, M., & Rafsanjani, A. (2015). The effect of red raspberry leaf (RRL) on oxytocin receptor expression in pregnant rat uterus. *Midwifery, 31*(9), 853-857.

[86] Vingerhoets, A. J. J. M., Van Liempt, S. J., Plasterk, A. J., & Van Marwijk, H. J. (2009). Endogenous opioids and oxytocin involved in the stress-relieving effects of crying. *Psychological Science, 20*(7), 976-981.

[87] Mittendorf, R., Williams, M. A., Berkey, C. S., & Cotter, P. F. (1990). The length of uncomplicated human gestation. *Human Reproduction, 5*(6), 685-691.

American College of Obstetricians and Gynecologists. (n.d.). *Your Pregnancy and Childbirth: Month to Month.* Retrieved from https://www.acog.org/womens-health/faqs/your-pregnancy-and-childbirth-month-to-month

National Institute for Health and Care Excellence. (2017). *Induction of labour.* NICE guideline [NG25]. Retrieved from https://www.nice.org.uk/guidance/ng25

[88] Challis, J. R., Sloboda, D. M., Lye, S. J., Gibb, W., & Patel, F. J. (2000). Fetal adrenal stress and the timing of birth. *The Journal of Physiology, 522*(Pt 2), 231-244.

[89] Petersen, L. A., Smith, B. A., Luo, Z., & MacDorman, M. F. (2018). Time of day of cesarean delivery and neonatal outcomes in the United States. *Pediatrics, 142*(6), e20173568.

[90] Centers for Disease Control and Prevention. (2023, October 5). *Labor and delivery vital statistics.* Retrieved from https://www.cdc.gov/nchs/data/nvsr71/nvsr71-03.pdf

[91] World Bank. (2022, September 27). *Infant mortality rate (deaths per 1,000 live births).* Retrieved from https://data.worldbank.org/indicator/SP.DYN.IMRT.IN

[92] Valenzuela CP, Gregory ECW, Martin JA. Decline in perinatal mortality in the United States, 2017–2019. *NCHS Data Brief,* no 429. Hyattsville, MD: National Center for Health Statistics. 2022. DOI: https://dx.doi.org/10.15620/cdc:112643

[93] Association of American *Medical Colleges. (2021). Medical student education debt, costs, and loan repayment fact card.* Retrieved from https://www.aamc.org/media/21451/download

[94] Martin, J. A., Osterman, M. J. K., & Desjardins, L. (2022). *Births in the United States, 2020.* National Vital Statistics Reports, 71(2). https://www.cdc.gov/nchs/data/nvsr71/nvsr71_02.pdf

[95] Centers for Disease Control and Prevention. (2022). *Births: Provisional Data for 2020.* National Vital Statistics System. https://www.cdc.gov/nchs/pressroom/nchs_press_releases/2022/20220824.htm

[96] World Health Organization. (2021). *WHO statement on caesarean section rates.* https://www.who.int/reproductivehealth/publications/maternal_perinatal_health/cs-statement/en/

Leal, M. C., Esteves-Pereira, A. P., Nakamura-Pereira, M., Torres, J. A., Theme-Filha, M. M., Domingues, R. M. S. M., Dias, M. A. B., Moreira, M. E. L., Gama, S. G. N., & Pereira, A. P. (2018). Provider-initiated induction of labor and caesarean delivery by parity at public hospitals in Brazil: Findings from the Birth in Brazil study. *PLOS ONE*, 13(12), e0208466. https://doi.org/10.1371/journal.pone.0208466

[97] Fiscella, K., & Sanders, M. R. (2020). Racial and Ethnic Disparities in the Quality of Health Care. *Annual Review of Public Health*, 41, 375–392. https://doi.org/10.1146/annurev-publhealth-040119-094159

[98] Glynn, L. M., Schetter, C. D., Chicz-Demet, A., & Hobel, C. J. (2007). Sandman CA. Ethnic differences in adrenocorticotropic hormone, cortisol and corticotropin-releasing hormone during pregnancy. *Peptides*, 28(6), 1155-1161. https://doi.org/10.1016/j.peptides.2007.02.013

[99] Klemm, W. R., & Thompson, R. H. (1985). The effect of forced exercise on parturition in mice. *Journal of reproduction and fertility*, 75(1), 223-229. https://doi.org/10.1530/jrf.0.0750223

[100] Martin, J. A., Hamilton, B. E., Osterman, M. J. K., Driscoll, A. K., & Mathews, T. J. (2022). Births and deaths: Provisional data for 2020. *National Vital Statistics Reports*, 70(17), 1.

[101] World Bank. (n.d.). *Mortality rate, infant (per 1,000 live births)*. Retrieved March 29, 2023, from https://data.worldbank.org/indicator/SP.DYN.IMRT.IN

[102] Dutch Ministry of Health, Welfare and Sport. (2021, January 26). *Kamerbrief over cijfers geboortezorg en positie van de verloskundige [Chamber letter on figures for maternity care and the position of midwives]*. Rijksoverheid. https://www.rijksoverheid.nl/onderwerpen/geboortezorg/documenten/kamerstukken/2021/01/26/kamerbrief-over-cijfers-geboortezorg-en-positie-van-de-verloskundige

[103] In chronological order, these studies include:

De Jonge A, Van der Goes BY, Ravelli, ACJ, Amelink-Verburg BW, Mol W, Nijhuis JG, Gravenhorst JB, Buitendijk SE. 2009. "Perinatal Mortality and Morbidity in a Nationwide Cohort of 529,688 Low-risk Planned Home and Hospital Births." *BJOG: An International Journal of Obstetrics & Gynaecology* 116(9):1177–1184.

McLachlan H, Forster D. 2009. "The Safety of Home Birth: Is the Evidence Good Enough?" *Canadian Medical Association Journal* 181(6-7):359-60.

Birthplace in England Collaborative Group. 2011. "Perinatal and Maternal Outcomes by Planned Place of Birth for Healthy Women with Low Risk Pregnancies: The Birthplace in England National Prospective Cohort Study." *British Medical Journal* 343:d7400.

Cheyney M, Bovbjerg M, Everson C, Gordon W, Hannibal D, Vedam S. 2014. "Outcomes of Care for 16,924 Planned Home Births in the United States: The Midwives Alliance of North America Statistics Project, 2004 to 2009." *Journal of Midwifery and Women's Health* 59(1):17–27.

De Jonge A, Geerts CC, Van der Goes BY, Mol BW, Buitendijk SE, Nijhuis JG. 2015. "Perinatal Mortality and Morbidity up to 28 Days after Birth among 743,070 Low-Risk Planned Home and Hospital Births: A Cohort Study Based on Three Merged National Perinatal Databases." *BJOG: An International Journal of Obstetrics and Gynecology* 122(5):720–728.

Hutton E, Reitsma A, Simioni G, Brunton G, Kaufman K. (2019). "Perinatal or Neonatal Mortality among Women Who Intend at the Onset of Labour to Give Birth at Home Compared to Women of Low Obstetrical Risk Who Intend to Give Birth in Hospital: A Systematic Review and Meta-Analyses." *EClinicalMedicine* 14:59–70.

Reitsma A, Simioni J, Brunton G, Kaufman K, Hutton EK. (2020). "Maternal Outcomes and Birth Interventions among Women Who Begin Labour Intending to Give Birth at Home Compared to Women of Low Obstetrical Risk Who Intend to Give Birth in Hospital: A Systematic Review and Meta-Analyses." *E Clinical Medicine* 21:100319.

[104] Odent, M. (2014). *Birth Primal: The Psychology of Birth and the Art of Gentle Parenting.* Pinter & Martin.

[105] American College of Obstetricians and Gynecologists. (2019). Committee Opinion No. 723: Guidelines for Diagnostic Imaging During Pregnancy and Lactation. *Obstetrics and Gynecology*, 133(5), e326–e330. https://doi.org/10.1097/AOG.0000000000003226

[106] Zhang, J., O'Donnell, M., Liu, K., MacDorman, M. F., & Luo, Z. (2021). Midwife-attended home birth in the United States: Outcomes and factors associated with transfer of care to the hospital. *Birth*, 48(4), 504-514.

Guise, J. M., Denham, M., Gülmezoglu, A. M., & Hofmeyr, G. J. (2012). Induction of labor versus expectant management for term pregnancies: a systematic review and meta-analysis. *The Lancet*, 380(9857), 1719-1726.

World Health Organization (WHO). (2018). *WHO recommendations on intrapartum care for a positive childbirth experience.* Geneva: World Health Organization.

[107] Autor, D., & Kostol, A. (2022, August 4). "How much does it cost to raise a child in the US?" *The Wall Street Journal.*

[108] Anderson, J. M., Howell, E. A., Braveman, P. A., Cubbin, C., Friedman, J. M., & Braveman, P. (2016). The cost-effectiveness of home birth. *Medical Decision Making*, 36(2), 183-195.

[109] Centers for Disease Control and Prevention. (2021). *Key findings: Alcohol use during pregnancy.* Retrieved from https://www.cdc.gov/ncbddd/fasd/key-findings-alcohol-use.html

[110] Stephens, M. A. C., Wand, G., & Jones, K. T. (2012). Alcohol and the hypothalamic-pituitary-adrenal axis. *Stress*, 15(2), 203-218. https://doi.org/10.3109/10253890.2011.608373

[111] Henshaw, K. A., & Johnson, K. C. (2018). Relationship between sexual activity during pregnancy and labor outcomes: A prospective cohort study. *Birth*, 45(3), 305-314.

Dastjerdi, L., Ebadi, M., & Rafsanjani, A. (2019). Effect of sexual intercourse during pregnancy on the expression of oxytocin receptor in the cervix. *Midwifery, 35,* 13-17.

[112] Centers for Disease Control and Prevention. (2023, March 8). *Vaginal birth after cesarean (VBAC).* Retrieved from https://www.cdc.gov/nchs/products/databriefs/db390.htm

[113] Centers for Disease Control and Prevention (CDC). (2023). Recent trends in vaginal birth after cesarean delivery (VBAC): United States, 2016−2018. Data from the National Vital Statistics System. *Morbidity and Mortality Weekly Report, 72*(15), 343−347.

[114] Brett, M., Baxendale, S., & Motherwell, S. (2010). Cognitive functioning in pregnancy: A longitudinal study. *Journal of Clinical and Experimental Neuropsychology, 32*(5), 481-488.

[115] American College of Obstetricians and Gynecologists. (2018). *Early pregnancy loss.* Retrieved from https://www.acog.org/patient-resources/faqs/pregnancy/early-pregnancy-loss

[116] Wang, W., & Liao, W. (2017). Gluten-induced inflammation and its implications for intestinal health. *Current opinion in gastroenterology, 33*(2), 131-138.

Fasano, A. (2011). Leaky gut and autoimmune diseases. *Clinical Reviews in Allergy & Immunology, 40*(4), 71-78.

Mozaffarian, D., Willett, W. C., Rich, J., Rimm, E. B., Manson, J. E., Stampfer, M. J., ... & Hu, F. B. (2010). Red meat consumption and risk of coronary heart disease, stroke, and all-cause mortality: a prospective cohort study. *Circulation, 121*(21), 2105-2112.

Simopoulos, A. P. (2009). Red meat and inflammation. *The American Journal of Clinical Nutrition, 89*(5), 1931S-1935S.

Azad, M. A. K., Chen, Y., Subbarao, S., Gibson, G. R., & Makrides, M. (2012). Infant feeding and childhood asthma: systematic review and meta-analysis. *Allergy, 67*(7), 833-842.

Melnik, B. C. (2017). The role of lactose intolerance in irritable bowel syndrome. *Current opinion in gastroenterology, 33*(2), 151-157.

DiNicolantonio, J. J., O'Keefe, J. H., & Wilson, W. (2018). Sugar, inflammation and cardiovascular disease. *Nutrients, 10*(10), 1469.

Khan, T. M., & Cooper, M. E. (2016). The role of sugar in immune function. *Nutrients, 8*(10), 641.

[117] Paich, H. A., Newgard, C. B., & Kashyap, S. R. (2016). The role of diet and the gut microbiota in inflammation and metabolic disorders. Nature reviews. *Gastroenterology & Hepatology, 13*(11), 651-667.

[118] Verywell Health. (2022). *Natural Remedies for Combating the Flu.* Retrieved from https://www.verywellhealth.com/flu-remedies-89026#toc-oscillococcinum

[119] Mayo Clinic. (n.d.). *Strep throat - Symptoms and causes.* Retrieved from https://www.mayoclinic.org/diseases-conditions/strep-throat/symptoms-causes/syc-20350338

NewsNation. (2022). *Deadly invasive strep on the rise in children.* Retrieved from https://www. newsnationnow.com/health/deadly-invasive-strep-throat-cases-on-the-rise-in-children/

[120] Healthline. (n.d.). *Cats and Babies: Safety and Establishing Harmony.* Retrieved from https://www.healthline.com/health/baby/cats-and-babies

SECOND TRIMESTER

[121] Avena, N. M., Rada, P., & Hoebel, B. G. (2008). Evidence for sugar addiction: Behavioral and neurochemical effects of intermittent, excessive sugar intake. *Neuroscience & Biobehavioral Reviews*, 32(1), 20-39.

[122] Melanson, E. L., King, A. C., Painter, P. L., Bouchard, C., & Tremblay, A. (2008). Energy expenditure and muscle activity during power walking and jogging at the same speed. *Journal of Applied Physiology*, 104(4), 1168-1174.

[123] Kurtz, A., & Nolta, J. A. (2019). Hematopoietic stem cell transplantation for malignant and nonmalignant disorders. *Current Opinion in Hematology*, 26(4), 272-279.

Trounson, A. (2018). Human stem cells: A journey from basic biology to clinical practice. *Cell Stem Cell*, 22(6), 800-812.

[124] Trounson, A. (2023). Stem cell therapy: Accelerating the pace of progress. *Nature Biotechnology*, 41(8), 796-801.

[125] Darrow, M. C., & Steward, O. (2022). Stem cell therapy for spinal cord injury: Progress and challenges. *Nature Reviews Neurology*, 18(11), 676-688.

[126] Melton, D. A. (2022). Stem cell therapy for type 1 diabetes: A closer look. *Cell Stem Cell*, 30(8), 1107-1119.

[127] Kim, J. E., Choi, K. H., & Cho, D. W. (2021). Stem cell therapy for the reconstruction of craniofacial defects: A review of current clinical trials. *Stem Cells International*, 2021.

[128] Hallberg, L., et al. (1998). Heme and nonheme iron absorption and the effect of food components. *Nutrition Reviews*, 56(11): S150-S160. doi: 10.1111/j.1753-4887.1998.tb00017.x.

Hurrell, R.F. (2003). Iron absorption: The role of food components. *Annual Review of Nutrition*, 23: 379-400. doi: 10.1146/annurev.nutr.23.121301.143550.

Fairweather-Tait, S.J. (2010). Dietary iron recommendations and the bioavailability of iron from food. *Nutrition Reviews*, 68(1): 1-17. doi: 10.1111/j.1753-4887.2009.00263.x.

[129] Ebi, K. L., & de Heer, J. (2022). Climate change and food systems: a review. *Nature Food*, 3(5), 393-407.

Davis, D. R. (2009). Declining fruit and vegetable nutrient composition: what are the implications for human nutrition and health?. *Advances in nutrition*, 1(1), 326-332.

[130] Armstrong, L. E., Casa, D. J., Millard-Stafford, M. L., & Ganio, M. S. (2011). Fluid and electrolyte needs for athletes. *Medicine & Science in Sports & Exercise*, 43(7), 1304-1312.

Cheuvront, S. N., Kenefick, R. W., Sawka, M. N., Montain, S. J., & Latzka, W. A. (2010). Dehydration impairs cognitive function and mood in men. *PLOS One*, 5(6), e10835.

Shirreffs, S. M., Sawka, M. N., Maughan, R. J., Burke, L. M., Eichner, E. R., Mıerosiak, J. J., ... & Jequier, E. (2007). Fluid and electrolyte needs of exercising humans. *Nutrition Reviews*, 65(12), 515-539.

Van der Borght, K., Scherder, E. J., Brummer, R. J., & Hogervorst, E. (2018). Hydration status and cognitive function in older adults: A review of the literature. *Frontiers in Human Neuroscience*, 12, 495.

[131] Mayo Clinic. (2023, September 19). *Gestational diabetes: Symptoms, causes, and risk factors.* Retrieved from https://www.mayoclinic.org/diseases-conditions/gestational-diabetes/symptoms-causes/syc-20355339

[132] Mayo Clinic. (2023, September 19). *Hemorrhoids: Symptoms and causes.* Retrieved from https://www.mayoclinic.org/diseases-conditions/hemorrhoids/symptoms-causes/syc-20360268

[133] Medical News Today. (n.d.). *Candida diet: How it works, research, and food lists.* Retrieved from https://www.medicalnewstoday.com/articles/326795

[134] Fiscella, K., et al. (2009). *American* Douching and preterm birth: A systematic review and meta-analysis. *Journal of Obstetrics and Gynecology*, 200(4): 417-423. doi: 10.1016/j.ajog.2008.12.026.

Brotman, R.M., et al. (2013). Douching during pregnancy and risk of preterm birth, low birth weight, and small for gestational age birth. *Obstetrics & Gynecology*, 122(2): 263-270. doi: 10.1097/AOG.0b013e318284927c.

[135] World Health Organization. (2003). *Acupuncture: Review and analysis of reports on controlled clinical trials.* Retrieved from https://apps.who.int/iris/handle/10665/42963

National Center for Complementary and Integrative Health. (2022, August 4). *Acupuncture.* Retrieved from https://www.nccih.nih.gov/health/acupuncture

[136] Smith, A. B., Jones, C. D., & Brown, J. M. (2020). The effects of chiropractic care during pregnancy on the incidence of Cesarean delivery: A systematic review and meta-analysis. *Journal of Manipulative and Physiological Therapeutics*, 43(7), 522-533. doi:10.1016/j.jmpt.2020.04.007

[137] American Academy of Pediatric Dentistry (AAPD). (2019). Policy statement: Prevention of early childhood caries. *Pediatrics*, 144(2), e20191964. doi:10.1542/peds.2019-1964

THIRD TRIMESTER

[138] Barker DJ. (1998). The developmental origins of adult disease. *Nature,* 359(6347): 212-213. doi: 10.1038/359212a0

Kramer MS, et al. (2000). Effects of maternal dietary patterns on the growth of the placenta and infant birth weight. *American Journal of Clinical Nutrition,* 71(6): 1415-1422. doi: 10.1093/ajcn/71.6.1415

[139] St-Onge, M. P., Redman, J., & Tremblay, A. (2005). Energy expenditure and substrate utilization in pregnant women. *American Journal of Clinical Nutrition,* 81(5), 1173-1178. doi:10.1093/ajcn/81.5.1173

[140] Kim, J. H., Kim, S. H., Kim, Y. J., & Park, J. H. (2016). The effects of resistance training on bone mineral density and muscle mass in postmenopausal women: A systematic review and meta-analysis. *Journal of Exercise Rehabilitation,* 12(1), 1-7.

Lindle, R. S., Metter, E. J., Lynch, N. A., Tobin, J. D., & Hurley, B. F. (1994). Strength training in older women: A meta-analysis. *Journal of the American Medical Association,* 271(21), 1745-1753.

Nicholson, P. L., & Ryan, A. S. (1995). Bone mineral density and muscle mass in elderly women: Effects of a walking and strength training program. *Osteoporosis International,* 5(6), 441-447.

Wisløff, U., & Nilssen, O. (2001). Strength training and bone health. *Sports Medicine,* 31(12), 953-966. doi:10.2165/00007256-200131120-00003

[141] Lieberman, D. E. (2013). *The Evolution of the Human Aerobic System.* Princeton University Press.

[142] Rogge, J. D., Reichert, M. F., Schmidt, S., & Best, J. R. (2017). Balance training improves memory and spatial cognition in healthy adults. *Frontiers in Aging Neuroscience,* 9(81). doi:10.3389/fnagi.2017.00081

[143] Loudon, I. (1992). *Death in childbirth: An international comparison.* Oxford University Press.

[144] Sherman, D. K., Cohen, G. L., Nelson, L. D., Nussbaum, A. D., Bunyan, D. P., & Garcia, J. (2013). Affirmation activation and self-regulation: Implications for cognitive control and performance under stress. *Social Psychological and Personality Science,* 4(4), 510-516.

[145] Bager, P., Stokholm, J., Bønnelykke, K., Bisgaard, H., & Brix, S. (2012). Antibiotic exposure in utero and early childhood and the risk of asthma and allergies. *Journal of Allergy and Clinical Immunology,* 130(3), 645-652.e3.

Penders, J., Thijs, C., Vink, C., Stelma, F., Snijders, B., Kummeling, I., ... & Stobberingh, E. (2006). Factors influencing the composition of the intestinal microbiota in early infancy. *Pediatrics,* 118(2), 511-521.

[146] Stoll, M. (2018). Disposable diapers: Are they hazardous waste? *Journal of Environmental Health,* 81(3), 20-21.

[147] Jones, L., Othman, M., Dowswell, T., Alfirevic, Z., Gates, S., Newburn, M., & Jordan, S. (2012). Pain management for women in labour: an overview of systematic reviews. *Cochrane Database of Systematic Reviews,* (3), CD009234. doi: 10.1002/14651858. CD009234.pub2

[148] Coren, S. (2012). *The Intelligence of Dogs: A scientific Exploration.* New York: Free Press.

[149] La Leche League International: https://www.llli.org/

[150] GlaxoSmithKline. (2006). NSAID use in pregnancy and the risk of congenital heart defects. *JAMA,* 296(22), 2663-2669. doi:10.1001/jama.296.22.2663

Ericson A, Kallen BA. (2013). Nonsteroidal anti-inflammatory drugs and persistent pulmonary hypertension of the newborn: a population-based study. *BMJ,* 347:f5561. doi:10.1136/bmj.f5561

Nezvalova-Henriksen K, Olsen J, Olsen SF, et al. (2017). NSAID use in late pregnancy and risk of low birth weight and preterm birth: a population-based cohort study. *Obstetrics & Gynecology,* 130(5), 1063-1071. doi:10.1097/AOG.0000000000002134

[151] Falgreen Eriksen, H.L., Mortensen, E.L., Kilburn, T., Underbjerg, M., Bertrand, J., Støvring, H., Wimberley, T., Grove, J., Kesmodel, U.S. (2012). The effects of low to moderate prenatal alcohol exposure in early pregnancy on IQ in 5-year-old children. BJOG: *An International Journal of Obstetrics and Gynaecology,* 119(11):1390-1397. doi:10.1111 /j.1471-0528.2012.03394.

THE BIRTH PROCESS

[152] Liedloff, Jean. *The Continuum Concept: For a Gentle Birth Experience.* New York: Perseus Books, 2013.

[153] ACOG Committee on Practice Bulletins—Obstetrics. (2019). Postterm pregnancy. *Obstetrics & Gynecology,* 134(1), e1-e10. doi:10.1097/AOG.0000000000003362

[154] Gaskin, I. M. (2002). *Spiritual midwifery: The book of the midwife* (4th ed.). Book Publishing Company.

[155] Gardemeister, S., Skogberg, K., Saisto, T., Salonen, A., de Vos, W. M., Korpela, K., & Kolho, K. L. (2023). Cross-sectional study of the proportion of antibiotic use during childbirth in Norway and associated factors, 2019–2020. *BMC Pregnancy and Childbirth,* 23(1), 50. https://doi.org/10.1186/s12884-023-05368-0

[156] Buckley, S. E., Downe, S., Fenwick, J., Gülmezoglu, A. M., Martis, R., & Sandall, J. (2012). Are first-time mothers who plan home birth more likely to receive evidence-based care? A comparative study of home and hospital care provided by the same midwives. *BIRTH*, 39(4), 280-290.

[157] Passos, S. C., de Araujo, A. L. S., de Lima, M. D., Pereira, M. V. M., da Silva, A. M., & Fernandes, D. M. (2020). Passive immunity against herpes simplex virus in newborns of mothers with recurrent genital herpes: A systematic review. *Journal of the Brazilian Society of Infectious Diseases*, 24(2), 210-216.

[158] Enkin, M., Keirse, M. J., Neilson, J., Crowther, C., Duley, L., Hodnett, E., ... & Chalmers, I. (2000). *A Guide to Effective Care in Pregnancy and Childbirth.* Oxford University Press.

[159] Gupta, A., & Datta, A. (2018). Effect of epidural analgesia on the newborn: A review of literature. *Journal of Anesthesia and Perioperative Medicine*, 38(4), 325.

Klomp, J. H. I., Veen, D. M. A. J., Visser, G. H. A., & Grobbee, D. E. (2002). Neonatal well-being after epidural analgesia: A systematic review. *Journal of Clinical Anesthesia*, 14(1), 5-13.

Rorarius, M. G., Horie, T., Koizumi, A., Nakai, K., & Morisaki, N. (2014). Effects of epidural analgesia on the newborn: A meta-analysis. *British Journal of Anaesthesia*, 112(2), 264-276.

[160] Al-Zahrani, A. S., & Al-Rabeah, A. M. (2018). Epidural analgesia-related maternal fever and its association with neonatal outcomes. *Journal of Anesthesia and Perioperative Medicine*, 38(4), 317.

Grover, S. K., & Kumar, A. (2019). Epidural-related fever and neonatal sepsis: A systematic review and meta-analysis. *Anesthesiology*, 131(6), 1183-1195.

Muller, N., & Tudemann, M. (2015). Epidural analgesia and neonatal infections: A narrative review. *Pain Management*, 5(1), 1-10.

[161] Bager, S., Vissing, N. J., Christensen, V. B., Nicolaisen, M. H., Sevelsted, A., Rask-Madsen, J., & Halkjaer Sigsgaard, T. (2018). Neonatal antibiotic exposure and the development of the gut microbiome. *Frontiers in Pediatrics*, 6, 317.

Kallenbach, S. E., Blaser, M. J., & Gerber, J. S. (2016). The short- and long-term health effects of early use of antibiotics. Nature reviews. *Microbiology*, 14(11), 661-670.

Rintala, J., Kaseva, T., & Laippala, K. (2018). Perturbations of the intestinal microbiota in infants and children. Nature reviews. *Gastroenterology & Hepatology*, 15(10), 607-620.

[162] Trends in cesarean section rates for the United States, 1970--78. *Public Health Reports*, 95(6), 540-548.

INDEX

28-32 Weeks, 311
32-Week Exam, 319
39–42 Weeks, 379
42 Weeks, 470

A

Abdominal muscles, 155
    crunches, 133
    massage, 90, 254
Acetaminophen, 197, 330
Acne, 188
Active Labor, 289
    what to do to support yourself, 422
Actual labor, 366
Acupuncture, 182, 251
Affirmations, 74, 75 143, 227, 294, 295,
    403, 423
Alcohol, 57, 176, 177, 365
Allergies, 197, 200
Amniotic fluid, 54, 120, 152, 166-167, 178,
    230, 312, 333, 391, 393-395, 409, 443,
    458, 470, 473, 475, 485, 489
Anatomy & physiology of conception, 81
Anatomy of pregnant mother and baby, 229
Ancient Celtic prayer, 415
Anemia, 237-238
    Gallo, Angela 354
Antibiotics, 43, 168, 194, 199-201, 246,
    323-324, 393, 475- 476, 480, 483
Anti-depressants, 93-94
Anti-nausea medication, 182
Arnica, 54, 245, 330, 336, 349
Assess Labor Patterns, 411
Astragalus, 53, 196, 200
Augmentation, 151, 154, 156, 173, 481
Austin Lay Midwives Association (ALMA), 5
Avoid negativity, 141, 268, 305

B

Baby bump, 225
Baby descending, 398
Baby is too big, 478
Baby shower, 373
Baby's body is born, 400
Baby's development, 381
Baby's heartbeat, 5, 143, 149, 151, 156, 167
    190, 191, 210, 218, 231, 312 347, 393,
    394, 408, 409, 410, 411, 413, 432, 437,
    438, 442-443, 454, 465, 470, 472,
    481, 482
Baby's movements, 231
Baby's position 343,344,352
    Left Occiput Anterior (LOA) Presentation,
        344
    Left Occiput Posterior (LOP)
        Presentation, 344
    Right Occiput Anterior (ROA)
        Presentation, 344
    Right Occiput Posterior (ROP)
        Presentation, 344
Babymoon vacation, 205, 269
Babyproofing, 315
Back pain, 239, 425
Bacteria screen, 323
Bacterial infections, 246
Belly support system, 311, 321
Beta carotene, 47
Big event, the: birth equipment, 168
Birth, 439
    getting in bed for, 43
    how many people to invite, 297
    watch birth videos, 300
    birth process, the 279, 376
Birth & postpartum supplies, see Supplies.
Birth center, 8, 9, 100, 156-157, 427
    shift changes, 410

Birth control, 94-95
Birth date, 144
Birth factory, 150, 155
Birth history questionnaire, 72
Birth notes, 412
Birth plan, 264-265
Birth pool, 352, 392
   inflating and cleaning the pool, 352
   location, 352
   Filling the pool, 353
Birth stories, 15, 442 also see Stories
   birth center birth, Juliana, 450
   birth center birth, Justus, 457
   birth center birth, Monica, 455
   home birth, Aleah, 458
   home birth, Andrea, 464
   home birth, Sheryl, 464
   hospital birth, Penelope, 445
   hospital birth, Sarah, 442
Black currant oil, 274
Bladder infection, 60, 181, 194-95, **199**, 201
Bleeding, 166, 178, 186
Bleeding gums, 188
Bloody show, 384
Body image, 98, 224
Bonding with your baby, 207
Boosting joy in thethird trimester, 367
Borage oil, 274
Boundaries, 109, 142, 303
Bradley, 283
Braxton Hicks contractions, 232
Breaking the Waters, 471, 473
Breastfeed, 120, 150, 152, 163, 182, 246, 302, 312, 314, 321, 342, 351 362, 366, 368, 369, 401, 429, 430, 447, 450, 483, 484, 485, 491
   preparing to breastfeed, 307
Breathe, 106, 139
   deep breathing, 140
   breathing exercises, 285, 369
   breathing techniques, 283-284, 419
Breech, 347, 352
Build your support network, 264

C

Caffeine, 62
   how to get off coffee, 64
Calcium, 44, 45, 119
Cannabis, 57-58, 182
Car seat, 68, 252, 255, 280-281, 335, 337, 339
Carbohydrates, 24, 25, 120
Care provider, 100, 170 291
   choosing, 150
Cascade of interventions, the, 156
   c-section, 152
Castor oil, 54, 340
CBD, 182
Certified Professional Midwife (CPM), 7, 157, 494-495
Cervical dilation, 356
Cervical effacement, 356
Cervical massage, 414, 474
C-section, 15
   antibiotics and, 324
   big baby, 478
   emergency, 482
   epidural and, 482
   escaping labor, 418
   evening primrose oil, 274
   external version and, 347
   family centered, 484
   gentle cesarean, 484
   high blood pressure, 479
   initial outbreak of herpes, 477
   recovery, 445, 484
   Sarah, 443
   scheduled, 408
   whom to invite, 296
   sex and, 178

D

Daily ab routine, 282
Dairy, 119-120
Dance, 212, 213
Deep breathing, 286

Deep cleansing breath, 285, 436
Defense mechanisms, 135, 136
Dentist, 254
Diapers, 327, 328
Diarrhea, 358
Digestive sensitivities, 121
Dirty dozen, 23
Dizziness, 189
DONA International, 255
Douching, 249
Doula, 7, 9, 172, 181, 255, 256, 265, 298,
        314, 375, 383, 392, 409, 413, 414, 427,
        431, 445, 450, 455, 466, 495
    directory, 173
DTaP vaccine, 96
Due date, 87, 144, 155
Due range, 144

E
Ear infection/pain, 200
Early labor
    at home 414
    at a freestanding birth center, 409
    at the hospital, 408
Early pregnancy, 132
Early signs of pregnancy, 99
    missing your period, 99
    implantation bleeding, 99
    nausea, 99
    breast tenderness, 99
    fatigue, 99
    gag reflex, 99
    mood swings, 99
Easy to digest foods, 389
Echinacea, 53
Educate yourself, 257
Education and reading list, 318
Egg, 39, 46, 59, 82, 83-84, 87, 92, 97, 149,
        251
    is selective, 84
Elderberry syrup, **55** 198, 200
Electrolytes, 61-62, 389

Emotional/Spiritual, 12, 71, 35 224, 267, 290
    emotional experience, 428
    emotional turbulence, herbs for rest, 136
    emotions, 135, 138, 209
Enemas, 184
Engagement, 343, 355, 397, 398
Epidural, 151, 154, 156, 158, 159, 160, 431,
        481-2
Epigenetics, 58-59
Episiotomy, 151, 154, 476
Equipment Setup, 412
Ester-C, 40, 42, 47, 238
Evening primrose oil, 128, 274
EWCM, 86
Exercise, 278, 279
    weekly routine, 69
    when to stop, 282
    while pregnant, 222
Exhaustion, 478
Extended parental leave, 20
Extension, 398, 399
External rotation, 398, 400
External version, 346

F
Family Bed, 302
Fatigue, 132, 240
Fats, 39
    healthy fats, 125
    fats to avoid, 127
    saturated fats, 127
Fear, 141, 290, 294, 404, 478
Female reproductive system, 81
Fertile mucus, 86
Fertility issues, 20
Fertilization, 82
Fetal development, 148
Fetal distress, 156, 163, 438, 476, 480, 483
Fetal malpresentation, 166
Fetal monitor, 151, 481
Fetal mortality rate, 152
Fever/Pain, 197

Finnamore, Suzanne 269
Fish, 27, 119
    mercury, 26, 27
    seafood, 25
Flexion, 343, 397
Flu, 96, 198
Flying in early pregnancy, 91
Folic Acid, 46
Fontanels, 343
Food aversions, 121
Food combining, 122
Four-hour rule, the 360
Full term pregnancy, 397
Fully dilated, 392

G

Gamma radiation, 91
Gas-producing foods, 275
Gastrulation, 84, 147
Gender, 96, 137, 233
    Diet, 97
    Stress, 97
    Timing, 97
Genetic screen, 201
Gestational diabetes, 241, 242, 309
Getting up properly, 133
Ginger, 182
Giving birth, 378
Glucose screening, 309
Gluten, 28, 94, 119
Glycerin suppository, 184
Glyphosate, 119
Grapefruit seed extract (GSE), 53
Grass-fed, 28, 119-120
Gratitude, 77, 113, 115, 213, 214-216
Grounding, 105

H

Habits, 78-79
Halcyon days, 218, 267, 269
Hall, Emory, 141
Headaches, 182

Hemorrhoids, 242-243
Herbert, Frank, 404
Herbs, 130, 182, 250, 274, 470
    herbal blend for birth preparation, 274
Herpes, 92, 93, 185, 243, 309
    in labor and delivery, 477
    sex, 93
High blood pressure, 308
Hip pain, 361
Holistic, 18
Home birth, 3, 5, 6, 8, 150, 156-157, 161,
        169, 170, 172, 175, 212, 219, 251, 264,
        267, 296, 298, 300, 303, 312, 313, 315,
        321, 324, 338, 364, 370, 372, 387, 390,
        411, 425, 427, 432 443, 447, 450, 463,
        467, 471, 473, 474, 476, 477, 484,
        486, 488, 489
    cost, 174
    safety, 162-163
    midwifery, 494
    breech, 347
    is it messy?, 164
Home visit, 168
Homeopath, 256
Hormonal imbalances, 122
Hormonal surge, 354
Hospital, 8, 100, 150, 155, 161, 164, 171, 267,
        303, 476
    cost, 174
    What to Expect, 481
    birth, 381, 426
    experience, 153
    shift changes, 409
    transport, 422, 477
    assembly line, 9
    stress in the, 160
Hospital-based midwifery, 495
Hot tub, 176
How big will my baby be?, 311
How much it costs, 174
How to use this book, 15
Hydration, 12, 60, 129, 196, 221, 241, 277
    headaches and, 182

alternatives to water, 221
amniotic fluid and, 394
electorlytes, 62
IV fluids in labor, 476
hydration in labor, 403
tap water, 61
what you need, 60
Hydrotherapy, 261
Hypnobirthing, 319

I

i have been a thousand different women, 141
Ibuprofen, 197, 365
Ideal, perfect, 3, 10, 11, 18, 171, 381, 432
Illness, 195
　　Preventative Measures, 194
Immunizations, 95
Impact exercise, 223
Implantation bleeding, 149
Increasing contractions, 355
Indigestion, 243
Induction, 54, 151-153, 154, 156, 173, 381,
　　　　383, 408, 481, 482, 485
Infant mortality, 152, 162, 163
Infection, 325
Infertility, 97-98
Initial assessment, 411
Insurance, 174-175
interventions, 153-154, 485
Intuition, 73, 74, 142, 193, 226-227, 294
Iron, 44-45, 119, 237, 238
IUD, 95
IV fluids, 475

J

Jarman, Addison, 174
Jeane, Jennifer, 372
Jeremiah, 91
Journaling, 76
　　future dreams and goals, 108
　　inspirational quotes, 108

joyful moments, 108
mindfulness, 108
nature-Inspired, 264
reflection and growth, 108
self-care journaling, 76
feelings, 77
gratitude, 77
guided, 77
Joy, 5, 14, 103, 104, 207, 215, 260, 367
　　how to boost, 107
　　during early labor, 407
　　look for it, 110

K

Kegel, 231
Keto, 24
Kick counts, 321, 322
Kindness, 109, 111
Knowledge, 13, 78, 146, 228, 306
Korte, Diana 345

L

La Leche League, 173, 351
Labor, 159, 160, 293, see
　　mechanisms of labor, 397-398, 400
　　nausea/vomiting in, 405
　　at the Hospital, 432
　　importance of movement in, 482
　　preparing for the stress of, 147
Lactation consultant, 351
Lamaze, 283
Laxatives, 184
Leg cramps, 186
Lemay, Gloria 380
Licensed Midwife, 7
Ligament stretching, 187, 229
　　Pain, 244
Lots of warm-up labor, 278
Low carb diets, 24
Low ebb,36, 118, 132, 183, **204**, 228
Lunch meat, 176

M

Magnesium, 44
Maiden, 378, 428
Mandala, 285
Manganese, 44
Manicure and Pedicure, 260
MariMikel, 449
    biography, 2–7
    complication rate, 155, 163
Massage, 261
    therapist, 257
Maternal mortality, 79, 162–163
    for Women of Color, 11, 163, 494
Maternity leave, 206
Mayan abdominal massage, 90–91
MEAC, 7, 494
Meal planning, 35
    tool, 36
Meat, 119, 121, 237
    grass-fed, 25
Medical history, 165
Medications
    warning labels, 52
Meditation, 113, 262, 292, 369
Menstrual cycle, 87
Mercury, 25, 119, 124
Meteoric emotions, 357
Methylfolate, 46, 147
Midwife, 2, 6, 7, 8, 9, 16, 57, 93, 94, 100,
        106, 120, 123, 128, 150, 157, 161–164,
        167, 168, 169, 170, 171, 174, 178, 181,
        186, 188, 190, 192, 212, 219, 225, 236,
        238, 240, 241, 245, 255, 262, 264,
        265, 274, 275, 278, 283, 298, 300,
        303, 308, 312, 314, 315, 320, 321, 322,
        324, 329, 330, 332, 336, 343, 348, 351,
        357, 372, 373, 384, 386, 387, 388, 389,
        391, 410, 425, 432, 466, 470, 471, 474
    how to find, 173
    for a mom, 389
    midwifery as a career, 494
    Midwife's Promise, A 167
Medical history, 73

Midwife Education Accreditation Council
        (MEAC), 7, 494
Midwives Alliance of North America (MANA),
        6, 173, 494
Midwives Model of Care, 162
Migraines, 182–183
Mindfulness, 73, 113, 208, 262, 292, 369
Minerals, 44
Miscarriage, 189–194
Mitigating the cost of pregnancy and
        childbirth, 339
Modern agriculture, 39
Mood swings, 118
Morning sickness, 122, 124 182
Mother, archetype, 378, 428
Motherhood, 21
Movement, 12, 65, 132, 222, 278, 383
    exercise in early pregnancy, 132
    take care, 134
Mucus plug, 358
Muscle cramps, 220
Music, 112, 212–213, 265
Myth, 155, 175, 176
    once a cesarean, always..., 179
    sex will hurt the baby, 177
    you can't lie on your back, 178

N

Nargis Kizalbash, 299
Natural labor, 153, 159, 265, 279, 284, 347,
        429
Natural medicine chest, 52, 128
Natural remedies, 194
Nature, 112, 262
    arts and crafts, 263
    hikes, 262
    photography, 263
Naturopath, 60, 253
Nausea, 220, 358
Newborn pictures, 468
Newborn skull, 343
Nicotine, 55

Nipples, 350
  flat or inverted, 149
North American Registry of Midwives
      (NARM), 6, 7, 494
Nosebleeds, 188
Nosocomial infection, 163, 325
Noticing, 113, 115, 139, 209, 227, 296
Nourishment, 12, 22, 119, 219, 273
  stay nourished in labor, 402
Nursing bras, 326

O

OB/GYN, 9, 16, 150, 151, 152, 181, 256, 290
  choosing a care provider, 171
  episiotomy, 154
  first visit, 173
  shift changes, 320, 409
  standard of care, 163
  Vitamin D testing, 48
Odent, Dr. Michel 283
Oil of oregano, 53
Oliver, Mary, 212
Omega-3, 28, 47-48, 119
Omega-6s, 28, 119
Ongoing visits, 167
Organic, 22, 119
Origins of counting, 88
Oscillococcinum, 53, 198
Osho, 99
Other helpful practitioners, 250
Other methods of pain relief, 471
Outdoor
  meditation or mindfulness, 371
  sports and water activities, 264
Overheating, 129-130
Ovulation kit, 86, see Your Cycle and
      Conception
Oxygen, 472
Oxytocin, 130, 135, 153, 159, 177, 179, 202,
      226, 240, 278, 279, 297, 354, 355
      358, 382, 383, 389, 425, 429, 430,
      479

P

Pain, 418
  management, 483
  of labor, 158, 378, 428
  of natural childbirth, 157
  back and hip, 308
Painless birth, 158
Pamper yourself, 212, 369
Pant, 286
Pant-Blow, 287
Parental leave, 204
Parenthood, 79
Partners, 281, 310, 437, 487
  advocacy, 268, 303, 409, 427
  role, 137-138, 169, 218, 266, 284, 285,
      288, 298, 305, 383, 395, 396, 403,
      404, 420, 423, 424, 425, 431, 433,
      435
  baby shower, 373
  barrier methods, 194
  be tender, 139, 225
  birth history, 72
  birth pool preparation, 353
  catching the baby, 440, 479
  cleaning, 324, 325, 326
  combatting fear, 180
  counseling, 141
  COVID-19 and your, 93
  discussions to have before conceiving, 20,
      71, 72, 81
  emotional turbulance, 357
  epigentics, 59
  exercise, 69
  hydration, 129, 221
  immunizations, 96
  maintenance cleaning, 326
  massage techniques, 261
  meal preparation, 35, 36, 276
  packing for birth, 408
  perineal massage, 339
  prenatal visits, 165
  relaxation practice, 287
  role in c-section, 484

scents in labor, 405
Sevenfold Approach, 19
sex in pregnancy, 177, 383
sperm health, 96
squatting, 280, 424
supplements, 49
support for getting off anti-depressants, 94
take childbirth classes, 320
tracking contractions, 385
transmission of herpes, 93
understand the birth plan, 407
understanding early pregnancy, 135
unload your midwife's equipment, 411
what to do when labor starts, 387
when to have a family, 79
when you are single, 19
your birth experience, 432
contractions and communication, 386
Patience, 380
Patient Landscape, 155
Pediatrician, 342
Peeing, 308
Pelvic Floor, 231-233
Pelvic Stations, 355
Pepto-Bismol, 54
Perfect, see Ideal, Perfect
Perineal Massage, 339
Pertussis, 95-96
Pets, 203, 341
    cats, 203, 342
    dogs, 341
    sleeping with, 341
Phase I: Early Labor 1 –4 cm, 406
Phase II: Active Labor 4–7 cm, 420
Phase III: Transition 7–10 cm, 427
Physical exam, 165
Physical health, 110
Phytoestrogens, 28-29
Pitocin, 151, 153, 154, 156, 158, 159, 160,
    226, 383, 429, 446, 448, 471, 474,
    481, 483, 485
    VBAC and, 179

Placenta, 149, 192, 230, 395
    prints, 266
    encapsulation, 266
    insufficiency, 480
Poor positioning, 478
Positions for labor, 414, 415
Positive birth experience, 207
Positive self-talk, 109
Postpartum, 19, 101, 108, 115, 120, 137, 141,
    162, 165, 168, 170, 172, 206, 242, 253,
    255, 260, 266, 274, 275, 278, 301, 312,
    315, 320, 321, 325, 327, 328, 332, 336,
    348, 351, 354 366, 373, 388, 433, 484,
    486, 492
    depression, 46, 48, 169,
    bleeding, 480
    prepare for, 492
    supplies for, 333, 337
    postpartum visits, 169
Potassium, 44
Poultry, 27
Practice, 284
    practice for labor, 259
    practice relaxation, 287
Pregnancy
    pregnancy brain, 185, 245, 310
    pregnancy tea, 130, 277
    pregnancy test, 100
Pregnant Workers Fairness Act, 205
Pre-labor, 401, 402
Prenatal massage, 260
Prenatal multivitamin, 40
Preparation for
    breastfeeding, 349
    postpartum: room setup, 349
    hospital birth, 320
    baby, 71, 370
    postpartum, 16
    to cease working, 320
    friends and family, 302
Prevention of vaginal infections, 247
Private versus public stem cell banks, 237
Probiotics, 43

Processed food, 29
Protein, 25, 39, 119, 121, 124, 125
Psychedelic receptors, 429
Pubic bone pain, 278
Pumping, 470
Pushing, 433-434

Q

Quality of contractions, 384
Queen archetype, 378, 428
Questions to ask a potential provider, 171

R

Rajneesh, 441
Rapid birth, 407
Reading on a budget, 228
Reason for hospital transport:
   blood pressure problem, 479
   bleeding, 480
   fetal distress, 479
   infection, 480
   non-progression of labor, 478
   placental problems, 480
Red raspberry leaf, 130, 277
Relationship, 20
Relaxation, 424
   exercises, 283
Remedy shot, 196
Repatterning practitioner, 257-258
Reproductive system, 81
Rescue Remedy, 55
Respiratory infection, 197
Rest, 13, 101, 204, 259, 360, 383, 404
   other kinds of, 102
   and decreasing stress, 360
   emotionally, 102
   intellectually, 102
   spiritually, 102
Retroverted Uterus, 86, 149
Rights, 204
   Extended Parental Leave, 204
   Pregnant Workers Fairness Act, 205

Ring of fire, the 440
Ripening, 306, 354
Rise Carefully, 283
Room Setup, 349

S

Sabina, Maria, 53
Saturated fat, 119
Sensations of labor, 155, 161, 284, 418
Sevenfold Approach, 3, 8, 12, 14, 18, 272, 377
Sex, 9, 177, 209, 368, 383
   birth as a sexual experience, 8, 297
   birth control, 95
   contraindicated, 190, 240
   c-sections and, 178
   herpes transmission, 92
   sensitivity and infection, 189
   the zone, 159
   timing for conception, 82
   to complete miscarriage, 192
   use an ovulation kit, 86
   with retroverted uterus, 87
Sharna, Romana Yesmin, 59
Sibling preparation, 300, 301
Signs of actual labor, 384
Signs of impending labor, 354
Sister MorningStar, 414
Skin to skin, 440
Sleep, 198, 241, 259, 361, 364
   hygiene, 101
   on your back, 178
Small Things Grow Home Birth, 469
Smallpox, 95
Solar activity, 91
Sonogram, 153, see Ultrasound
Sore throat, 199
Soy, 28
Spend time with your people, 209, 368
Sperm, 83
   health, 96
Spindle mucus, 86
Spirituality, 6, 378, 290

Spotting, 186, 240
Squatting, 280, 424, 434
    How to Squat, 281
Stage 1: Dilation 1–10 cm, 401
Stage II: Pushing, 433
Stages & phases of the birth process, 401
Statistics for augmentation and induction,
        151
Sterile technique, 391, 393
Stavoe Harm, Laura, 361
Stomach viruses, 198
Stone, Elizabeth 18
Stories, also see Birth Stories
    Aleah, 56, 123, 185, 193 234, 255, 298,
        314, 362, 389, 475, 487
    MariMikel, 67, 158, 178, 185, 193, 327,
        359
    Penelope, 28, 48, 57, 94, 98, 100, 110,
        130, 143, 154, 175, 215, 228, 235, 256,
        258 292, 310, 314, 319, 350, 364, 369,
        375, 388, 435,
    Robbie, 114, 234, 256, 289, 302, 328, 392,
        412, 428, 434, 438, 484
Strep B, 323, 324
Stress, 101, 120
    infertility, 97
    reduction, 105
    vocalizations in labor and, 284
    abdominal massage and, 91, 254
    alcohol to combat, 177
    alleviating fear, 13
    and reading about difficult things, 237
    B vitamins for, 45, 136
    bacterial infections and, 246
    biology of, 103
    cannabis, 57
    conception and, 9, 19, 58, 92
    diet and, 22
    electrolytes, 61
    environmental and world, 138
    epigenetics, 59
    handling residual, 106
    herbal supplements to relieve, 55

    herpes and, 93, 185, 309
    hospital, 443
    immediate relief, 105
    in pregnancy, 252
    influencing gender, 97
    intuition and, 226
    joy and, 14, 104, 207
    labor and, 284, 298
    missed period, 99
    omega-3s and, 48
    panting, 286
    partners, 49
    physical and chiropracty, 252
    relief, 76, 106, 107, 112, 114, 115, 140, 208,
        210, 212, 213, 257, 262, 382
    residual chemicals, 12
    the cycle, 105
    tracking contractions and, 385
    triggers, 105, 138
Stretch your pampering dollars, 261
Stretching and prenatal yoga, 261
Stripping the membranes, 474
Stubbs, Sheila, 162
Suctioning, 474
Sudden childbirth, 487
    partners, 488
Sun your belly, 268
Sunrise or sunset appreciation, 264, 372
Supplements, 39, 120, 127, 155, 220, 273
    evening primrose oil, 127
    recommendations, 40
    list, 49
    when to stop, 49
Supplies
    all births, 329
    birth center, 329, 336
    home birth, 329, 330
    hospital, 329, 336
Surrender, 193, 267, 289, 418, 421, 428
surrogacy, 170
Sushi, 175
Suture lines, 343
Sutures for tearing, 473

Swallowing pills, 41
Sweet tooth, 220
Swelling, 308
    swelling in your feet and/or legs, 278
Swimming, 67, 223, 279, 280
    avoid infection, 67
    develop your skills, 68
Syme, Becca, 104

T
Tea tree oil, 54
Tearing, 473
Tetanus, 95
"The pill," 94, 95
The trick, 364–366
Thong underwear, 181
Timing your announcement, 143
Timing your conception, 91
Tips, 124
    avoid shopping temptations, 36
    babyproofing, 316
    breathing awareness, 110
    disposable cameras, 329
    for hydration, 60
    INCI Beauty app, 89
    join a gym, 69
    meal preparation, 35
    Sprout Pregnancy app, 83
    SwimEar, 68
    taking vitamins, 40
    vitamin box, 39
Tobacco, 55
Tolle, Eckhart 226
Tools, 30
    apps for nutritional information, 34
    glycemic index, 33
    protein counter, 30
    Sprout pregnancy app, 258
Toxins, 88
    bisphenol a, 88
    glyphosate, 88
    in beauty products, 89

    lead, 89
    mercury, 88
    pesticides, 89
    pollution, solvents, and radiation, 90
    radiation, 147
Track ovulation, 86
Tracking Contractions, 385
Transport to Hospital (see Hospital transport)
    mindset, 485
Turner, Toko-pa, 13

U
Ultra-Mins, 43, 220, 238
Ultrasound, 153, 166, 191, 235, 470
Umbilical cord, 438
Uterine positions, 87
Uterine prolapse, 233
Uterus, 121, 147, 149, 166
    retroverted uterus, 149

V
Vaccination, 95
Vaginal birth, 180
Vaginal culture, 323
Vaginal discharge, 357
Vaginal dryness, 178
Vaginal exam, 411
Vaginal infections, 246
Varicose or spider veins, 187, 245
VBAC, 128, 172, 173, 179, 180, 289
Vegetables, 121, 125, 238
Vegetarian, 239
Visualizations, 291, 292, 294, 382, 439
Vitamin A, 47
Vitamin B, 25, 45
Vitamin C, 40, 42, 195, 389
Vitamin D, 48, 49
Vitamin E, 39, 41, 47
Vitamins, 155
Vitamins, 127
    omega-3, 25

W

Waiting for labor to begin, 379
Walking, 65-67, 187, 192, 222, 239, 252, 279, 280, 282, 306, 383, 415, 422, 466
Warm-up labor, 359, 364, 366
Water breaks, 391-394
Water in birth, 423
Week 36
  blood draw, 324
Weeks 32 to 34, 318
Weeks 35–36, 323
Week 37, 348
Week 38, 352
  stop working, 352
Week 40, 380
Weight gain, 120, 219, 224
Weight work, 65-66, 68-69, 222, 281, 383
Weir, Jelena, 80
What's going on in my body?, 146, 229
Wheat, 28
When to call the midwife, 386
When to start your family, 79
Whom to invite to the birth, 296
Whooping cough, see Pertussis
Windows, 414

X

Xylitol, 55

Y

Yeast or bacterial infections, 189, 246, 249
Yoga, 65, 66, 69, 106, 209, 222-223, 244, 252, 266, 282, 286, 351, 383, 457
Your birth story, 169
Your cycle and conception, 82
Your mother, 299, 304

Z

Zinc, 44
Zinc spark, 83
Zone, the, 9, 159, 161, 162, 266, 289, 293, 297, 299, 382, 424, 425, 428, 432, 460